Bentham Briefs in Biomedicine and Pharmacotherapy

Oxidative Stress and Natural Antioxidants

(Volume 1)

Edited by

Pardeep Kaur
Department of Botanical & Environmental Sciences
Guru Nanak Dev University
Amritsar, Punjab
India

Rajendra G. Mehta
IIT Research Institute and Illinois Institute of Technology
Chicago, Illinois
USA

Robin
Khalsa College for Women, Amritsar and Department of
Botanical & Environmental Sciences
Guru Nanak Dev University
Amritsar, Punjab
India

Tarunpreet Singh Thind
Govt. College for Girls Ludhiana
Punjab
India

&

Saroj Arora
Department of Botanical & Environmental Sciences
Guru Nanak Dev University
Amritsar, Punjab
India

Bentham Briefs in Biomedicine and Pharmacotherapy
Oxidative Stress and Natural Antioxidants

(Volume 1)

Editors: Pardeep Kaur, Rajendra G. Mehta, Robin, Tarunpreet Singh Thind and Saroj Arora

ISBN (Online): 978-981-4998-87-1

ISBN (Print): 978-981-4998-88-8

ISBN (Paperback): 978-981-4998-89-5

©2021, Bentham Books imprint.

Published by Bentham Science Publishers Pte. Ltd. Singapore. All Rights Reserved.

need for a court order if at any point you breach any terms of this License Agreement. In no event will any delay or failure by Bentham Science Publishers in enforcing your compliance with this License Agreement constitute a waiver of any of its rights.

3. You acknowledge that you have read this License Agreement, and agree to be bound by its terms and conditions. To the extent that any other terms and conditions presented on any website of Bentham Science Publishers conflict with, or are inconsistent with, the terms and conditions set out in this License Agreement, you acknowledge that the terms and conditions set out in this License Agreement shall prevail.

Bentham Science Publishers Pte. Ltd.
80 Robinson Road #02-00
Singapore 068898
Singapore
Email: subscriptions@benthamscience.net

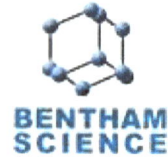

BENTHAM SCIENCE

CONTENTS

FOREWORD

I am pleased to write this foreword for the e-book entitled 'Oxidative Stress and Natural Antioxidants'. This outstanding endeavor by the co-editors represents a multi-disciplinary coverage of all aspects of oxidative stress and the role of anti-oxidants in this fundamental phenomenon. This e-book represents an effective compilation of chapters on the fundamentals of oxidative stress and the role of anti-oxidants in health and disease. The authors deserve credit for their time and effort to contribute excellent chapters relevant to their individual expertise. These chapters include excellent discussions on oxidative stress in human physiology, redox homeostasis, functions of free radicals and intrinsic cellular mechanisms for naturally occurring anti-oxidants. I am confident that this book will be a valuable addition to the bookshelves of teaching faculty, established investigators and young graduate students. I wish all, the success for the launch of this book.

Nitin Telang
Cancer Prevention Research Program
Palindrome Liaisons Consultants
Montvale
New Jersey
USA

PREFACE

"*Oxidative Stress and Natural Antioxidants*" presents the one pot solution for the interested readers ranging from an understanding of oxidative stress, recent advances in preparation methods, characterization, and applications of antioxidants. Taken altogether, the gathered information in this volume will cover an array of topics highlighting the importance of natural antioxidants in various oxidative stress associated diseases.

The scientific framework of this e-book contains chapters by eminent experts with in-depth knowledge of antioxidants and oxidative stress. The chapters comprise the role of reactive oxygen species and environmental contaminants in redox homeostasis with cellular mechanisms in oxidative stress that trigger the development and progression of many diseases. The literature includes the extraction, profiling, and characterization of antioxidants *via* different procedures and screening assays. Further, the chapters deliberate the role of antioxidants in human physiology, redox homeostasis, intrinsic cellular mechanisms, and their therapeutic potential with industrial prospects. Authors whose names appear on the chapters have remarkably contributed to the scientific work in this ebook and are responsible and accountable for any scientific queries or questions.

We believe that the chapters published in this volume will enrich the understanding of interdisciplinary domains of natural products as well as offer insights into emerging avenues in drug discovery trends.

Pardeep Kaur
Department of Botanical & Environmental Sciences
Guru Nanak Dev University
Amritsar, Punjab
India

Rajendra G. Mehta
IIT Research Institute and Illinois Institute of Technology
Chicago, Illinois
USA

Robin
Khalsa College for Women
Amritsar and Department of Botanical & Environmental
Sciences
Guru Nanak Dev University
Amritsar, Punjab
India

Tarunpreet Singh Thind
Govt. College for Girls Ludhiana
Punjab
India

Saroj Arora
Department of Botanical & Environmental Sciences
Guru Nanak Dev University
Amritsar, Punjab
India

List of Contributors

Agnieszka Bilak	Department of Molecular Biology, Faculty of Biology, University of Gdansk, Wita Stwosza 59, 80-308 Gdansk, Poland
Ajay Kumar	Department of Botanical and Environmental Sciences, Guru Nanak Dev University Amritsar, Punjab, 143005, India
Amandeep Kaur	Faculty of Applied Medical Sciences, Lovely Professional University, Phagwara, India
Anna Aleena Paul	Food Technology and Nutrition, School of Agriculture, Lovely Professional University, Phagwara, Punjab-144411, India
Atsadang Theerasri	Age-Related Inflammation and Degeneration Research Unit, Department of Clinical Chemistry, Faculty of Allied Health Sciences, Chulalongkorn University, Bangkok 10330, Thailand
Avinash Kumar	Department of Botanical and Environmental Sciences, Guru Nanak Dev University, Amritsar, Punjab, India
Balbir Singh	Department of Pharmaceutical Sciences, Guru Nanak Dev University, Amritsar, Punjab, India
Basharat A Bhat	Department of Bioresources, School of Biological Sciences, University of Kashmir, Srinagar 190006, India
Bashir Ahmad Sheikh	Department of Bioresources, School of Biological Sciences, University of Kashmir, Srinagar 190006, India
Davinder Singh	Department of Botanical and Environmental Sciences, Guru Nanak Dev University, Amritsar, Punjab, India
Diksha Sharma	Department of Biotechnology, CT Institute of Pharmaceutical Sciences, CT Group of Institutions, Jalandhar, Punjab, India
Dona Sinha	Department of Receptor Biology and Tumor Metastasis, Chittaranjan National Cancer Institute, 37, S.P. Mukherjee Road, Kolkata-700026, India
Drishtant Singh	Department of Molecular Biology and Biochemistry, Guru

	Nanak Dev University Amritsar, Punjab, 143005, India
Estera Rintz	Department of Molecular Biology, Faculty of Biology, University of Gdansk, Wita Stwosza 59, 80-308 Gdansk, Poland
Farhana Rashid	Department of Botanical and Environmental Sciences, Guru Nanak Dev University, Amritsar, Punjab, India
Ginpreet Kaur	Shobhaben Pratapbhai Patel School of Pharmacy and Technology Management, SVKM's NMIMS, Mumbai-56, Maharashtra, India
Grzegorz Węgrzyn	Department of Molecular Biology, Faculty of Biology, University of Gdansk, Wita Stwosza 59, 80-308 Gdansk, Poland
Gülşen Kaya	Scientific and Technology Research Centre, Inonu University, Turkey
Harneetpal Kaur	Department of Botanical and Environmental Sciences, Guru Nanak Dev University, Amritsar, Punjab, India
Harpal S. Buttar	Department of Pathology and Laboratory Medicine, University of Ottawa, School of Medicine, Ottawa, Canada
Hina Qayoom	Department of Bioresources, School of Biological Sciences, University of Kashmir, Srinagar 190006, India
Hiral K. Mistry	Shobhaben Pratapbhai Patel School of Pharmacy and Technology Management, SVKM's NMIMS, Mumbai-56, Maharashtra, India
Jagoda Mantej	Department of Molecular Biology, Faculty of Biology, University of Gdansk, Wita Stwosza 59, 80-308 Gdansk, Poland
Julian Guzowski	Department of Molecular Biology, Faculty of Biology, University of Gdansk, Wita Stwosza 59, 80-308 Gdansk, Poland
Jyoti Lakhanpal	Faculty of Applied Medical Sciences, Lovely Professional University, Phagwara, India
Karolina Pierzynowska	Department of Molecular Biology, Faculty of Biology, University of Gdansk, Wita Stwosza 59, 80-308 Gdansk, Poland

Khadiga S. Ibrahim

Environmental & Occupational Medicine Department - National Research Centre, El-Bohouth St. (Tahrir St.Prev.) Dokki, Cairo 12622, Egypt

Kirandeep Kaur

Department of Pharmaceutical Sciences, Guru Nanak Dev University, Amritsar, Punjab, India

Kritika Pandit

Department of Botanical and Environmental Sciences, Guru Nanak Dev University Amritsar, Punjab, 143005, India

Lidia Gaffke

Department of Molecular Biology, Faculty of Biology, University of Gdansk, Wita Stwosza 59, 80-308 Gdansk, Poland

Magdalena Bałuch

Department of Molecular Biology, Faculty of Biology, University of Gdansk, Wita Stwosza 59, 80-308 Gdansk, Poland

Magdalena Podlacha

Department of Molecular Biology, Faculty of Biology, University of Gdansk, Wita Stwosza 59, 80-308 Gdansk, Poland

Manju

Faculty of Applied Medical Sciences, Lovely Professional University, Phagwara, India

Manzoor A Mir

Department of Bioresources, School of Biological Sciences, University of Kashmir, Srinagar 190006, India

Marta Bednarek

Department of Molecular Biology, Faculty of Biology, University of Gdansk, Wita Stwosza 59, 80-308 Gdansk, Poland

Maushmi S. Kumar

Shobhaben Pratapbhai Patel School of Pharmacy and Technological Management, SVKM's NMIMS, V. L. Mehta Road, Vile Parle (west), Mumbai- 400056, India

Meena Chintamaneni

Shobhaben Pratapbhai Patel School of Pharmacy and Technology Management, SVKM's NMIMS, Mumbai-56, Maharashtra, India

Merve Keskin

Vocational School of Health Services, Bilecik Şeyh Edebali University, Turkey

Neena Bedi

Department of Pharmaceutical Sciences, Guru Nanak Dev University, Amritsar, Punjab, India

Neha Sharma

Department of Botanical and Environmental Sciences, Guru

	Nanak Dev University Amritsar, Punjab, 143005, India

Patrycja Bielańska   Department of Molecular Biology, Faculty of Biology, University of Gdansk, Wita Stwosza 59, 80-308 Gdansk, Poland

Poonam Jaglan   Food Technology and Nutrition, School of Agriculture, Lovely Professional University, Phagwara, Punjab-144411, India

Prabhjot Kaur   Department of Botanical and Environmental Sciences, Guru Nanak Dev University, Amritsar, Punjab, India

Priyanka Saha   Department of Receptor Biology and Tumor Metastasis, Chittaranjan National Cancer Institute, 37, S.P. Mukherjee Road, Kolkata-700026, India

Priyanka Suthar   Food Technology and Nutrition, School of Agriculture, Lovely Professional University, Phagwara, Punjab-144411, India

Priyankshi Thakkar   Shobhaben Pratapbhai Patel School of Pharmacy and Technology Management, SVKM's NMIMS, Mumbai-56, Maharashtra, India

Priyanshi S. Desai   Shobhaben Pratapbhai Patel School of Pharmacy and Technological Management, SVKM's NMIMS, V. L. Mehta Road, Vile Parle (west), Mumbai- 400056, India

Rohit Rai   Faculty of Applied Medical Sciences, Lovely Professional University, Phagwara, India

Safura Nisar   Department of Bioresources, School of Biological Sciences, University of Kashmir, Srinagar 190006, India

Sakawrat Janpaijit   Age-Related Inflammation and Degeneration Research Unit, Department of Clinical Chemistry, Faculty of Allied Health Sciences, Chulalongkorn University, Bangkok 10330, Thailand

Samiksha   Department of Zoology, Guru Nanak Dev University Amritsar, Punjab, 143005, India

Sandeep Kaur   Department of Botanical and Environmental Sciences, Guru Nanak Dev University Amritsar, Punjab, 143005, India

Sandeep Kumar   Pharmacology and Toxicology Lab, Block-J, CSIR-IHBT Palampur-176061, India

Saraswathy Nagendran   Department of Pathology and Laboratory Medicine, University of Ottawa, School of Medicine, Ottawa, Canada

Saroj Arora — Department of Botanical and Environmental Sciences, Guru Nanak Dev University, Amritsar, Punjab, India

Satish Kumar — Food Technology and Nutrition, School of Agriculture, Lovely Professional University, Phagwara, Punjab-144411, India College of Horticulture and Forestry, Thunag- Mandi, Dr. Y. S. Parmar University of Horticulture and Forestry, Nauni, Solan (HP)-173230, India

Satwinder Kaur Sohal — Department of Zoology, Guru Nanak Dev University Amritsar, Punjab, 143005, India

Satwinderjeet Kaur — Department of Botanical and Environmental Sciences, Guru Nanak Dev University Amritsar, Punjab, 143005, India

Sharad Thakur — Department of Molecular Biology and Biochemistry, Guru Nanak Dev University & PG Department of Agriculture, Khalsa College, Amritsar- 143005, Punjab, India

Shivani Attri — Department of Botanical and Environmental Sciences, Guru Nanak Dev University, Amritsar, Punjab, India

Siddhi Bagwe-Parab — Shobhaben Pratapbhai Patel School of Pharmacy and Technology Management, SVKM's NMIMS, Mumbai-56, Maharashtra, India

Suchisnigdha Datta — Department of Receptor Biology and Tumor Metastasis, Chittaranjan National Cancer Institute, 37, S.P. Mukherjee Road, Kolkata-700026, India

Suman Kumari — Faculty of Applied Medical Sciences, Lovely Professional University, Phagwara, India

Tewin Tencomnao — Age-Related Inflammation and Degeneration Research Unit, Department of Clinical Chemistry, Faculty of Allied Health Sciences, Chulalongkorn University, Bangkok 10330, Thailand

Umar Mehraj — Department of Bioresources, School of Biological Sciences, University of Kashmir, Srinagar 190006, India

Vikas Kumar — Department of Food Science and Technology, Punjab Agricultural University, Ludhiana, Punjab-141004, India

Wajahat R Mir — Department of Bioresources, School of Biological Sciences, University of Kashmir, Srinagar 190006, India

Yogendra Padwad   Pharmacology and Toxicology Lab, Block-J, CSIR-IHBT
                             Palampur-176061, India

Zeinab A. Saleh   Nutrition and Food Science Department - National Research
                             Centre, El-Bohouth St. (Tahrir   St.Prev.) Dokki, Cairo 12622,
                             Egypt

Zuzanna Cyske   Department of Molecular Biology, Faculty of Biology,
                             University of Gdansk, Wita Stwosza 59, 80-308 Gdansk,
                             Poland

Level of Oxidative Stress: A Fate-Determiner of Carcinogenesis and Anti-Carcinogenesis

Suchisnigdha Datta[1], Priyanka Saha[1] and Dona Sinha[1,*]

[1] *Department of Receptor Biology and Tumor Metastasis, Chittaranjan National Cancer Institute, 37, S.P. Mukherjee Road, Kolkata-700026, West Bengal, India*

Abstract: Molecular oxygen, a double-edged sword, is both a boon and a curse for the existence of life. Oxidative stress is the disequilibrium between reactive oxygen (ROS)-generation and elimination that inflicts cellular damage. Living cells can adapt to the ever-changing internal or external stresses. However, they gradually lose their radical-scavenging adaptability with persistent stress, which further increases during neoplasia. Cancer cells, well adapted in pro-oxidative milieu, drive metabolic and genomic reprogramming, which further escalates the oxidative load. This vicious cycle promotes further carcinogenic alterations. Contrastingly, the same ROS is essential for the oxidative-burst mediated anticancer host-defense. To sustain this redox pressure, cancer cells hijack the intracellular antioxidants. Therefore, redox reorientation towards enhanced responsiveness may selectively target malignant cells by ROS-enhancement beyond tolerance leading to mortality. Carcinogenesis, a multistep process, requires ROS during initiation, promotion and progression. However, supraphysiological ROS may induce apoptosis in unmanageable malignancies. Interestingly cells possess an evolutionary-conserved nature to get hormetically pre-conditioned by a transient ultra-low exposure of a stressor, which in higher dose may show the opposite effect. Antioxidants are excellent chemopreventives and chemotherapeutics. Here, we have condensed the possible anticancer modulation of oxidative stress by phytochemicals, aiming at an insight for future strategies in cancer management.

Keywords: Anticancer Therapy, Antioxidant, Carcinogenesis, Dietary Phytochemicals, Hormesis, Nuclear Factor (Erythroid-Derived 2)-Like 2 (Nrf2), Oxidative Stressor, Prooxidant, Reactive Oxygen Species, Xenobiotic Metabolism.

* **Corresponding author Dona Sinha:** Department of Receptor Biology and Tumor Metastasis, Chittaranjan National Cancer Institute, 37, S.P. Mukherjee Road, Kolkata-700026, West Bengal, India; E-mails: dona.sinha@cnci.org.in and donasinha2012@gmail.com

OXIDATIVE STRESS: ORIGIN, DEFINITION AND FEATURES

Oxygen, which is indispensable for existence of all aerobic life forms, becomes lethal when in excess. ROS are oxygen-containing highly reactive species that are produced due to cellular metabolism or environmental stress and can damage nucleic acids, lipids, and proteins structurally and functionally (Jelic *et al.* 2019). ROS are a broad class of chemicals that includes partially oxidized radicals with unpaired electrons, such as superoxide ion ($O_2^{\cdot-}$) and hydroxyl radical ($OH^{\cdot}$), and non-radicals, such as singlet oxygen ($^1O_2$), hydrogen peroxide (H_2O_2) and hypochlorous acid (HOCl).

The origin and evolution of aerobic life on Earth was accompanied by ROS and oxidative stress, which has emerged as a concept in redox biology in the past 60-odd years. Oxidative stress was defined by Jones as "an imbalance between oxidants and antioxidants in favour of the oxidants, leading to a disruption of redox signaling and control and/or molecular damage" (Sies 2017). The endogenous sources of oxidants are inflammatory cells, mitochondria, and peroxisomes which produce mostly H_2O_2 and $O_2^{\cdot-}$ as ROS molecules (Jelic *et al.* 2019). Exposomes, which include all the exogenous sources, can be direct environmental oxidants such as pollution, cigarette smoke, microbes, allergens, pesticides and ionizing or solar (UV, visible, infrared-A) radiations. Oxidative stress can be stratified according to intensity ranging from physiological oxidative stress (eustress) essential for redox signaling to supraphysiological oxidative burden (distress), which damages biomolecules (Sies 2017).

Oxidative stress markers can be divided into three categories (Valadez-Vega *et al.* 2013):

1. Modified molecules (nucleotide, protein, lipid) formed by the action of free radicals
2. Antioxidant molecules or enzymes
3. Second messengers and transcription factors

When the ROS production or accumulation exceeds the antioxidant defence, redox imbalance becomes inevitable, which leads to toxic effects on the structural and functional integrity of biological tissues. This imbalance can either arise because of the rise in the ROS production or fall in the antioxidant defence or both. Therefore the main mechanism of antioxidant action is either a) suppression of ROS production b) scavenging free radicals c) upregulation of antioxidative defence or a combination of all these (Valadez-Vega *et al.* 2013). To counteract this inevitable exposure to free radicals from several sources, our physiological system has evolved to develop following mechanisms:

1. Preventive mechanisms
2. Repair mechanisms
3. Physical defences
4. Antioxidant defences

Effect of Oxidative Stress on Life and Disease

Though the average age has increased over the past few decades, simultaneously, the cancer burden has also risen to 19.3 million new cases and 10 million cancer deaths in 2020 (Sung *et al.* 2021). Persistently elevated ROS causes oxidative stress, which plays a vital role in the development of many age-associated diseases, including cancer. Even in the presence of the cell's defence system, oxidative damage acquires throughout the life (Arsova-Sarafinovska and Dimovski 2013). Though the production of ROS enhances during aging, proper ROS signaling is an essential requirement for healthy aging as it can regulate the lifespan directly. Endogenous and exogenous antioxidants can prevent and repair damage caused by ROS. Therefore, they can lower the risk of chronic-ROS driven diseases, including cancer or may even improve its prognosis.

Enzymatic antioxidants, like superoxide dismutase (SOD), glutathione peroxidase (GPx), NADPH quinone dehydrogenase (NQO) and catalase (CAT), act by chelating superoxide and other peroxides. In addition, non-enzymatic antioxidants (flavonoids, alkaloids, thiols, vitamins E and C, coenzyme Q, histidine, carotene, retinoic acid and glutathione) serve as an important biological defence against ROS attack (Sies 2017). In fact, the process of carcinogenesis is intricately linked with the inherited or acquired defects in enzymes responsible for the redox-mediated signaling axis (Tan *et al.* 2018). Therefore, the efficacy of antioxidant molecules that promote chemoprevention or chemotherapy by counteracting oxidative stress is of prior importance. In this chapter, we have highlighted the molecular mechanisms of antioxidants/prooxidants associated with anticancer management.

PHYSIOLOGICAL IMPORTANCE OF ROS

ROS can stimulate pro-inflammatory cytokine secretion from phagocytic cells, fibroblasts, and chondrocytes which can lead to acute disease conditions like, systemic inflammatory response, acute respiratory/renal insufficiencies, ischemia/reperfusion, and acute intestinal/ renal/ arthritic/ cardiac inflammation (Roy *et al.* 2017). However, it has some essential role too for the healthy maintenance of the body. $O_2^{\cdot-}$ due to its highly energized aggressive nature is detrimental and destroys biological macromolecules (protein, nucleotide and lipid). H_2O_2 has a role in regulating protein functioning as a second messenger or as a signaling molecule when its level is within a physiological range (Helfinger and Schröder 2018). The first role of ROS as a signaling molecule is to sense unfavourable environmental conditions. Therefore, the aim of the cellular antioxidant system is to keep the stress-sensor ROS molecules at a threshold level and any imbalance can trigger the ROS signaling cascade (Mittler 2017). A fine and dynamic balance between the ROS producing enzymes, NADPH oxidases (NOX), NO synthases, cytochrome P-450 (cyt P450) and ROS scavenging enzymes such as SOD, GPx, NQO, and CAT determine the regulation of redox signaling.

Under tight physiological control, a regulated release of ROS is essential for the fundamental life processes. Low basal levels of ROS are required for normal movement of skeletal muscles by stimulating the sarcoplasmic reticulum ATPase activity (Oyagbemi *et al.* 2009). Another important role of ROS-mediated signaling is the innate immune machinery. Receptor activation of immune-surveillance is promoted by increased ROS production which helps in the release of the pro-inflammatory cytokines interleukin (IL) 1β, tumour necrosis factor α (TNFα) and interferon γ (IFN γ) which all lead to T-cell activation and maturation (Chen *et al.* 2016). Low ROS levels can cause immunosuppression, whereas high ROS levels mediate autoimmune reactions (Roy *et al.* 2017). ROS acts as the signaling messenger of the Mitogen-activated protein kinase (MAPK) pathway regulation. Maintenance of normal vascular tone is another typical example of radical-mediated signaling (Oyagbemi *et al.* 2009). A basal level of ROS maintained by NOX or mitochondria is required for normal cellular proliferation, stem cell renewal and terminal differentiation. Highly-oxidizing environment is a pre-requisite for several types of stem cell growth (Roy *et al.* 2017).

Pathological Significance of ROS

The beneficial effects of ROS can be confiscated by cancer cells that tilt the ROS status in their favour and sustain an escalated ROS level that favours cancer cell proliferation (Schieber and Chandel 2014). Cancer cells and some stem cells harbour a moderately higher ROS level (below cytotoxic level) that redirects redox-signaling reactions in favour of uncontrolled growth *via* pro-oncogenic pathways involving hypoxia-inducible factors (HIFs), phosphoinositide3-kinase (PI3K), nuclear factor κ light chain enhancer of activated B cells (NF-κB), MAPK, JUN N-terminal kinase (JNK), cyclin D1, and extracellular signal-regulated kinase (ERK) (Roy *et al.* 2017). ROS can induce tumorigenicity by, introducing genomic alterations and DNA instability during the initial stages of tumorigenesis, increasing cell proliferation, deregulating cell cycle check-point and apoptosis, and causing abnormal gene expression during cancer progression (Yao *et al.* 2014).

ROS and Carcinogenesis

One of the prominent features of cancer cells, in comparison to their normal counterparts, is a continuous pro-oxidant status due to metabolic stress and hyperactivation of oxidase enzymes (Martinez-Outschoorn *et al.* 2010). One of the initial steps in oncogenesis is DNA damage leading to mutation and destabilization which is favoured by increased oxidative load and these altered genes further increase ROS production (Helfinger and Schröder 2018). Moreover, it is reported that the OH$^{.-}$ can bind with whole DNA molecule, and consequently, damage the deoxyribose backbone, including nucleotide bases (Saha *et al.* 2017). These genomic alterations are primarily represented by 8-hydroxydeoxyguanosine (8-OHdG), an oxidation-product of nucleoside. It is a predominant oxidative lesion and a proportional indicator of ROS-induced carcinogenesis which has been found to be increased in primary tumors compared to neighbouring non-malignant tissue thus promoting neoplastic transformation (Reuter *et al.* 2010). 8-OHdG causes transcriptional repression by introducing methylation. This global DNA hypomethylation is considered to induce downregulation of tumor suppressor genes and also upregulation of oncogenes (Perillo *et al.* 2020).

ROS may also deregulate DNA repair, resulting in the production of altered tumor-progenitor cells in a stress-dependent manner (Martinez-Outschoorn *et al.* 2010). In the promotion stage, the oxidative load may accelerate the abnormal gene expression especially the inactivation of tumor suppressor genes, activation of oncogenes or deregulation of cell-cycle vigilance, modification of second messenger systems, thus culminating in increased cell proliferation or decreased cell-death of the initiated tumor cell population. Finally, oxidative stress may also facilitate the cancer progression by accelerating further DNA abnormalities to the initiated cell population which evades the dependence on cell-cell or cell-matrix interaction (Reuter *et al.* 2010).

ROS in Cancer Signaling

It is well reported that malignant cells or even some cancer stem cells compared to benign cells show a persistently oxidizing environment with elevated ROS levels (Jelic *et al.* 2019). To thrive in such sustained redox deregulated environment, cancer cells, optimally utilize the cellular enzymatic and non-enzymatic antioxidant machinery. Oncogenic activation of Kirsten Rat Sarcoma virus (KRas), v-Raf murine sarcoma viral oncogene homolog B (Braf) and v-Raf murine sarcoma viral oncogene homolog B (c-Myc) increase the activity of the main redox regulator of human nuclear factor (erythroid-derived 2)-like 2 (Nrf2), which in turn enhances the expression of the oxidative defence program for maintaining ROS and thereby positively regulates tumor cell proliferation and tumorigenicity (Helfinger and Schröder 2018).

Once the tumorigenesis has well initiated, a chronic but moderate concentration of ROS, acts as a pro-neoplastic factor. It helps in activation of proto-oncogenes such as protein kinase C (PKC), FBJ murine osteosarcoma viral oncogene homolog or cellular oncogene fos (c-Fos), V-jun avian sarcoma virus 17 oncogene homolog (c-jun), c-myc (Surabhi 2019) and inactivation of tumour suppressor genes such as - phosphatase and tensin homolog (PTEN), forkhead box protein O (FOXO)-p53 (Strzelczyk and Wiczkowski 2012) or activation of the cancer cell survival signaling cascade involving MAPK/ERK1/2, p38, JNK, Nrf2 and PI3K / protein kinase B (Akt) (Aggarwal *et al.* 2019).

Akt revolves at the center of several signaling networks that connect multiple potentially oncogenic molecules. ROS activates Akt by inhibiting PTEN which has been proved to impair antioxidant defences and favour cancer cell survival (Reuter *et al.* 2010). Akt directly inhibits apoptosis by inactivating pro-apoptotic factors, including the Bcl-2 homology 3 (BH3)-only protein Bcl-XL/Bcl-2-associated death promoter (Bad), Bcl-2 associated X protein (Bax), caspase-9, Bcl-2-like protein 11 or Bcl2-interacting mediator of cell death (Bim) or FOXO (Rahmani *et al.* 2009). ROS activate transcription factor NF-κB, gelatinolytic enzymes matrix metalloproteinases (MMPs), and vascular endothelial growth factor (VEGF). In addition, Akt promotes nuclear translocation of the ubiquitin ligase mouse double minute 2 homolog (MDM2), which counterbalances p53-mediated apoptosis (Reuter *et al.* 2010).

ROS can directly inactivate p53 by oxidation of cysteine residues in the DNA-binding domain, whereas, constant oxidative stress promotes a selection of cell clones lacking wild-type p53 which favours resistant to apoptosis (Liou and Storz 2010). Negligible to mild oxidative stress causes p53 to activate antioxidant enzymes like SOD, GPx. This rise in the p53 activity is proportional to the ROS level up to a range but subsequently the excess ROS inhibit p53 which in turn prevents apoptosis (Strzelczyk and Wiczkowski 2012). Thus, by avoiding apoptosis and favouring oxidative metabolism, redox stress, and NF-κB upregulation, ROS facilitate neoplastic cell transformation, proliferation, and angiogenesis (Reuter *et al.* 2010).

ROS in Cancer Metabolism

All cancerous cells show a thorough alteration of their metabolic status by ROS during cancer initiation, promotion, epithelial–mesenchymal transition (EMT), angiogenesis, cell migration, invasion, metastasis, and acquisition of cancer stemness (Lee *et al.* 2017). These metabolic processes lower cellular dependency on oxygen allowing proliferation in hypoxic interior of solid tumors even in presence of sufficient molecular oxygen (Martinez-Outschoorn *et al.* 2010). Initiated cells with decreased oxidative phosphorylation favour aerobic glycolysis. Increased oxidative burden and anaerobic glycolysis in the cancer microenvironment can influence tumor cell behaviour. ROS have been indicated in the metabolic rearrangement of both cancer cells and cancer associated fibroblasts (CAFs), allowing an adaptation to oxidative stress that subsequently promotes carcinogenesis and chemoresistance (Costa *et al.* 2014).

Not only the imbalance in intracellular energy maintenance and stress signaling but also a deregulated production of mitochondrial ROS (mtROS) and other metabolic by-products, disruption in ROS scavenging by the mitochondrial antioxidant machineries [manganese superoxide dismutase (MnSOD), glutaredoxin-2 (Grx2), GPx1, thioredoxin (TRX), and peroxiredoxin] play coordinated roles in carcinogenesis (Idelchik *et al.* 2017). Increased mtROS generation and mitochondrial DNA (mtDNA) instability due to lack of histone protection is another mechanism that contributes to tumorigenic phenotype in a canonical Wnt/β-catenin independent pathway (Idelchik *et al.* 2017). Mutations of mtDNA in tumor cells result in a derailment in respiratory complex chains and the aberrant oxidative phosphorylation which contribute to the overproduction of ROS (Chen *et al.* 2016). The balance of mtROS as a beneficial death-inducer of cancer cells and detrimental activator of cancer cells determines the process of cancer pathophysiology (Sabharwal and Schumacker 2014).

ROS Mediated Inflammation

In the course of inflammation, neutrophils and macrophages usually release large amount of $O_2^{\cdot-}$, H_2O_2, and $^{\cdot}OH$. Under chronic inflammatory condition, these ROS are produced from inflammatory and epithelial cells (Kawanishi *et al.* 2017). Numerous carcinogens exert their deleterious inflammatory action through ROS production. This inflammatory microenvironment promotes carcinogenesis. Inflammatory cells can encourage DNA damage by converting procarcinogens to DNA-damaging species by robust generation of ROS (Ohnishi *et al.* 2013). Chronic inflammation is a typical example of the impact of cellular microenvironment on neoplastic transformation. ROS can further activate cancer and inflammatory cells to secrete pro-inflammatory cytokines like TNF, NOX2, IL-6, IL-2 and IL-8, which aggravate cancer stem cell (CSC) renewal and ultimately maintains progressive tumor microenvironment (Gu *et al.* 2018).

ROS Facilitate EMT, Migration and Invasion

NOX1-derived ROS generation promotes cancer cell invasion by enhancing nuclear translocation of NF-κB *via* pyruvate dehydrogenase kinase 1 (PDK1) which helps proliferative effect of epithelial growth factor receptor (EGFR) and subsequent expression of the MMP-9 (Helfinger and Schröder 2018). During EMT, NOX-mediated ROS formation induces histone H3 acetylation of the slug promoter region and expressional induction (Kamiya *et al.* 2016). ROS downregulates E-cadherin *via* hypermethylation of its promoter. This promoter hypermethylation is mediated by a snail-dependent recruitment of DNA methyltransferase 1 (DNMT1) and histone deacetylase 1 (HDAC1) which two are further upregulated by the same factor, ROS (Helfinger and Schröder 2018). ROS mediates hypoxia-induced EMT by stabilizing HIF-1α and encouraging cancer cells to produce angiogenic factors (Lv *et al.* 2017).

ROS promote aberrant MMPs-mediated increase in cell migration and invasion by inducing the Ras-Erk1/2, Rac-1-JNK, activating protein-1 (AP-1) or p38 signaling pathways (Liou and Storz 2010). ROS not only activate the MMPs directly by reacting with the thiol groups of the protease catalytic domain but also suppress their inhibitor, tissue inhibitor of metalloproteinases (TIMPs) (Reuter *et al.* 2010). Smad2, p38 and phosphorylated ERK1/2, along with α-smooth muscle actin (α-SMA) and fibronectin upregulation, and E-cadherin repression trigger ROS dependent induction of transforming growth factor β (TGF-β) signaling. This in turn facilitates EMT, migration, invasion and metastasis. Integrin activation causes altered mitochondrial metabolism and enhances ROS production by activating many oxidases including lipoxygenase, NOX and cyclooxygenase (COX)-2 (Goitre *et al.* 2012). A synergistic signaling between integrins and growth factors results into an oxidative burst through ras-related C3 botulinum toxin substrate 1 (Rac1). Rac1-ROS signal transduction is engaged in proto-oncogene tyrosine-protein kinase Src and protein-tyrosine kinase (Pyk2) mediated phosphorylation of β-catenin and p120-catenin, which in turn increases cell adhesion to extra-cellular matrix, cell spreading and proliferation. Anchorage free proliferation or resistance to anoikis takes place most probably *via* the increased generation of intracellular ROS (Liou and Storz 2010).

ROS in Angiogenesis

ROS-dependent angiogenesis initiates through secretion of angiogenic modulators in the tumor microenvironment. Rac1, an upstream regulator of NOX, elicits ROS, which is involved in dismantling of vascular-endothelial cadherin cell-cell and cell-matrix junction and interaction between endothelial cells. This phenomenon is associated with vascular dysfunctions such as increased permeability, angiogenesis and endothelial migration (Helfinger and Schröder 2018). Endothelial cells derived NOX elevate cellular ROS by upregulation of HIF-1α and receptor phosphorylation of its major downstream VEGF signalling protein (Xia *et al.* 2007). Along with VEGF, growth factors like fibroblast growth factor (FGF) and platelet-derived growth factor (PDGF) are secreted into the tumor microenvironment in response to several stimuli including ROS which ultimately helps in angiogenesis (Reuter *et al.* 2010).

ROS in Cell Cycle Surveillance

Oxidative DNA lesions identified by ataxia telangiectasia-mutated protein (ATM), ATM- and Rad3-related (ATR) and DNA-dependent protein kinase catalytic subunit (DNA-PKs) contribute to several redox signaling pathways and act *via* modulation of DNA damage repair (DDR) pathways (Davalli *et al.* 2018). DDR, Cdc25 phosphatases (Cdc25s) and the cyclin dependent kinases (CDKs) are regulated by the intracellular redox environment and ROS induced damaged DNA lesions (Shackelford *et al.* 2000). ROS induces AP-1 activity in a JNK/MAPK-dependent way leading to increased expression of growth-stimulatory genes including cyclin D1, inhibition of the cell cycle repressor p21 as well as upregulation of MMPs and metastasis (Helfinger and Schröder 2018). ROS can upregulate the mRNA levels of cyclins including cyclin B2, cyclin D3, cyclin E1 and cyclin E2 which regulate the cell cycle to expedite G1 to S phase transition, ultimately leading into aberrant proliferation (Hardwick 2015).

ROS in Cancer Stemness

Contrary to cancer cells, which maintain a high ROS levels throughout stages of malignancy, cancer stem cells have an extraordinary antioxidant capacity (Liou and Storz 2010). CSCs that attribute aggressiveness, resistance and relapse have a strong antioxidant protection against ROS enabling them against conventional chemotherapy and radiotherapy, which functions by elevating ROS level. The stemness marker of CSCs *e.g.* aldehyde dehydrogenase 1 (ALDH1) and ATP-binding cassette sub-family G member 2 (ABCG2) work by protecting the CSCs from intracellular ROS-induced death (Hatem and Azzi 2016). Redox equilibrium plays an important role in the maintenance of stem cell survival, self-renewal, differentiation (Reuter *et al.* 2010) through the antioxidative measure and/or anti-inflammatory response and this niche can provide mutation signals. Stem cells that accumulate these mutation signals may become more tumorigenic, resulting in CSCs (Franco *et al.* 2015).

ROS in Tumor Microenvironment

Cancer cells exploit "oxidative stress" in nearby cancer associated fibroblasts (CAFs) to drive tumor-stroma co-evolution as a "metabolic engine" to fuel their own survival. This process is influenced by stromal production of nutrients to stimulate their mitochondrial biogenesis (Cuyàs *et al.* 2014). The oxidative burst is used by cancer cells in promoting DNA damage, aneuploidy and genomic instability to progress their own mutagenic evolution towards a more robust phenotype *via* a bystander effect (Martinez-Outschoorn *et al.* 2010). Other than the tumor cells, CAFs also release H_2O_2 extracellularly that induce oxidative stress in normal fibroblasts, initiating the reprogramming to CAFs and promoting cancerization of that field, EMT, invasion and cancer aggressiveness. Immune cells, such as myeloid-derived suppressor cells, tumor-associated macrophages, regulatory T cells (Treg), neutrophils, eosinophils, and mononuclear phagocytes, can also generate ROS (mostly H_2O_2) into the tumor microenvironment (Snezhkina *et al.* 2020).

ROS Prevention as a Part of Chemoprevention

It is an estimate that, more than 30% of human cancers might be prevented through appropriate lifestyle modification. About 10–70% (average 35%) of human cancer is not solely dependent on inherited genetic background but is highly attributable to diet which can be called as human carcinogens (Russo 2007). Phytochemicals are considered as the non-nutritive bio-active components of the diet based on plants and possess multi-modal or pleotropic antimutagenic and anticarcinogenic properties (Russo 2007). Increased consumption of antioxidative fruits and vegetables containing several anticancer compounds have been always more effective than a single agent (Russo 2007). 'Chemoprevention' by its definition is the strategy of stopping or retarding the onset of malignant changes with relatively nontoxic natural or (semi)synthetic chemical substances. The National Cancer Institute (NCI) is investigating several hundreds of potential agents out of more than 5000 phytochemicals and is also sponsoring a significant portion of it for Phase I, II and III chemoprevention trials (Surh 2003).

Nature and Types of Chemopreventive Agents

According to the origin and mode of synthesis, chemopreventive antioxidants are of two types- pharmacological and dietary chemopreventives. Pharmacological chemopreventives are chemically synthesized or derived from natural precursors and alone or in combination can work in a synergistic manner like (1) by blocking the cancer initiation *via* induction of antioxidant enzymes in high risk healthy individuals; (2) by inhibiting the cancer progression *via* the activation of the apoptotic pathway and cell cycle arrest in individuals already with pre-malignant lesions; (3) by escalating aberrant epigenetic alterations as an anti-cancer mechanism in patients with primary cancer; and (4) by eliminating the self-renewal potential of CSCs in case of relapse after an initial cancer-reduction (Lee *et al.* 2013b). Anthracyclines, platins, antagonistic antibodies, taxanes, anticancer antibiotics, cyclophosphamides *etc.* are some well-used pharmacological chemopreventives.

Dietary chemopreventives, which are present in a regular diet but as a non-nutritive part are again of two major types- blocking agents and suppressing agents (Russo 2007). Blocking agents are those, which prevent carcinogens from reaching the target sites or promote rapid detoxification, inhibit carcinogens from undergoing metabolic activation or from subsequent interaction with crucial biomolecules. On the other hand, suppressing agents are those which inhibit the malignant transformation of already initiated cells, either in the promotion or in the progression stage by controlling deregulated cell cycle, tumor-suppressive signal transduction and apoptotic induction (Tanaka and Sugie 2007). Carotenoids, alkaloids, polyphenols, nitrogen-containing and organosulfur compounds are the dietary agents with prominent chemopreventive properties (Russo 2007). The anticancer properties of the major classes of phytochemicals are enlisted in Table **1**.

Each chemopreventive compound, within every class, has its own set of adverse reactions. One of the major causes of adverse reactions is the excessive production of ROS and subsequent accumulation of oxidative stress. To curb these unwanted side effects, several dietary supplements have been investigated, amongst which antioxidants have gained increasing acceptability as adjuvant in cancer chemotherapy (Singh *et al.* 2018). The induction of oxidative stress as the mechanism of action of many anticancer drugs has been well reported (Rigas and Sun 2008). Since, antioxidants may save the malignant cells from ROS-induced toxicity, success of anticancer therapy may be conditioned by maintaining the level of antioxidants in our body, which can be produced de novo (endogenous) or can be ingested through the diet and nutritional supplements (exogenous) (Rodríguez-Serrano *et al.* 2015). Antioxidants have shown to exert beneficial effect when used along with chemotherapeutic drugs against initiation, promotion and progression of carcinogenesis (Valadez-Vega *et al.* 2013).

The synergistic and pleiotropic action of low dose endogenous and exogenous antioxidants may neutralize free radicals more effectively during the process of multistep carcinogenesis (Sonam and Guleria 2017, Kaur *et al.* 2019). The anticancer properties of the antioxidative phytochemicals have therapeutic evidence during early initiation, promotion, local progression even up to distant metastasis. They can work by (Amin *et al.* 2015).

Table 1. Anticancer properties of major classes of dietary phytochemicals.

Class of dietary phytochemical	Characteristics	Source	Compounds	Anticancer Action	References
Phenolics	• One or more aromatic ring with one or more –OH group • Fruit secondary metabolites • Phenolic acids and flavonoids are major subtypes	Soybean, Wine, Tea, Coffee, Fruits, Vegetables Turmeric	Genistein, Resveratrol, Epigallo-catechingallate (EGCG), Caffeic acid, Anthocyanin, Quercetin, Curcumin	• Reduction of chemical carcinogens and electrophiles • Inhibition of promotion and hyperproliferation	(Tuli *et al.* 2019), (Ulrich *et al.* 2005), (Yang *et al.* 2011), (Espíndola *et al.* 2019), (Wang and Stoner 2008), (Wu *et al.* 2020), (Liao *et al.* 2017) (Tanaka *et al.* 2012), (Sahin and Kucuk 2013) (Su *et al.* 2015), (Rather and Bhagat 2018), (Choi 2017), (Jiang *et al.* 2018)
Carotenoids	• 40-C long double H-bonded all-trans cyclic isoprene • Natural pigment with provitamin property • Diverse level of hydrogenation, & oxygen-containing functional groups	Carrots, Tomato	β-Carotene, Lycopene	• Induces cancer cell differentiation • Inhibit lipid peroxidation	
Alkaloids	• Basic nitrogen-containing organic ring-structure originating from amino acids • Diverse pharmacological effects • True-, proto-, cyclo- & pseudo-alkaloids are the major sub-types	Bacteria Fungi, Plants, Animals	Tetrachloro-benzoquinon, Vinblastine, Vincristine	• Modification of carcinogen and tumor metabolism • Retardation of tumor growth	
Organo-Sulfur compounds	• Sulphur-containing organic compounds • Mono-, di-, poly-sulfides, thiols, sulfuranes, isothiocynates are the key groups	Allium, Broccoli, Cabbage	Diallyl Disulfide, Sulforaphane	• Detoxification of free radicals and carcinogens • Repression of DNA adduct formation • Initiation of cell cycle arrest	

(Table 1) cont.....

Class of dietary phytochemical	Characteristics	Source	Compounds	Anticancer Action	References
Nitrogen-containing compounds	• Both organic and inorganic nitrogen-containing compound • Amino acids, proteins, vitamins and hormones are the key types	Bacteria Fungi, Plants, Animals	Proline, Arginine, Histidine, Melatonin, Bilirubin	• Inhibition of tumor metabolic activation	(Mansour 2000)

• Modulating Hormones/Growth Factors Receptors

[Oestrogen, progesterone and their receptors, VEGF, epidermal growth factor (EGF), PDGF, FGF and their respective receptors]

• Phase 1 and 2 Metabolizing Enzyme Mediated Depletion of Potential Carcinogens

[↓SOD, ↓CAT, ↓glutathione, ↓GPx, ↓GSH and ↓cyt P450]

• Inhibiting Oncogenes and Activating Tumour Suppressor Genes

[↓KRas, ↓BRaf, ↓cMyc, ↓EGFR, PI3K/AKT, ↓Cyclins and ↑p53, ↑p27, ↑PTEN, ↑FOXO, ↑poly(ADP) ribose polymerase (PARP), ↑ATM]

• Inducing Terminal Differentiation

[↑IkB kinase α (IKKα), ↑all-trans retinoic acid, ↑retinoid receptors, ↑histone deacetylase inhibitors (HDACI), peroxisome proliferator-activator receptor γ agonists, independent of p53]

• Activating Checkpoints and Apoptosis

[↓Cyclin B, ↓B1, ↓D1, ↓CDK A, ↓E, ↓CDK 1, ↓2, ↓4 and ↑p53, ↑p21, ↑pRb, ↑p57]

• Restoring Immune-Response

[↓cytotoxic T lymphocyte antigen 4, ↓programmed death ligand 1, ↓Treg and ↑Helper T cells, ↑natural killer (NK) cells, ↑macrophage, ↑antibody dependent cellular cytotoxicity]

• **Inhibiting EMT and Angiogenesis**

[↓snail, ↓twist, cadherins, integrins, ↓MMPs and ↓TGF-β, ↓VEGF, ↓PDGF, ↓FGF, ↓HIF1-α]

• **Avoiding the Adverse Effects Associated with the High Drug Doses**

[↓immune suppression, ↓mucositis, ↓alopecia, ↓nausea, ↓anorexia]

DEFINITION, TYPES AND FEATURES OF ANTIOXIDANTS

The first definition of antioxidant was proposed by Halliwell *et al.* in 1989 as "any substance that, present in low concentrations compared to oxidizable substrates (carbohydrates, lipids, proteins or nucleic acids), significantly delays or inhibits the oxidation of the mentioned substrates" or later "any substance that can eliminate ROS directly or indirectly, acting as a regulator of the antioxidant defence, or inhibiting the production of those species" (Rodríguez-Serrano *et al.* 2015). Antioxidants neutralize free radicals by donating one of their own electrons and ending the electron "stealing" reaction (Singh *et al.* 2018).

Antioxidants can be differentiated into three types of defence according to their mechanism of action. The first type includes antioxidants that prevent the formation of free radicals such as SOD (IUPAC Enzyme Commission No. 1.15.1.1), CAT (IUPAC Enzyme Commission No. 1.11.1.6), and GPX, (IUPAC Enzyme Commission No.1.11.1.9) (Wiecek *et al.* 2018).

The second group of antioxidants is responsible for capturing free radicals, and thus they prevent oxidative chain reactions. This group includes metabolic antioxidants, such as lipoic acid, glutathione, L-ariginine, histidine, coenzyme Q, melatonin, uric acid, albumin, bilirubin, metal-chelating proteins, transferrin, *etc.*, and dietary antioxidants, such as vitamin E, vitamin C, flavonoids, carotenoids, trace metals (selenium, manganese, zinc), omega-3 and omega-6 fatty acids (Arsova-Sarafinovska and Dimovski 2013).

The third line of defence includes antioxidant enzymes that are involved in the repair mechanism of the damage caused by free radicals, such as lipases, transferases, proteases, DNA repair enzymes, and methionine-sulfoxide reductases. The antioxidant consumption seems to influence the effectiveness of antitumor therapy depending on the type of cancer, the mechanism of action of the drug used in the treatment, dose and timing of treatment and also on the type of antioxidants and basal antioxidant status (Rodríguez-Serrano *et al.* 2015). Recent findings reported that antioxidant when given concurrently (a) do not interfere with chemotherapy, (b) enhance the cytotoxic effect of chemotherapy,

(c) protects normal tissue and (d) increases patient survival and therapeutic response (Simone *et al.* 2007).

Two Sides of a Coin: Antioxidants or Pro-oxidants?

"All substances are poisons, the right dose differentiates a poison from a remedy" was an appropriate paraphrase of the great ancient physician, Paracelsus (Russo 2007). Usually preventive dose is a lower dose and a therapeutic dose is a higher dose. Preventive dose has shown protection of benign and malignant cells whereas therapeutic dose has shown inhibition of the growth of cancer cells but not that of normal cells (Singh *et al.* 2018). High-dose antioxidative supplements may cause hazardous health effects as it may negatively interact with some anti-cancer medications. It has also been seen that continuous use of ROS-scavenging enzymes may work as the barrier against effective apoptosis by excessively reducing ROS beyond a necessary threshold (Asadi-Samani *et al.* 2019). Dose and exposure duration of an administered compound play the crucial fate-determining role in cancer. The concept of hormesis, a biphasic dose-response relationship in which a chemical exerts opposite effects dependent on the dose, has become effective in the field of cancer management.

An antioxidant is present at low concentrations in the cell and significantly reduces oxidation of the oxidizable substrates, decreases levels of cells' oxidants like ROS, causes increase in apoptosis and therefore can be considered as an approach to treat fatal cancers. Phytochemical derived antioxidants often exhibit their chemopreventive effects in a prooxidant manner (Block *et al.* 2008). This dual nature of phytochemicals depends on their concentration, pH and solubility but ultimately lead to promotion of antiproliferative process and apoptosis (Babich *et al.* 2011). Antioxidant treatment may be more fruitful during the initiation phase, when a mild increase in ROS concentrations over the physiological threshold can cause genotoxic damage (Russo 2007). Much of the late-stage cancer's inertness may be due to its possession of excess antioxidants where prooxidative measures may give fruitful outcome (Watson 2013).

Important Phytochemicals with Anti-Oxidant and Pro-Oxidant Effect in Cancer Prevention

Free radicals increase oxidative stress that induce chronic inflammation, reduce apoptosis, promote abnormal cell proliferation, angiogenesis and metastasis *via* DNA damage and activation of oncogenes and transcriptional factors. Dietary phytochemicals on the other hand show anti-cancer properties through both pro-oxidant and anti-oxidant properties (Kaur *et al.* 2018). Innumerable studies have been done on antioxidative effect of phytochemicals. An in-depth discussion of the dose and mechanisms of antioxidants responsible for redox regulation of cancer and their mode of anticancer efficacies might provide a detailed approach for potential anticancer mechanisms (Fig. **1**). Some of the selected dietary phytochemicals that elicited anti-cancer properties by virtue of anti-oxidant properties have been depicted in Table **2** and those by pro-oxidant properties in Table **3**.

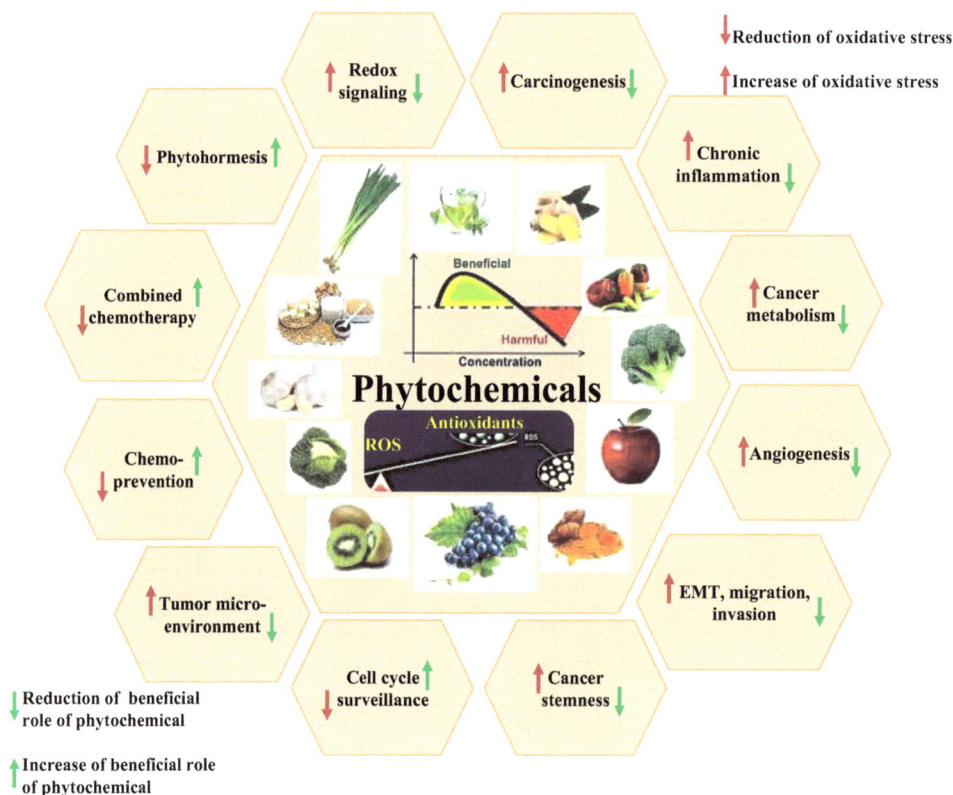

Fig. (1). Modulation of carcinogenic process by phytochemicals: Some globally used phytochemicals like, curcumin, resveratrol, EGCG, genistein, diallyldisulphide, quercetin, lycopene, sulforaphane obtained from plant sources of our daily diets like- turmeric, grapes, green tea, soy bean, garlic, broccoli, tomato *etc.* have shown wide anticancer properties by modulating the cancer signaling, metabolism, EMT, angiogenesis, microenvironment and stemness with their unique redox regulating property. Phytochemicals may be both beneficial and harmful depending on concentration and duration of exposure.

Curcumin

The polyphenol curcumin, derived from the plant *Curcuma longa*, of family *Zingiberaceae* is the principal constituent of Indian spice turmeric (Pubchem CID 969516). It exhibited both anti-oxidant and pro-oxidant properties along with chemopreventive, anti-inflammatory and anti-cancer effects. In benzo(a)pyrene (BaP) induced lung carcinoma of swiss albino mice curcumin exhibited antioxidant property, reduced lipid peroxidation and upregulated anti-oxidative enzymes such as SOD, GPx, CAT and glutathione S transferase (GST) (Sehgal *et al*. 2012). Another study reported that in human pancreatic cancer (BxPC-3 and Panc-1) cells curcumin reduced oxidative stress by quenching ROS and H_2O_2 and retarded EMT and cell migration (Li *et al*. 2018). On the other hand, curcumin by virtue of pro-oxidant nature increased ROS level, induced apoptosis and sub G0/G1 phase growth arrest in human papillary thyroid carcinoma (PTC)-[BCPAP and TPC-I] cells. The study has shown induced expression of cleaved caspase-3, -8 and -9 along with reduced expression of cell cycle molecules (Khan *et al*. 2020). Curcumin has been reported to induce apoptosis in A375 melanoma cells along with upregulated ROS production (Liao *et al*. 2017).

Epigallocatechin Gallate (EGCG)

EGCG is a phenolic tea phytochemical extracted from green and black tea plants (Pubchem CID 65064). EGCG was found to have anti-oxidant effect along with chemopreventive and anti-cancer effects but several studies have shown pro-oxidant effect of EGCG. In human cervical cancer (HeLa) cells and tumor biopsy samples, EGCG was found to induce expression of anti-oxidant enzymes which promoted anti-cancer effect (Hussain 2017). In lung adenocarcinoma (NCI-H23 and A549) cells, EGCG exhibited antioxidant effect in NCI-H23 and pro-oxidant effect in A549 through differential modulation of Nrf2 at a high and low doses respectively (Datta and Sinha 2019). In another study EGCG was found to induce pro-oxidant effect in human colon cancer (HT-20) cells through increased ROS generation, apoptosis and reduced expression of pro-survival genes (Hwang *et al*. 2007). In human endometrial Ishikawa cancer cells and normal HEK-293 cells, EGCG showed anti-cancer effect by elevated ROS generation, reduced anti-oxidant enzymes and increased Bax/caspase-3 mediated apoptosis (Manohar *et al*. 2013). EGCG induced ROS production and upregulated apoptosis signal-regulating kinase 1 (ASK1)-p38/JNK signaling pathway along with apoptosis in human chondrosarcoma (JJ012) cells (Yang *et al*. 2011).

Resveratrol

Resveratrol is a phytoalexin belonging to polyphenolic group which is extracted from grapes, nuts, fruits, and red wine (Pubchem CID 445154). Resveratrol exhibited anti-inflammatory, anti-cancer activity along with anti-oxidative and pro-oxidative properties. Anti-oxidative properties of resveratrol exhibited in human pancreatic cancer (BxPC-3 and Panc-1) cells where it curtailed ROS production along with reduction in cancer cell invasion due to hypoxia (Li *et al*. 2016). On the other hand, resveratrol inflicted ROS production in human colon carcinoma (HCT116) cells along with G1 phase and senescence like cell growth arrest (Heiss *et al.* 2007). Pro-oxidant behaviour of resveratrol was also observed in human gastric adenocarcinoma (SGC7901) cells along with induction of apoptosis and reduction of cell proliferation (Wang *et al.* 2012).

Quercetin

Quercetin is a flavonoid belonging to polyphenolic group, derived from apples, onions, and green tea (Pubchem CID 5280343). It exhibited chemopreventive, anti-inflammatory and anti-allergic effects along with anti-oxidative and pro-oxidative properties. In human fibrosarcoma (HT1080) cells, quercetin inhibited phenazinemethosulfate (PMS) induced ROS production and also abated cell motility through reduced expression of MMP-2 and -9 (Lee *et al.* 2013a). On the other hand, in several other studies quercetin was found to have pro-oxidative properties. In HA22T/VGH and HepG2 hepatoma cells, quercetin aggravated ROS production and malondialdehyde along with inhibition in cell growth (Chang *et al.* 2006). In rat hepatoma (H4IIE) cells, quercetin downregulated gene expression of anti-oxidative enzymes dose dependently (Röhrdanz *et al.* 2003). Quercetin induced autophagy through increased expression of nuclear protein1 (NUPR1) which is needed for the expression of stress-response genes along with ROS production in osteosarcoma (MG-63) cells (Wu *et al.* 2020).

Fisetin

Fisetin, a flavonoid belonging to polyphenolic group, derived from edible vegetables, fruits, and wine, exhibited anti-inflammatory, anti-cancer, anti-oxidant and pro-oxidant properties (Pubchem CID 5281614). In Aflatoxin-B1 (AFB1)-induced hepatocarcinogenesis of rats, fisetin elicited anti-cancer effect through reduced ROS production and increased expression of anti-oxidative enzymes (Maurya and Trigun 2016). Fisetin also showed anti-oxidant properties through increased antioxidant enzyme mediated free radical in BaP-induced lung carcinogenesis in male Swiss albino mice (Ravichandran *et al.* 2011). On the other hand, fisetin was found to have pro-oxidant effect along with ROS-induced apoptosis and elevated expression of pro-apoptotic molecules in human non-small cell lung cancer (NCI-H460) cells (Kang *et al.* 2015). Fisetin triggered ROS production along with apoptotic and necroptosis signaling in HepG2 cells (Sundarraj *et al.* 2020).

Genistein

Genistein is an isoflavone, derived from soybeans and soy products like tofu, with anti-inflammatory, anti-proliferative and anti-cancer effect along with anti-oxidant and pro-oxidant effect (Pubchem CID 5280961). In prostate cancer (DU145 and PC3) cells, it was found to have anti-oxidant effect through reduced

ROS production and increased anti-oxidant enzymes (Park *et al.* 2010) whereas in breast cancer (MDA-MB-231, and MDA- MB-468) cells it was found to have pro-oxidant effect through increased ROS and pro-apoptotic signaling (Ullah *et al.* 2011). Genistein in bladder cancer (T24) cells induced G2/M growth arrest and apoptosis along with ROS generation (Park *et al.* 2019).

Mangiferin

Mangiferin (Pubchem CID 5281647), a xanthonoid derived from *Mangifera indica*, exhibited anti-viral, anti-bacterial, analgesic and anti-inflammatory properties (Rajendran *et al.* 2008). Mangiferin exhibited anti-oxidant and anti-tumor properties against diethynitrosamine (DEN)-induced hepatocellular carcinoma in male Sprague-Dawley rats through reduced 8-OHdG, ROS production and induction of enzymatic and non-enzymatic antioxidants along with reduced expression of liver enzymes (Yang *et al.* 2019). In embryonic rhabdomyosarcoma (RD) cells mangiferin induced cytotoxicity and apoptosis along with oxidative stress through ROS generation (Padma *et al.* 2015).

Baicalein

Baicalein (Pubchem CID 5281605), a flavonoid derived from the roots of *Scutellaria baicalensis* Georgi, exhibited anti-hepatotoxicity, anti-inflammatory and anti-viral properties (Naveenkumar *et al.* 2013). Baicalein reduced lung carcinogenesis induced by BaP in male Swiss albino mice through depletion of ROS and activation of anti-oxidant enzymes along with apoptosis (Naveenkumar *et al.* 2013). In human bladder cancer (5637) cells, baicalein exhibited ROS dependent activation of apoptosis through upregulation of pro-apoptotic signaling (Choi *et al.* 2016).

Luteolin

Luteolin is a flavonoid, which is present in different types of vegetables, fruits and herbs. It exhibited anti-neoplastic, anti-inflammatory, anti-oxidant and pro-oxidant properties (Pubchem CID 5280445). In BaP-induced lung carcinogenesis in male swiss albino mice, luteolin exhibited anti-oxidant properties through reduced lipid peroxidation, increased enzymatic and non-enzymatic antioxidants along with curtailed cell proliferation (Kasala *et al.* 2016). In lung cancer (H23, H2009, H460, and A549) cells luteolin influenced apoptosis along with ROS generation (Ju *et al.* 2007).

Apigenin

Apigenin, a dietary flavone present in many fruits and vegetables, exhibited anti-inflammatory, anti-metastatic and anti-proliferative properties (Pubchem CID 5280443). Apigenin exhibited anti-oxidant effect in oral carcinogenesis induced by DMBA in golden Syrian hamsters *via* upregulation of enzymatic and non-enzymatic antioxidants (Silvan *et al.* 2011). Apigenin elicited pro-oxidant properties through ROS production and apoptosis in promyelotic leukemia (HL-60) cells (Miyoshi *et al.* 2007) and in hepatocarcinoma (Hep3B and HepG2) cells (Kang *et al.* 2018).

Capsaicin

Capsaicin is an alkaloid, extracted from hot red chili peppers and capsicum, and belong to family *Solanaceae* (Pubchem CID 1548943). It exhibited anti-cancer, chemopreventive, analgesic, anti-inflammatory, anti-oxidant and pro-oxidant properties. Capsaicin showed anti-oxidant properties through decreased lipid peroxidation and increased expression of enzymatic antioxidants like SOD, GPx, GST and non-enzymatic antioxidants like reduced glutathione and vitamin A, E and C in BaP-induced lung carcinoma in male Swiss albino mice (Jang *et al.* 2008). On the other hand, capsaicin exhibited pro-oxidant effect through increased ROS production, apoptosis and cell cycle arrest in human bladder cancer (T24, 5637) cells, NOD/SCID mice (Qian *et al.* 2016) and also in human hepatoma cancer (SMMC-7721) cells (Lee and Song 2013). Capsaicin also exhibited pro-oxidant effect in renal 789-O cells along with apoptosis (Liu *et al.* 2016).

Piperine

Piperine, an alkaloid extracted from black pepper (*Piper nigrum*) and long pepper (*Piper longum*), has been reported with anti-cancer effect along with anti-oxidant and pro-oxidant properties (Pubchem CID 638024). In BaP-induced lung carcinogenesis in male Swiss albino mice (Selvendiran *et al.* 2004) and 7,12-dimethylbenz[a]anthracene (DMBA) induced skin carcinogenesis in male Swiss albino (Vellaichamy *et al.* 2009), piperine exhibited anti-oxidant effect through suppression of lipid peroxidation and elevated expression of enzymatic and non-enzymatic antioxidants. Piperine evoked pro-oxidant effect through increased ROS formation and apoptosis through upregulation of cleaved caspase-3 in human KB oral squamous carcinoma (Siddiqui *et al.* 2017) and HeLa (Jafri *et al.* 2019) cells.

Lycopene

Lycopene is a carotenoid found in fruits such as tomatoes, red oranges, apricots, watermelon and guava and is essential in animal diet (Pubchem CID 446925). Lycopene has potent anti-cancer effect along with anti-oxidant and pro-oxidant properties. In human pancreatic cancer (PANC-1) cells, it was found to have anti-oxidant effect through minimized ROS production and augmented apoptosis (Jeong *et al.* 2019). Treatment of N-Methyl-N′-nitro-nitrosoguanidine (MNNG)-induced gastric carcinoma with lycopene led to the suppression of oxidative stress through induction of anti-oxidant enzymes and immunity markers in male Wister rats, (Luo and Wu 2011). Lycopene increased oxidative stress through enhanced lipid peroxidation and 8-OHdG formation in human prostate cancer (LNCaP) cells leading to DNA damage and reduced cell proliferation (Hwang and Bowen 2005).

Table 2. Role of phytochemicals as antioxidants in cancer prevention.

Phyto-chemical	Nature	Model	Dose of phyto-chemical	Effect	Mode of action	Reference
Curcumin	Polyphenol	6-8 weeks male Swiss albino mice	100 mg/kg	↓Oxidative stress in lung carcinoma induced by B(a)P	↓LPO ↑GR ↑GST ↑SOD ↑GPx ↑CAT	(Sehgal *et al.* 2012)
		BxPC-3 and Panc-1 cells	20 µM	↓Cell migration ↓EMT	↓ROS ↓H$_2$O$_2$ ↓p-Akt ↓p-NF-κB ↑E-cadherin ↓N-cadherin ↓Vimentin	(Li *et al.* 2018)
EGCG	Polyphenol	HeLa cells, cervical cancer biopsy	0, 10, 20, 30, 40, and 50 µg/ml	↓Cell proliferation	↑SOD ↑GPx	(Hussain 2017)
		NCI-H23 cells	50 µM	↑DNA damage	↑SOD1 ↑Nrf2 ↓Keap1 ↓FOXO3 ↓RAR ↑RXR ↓p-53 ↑p-21	(Datta and Sinha 2019)
Resveratrol	Flavonoid	BxPC-3 and Panc-1 cells	12.5, 25 and 50 µM	↓Cell invasion induced by hypoxia	↓ROS ↓HIF-1α ↓uPA ↓MMP-2 ↓SHH ↓SMO ↓GLI1	(Li *et al.* 2016)
Quercetin	Flavonoid	HT1080 cells	Upto 10 µg/ml	↓PMS induced cell motility	↓ROS ↓MMP2 ↓MMP9	(Lee *et al.* 2013a)

(Table 2) cont.....

Phyto-chemical	Nature	Model	Dose of phyto-chemical	Effect	Mode of action	Reference
Fisetin	Flavonoid	18–20 weeks male Charles foster rats	20 mg/kg	↓Hepato-carcino-genesis induced by AGB1	↓TNFα ↓IL1β ↓ROS ↑SOD1 ↑GPx ↑GSH ↑CAT	(Maurya and Trigun 2016)
		Male Swiss albino mice of 6–8 weeks	25 mg/kg	↓Lung carcino-genesis induced by B(a)P	↓ROS ↑SOD ↑CAT ↑GPx ↑GST ↑GR ↓LPO ↓PCNA	(Ravich-andran *et al.* 2011)
Genistein	Isoflavone	DU145 and PC3 cells	5, 10, and 25 μM	↑Tumor suppression	↓ROS ↑CAT ↑MnSOD ↑PTEN ↑pAMPK ↓p-ERK	(Park *et al.* 2010)
Mangiferin	Xanthonoid	Male Sprague-Dawley rats	50 mg/kg	↓Hepato cellular carcinoma induced by DEN	↓8-OHdG ↓ROS ↑SOD ↑CAT ↑GPx ↑GR ↑GSH ↑Vit E,C ↑caspase-3 ↑Bax ↓Bcl-2 ↓ALT ↓AST ↓ALP ↓GGT ↓LDH	(Yang *et al.* 2019)
Baicalein	Flavanoid	Male Swiss albino mice of 8-10 weeks	12 mg/kg	↓BaP induced lung carcino-genesis ↑Apoptosis	↓ROS ↓LPO ↑SOD ↑CAT ↑GPx ↑GST ↑GR ↑GSH ↑Vit E,C ↑Bid ↑Bim ↓Bcl-xL	(Naveen-kumar *et al.* 2013)

(Table 2) cont.....

Phyto-chemical	Nature	Model	Dose of phyto-chemical	Effect	Mode of action	Reference
Luteolin	Flavanoid	Male Swiss albino mice of 6-8 weeks	15 mg/kg	↓Lung carcino-genesis induced by BaP	↓LPO ↑SOD ↑GST ↑GR ↑CAT ↑GPx ↑GSH ↑Vit E,C ↓NF-kB ↓PCNA ↓CYP1A1	(Kasala *et al.* 2016)
Apigenin	Flavone	Hamsters	2.5 mg/kg	↓DMBA induced oral carcino-genesis	↑SOD ↑GST ↑GSH ↑CAT ↑GPx ↑GR ↑Vit E,C ↓CytP450 ↓Cyt b5	(Silvan *et al.* 2011)
Capsaicin	Alkaloid	Male Swiss albino mice of 8-10 weeks	10 mg/kg	↓Lung carcinoma induced by B(a)P	↓LPO ↑SOD ↑GR ↑GST ↑CAT ↑GSH ↑GPx ↑Vit A,C,E	(Jang *et al.* 2008)
Piperine	Alkaloid	17–20 grams male Swiss albino mice	50 mg/kg	↓Lung carcino-genesis induced by B(a)P	↓LPO ↑CAT ↑GPx ↑SOD ↑GSH ↑Vit C,E	(Selvendiran *et al.* 2004)
		4–6 weeks old male Swiss albino mice	50 mg/kg	↓Skin carcino-genesis induced by DMBA	↓LPO ↑SOD ↑CAT ↑GPx ↑GSH ↑GST ↑GR ↓cytP450	(Vellaichamy *et al.* 2009)

(Table 2) cont.....

Phyto-chemical	Nature	Model	Dose of phyto-chemical	Effect	Mode of action	Reference
Lycopene	Carotenoid	PANC-1 cells	0, 0.25 and 0.5 μM	↓Oxidative stress ↑Apoptosis	↓ROS ↓NF-κB ↓cIAP1,2 ↓survivin ↑caspase-3	(Jeong *et al.* 2019)
		6-week-old male Wistar rats	100, 200 and 300 mg/kg	↓Gastric carcinoma induced by MNNG	↓MDA ↑SOD ↑CAT ↑GSH-Px ↑IL-2 ↑IL-10 ↑IL-4 ↑TNF-α	(Luo and Wu 2011)
Vitamin C /Ascorbic acid	Micro-nutrient	Human gastric cancer patients	Median values: Vitamic C-106 μg/g and Ascorbic acid-85.9 μg/g	↓Radical mediated DNA damage	↓oxygen radical	(Drake *et al.* 1996)
Diallyl sulfide	Organo-sulphur compound	170-200 g male Wistar albino rats	80 mg/ml	↓Liver carcino-genesis induced by NDEA	↓NO ↓MDA ↑G6Pase ↓GST ↓AR ↑LDH ↑G6PD ↑AST ↑ALP ↑GGT ↑Cyt c	(Ibrahim and Nassar 2008)
Sulfora-phane	Isothio-cyanate	4-6 weeks old female Swiss albino mice	9 μM/ mouse/ day	↓Lung carcino-genesis induced by B(a)P	↑SOD ↑GPx ↑GSH ↓LPO	(Priya *et al.* 2011)

Abbreviations: 8-OHdG-8-hydroxydeoxyguanosine; **Akt-** protein kinase B; **ALP-** alkaline phosphatase; **ALT-** alanine transaminase; **AMPK-** AMP-activated protein kinase; **AR-** aldose reductase; **AST-** aspartate transaminase; **Bax -** Bcl-2-associated X protein; **Bcl-2-** B-cell lymphoma 2; **CAT** – catalase; **cIAP1-** cellular inhibitor of apoptosis protein 1; **CYP1A1-** cytochrome P450 1A1; **ERK-** extracellular signal-regulated kinase; **FOXO** - forkhead box protein O; **G6Pase** - glucose-6-phosphatase; **GGT-** gamma-glutamyl trans-peptidase**; GPx** - glutathione peroxidase; **GR-** glutathione reductase; **GSH-** glutathione; **GST-** glutathione S-transferase; **H2AX-** histone family member X; $\mathbf{H_2O_2}$**-** hydrogen peroxide; **HIF-1α** - Hypoxia-inducible factor 1-alpha; **Keap1** - Kelch like ECH associated protein; **LDH-** lactate dehydrogenase; **LPO-** lipid Peroxidation; **MDA-** malondialdehyde; **MMP-** matrix metalloproteinases; **MnSOD -** manganese superoxide dismutase; **Nrf2** - nuclear factor erythroid2-related factor2 ; **NF-κB-** nuclear factor kappa-light-chain-enhancer of activated B cells; **NO-** nitric Oxide; **PCNA-** proliferating cell nuclear antigen; **PTEN -** phosphatase and tensin homolog; **RAR-** retinoid acid receptor; **ROS -** reactive oxygen species; **RXR-** retinoid X receptor; **SHH-** sonic hedgehog; **SMO-** smoothened; **SOD -** superoxide dismutase; **TNFα** -Tumor Necrosis Factor α; **uPA-** Urokinase-type plasminogen activator

Vitamin C

Ascorbic acid (Vitamin C), found in green vegetables and citrus fruits, acts as a potent anti-oxidant agent (Pubchem CID 54670067). It exhibited anti-bacterial, anti-cancer and anti-oxidant properties. Ascorbic acid was found to scavenge free oxygen radicals in the gastric mucosa of human gastric cancer patients (Drake *et al.* 1996). It also caused oxidative stress-induced cytotoxicity in male Wistar rats and female Sprague-Dawley rats through increased production of ascorbate radical and hydrogen peroxide (Chen *et al.* 2007).

Organosulphur Compounds

Diallyl sulfide, constituent of garlic (*Allium sativum*) (Pubchem CID 11617) reduced malondialdehyde and nitric oxide levels and increased anti-oxidant enzymes in N-nitrosodiethylamine (NDEA)-induced liver carcinogenesis in Wistar rats (Ibrahim and Nassar 2008). In adenocarcinoma (Colo 320 DM) cells, diallyl sulfide induced ROS production, apoptosis and increased G2/M phase growth arrest (Sriram *et al.* 2008). Diallyl trisulfide also exhibited pro-oxidant effect in gastric cancer (AGS) cells along with induction of G2/M phase arrest and apoptosis (Choi 2017).

Sulforaphane, an isothiocyanate present in cruciferous vegetables like cabbage and broccoli (Pubchem CID 5350) showed anti-oxidant properties in B(a)P induced lung carcinoma in female Swiss albino mice through induced expression of anti-oxidant enzymes (Priya *et al.* 2011). In osteosarcoma (MG-63) cells, sulforaphane inflicted oxidative stress through ROS production (Ferreira De Oliveira *et al.* 2014).

Table 3. Role of phytochemicals as pro-oxidants against cancer.

Phyto-chemical	Nature	Model	Dose of phyto-chemical	Effect	Mode of action	References
Curcumin	Polyphenol	PTC, BCPAP and TPC-I cells	10, 20 and 40 µM	↑Apoptosis ↑Sub G0/G1 phase of cell cycle	↑ROS ↑cleaved caspase-3,8,9 ↑PARP ↑p-H2AX ↓p-STAT3 ↓p-Jak2 ↓p-CXCR4 ↓Cyclin D1	(Khan *et al.* 2020)
		A375 cells	0, 20, 40 and 80 µM	↑Apoptosis	↑ROS ↓GSH ↓MMP ↓cyclin D ↓G6PD ↑HIF1α ↑Bax ↓Bcl-2	(Liao *et al.* 2017)

(Table 3) cont.....

Phyto-chemical	Nature	Model	Dose of phyto-chemical	Effect	Mode of action	References
EGCG	Polyphenol	A549	0.5 μM	↑DNA damage	↓SOD1 ↓Nrf2 ↑Keap1 ↑FOXO3 ↑RAR ↑RXR ↑p53 ↓p21	(Datta and Sinha 2019)
		HT-29 cells	50, 100, 200 and 400 μM	↑Apoptosis ↓Cell growth	↑ROS ↑AMPK ↓COX-2 ↓ Glut-1 gene ↓VEGF	(Hwang *et al.* 2007)
		Ishikawa cells	50, 75, 100, 125 and 150 μM	↓Cell viability ↑Apoptosis	↑ROS ↓GSH ↓ER-α ↓PR ↓cyclin D1 ↓PCNA ↑p-38 ↓p-ERK ↓c-jun ↓c-fos ↓Bcl-2 ↑Bax ↑caspase-3 ↑cleaved PARP	(Manohar *et al.* 2013)
		JJ012 cells	25, 50, 100, 200 and 400 μM	↑Apoptosis	↑ROS ↑Bax ↑Bak ↓Bcl-2 ↑ASK1-p38/ JNK pathway	(Yang *et al.* 2011)
Resveratrol	Flavonoid	HCT 116 cells	30 μM	↑Senescence ↑S-phase growth arrest	↑ROS ↑ATM ↑p38 MAPK ↑p-p53 ↑p21	(Heiss *et al.* 2007)
		SGC 7901 cells	0, 25, 50, 100 and 200 μM/l	↓Cell growth ↑Apoptosis	↑ROS ↑caspase-3 ↑γH2AX ↓Ku70	(Wang *et al.* 2012)

(Table 3) cont.....

Phyto-chemical	Nature	Model	Dose of phyto-chemical	Effect	Mode of action	References
Quercetin	Flavonoid	HA22T/VGH and HepG2 cells	40, 60, or 80 μM	↓Cell growth ↑Apoptosis	↑ROS ↑MDA	(Chang *et al.* 2006)
		Rat hepatoma H4IIE cell	5, 10, 50 and 100 μM	↓Antioxidant enzyme mRNA expression	↓Mn-SOD ↓CuZn-SOD ↓GPx	(Röhrdanz *et al.* 2003)
		MG-63 cells	50, 100 and 200 μM	↑Autophagy	↑ROS ↑LC3B-II/LC3B-I ↓P62/SQSTM1 ↑NUPR1	(Wu *et al.* 2020)
Fisetin	Flavonoid	NCI-H460 cells	75 μg/ml	↑Apoptosis	↑ROS ↓Bcl-2 ↑Bax ↑caspase-3,9	(Kang *et al.* 2015)
		HepG2 cells	25, 50 and 100 μM	↑Apoptosis ↑Necroptosis	↑ROS ↑TNFα ↑IKκB ↓NF-κB ↓pNF-κB ↓pIKκB ↓Bcl2 ↑Bax ↑caspase-3 ↑RIPK1 ↑RIPK3 ↑MLKL	(Sundarraj *et al.* 2020)
Genistein	Isoflavone	MDA-MB-231, and MDA-M--468 cells	50 μM	↓Cell growth ↑Apoptosis	↑ROS ↓Bcl-2 ↑Bax ↑caspase-3,9	(Ullah *et al.* 2011)
		T24 cells	40, 80, 120 and 160 μM	↑G2/M phase arrest ↑Apoptosis	↑p21 ↓cyclin A,B1 ↑Bax ↓Bcl-2 ↓p-PI3K ↓p-Akt ↑ROS	(Park *et al.* 2019)
Mangiferin	Xanthonoid	RD cells	50, 70 and 90 μM	↑Cytotoxicity ↑Apoptosis	↑ROS ↑LDH ↑NO ↓GSH ↓SOD ↓CAT ↓GST	(Padma *et al.* 2015)

(Table 3) cont.....

Phyto-chemical	Nature	Model	Dose of phyto-chemical	Effect	Mode of action	References
Baicalein	Flavonoid	5637 cells	0, 50, 150 and 250 μM	↑Apoptosis	↑ROS ↑Bax ↑caspase-3,8,9 ↓Bcl-2 ↑PARP ↓cIAP-1 and cIAP-2 ↑TRAIL ↑FasL	(Choi *et al.* 2016)
Luteolin	Flavonoid	H23, H2009, H460, and A549 cells	40 μM	↑Apoptosis	↑ROS ↓SOD ↑p-JNK ↓NF-κB	(Ju *et al.* 2007)
Apigenin	Flavone	HL-60 cells	50 μM	↑Apoptosis ↑Autophagy	↑ROS ↑caspase-3	(Miyoshi *et al.* 2007)
		Hep3B and HepG2 cells	20 μM	↑TRAIL-induced apoptosis, ↑Autophagy	↑ROS ↑caspase-3 ↓Bcl-2 ↑DR5	(Kang *et al.* 2018)
Capsaicin	Alkaloid	T24, 5637 cells and NOD/SCID mice	0, 150 and 300 μM	↓Cell growth and migration ↑G0/G1 phase arrest	↑ROS ↑FOXO3a ↑MnSOD ↓CDK2/4/6 ↓cyclin D1	(Qian *et al.* 2016)
		SMMC-7721 cells	0, 150, 200 and 250 μM	↑Apoptosis	↑ROS ↑JNK ↑p38 MAPK	(Lee and Song 2013)
		786-O cell	0 to 400 μM	↑Apoptosis, ↓Proliferation	↑ROS ↑caspase-3,8,9 ↑c-myc ↑FADD ↑Bax ↓Bcl-2 ↓p-ERK1/2 ↑p-P38 ↑p-JNK	(Liu *et al.* 2016)

(Table 3) cont.....

Phyto-chemical	Nature	Model	Dose of phyto-chemical	Effect	Mode of action	References
Piperine	Alkaloid	KB cells	25, 50, 100, 200 and 300 mM	↑Cell death ↑Nuclear condensation ↑Apoptosis	↑caspase-3,9 ↓Cyclin B1 ↑ROS	(Siddiqui *et al.* 2017)
		HeLa cells	10, 25, 50, 100 and 200 μM	↑Nuclear condensation, ↓MMP ↑Apoptosis ↑G2/M phase growth arrest ↓Cell motility and invasion	↑ROS ↑caspase-3 ↓MMP	(Jafri *et al.* 2019)
Lycopene	Carotenoid	LNCaP cells	> 5 μM	↓Cell growth ↑DNA damage	↑8-OHdG ↑LPO	(Hwang and Bowen 2005)
Vitamin C	Micro-nutrient	Male Wistar rats and female Sprague Dawley rats	0.25–5 mg/g	↑Pro-oxidant	↑Asc· radical ↑H$_2$O$_2$	(Chen *et al.* 2007)
Diallyl sulfide	Organo-sulfur compound	Colo 320 DM cells	50 μM	↓Cell growth ↑Apoptosis ↑G2/M phase arrest	↑ROS ↓LDH ↓ERK-2 ↑caspase-3 ↑NFκB	(Sriram *et al.* 2008)
Diallyl trisulfide	Organo-sulfur compound	AGS cells	50 μM	↑G2/M arrest ↑Apoptosis	↑p-AMPK ↑p-ACC ↑ROS	(Choi 2017)
Sulfo-raphane	Isothio-cyanate	MG-63 cells	0, 5, 10, and 20 μM	↑Apoptosis ↑DNA damage	↑ROS ↓GSH ↓SOD ↓CAT ↓GPx ↓GR	(Ferreira de Oliveira *et al.* 2014)

Abbreviations: 8-OHdG-8-hydroxydeoxyguanosine; **Akt**- protein kinase B; **AMPK**- AMP-activated protein kinase; **Asc•**- radical- ascorbate radical; **ASK1** - apoptosis signal-regulating kinase 1; **ATM** - Ataxia Telangiectasia-mutated; **Bax** - Bcl-2-associated X protein; **Bcl2** - B-cell lymphoma 2; **CAT** – catalase; **CDK**-cyclin-dependent kinases; **cIAP-1**- cellular inhibitor of apoptosis protein 1; **COX-2**- cyclooxygenase-2 ; **CuZn-SOD**- copper, zinc superoxide dismutase; **CXCR4**- C-X-C chemokine receptor type 4; **DR5**- death receptor 5; **ERK** - extracellular signal-related kinase; **ER-α**- estrogen receptor alpha; **FADD**- Fas-associated death domain; **FOXO3** - forkhead box protein O; **G6PD**- glucose 6 phosphate dehydrogenase; **Glut-1** - glucose transporters 1; **GPx** - glutathione peroxidase; **GSH** - glutathione; **GST** - glutathione S-transferase; **H2AX** - histone family member X (p-H2AX); **H$_2$O$_2$**- hydrogen peroxide; **HIF1α** - hypoxia-inducible factor 1-alpha; **IKκB** – inhibitor of kappa B kinase; **JNK** - c-Jun NH2-terminal kinase; **Keap1**- Kelch like ECH associated protein 1; **LC3**- microtubule-associated proteins 1A/1B light chain 3B; **LDH** – lactate dehydrogenase; **LPO**- lipid Peroxidation; **MAPK** - mitogen-activated protein kinase; **MDA** – malondialdehyde; **MLKL** - mixed lineage kinase domain-like protein; **MMP** - matrix metalloproteinases; **MnSOD** - manganese superoxide dismutase; **NF-κB**- nuclear factor kappa-light-chain-enhancer of activated

B cells; **Nrf2** - nuclear factor erythroid2-related factor2 ; **NUPR1** - nuclear protein 1; **p-ACC**- phospho-acetyl CoA carboxylase; **PARP** – poly (ADP-ribose) polymerase; **PCNA** - proliferating cell nuclear antigen; **p-H2AX** - phosphor-histone family member X; **PI3K** - phosphatidylinositol-3-kinase; **RAR** - retinoic acid receptors; **RIPK**- receptor-interacting serine/threonine-protein kinase; **ROS** - reactive oxygen species; **RXR** - retinoid X receptors; **SOD** - superoxide dismutase; **STAT3** - signal transducer and activator of transcription; **TNFα** – tumor Necrosis Factor- alpha; **TRAIL**- TNF-related apoptosis-inducing ligand; **VEGF** - vascular endothelial growth factor

Phytochemicals and Chemotherapy

Phytochemicals with chemotherapeutic drugs and their synergistic anticancer ROS mediated effect are listed in Table **4**. Curcumin (0-50 μM) induced apoptosis and cell cycle arrest at G2/M growth phase along with increase in antioxidant enzymes SOD and GSH in cisplatin (5 μg/ml) resistant human ovarian cancer cells (Weir *et al.* 2007). In colorectal cancer (LoVo and HT-29) cells, curcumin at 10 and 6 μg/ml dose induced anti-cancer effect along with irinotecan at 6 and 12 μg/ml dose on LoVo and HT-29 cells respectively, through upregulation of endoplasmic reticulum (ER) stress signaling pathway, S-phase arrest and apoptosis (Huang *et al.* 2017).

Leptomycin B is an antibiotic drug derived from *Streptomyces sp.* that shows several anti-tumor effects. EGCG (20 μM) reduced cell survivability and increased cytotoxicity in human lung adenocarcinoma (A549) cells when treated with leptomycin B (0–10 nM) through increased production of ROS and modulating p21/surviving pathway (Cromie and Gao 2015).

Resveratrol (100 μM), induced chemosensitization of 5-fluorouracil (10 μM) in colorectal carcinoma (HT-29 and SW-620) cells. The cell viability was inhibited due to reduced p-STAT3 /p-Akt along with increased ROS and lipid peroxidases (Santandreu *et al.* 2011).

Quercetin (40 μM), sensitized human laryngeal (HeP2) cells towards cisplatin (2.5 μg/ml) in head and neck cancer *via* increased pro-apoptotic signaling and decreased anti-apoptotic gene expression along with reduction in NOS and Cu-Zn SOD (Sharma *et al.* 2005).

Capsaicin (100 μM) induced G0/G1 cell cycle, inflicted autophagy, increased ROS generation, apoptosis and in turn sensitized osteosarcoma (MG63, 143B and HOS) cells towards cisplatin (16.7 μM) (Wang *et al.* 2018).

Ascorbic acid (0.125 mM), induced chemosensitization of BCR/ABL+ cell line KCL22 towards imatinib (0.5 mM) by reduced binding of Nrf2 to DNA along with reduction in GSH (Tarumoto *et al.* 2004). Ascorbic acid (100 μg/ml) also induced chemosensitization towards cisplatin (100 μM) through increased apoptosis, DNA damage and oxidative stress due to reduced expression of anti-oxidant enzymes (Leekha *et al.* 2016).

Genistein (100 µM) induced apoptosis and reduced survivability with 5-fluorouracil (50 µM) in human colon cancer (HT-29) cells, cervical cancer (HeLa) cells and breast cancer (MCF-7) cells through induction of oxidative stress, pronounced expression of apoptosis inducing genes and reduced expression of cell survival genes (Hwang *et al.* 2005).

Sulforaphane (20 µM) sensitized human malignant mesothelioma (H-28) cells towards cisplatin (40 µM) through apoptosis and G2/M phase arrest. Upregulation of ROS, and pro-apoptotic signaling was evident in this study (Lee and Lee 2017).

Synergistic effect of co-encapsulated baicalein (2 and 5 mg/ml) and paclitaxel (2 and 5 mg/ml) in nanoemulsions, upregulated chemosensitivity towards paclitaxel through reduction of anti-oxidant enzymes and induction of ROS along with apoptosis in human breast cancer (MCF-7) cell and its taxol-resistant MCF-7/Tax cells (Meng *et al.* 2016).

Apigenin (4 µmol/l and 20 mg/kg) in hepatocellular carcinoma (SK-Hep-1 and BEL-7402) cells and in xenograft model of nude mice, exhibited chemosensitization towards 5-Fluorouracil (100 µg/ml) through pro-oxidant properties and mitochondrial dependent apoptosis (Hu *et al.* 2015). Apigenin (15 µM) also exhibited chemosensitivity towards paclitaxel (4 nM) in epithelial carcinoma (HeLa) cells, negroid hepatocyte carcinoma (Hep3B), lung carcinoma (A549), and human embryonic kidney 293A (HEK293A) cells by inducing oxidative stress and apoptosis (Xu *et al.* 2011).

Table 4. Synergistic effect of phytochemical and chemotherapeutic drug.

Phyto-chemical	Chemo-therapeutic Drug	Model	Drug Dose	Oxidant Nature	Effect	Mode of Action	References
Curcumin	Cisplatin	Cisplatin-resistant (CR) and cisplatin-sensitive (CS) ovarian cancer cells	50 µM	Anti-oxidant	↑G2/M phase arrest ↑Apoptosis	↑SOD ↑GSH ↓p-Akt ↑p38 MAPK ↑p-p53	(Weir *et al.* 2007)
	Irinotecan	LoVo and HT-29 cells	10 µg/ml on LoVo and 6 µg/ml on HT-29 cells	Pro-oxidant	↑Apoptosis ↑ER stress pathway ↑S-phase arrest	↑ROS ↑BIP ↑PDI ↑CHOP	(Huang *et al.* 2017)

(Table 4) cont.....

Phyto-chemical	Chemo-therapeutic Drug	Model	Drug Dose	Oxidant Nature	Effect	Mode of Action	References
EGCG	Leptomycin B	A549	20 μM	Pro-oxidant	↓Cell survival	↑ROS ↓CYP3A4 ↓SOD ↓GPX1 ↑p21 ↓survivin	(Cromie and Gao 2015)
Resveratrol	5-fluorouracil (5-FU)	HT-29 and SW-620 cells	100 μM	Pro-oxidant	↓Cell survival ↑Chemo-sensiti-zation	↑ROS ↑LPO ↓p-STAT3 ↓p-Akt	(Sant-andreu *et al.* 2011)
Quercetin	Cisplatin	HeP2 cells	40 μM	Pro-oxidant	↑Apoptosis ↑Chemo-sensiti-zation	↓Cu-Zn SOD ↓Bcl-xl ↓Bcl-2 ↑Bax ↑caspase-8,9 ↑cyt-c ↓NOS ↓survivin	(Sharma *et al.* 2005)
Capsaicin	Cisplatin	MG63, 143B and HOS cells	100 μM	Pro-oxidant	↑G0/G1 phase arrest, ↓cell invasion, ↑autophagy, ↑apoptosis	↑ROS ↓CyclinD1,D3 ↓(CDK2, 4,6) ↑(p18, p21,p27) ↓MMP-2,9 ↑Beclin 1, Atg3, Atg16, Atg5 ↑caspase-3	(Wang *et al.* 2018)
Ascorbic acid (Vitamin C)	Imatinib	KCL22 is a BCR/ABL+ cells	0.125 mM	Pro-oxidant	↑Chemo-sensiti-zation	↓GSH ↓Nrf2-DNA binding	(Tarumoto *et al.* 2004)
	Cisplatin	HEK and SiHa cells	100 μg/ml	Pro-oxidant	↑Apoptosis ↑DNA damage	↑ROS ↓GSH ↓SOD ↓GPx ↑p-53	(Leekha *et al.* 2016)
Genistein	5-fluorouracil	HT-29, MCF-7 and HeLa cells	100 μM	Pro-oxidant	↑Apoptosis	↑p53 ↑p21 ↑Bax ↓Glut-1 ↓COX-2 ↓PGE2 ↑AMPK ↑ROS	(Hwang *et al.* 2005)
Sulfora-phane	Cisplatin	H-28 cells	20 μM	Pro-oxidant	↑Apoptosis, ↑G2/M phase arrest	↑ROS ↑p53 ↑Bax ↑caspase-3 ↑PARP ↓Bcl-2 ↑p-Cdc2Tyr15 ↑cyclin B1 ↓p21WAF1/CIP1 ↓cyclin D1	(Lee and Lee 2017)
Baicalein	Paclitaxel	MCF-7 and MCF-7/Tax cells	2,5 mg/ml	Pro-oxidant	↑Apoptosis ↓MDR	↑ROS ↓GSH ↑caspase-3	(Meng *et al.* 2016)

(Table 4) cont.....

Phyto-chemical	Chemo-therapeutic Drug	Model	Drug Dose	Oxidant Nature	Effect	Mode of Action	References
Apigenin	5-Fluorouracil	*In vitro-* SK-He-1 and BEL-7402 cells *In vivo-* nude mice	*In vitro-* 4 μmol/l *In vivo-* 20 mg/kg	Pro-oxidant	↑Chemo-sensiti-zation, ↑Apoptosis	↑ROS ↓ΔΨm ↑caspase-3 ↓Bcl-2	(Hu *et al.* 2015)
	Paclitaxel	HeLa, A549, Hep3B and HEK293A cells	15 μM	Pro-oxidant	↑Apoptosis ↑Chemo-sensiti-zation	↑ROS ↓SOD ↑caspase-3 ↑PARP	(Xu *et al.* 2011)

Abbreviations: **ΔΨm-** mitochondrial membrane potential; **Akt-** protein kinase B; **AMPK-** AMP-activated protein kinase; **Atg-** autophagy related; **Bax** - Bcl-2-associated X protein; **Bcl2** - B-cell lymphoma 2; **BIP-GRP78,** an HSP family protein is referred as immunoglobulin heavy chain-binding protein.; **CDK-** Cyclin-dependent kinases; **CHOP-** CCAAT/enhancer-binding protein homologous protein; **COX-2-** cyclooxygenase-2; **CuZn-SOD-** copper, zinc superoxide dismutase; **CYP3A4-** Cytochrome P450 3A4; **Glut-1** - Glucose transporters 1; **GPx** - glutathione peroxidase; **GSH** – Glutathione; **MAPK** - mitogen-activated protein kinase; **NOS-** nitric oxide synthase; **Nrf2** - Nuclear factor erythroid2-related factor 2; **PARP** - poly (ADP-ribose) polymerase; **PDI-** protein disulfide isomerase; **PGE2-** prostaglandin E2; **ROS** - reactive oxygen species; **SOD** - superoxide dismutase; **STAT3** - signal transducer and activator of transcription

CANCER IN THE LIGHT OF STRESS RESPONSE: FROM HOMEOSTASIS TO HORMESIS

Genotoxic and non-genotoxic agents cause carcinogenesis either genetically by DNA damage (by covalently binding to DNA and causing mutations) or by epigenetic processes like transcriptional activation/suppression, post translational modification which ultimately destabilizes the balance of oncoproteins and tumor suppressor proteins (Chappell *et al.* 2016). An altered growth factor/hormonal status may enhance the rate of cell proliferation by involving receptor-mediated processes without genetic involvement and can also increase the population of destabilized cells (Narayanan *et al.* 2015). An initial adaptive response is elicited by the biologically effective doses that maintain homeostasis by detoxification. On the contrary, harmful effects of persistent severe doses often involve irreversible cellular processes such as DNA or proteins alterations and result in interruption of homeostasis. At extreme low doses, cellular activities in target cells might be regulated such that not just a threshold dose is achieved but also a reduction in lesion occurs, which is not more than 30-60% greater than the control (Fukushima *et al.* 2005).

ROS production is one such endogenous compensatory mechanism existing in our body, which may lead to non-linear dose effects and lead to the J-or U- or inverted-U shaped response curves. The example for the resistance to high H_2O_2 levels depends on the formation of low levels of $O_2^{\cdot-}$ which co-ordinate an adaptive program (Zimmermann *et al.* 2014). Physiological mechanisms like adaptive mitochondrial ROS signaling, low doses of endoplasmic reticulum (ER)-stress, activation of ion-channels, heat-shock proteins, anti-apoptotic families, unfolded protein response (UPR) induce euproteomic state and cytoprotective autophagy which converge on enhanced stress tolerance (Lin *et al.* 2019). In the context of anticancer therapies, underdosing might favour the survival of neoplastic cells in the organism. As for instance, the sub-lethal application of anti-neoplastics can cause multi drug resistance (MDR) thus facilitating ROS-induced mutagenesis (Kohanski *et al.* 2010). Persistence of hormetically active low doses also result in a similar outcome (Zimmermann *et al.* 2014). Moreover the initial stressor elicits combating responses not only against higher doses of the same stressor, but also against other similar stressors or even less specific agents including oxidative metabolic products (Son *et al.* 2008).

Phytohormetins: Role in Cancer Prevention

Dietary phytochemicals, with their low-dose stress-inducing properties, are potential biological and nutritional hormetins (Zimmermann *et al.* 2014). Instead of following a linear and threshold response, they often follow a self-contradictory biphasic dose response (Calabrese 2016). One adaptive mechanism of action of phytochemicals is activation of mild cellular stress response by their low doses. This preconditioning or hormetic effect of these subtoxic concentrations involves the induction of phase-I and II antioxidant enzymes mediated by ROS-sensitive transcription factor Nrf2 (Oliveira *et al.* 2018). Although some phytochemicals maintain direct ROS-scavenging capacities at high concentrations, in lower doses (as found in the diet), phytochemicals like curcumin, EGCG, resveratrol, genistein, sulforaphane *etc.* may activate multiple adaptive stimulating stress responses pathways. Particular examples of such signaling include the Nrf-2/ARE sirtuin–FOXO, NF-κB, and the HIF-1α pathway (Son *et al.* 2008). The mechanisms of action of major phytochemicals and their respective stress response strategies have been summarized below Table **5**.

Curcumin has shown a hormetic effect by downregulating the heat shock proteins (HSPs), and upregulating sirtuin pathway and the antioxidative system. Resveratrol inhibited the autophagic signaling but activated the HSP and antioxidants. EGCG and leuteolin primarily acted on the Nrf2 signaling. NF-κβ activation was shown by sulforaphane. Genistein and phenyl-isothiocyanate typically showed a low dose stimulation and high-dose activation pattern as shown in Table **5**.

Table 5. Hormetic phytochemicals with adaptive stress response signaling against cancer.

(Table 5) cont.....

Dietary Phytochemicals	Stress Adopting Pathways	Transcription Factors	Biological Outcomes	References
Curcumin	NFκB inflammatory pathway	NFκB	↑SOD-2 ↑Hsp60	
	HSP response	HSF-1	↓Hsp27 ↓Hsp70 ↓Hsp90 ↑Hsp27 ↑Hsp70↑	
	Sirtuin response pathway	-	↑SIRT3	
	Antioxidant signaling	Nrf2	↑GSH ↑HO-1	
Resveratrol	NFκB inflammatory pathway	NFκB	↓TNF-α ↓ IL-6 ↓iNOS	
	HSP response	HSF-1	↑Hsp25 ↑Hsp70	
	Autophagic activation	_	mTOR inhibition	
	Sirtuin response pathway	_	↑SIRT1	
	Antioxidant signaling	Nrf2	↑GST ↑NQO1 ↑HO-1	
EGCG	NFκB inflammatory pathway	NFκB	↓IL-12p40 ↓IL-6	(Shehzad and Lee 2013) (Ulrich *et al.* 2005) (Yang *et al.* 2011) (Lin *et al.* 2008) (Wu *et al.* 2020) (Jiang *et al.* 2018) (Park *et al.* 2019) (Gupta *et al.* 2014) (Gezer 2018) & (Bhakta-Guha and Efferth 2015)
	HSP response	HSF-1	↓Overexpressed Hsp90	
	Autophagic activation	_	HIF-1α, mTOR inhibition	
	Antioxidant signaling	Nrf2	↑HO-1 ↑CYP1A1 ↑NQO1 ↑GST-P1 ↑GCLC ↑GCLM	
Luteolin	NFκB inflammatory pathway	NFκB	↓TNF-α ↓NO	
	Autophagic activation	--	↓HIF-1α	
	Sirtuin response pathway	_	↑SIRT1	
	Antioxidant signaling	Nrf2	↑GSH ↑GPx ↑GR ↑GST, ↑GCLC ↑GCLM ↑HO-1	
Quercetin	NFκB inflammatory pathway	NFκB	↓COX-2	
	HSP response	HSF-1	↓Hsp27 ↓Hsp70	
	Autophagic activation	-	HIF-1, mTOR inhibition	
	Antioxidant signaling	Nrf2	↑HO-1 ↑SOD-1 ↑NQO1	
Sulforaphane	NFκB inflammatory pathway	NFκB	↓TNF-α ↓IL-6	
	Autophagic response pathway	_	HIF-1α inhibition	
Genistein	Low dose proliferation, high dose inhibition	_	↑Cleaved PARP ↓NFκB ↓Akt	
Phenyl-Isothiocyanate	Low dose proliferation, high dose suppression	_	Alters cell growth and migration	

Abbreviations: Akt- protein kinase B; **CYP1A1-** cytochrome P450 1A1; **GCLC-** glutamate-cysteine ligase catalytic subunit; **GCLM-** glutamate-cysteine ligase modifier subunit; **GPx-** glutathione peroxidase; **GR-** glutathione reductase; **GSH-** glutathione; **GST-** glutathione S-transferase; **HIF-1α-** Hypoxia-inducible factor 1-alpha; **HO-1-** hemoxygenase 1; **Hsp-** heat shock protein; **iNOS-** inducible nitric oxide synthase; **mTOR-** mammalian target of rapamycin; **NFκB-** Nuclear factor erythroid2-related factor2; **PARP-** poly (ADP-ribose) polymerase; **TNF- α-** Tumor Necrosis Factor α

Duality as a trait is confined not only to signaling pathways, but also among chemical compounds. In fact most of the stressors (endogenous or exogenous) show a duality in response, where a proliferative low dose is contradictory to the inhibitory high dose (Bhakta-Guha and Efferth 2015). Hormesis is an evolutionary conserved adaptive measure of a cell or an individual as to restabilize any imbalance in homeostasis caused by the stressor. There are endogenous (human and dietary) or exogenous (environmental and synthetic) compounds which owing to their hormetic property at their 'optimal concentration', confer protection to healthy cells, as well as induce signaling that converge to death of cancer cells (Gopalakrishnan and Tony Kong 2008).

Due to the availability of plenty of tumor cell lines the study of the effects of various endogenous antioxidants like vitamins and their analogues, dietary plant extracts and their secondary metabolites, environmental and pharmaceutical stressor agents including antineoplastic drugs and other chemical groups has great experimental and clinical implications. In this scenario, the following Table **6** describes the tissue specific studies of the effect of several hormetic agents of different origin [phytochemicals (P), antineoplastic drugs (D), endogenous agents (E), environmental toxicants (T)] on the different tumor cell lines.

Hormetic response has been shown by various phytochemicals (genistein, quercetin, Vit D3 analogs and resveratrol) in different breast cancer cell lines like MCF-7 and MDA-MB231. Resveratrol indicated hormetic response against K562, CEM-C7H2, and U937 leukemia cell lines. Genistein, EGCG, quercetin responded hormetically against SCC-25 oral cancer cell line. Anti-cancer drug, dexamethasone also possesses hormetic effect in neuro-epithelial cell lines such as U373, KNS42, and SF268. Other than the different categories of exogenous agents (natural or synthetic), several endogenous substances are also found to show hormetic type of response in cancer.

Table 6. Phytochemicals displaying hormetic effects against varied cancers.

(Table 6) cont.....

Tumor Tissue	Example	Hormetic chemicals	References
Breast	MCF-7, SKBR-3, MDA-MB231	Genistein (P)	(Jiang *et al.* 2018)
		Quercetin (P)	(Leon-Galicia *et al.* 2018)
		Retinoic acid (P)	(Alam *et al.* 2018)
		Vit D3 analogs (P)	(Frazzi and Guardi 2017)
		Resveratrol (P)	(Fuggetta *et al.* 2004)
Neuro-epithelial	U373, KNS42, SF268	Dexamethasone (D)	(Akhtar and Swamy 2018)
Ovarian	A2780, OVCAR-3, SK-OV-3	GnRH (E)	(Vourtsis *et al.* 2013)
		EGF (E)	(Leone *et al.* 2017)
		Progesterone (E)	(Kim and Kim 2014)
Melanoma	SK-MEL, H1144, B16	Resveratrol (P)	(Calabrese 2005)
		Thrombin (E)	
Colon	HT29, Colo-205, HCT-116	Catechin (P)	
		Genistein (P)	
		Doxorubicin (D)	
		Cisplatin (D)	
Myeloma	RPMI 8226, SK-MEI-28	-	
Leukemia	K562, CEM-C7H2, U937	Resveratrol (P)	
		NO$_2$ (E)	
Osteosarcoma	U-20S, G-292, OS 1	GM-CSF (E)	
Lung	NCI-H187, A-549, HL60	Caffeine (P)	
		Doxorubicin (D)	
Thyroid	FRO, FTC-236, FTC-UC1	TSH (E)	
Liver	HepG2, SMMC-7721	TNF-α (E)	
Sarcoma	AG73, SK-UT1	-	
Leydig	MA-10, MLTC-1	Prolactin (E)	
Neuroblastoma	IMR, Neuro-2a	Cycloheximide (D)	
		NaAsO$_2$ (T)	
Pancreatic	SW-1990	CCK-8 (E)	
Prostate	PC3, LNCap	Retinoic acid (P)	
		Morphine (D)	
Bladder	KK-47, G47V	Sulforaphane (E)	
Lymphoma	Jurkat	α-Fetoprotein (E)	
Head and neck	Cal 27, Cal 33	-	
Pituitary	NTU-G	2 ME (E)	
Endometrial	AN3 CA, HELA CA	TNFα (E)	
		Radiation (T)	
Cervical	SiHa	Cisplatin (D)	
Oral	SCC-25	Genistein (P)	
		EGCG (P)	
		Quercetin (P)	
Renal	SN12-C	IL-3 (E)	
Gasric	AGS	Gastrin (E)	

Hormones or growth factors like GnRH, EGF, and progesterone elicited hormetic response against A2780, OVCAR-3, and SK-OV-3 ovarian cell lines. A pleotropic effect of different types of endogenous (hormones, growth factors) and exogenous (natural or synthetic) compounds has also been observed. Resveratrol, a phytochemical and endogenous thrombin were observed with hormetic response against melanoma cell lines like SK-MEL, H1144, and B16. Phytochemicals such as catechin and genistein and drugs like doxorubicin and cisplatin exhibited hormetic response against SK-MEL, H1144, and B16 colon cancer cell lines. Caffeic acid and doxorubicin elicited hormetic response against NCI-H187, A-549 and HL60 lung cancer cell lines. Retinoic acid and morphine have hormetic response against PC3 and LNCap prostate cancer cell lines as shown in Table **6**.

Maintenance of Redox Homeostasis in Cancer Cells by Phytochemicals

Antioxidant supplements, as adjuvant during chemotherapy can protect normal adjacent tissue without interrupting tumor management, decreasing the side effects and increasing the disease-free survivability (Singh *et al.* 2018). The use of antioxidants at supraphysiological doses has attracted increasing importance as a possible primary and secondary cancer deterrence strategy (Donaldson 2004). Higher levels of endogenous antioxidant may prevent chemotherapy induced oxidative stress especially in those patients having impaired capacity to fight against oxidative insult (Singh *et al.* 2018).

The mode of action of several antineoplastic agents involves formation of free radicals further leading to cellular damage and necrosis of malignant cells (Singh *et al.* 2018). Therefore, cancer cells may be more sensitive to agents that generate large amount of ROS, or drugs that damage the ROS scavenging efficiency of cells, leading to apoptosis. Therefore ROS can predict the prognostic value of an anticancer drug (Zaidieh *et al.* 2019). Administration of excessive antioxidants cause little surge in free radicals which may promote the proliferation of harmful cells in the neoplastic state, promoting carcinogenesis rather than interrupting it which may require new anticancer therapies to eliminate tumor cells selectively using ROS-mediated mechanisms (Rodríguez-Serrano *et al.* 2015).

As one of the most promising mechanism, oxidative stress slows the process of cell replication, but it is during cell replication that chemotherapy actually kills metabolically active cancer cells. Therefore, slower cell replication imply lower effectiveness of chemotherapy because- (i) the neoplastic cells may not only survive but may also become resistant (ii) even if they respond, the death becomes more necrotic than apoptotic (Block *et al.* 2008). Whereas addition of certain antioxidants at specific dosages reduce oxidative stress, thus making the chemotherapy treatment more effective (Singh *et al.* 2018). Structural and functional chemistry of antioxidants and chemotherapy drugs suggests that antioxidants might improve therapeutic efficacy of antineoplastics by counteracting aldehydes that impede the passage of cells through the regular cell cycle (Block *et al.* 2008). Some antioxidants have been found to be useful for restoring the natural antioxidants in the body, which are often depleted after the completion of chemotherapy, resulting in decreased side effects and increased survival time (Singh *et al.* 2018).

In the ROS-sensitive malignant cells, natural phytochemical-derived Nrf2-inhibitors can induce ROS that may result in cell death. Many polyphenolic antioxidants such as EGCG, PEITC, sulforaphane, curcumin are significant groups of Nrf2 inhibitors which induce apoptosis (Lee *et al.* 2013b). Contrasting activities of dietary herbs such as antioxidants in cancer prevention and treatment depend on their dosing. At low concentration, they mostly promote cells' antioxidant properties *via* activating Nrf2-dependent signaling and enhancing ROS scavenging capability. Whereas, higher doses can inhibit antioxidant defence and induce oxidative stress (Tan *et al.* 2018). Constitutive upregulation of Nrf2 is common in human cancer and most of the antioxidants possess the property to increase Nrf2 activity, which is further necessary for proliferation of cancer cells. The usage of antioxidants was considered as gold standard to reduce the inevitable adverse effects of treatment-related chemotoxicities or radiotoxicities, (Block *et al.* 2008). Many natural chemopreventive phytochemicals like curcumin, EGCG, resveratrol, genistein *etc.* have been shown to suppress COX-2 ad MAP Kinase mediated NF-κβ activation and FOS, JUN derived AP1 activation in malignant cells (Surh 2003).

Limitations of Chemopreventive Phytochemicals

With the exception of issues with bioavailability and pharmacokinetics, dietary phytochemicals fulfil all the essential criteria of a good chemopreventive agent like little or zero toxicity, high efficacy in multiple sites *via* multiple mechanisms, orally consumable, inexpensive, and globally accessible which makes them an effective approach against cancer control and management (Meybodi *et al.* 2017). However, the efficacy is mostly achieved at excessively higher doses and such supraphysiological concentrations might not be achieved when the phytochemicals are administered as part of diet. The main reasons behind poor bioavailability are quick metabolism, indigestibility, mutual interactions between phytochemicals and cargo molecules, epithelial barrier of intestinal mucosa and nonspecific distribution in the body (Kaur *et al.* 2018).

Anticancer Phyto-nanoformulations

Different types of modifications like liposome, micelle, nano-carrier *etc.* have been planned for the improvement of bioavailability of the phytochemicals and nano formulations are one of the most notable approaches among them (Davatgaran-Taghipour *et al.* 2017). Nanotechnology emerges as a promising field for the development of new applications in anticancer drug designing. Silver, gold, zinc oxide, iron oxide, copper oxide, and aluminum oxide are the most commonly used metallic nanoparticles for the green synthesis of nano-compounds from phytochemicals (Visweswara Rao *et al.* 2016). Nanoformulations of bioactive agents from natural phytochemicals, including vitamins, resveratrol, curcumin, genistein, quercetin, EGCG, sulforaphane, luteolin, and coumarin derivatives, in a dose-dependent manner, result in better efficacy for the prevention and treatment of cancer. Application of nano-formulated bio-compounds not only deals with the issue of bioavailability but also improves the selective targeting of the anticancer compound singly or when in combination and enhances its *in vitro* stability and sustained release (Li *et al.* 2015).

FUTURE PERSPECTIVES OF ROS-DEPENDENT PHYTO-REMEDIATION IN CANCER

Huge amount of studies supporting the antioxidant hypothesis as the anticancer strategy are based on cell lines or on animal model where tumors were experimentally induced by high doses of chemical carcinogens (Russo 2007). However, due to lack of tissue or organ grade complexity, it is not possible to deduce the mechanism of those compounds acting in the tumour microenvironment (Bregenzer *et al.* 2019). Furthermore, phenolic phytochemicals are often found as glycosides or are converted to other conjugated products after absorption, which might further lower the bioavailablity. The two limitations *i.e.* the uptake of a particular antioxidant cannot be defined as a consequence of the distribution and processing of the original food and metabolic conjugations like methylation, sulfation, glucoronidation are inevitable (Russo 2007). The limitations of bioavailability and pharmacokinetics can be resolved by (i) *in vitro* syntheses of pharmaceutical analogues, (ii) tissue specific targeted delivery and (iii) formulation of novel delivery systems (Kaur *et al.* 2018). Tailored supplementation with designer foods that consist of cocktails of chemopreventive phytochemicals each having their own distinct anticancer mechanisms will be another available option in the near future (Surh 2003).

CONFLICT OF INTEREST

The authors declare no conflict of interest.

ACKNOWLEDGEMENT

The authors are thankful to Director, Chittaranjan National Cancer Institute for granting the fellowship to SD and PS and for providing the infrastructural facilities.

CONSENT FOR PUBLICATION

None

REFERENCES

Aggarwal, V, Tuli, HS, Varol, A, Thakral, F, Yerer, MB, Sak, K, Varol, M, Jain, A, Khan, MA & Sethi, G (2019) Role of reactive oxygen species in cancer progression: Molecular mechanisms and recent advancements. *Biomolecules,* 9, 735.
[http://dx.doi.org/10.3390/biom9110735] [PMID: 31766246]

Akhtar, MS, Swamy, MK (2018). *Anticancer plants: Natural products and biotechnological implements, Anticancer Plants: Natural Products and Biotechnological Implements.*

Alam, MN, Almoyad, M & Huq, F (2018) Polyphenols in colorectal cancer: Current State of knowledge including clinical trials and molecular mechanism of action. *BioMed Res Int,* 20184154185
[http://dx.doi.org/10.1155/2018/4154185] [PMID: 29568751]

Amin, ARMR, Karpowicz, PA, Carey, TE, Arbiser, J, Nahta, R, Chen, ZG, Dong, JT, Kucuk, O, Khan, GN, Huang, GS, Mi, S, Lee, HY, Reichrath, J, Honoki, K, Georgakilas, AG, Amedei, A, Amin, A, Helferich, B, Boosani, CS, Ciriolo, MR, Chen, S, Mohammed, SI, Azmi, AS, Keith, WN, Bhakta, D, Halicka, D, Niccolai, E, Fujii, H, Aquilano, K, Ashraf, SS, Nowsheen, S, Yang, X, Bilsland, A & Shin, DM (2015) Evasion of anti-growth signaling: A key step in tumorigenesis and potential target for treatment and prophylaxis by natural compounds. *Semin Cancer Biol,* 35 (Suppl.), S55-77.
[http://dx.doi.org/10.1016/j.semcancer.2015.02.005] [PMID: 25749195]

Arsova-Sarafinovska, Z & Dimovski, AJ (2013) Natural antioxidants in cancer prevention. *Macedonian Pharmaceutical Bulletin,* 59, 3-14.
[http://dx.doi.org/10.33320/maced.pharm.bull.2013.59.001]

Asadi-Samani, M, Kaffash Farkhad, N, Reza Mahmoudian-Sani, M & Shirzad, H (2019) *Antioxidants as a double-edged sword in the treatment of cancer.* https://www.intechopen.com/books/antioxidants
[http://dx.doi.org/10.5772/intechopen.85468]

Babich, H, Schuck, AG, Weisburg, JH & Zuckerbraun, HL (2011) Research strategies in the study of the pro-oxidant nature of polyphenol nutraceuticals. *J Toxicol,* 2011467305
[http://dx.doi.org/10.1155/2011/467305] [PMID: 21776260]

Bhakta-Guha, D & Efferth, T (2015) Hormesis: Decoding two sides of the same coin. *Pharmaceuticals (Basel),* 8, 865-83.
[http://dx.doi.org/10.3390/ph8040865] [PMID: 26694419]

Block, KI, Koch, AC, Mead, MN, Tothy, PK, Newman, RA & Gyllenhaal, C (2008) Impact of antioxidant supplementation on chemotherapeutic toxicity: a systematic review of the evidence from randomized controlled trials. *Int J Cancer,* 123, 1227-39.
[http://dx.doi.org/10.1002/ijc.23754] [PMID: 18623084]

Bregenzer, ME, Horst, EN, Mehta, P, Novak, CM, Raghavan, S, Snyder, CS & Mehta, G (2019) Integrated cancer tissue engineering models for precision medicine. *PLoS One,* 14e0216564
[http://dx.doi.org/10.1371/journal.pone.0216564] [PMID: 31075118]

Calabrese, EJ (2005) Cancer biology and hormesis: human tumor cell lines commonly display hormetic (biphasic) dose responses. *Crit Rev Toxicol,* 35, 463-582.
[http://dx.doi.org/10.1080/10408440591034502] [PMID: 16422392]

Calabrese, EJ (2016) The emergence of the dose-response concept in biology and medicine. *Int J Mol Sci,* 17, 2034.

[http://dx.doi.org/10.3390/ijms17122034] [PMID: 27929392]

Chang, YF, Chi, CW & Wang, JJ (2006) Reactive oxygen species production is involved in quercetin-induced apoptosis in human hepatoma cells. *Nutr Cancer,* 55, 201-9.
[http://dx.doi.org/10.1207/s15327914nc5502_12] [PMID: 17044776]

Chappell, G, Pogribny, IP, Guyton, KZ & Rusyn, I (2016) Epigenetic alterations induced by genotoxic occupational and environmental human chemical carcinogens: A systematic literature review. *Mutat Res Rev Mutat Res,* 768, 27-45.
[http://dx.doi.org/10.1016/j.mrrev.2016.03.004] [PMID: 27234561]

Chen, Q, Espey, MG, Sun, AY, Lee, JH, Krishna, MC, Shacter, E, Choyke, PL, Pooput, C, Kirk, KL, Buettner, GR & Levine, M (2007) Ascorbate in pharmacologic concentrations selectively generates ascorbate radical and hydrogen peroxide in extracellular fluid *in vivo. Proc Natl Acad Sci USA,* 104, 8749-54.
[http://dx.doi.org/10.1073/pnas.0702854104] [PMID: 17502596]

Chen, X, Song, M, Zhang, B & Zhang, Y (2016) Reactive oxygen species regulate T cell immune response in the tumor microenvironment. *Oxid Med Cell Longev,* 20161580967
[http://dx.doi.org/10.1155/2016/1580967] [PMID: 27547291]

Choi, EO, Park, C, Hwang, HJ, Hong, SH, Kim, GY, Cho, EJ, Kim, WJ & Choi, YH (2016) Baicalein induces apoptosis *via* ROS-dependent activation of caspases in human bladder cancer 5637 cells. *Int J Oncol,* 49, 1009-18.
[http://dx.doi.org/10.3892/ijo.2016.3606] [PMID: 27571890]

Choi, YH (2017) Diallyl trisulfide induces apoptosis and mitotic arrest in AGS human gastric carcinoma cells through reactive oxygen species-mediated activation of AMP-activated protein kinase. *Biomed Pharmacother,* 94, 63-71.
[http://dx.doi.org/10.1016/j.biopha.2017.07.055] [PMID: 28753455]

Costa, A, Scholer-Dahirel, A & Mechta-Grigoriou, F (2014) The role of reactive oxygen species and metabolism on cancer cells and their microenvironment. *Semin Cancer Biol,* 25, 23-32.
[http://dx.doi.org/10.1016/j.semcancer.2013.12.007] [PMID: 24406211]

Cromie, MM & Gao, W (2015) Epigallocatechin-3-gallate enhances the therapeutic effects of leptomycin B on human lung cancer a549 cells. *Oxid Med Cell Longev,* 2015217304
[http://dx.doi.org/10.1155/2015/217304] [PMID: 25922640]

Cuyàs, E, Corominas-Faja, B & Menendez, JA (2014) The nutritional phenome of EMT-induced cancer stem-like cells. *Oncotarget,* 5, 3970-82.
[http://dx.doi.org/10.18632/oncotarget.2147] [PMID: 24994116]

Datta, S & Sinha, D (2019) EGCG maintained Nrf2-mediated redox homeostasis and minimized etoposide resistance in lung cancer cells. *J Funct Foods,* 62103553
[http://dx.doi.org/10.1016/j.jff.2019.103553]

Davalli, P, Marverti, G, Lauriola, A & D'Arca, D (2018) Targeting oxidatively induced DNA damage response in cancer: Opportunities for novel cancer therapies. *Oxid Med Cell Longev,* 20182389523
[http://dx.doi.org/10.1155/2018/2389523] [PMID: 29770165]

Davatgaran-Taghipour, Y, Masoomzadeh, S, Farzaei, MH, Bahramsoltani, R, Karimi-Soureh, Z, Rahimi, R & Abdollahi, M (2017) Polyphenol nanoformulations for cancer therapy: experimental evidence and clinical perspective. *Int J Nanomedicine,* 12, 2689-702.
[http://dx.doi.org/10.2147/IJN.S131973] [PMID: 28435252]

Donaldson, MS (2004) Nutrition and cancer: a review of the evidence for an anti-cancer diet. *Nutr J,* 3, 19.
[http://dx.doi.org/10.1186/1475-2891-3-19] [PMID: 15496224]

Drake, IM, Davies, MJ, Mapstone, NP, Dixon, MF, Schorah, CJ, White, KLM, Chalmers, DM & Axon, ATR (1996) Ascorbic acid may protect against human gastric cancer by scavenging mucosal oxygen radicals. *Carcinogenesis,* 17, 559-62.
[http://dx.doi.org/10.1093/carcin/17.3.559] [PMID: 8631145]

Espíndola, KMM, Ferreira, RG, Narvaez, LEM, Silva Rosario, ACR, da Silva, AHM, Silva, AGB, Vieira, APO & Monteiro, MC (2019) Chemical and pharmacological aspects of caffeic acid and its activity in hepatocarcinoma. *Front Oncol,* 9, 541.
[http://dx.doi.org/10.3389/fonc.2019.00541] [PMID: 31293975]

Ferreira de Oliveira, JMP, Costa, M, Pedrosa, T, Pinto, P, Remédios, C, Oliveira, H, Pimentel, F, Almeida, L & Santos, C (2014) Sulforaphane induces oxidative stress and death by p53-independent mechanism: implication of impaired glutathione recycling. *PLoS One,* 9e92980
[http://dx.doi.org/10.1371/journal.pone.0092980] [PMID: 24667842]

Santos Franco, S, Raveh-Amit, H, Kobolák, J, Alqahtani, MH, Mobasheri, A & Dinnyes, A (2015) The crossroads between cancer stem cells and aging. *BMC Cancer,* 15 (Suppl. 1), S1.
[http://dx.doi.org/10.1186/1471-2407-15-S1-S1] [PMID: 25708542]

Frazzi, R & Guardi, M (2017) Cellular and molecular targets of resveratrol on lymphoma and leukemia cells. *Molecules,* 22, 885.
[http://dx.doi.org/10.3390/molecules22060885] [PMID: 28555002]

Fuggetta, MP, D'Atri, S, Lanzilli, G, Tricarico, M, Cannavò, E, Zambruno, G, Falchetti, R & Ravagnan, G (2004) *In vitro* antitumour activity of resveratrol in human melanoma cells sensitive or resistant to temozolomide. *Melanoma Res,* 14, 189-96.
[http://dx.doi.org/10.1097/01.cmr.0000130007.54508.b2] [PMID: 15179187]

Fukushima, S, Kinoshita, A, Puatanachokchai, R, Kushida, M, Wanibuchi, H & Morimura, K (2005) Hormesis and dose-response-mediated mechanisms in carcinogenesis: evidence for a threshold in carcinogenicity of non-genotoxic carcinogens. *Carcinogenesis,* 26, 1835-45.
[http://dx.doi.org/10.1093/carcin/bgi160] [PMID: 15975961]

Gautam Surabhi, BS (2019) The Link between Oxidative Stress and Cancer: Prevention through Yoga. *Cell Med Press,* 8, 258-66.

Gezer, C (2018) *Stress response of dietary phytochemicals in a hormetic manner for health and longevity.* https://www.intechopen.com
[http://dx.doi.org/10.5772/intechopen.71867]

Goitre, L, Pergolizzi, B, Ferro, E, Trabalzini, L & Retta, SF (2012) Molecular crosstalk between integrins and cadherins: Do reactive oxygen species set the talk? *J Signal Transduct,* 2012807682
[http://dx.doi.org/10.1155/2012/807682] [PMID: 22203898]

Gopalakrishnan, A & Tony Kong, AN (2008) Anticarcinogenesis by dietary phytochemicals: cytoprotection by Nrf2 in normal cells and cytotoxicity by modulation of transcription factors NF-κ B and AP-1 in abnormal cancer cells. *Food Chem Toxicol,* 46, 1257-70.
[http://dx.doi.org/10.1016/j.fct.2007.09.082] [PMID: 17950513]

Gu, H, Huang, T, Shen, Y, Liu, Y, Zhou, F, Jin, Y, Sattar, H & Wei, Y (2018) Reactive oxygen species-mediated tumor microenvironment transformation: The mechanism of radioresistant gastric cancer. *Oxid Med Cell Longev,* 20185801209
[http://dx.doi.org/10.1155/2018/5801209] [PMID: 29770167]

Gupta, P, Wright, SE, Kim, SH & Srivastava, SK (2014) Phenethyl isothiocyanate: a comprehensive review of anti-cancer mechanisms. *Biochim Biophys Acta,* 1846, 405-24.
[PMID: 25152445]

Hardwick, JP (2015) Cytochrome P450 function and pharmacological roles in inflammation and cancer. Preface. *Adv Pharmacol,* 74, xv-xxxi.
[http://dx.doi.org/10.1016/S1054-3589(15)00047-2] [PMID: 26233914]

Hatem, E & Azzi, S (2016) Oxidative stress in carcinogenesis and therapy. *Journal of Cell Signaling,* 11000102
[http://dx.doi.org/10.4172/2576-1471.1000102]

Heiss, EH, Schilder, YDC & Dirsch, VM (2007) Chronic treatment with resveratrol induces redox stress- and

ataxia telangiectasia-mutated (ATM)-dependent senescence in p53-positive cancer cells. *J Biol Chem,* 282, 26759-66.
[http://dx.doi.org/10.1074/jbc.M703229200] [PMID: 17626009]

Helfinger, V & Schröder, K (2018) Redox control in cancer development and progression. *Mol Aspects Med,* 63, 88-98.
[http://dx.doi.org/10.1016/j.mam.2018.02.003] [PMID: 29501614]

Hu, XY, Liang, JY, Guo, XJ, Liu, L & Guo, YB (2015) 5-Fluorouracil combined with apigenin enhances anticancer activity through mitochondrial membrane potential ($\Delta\Psi$m)-mediated apoptosis in hepatocellular carcinoma. *Clin Exp Pharmacol Physiol,* 42, 146-53.
[http://dx.doi.org/10.1111/1440-1681.12333] [PMID: 25363523]

Huang, YF, Zhu, DJ, Chen, XW, Chen, QK, Luo, ZT, Liu, CC, Wang, GX, Zhang, WJ & Liao, NZ (2017) Curcumin enhances the effects of irinotecan on colorectal cancer cells through the generation of reactive oxygen species and activation of the endoplasmic reticulum stress pathway. *Oncotarget,* 8, 40264-75.
[http://dx.doi.org/10.18632/oncotarget.16828] [PMID: 28402965]

Hussain, S (2017) Comparative efficacy of epigallocatechin-3-gallate against H_2O_2-induced ROS in cervical cancer biopsies and HeLa cell lines. *Contemp Oncol (Pozn),* 21, 209-12.
[http://dx.doi.org/10.5114/wo.2017.70110] [PMID: 29180927]

Hwang, ES & Bowen, PE (2005) Effects of tomato paste extracts on cell proliferation, cell-cycle arrest and apoptosis in LNCaP human prostate cancer cells. *Biofactors,* 23, 75-84.
[http://dx.doi.org/10.1002/biof.5520230203] [PMID: 16179749]

Hwang, JT, Ha, J & Park, OJ (2005) Combination of 5-fluorouracil and genistein induces apoptosis synergistically in chemo-resistant cancer cells through the modulation of AMPK and COX-2 signaling pathways. *Biochem Biophys Res Commun,* 332, 433-40.
[http://dx.doi.org/10.1016/j.bbrc.2005.04.143] [PMID: 15896711]

Hwang, JT, Ha, J, Park, IJ, Lee, SK, Baik, HW, Kim, YM & Park, OJ (2007) Apoptotic effect of EGCG in HT-29 colon cancer cells *via* AMPK signal pathway. *Cancer Lett,* 247, 115-21.
[http://dx.doi.org/10.1016/j.canlet.2006.03.030] [PMID: 16797120]

Ibrahim, SS & Nassar, NN (2008) Diallyl sulfide protects against N-nitrosodiethylamine-induced liver tumorigenesis: role of aldose reductase. *World J Gastroenterol,* 14, 6145-53.
[http://dx.doi.org/10.3748/wjg.14.6145] [PMID: 18985804]

Idelchik, MDPS, Begley, U, Begley, TJ & Melendez, JA (2017) Mitochondrial ROS control of cancer. *Semin Cancer Biol,* 47, 57-66.
[http://dx.doi.org/10.1016/j.semcancer.2017.04.005] [PMID: 28445781]

Jang, MH, Piao, XL, Kim, JM, Kwon, SW & Park, JH (2008) Inhibition of cholinesterase and amyloid-beta aggregation by resveratrol oligomers from Vitis amurensis. *Phytother Res,* 22, 544-9.
[http://dx.doi.org/10.1002/ptr.2406] [PMID: 18338769]

Jafri, A, Siddiqui, S, Rais, J, Ahmad, MS, Kumar, S, Jafar, T, Afzal, M & Arshad, M (2019) Induction of apoptosis by piperine in human cervical adenocarcinoma *via* ROS mediated mitochondrial pathway and caspase-3 activation. *EXCLI J,* 18, 154-64.
[PMID: 31217779]

Jelic, M, Mandic, A, Maricic, S & Srdjenovic, B (2019) Oxidative stress and its role in cancer. *J Cancer Res Ther* Epub ahead of print
[http://dx.doi.org/10.4103/jcrt.JCRT_862_16] [PMID: 33723127]

Jeong, Y, Lim, JW & Kim, H (2019) Lycopene inhibits reactive oxygen species-mediated NF-kB signaling and induces apoptosis in pancreatic cancer cells. *Nutrients,* 11, 762.
[http://dx.doi.org/10.3390/nu11040762]

Jiang, H, Fan, J, Cheng, L, Hu, P & Liu, R (2018) The anticancer activity of genistein is increased in estrogen receptor beta 1-positive breast cancer cells. *OncoTargets Ther,* 11, 8153-63.

[http://dx.doi.org/10.2147/OTT.S182239] [PMID: 30532556]

Jiang, X, Liu, Y, Ma, L, Ji, R, Qu, Y, Xin, Y & Lv, G (2018) Chemopreventive activity of sulforaphane. *Drug Des Devel Ther,* 12, 2905-13.
[http://dx.doi.org/10.2147/DDDT.S100534] [PMID: 30254420]

Ju, W, Wang, X, Shi, H, Chen, W, Belinsky, SA & Lin, Y (2007) A critical role of luteolin-induced reactive oxygen species in blockage of tumor necrosis factor-activated nuclear factor-kappaB pathway and sensitization of apoptosis in lung cancer cells. *Mol Pharmacol,* 71, 1381-8.
[http://dx.doi.org/10.1124/mol.106.032185] [PMID: 17296806]

Kamiya, T, Goto, A, Kurokawa, E, Hara, H & Adachi, T (2016) Cross Talk Mechanism among EMT, ROS, and histone acetylation in phorbol ester-treated human breast cancer MCF-7 cells. *Oxid Med Cell Longev,* 20161284372
[http://dx.doi.org/10.1155/2016/1284372] [PMID: 27127545]

Kang, CH, Molagoda, IMN, Choi, YH, Park, C, Moon, DO & Kim, GY (2018) Apigenin promotes TRAIL-mediated apoptosis regardless of ROS generation. *Food Chem Toxicol,* 111, 623-30.
[http://dx.doi.org/10.1016/j.fct.2017.12.018] [PMID: 29247770]

Kang, KA, Piao, MJ & Hyun, JW (2015) Fisetin induces apoptosis in human nonsmall lung cancer cells *via* a mitochondria-mediated pathway. *In vitro Cell Dev Biol Anim,* 51, 300-9.
[http://dx.doi.org/10.1007/s11626-014-9830-6] [PMID: 25381036]

Kasala, ER, Bodduluru, LN, Barua, CC & Gogoi, R (2016) Antioxidant and antitumor efficacy of Luteolin, a dietary flavone on benzo(a)pyrene-induced experimental lung carcinogenesis. *Biomed Pharmacother,* 82, 568-77.
[http://dx.doi.org/10.1016/j.biopha.2016.05.042] [PMID: 27470398]

Kaur, P, Robin, , Mehta, RG, Singh, B & Arora, S (2019) Development of aqueous-based multi-herbal combination using principal component analysis and its functional significance in HepG2 cells. *BMC Complement Altern Med,* 19, 18.
[http://dx.doi.org/10.1186/s12906-019-2432-9] [PMID: 30646883]

Kaur, V, Kumar, M, Kumar, A, Kaur, K, Dhillon, VS & Kaur, S (2018) Pharmacotherapeutic potential of phytochemicals: Implications in cancer chemoprevention and future perspectives. *Biomed Pharmacother,* 97, 564-86.
[http://dx.doi.org/10.1016/j.biopha.2017.10.124] [PMID: 29101800]

Kawanishi, S, Ohnishi, S, Ma, N, Hiraku, Y & Murata, M (2017) Crosstalk between DNA damage and inflammation in the multiple steps of carcinogenesis. *Int J Mol Sci,* 18, 1808.
[http://dx.doi.org/10.3390/ijms18081808] [PMID: 28825631]

Khan, AQ, Ahmed, EI, Elareer, N, Fathima, H, Prabhu, KS, Siveen, KS, Kulinski, M, Azizi, F, Dermime, S, Ahmad, A, Steinhoff, M & Uddin, S (2020) Curcumin-mediated apoptotic cell death in papillary thyroid cancer and cancer stem-like cells through targeting of the JAK/STAT3 signaling pathway. *Int J Mol Sci,* 21, 438.
[http://dx.doi.org/10.3390/ijms21020438] [PMID: 31936675]

Kim, YS & Kim, C-H (2014) Chemopreventive role of green tea in head and neck cancers. *Integr Med Res,* 3, 11-5.
[http://dx.doi.org/10.1016/j.imr.2013.12.005] [PMID: 28664073]

Kohanski, MA, DePristo, MA & Collins, JJ (2010) Sublethal antibiotic treatment leads to multidrug resistance *via* radical-induced mutagenesis. *Mol Cell,* 37, 311-20.
[http://dx.doi.org/10.1016/j.molcel.2010.01.003] [PMID: 20159551]

Lee, DE, Chung, MY, Lim, TG, Huh, WB, Lee, HJ & Lee, KW (2013) Quercetin suppresses intracellular ROS formation, MMP activation, and cell motility in human fibrosarcoma cells. *J Food Sci,* 78, H1464-9. a
[http://dx.doi.org/10.1111/1750-3841.12223] [PMID: 23902346]

Lee, JH, Khor, TO, Shu, L, Su, ZY, Fuentes, F & Kong, ANT (2013) Dietary phytochemicals and cancer

prevention: Nrf2 signaling, epigenetics, and cell death mechanisms in blocking cancer initiation and progression. *Pharmacol Ther,* 137, 153-71. b
[http://dx.doi.org/10.1016/j.pharmthera.2012.09.008] [PMID: 23041058]

Lee, SY, Jeong, EK, Ju, MK, Jeon, HM, Kim, MY, Kim, CH, Park, HG, Han, SI & Kang, HS (2017) Induction of metastasis, cancer stem cell phenotype, and oncogenic metabolism in cancer cells by ionizing radiation. *Mol Cancer,* 16, 10.
[http://dx.doi.org/10.1186/s12943-016-0577-4] [PMID: 28137309]

Lee, YH & Song, GG (2013) Induction of apoptosis by capsaicin in hepatocellular cancer cell line SMMC-7721 is mediated through ROS generation and activation of JNK and p38 MAPK pathways H. *Neoplasma,* 60, 607-16.

Lee, YJ & Lee, SH (2017) Pro-oxidant activity of sulforaphane and cisplatin potentiates apoptosis and simultaneously promotes autophagy in malignant mesothelioma cells. *Mol Med Rep,* 16, 2133-41.
[http://dx.doi.org/10.3892/mmr.2017.6789] [PMID: 28627624]

Leekha, A, Gurjar, BS, Tyagi, A, Rizvi, MA & Verma, AK (2016) Vitamin C in synergism with cisplatin induces cell death in cervical cancer cells through altered redox cycling and p53 upregulation. *J Cancer Res Clin Oncol,* 142, 2503-14.
[http://dx.doi.org/10.1007/s00432-016-2235-z] [PMID: 27613187]

Leon-Galicia, I, Diaz-Chavez, J, Albino-Sanchez, ME, Garcia-Villa, E, Bermudez-Cruz, R, Garcia-Mena, J, Herrera, LA, García-Carrancá, A & Gariglio, P (2018) Resveratrol decreases Rad51 expression and sensitizes cisplatin&-resistant MCF&-7 breast cancer cells. *Oncol Rep,* 39, 3025-33.
[http://dx.doi.org/10.3892/or.2018.6336] [PMID: 29620223]

Leone, A, Diorio, G, Sexton, W, Schell, M, Alexandrow, M, Fahey, JW & Kumar, NB (2017) Sulforaphane for the chemoprevention of bladder cancer: molecular mechanism targeted approach. *Oncotarget,* 8, 35412-24.
[http://dx.doi.org/10.18632/oncotarget.16015] [PMID: 28423681]

Li, C, Zhang, J, Zu, YJ, Nie, SF, Cao, J, Wang, Q, Nie, SP, Deng, ZY, Xie, MY & Wang, S (2015) Biocompatible and biodegradable nanoparticles for enhancement of anti-cancer activities of phytochemicals. *Chin J Nat Med,* 13, 641-52.
[http://dx.doi.org/10.1016/S1875-5364(15)30061-3] [PMID: 26412423]

Li, W, Cao, L, Chen, X, Lei, J & Ma, Q (2016) Resveratrol inhibits hypoxia-driven ROS-induced invasive and migratory ability of pancreatic cancer cells *via* suppression of the Hedgehog signaling pathway. *Oncol Rep,* 35, 1718-26.
[http://dx.doi.org/10.3892/or.2015.4504] [PMID: 26707376]

Li, W, Jiang, Z, Xiao, X, Wang, Z, Wu, Z, Ma, Q & Cao, L (2018) Curcumin inhibits superoxide dismutase-induced epithelial-to-mesenchymal transition *via* the PI3K/Akt/NF-κB pathway in pancreatic cancer cells. *Int J Oncol,* 52, 1593-602.
[http://dx.doi.org/10.3892/ijo.2018.4295] [PMID: 29512729]

Liao, W, Xiang, W, Wang, FF, Wang, R & Ding, Y (2017) Curcumin inhibited growth of human melanoma A375 cells *via* inciting oxidative stress. *Biomed Pharmacother,* 95, 1177-86.
[http://dx.doi.org/10.1016/j.biopha.2017.09.026] [PMID: 28926928]

Lin, Y, Jiang, M, Chen, W, Zhao, T & Wei, Y (2019) Cancer and ER stress: Mutual crosstalk between autophagy, oxidative stress and inflammatory response. *Biomed Pharmacother,* 118109249
[http://dx.doi.org/10.1016/j.biopha.2019.109249] [PMID: 31351428]

Lin, Y, Shi, R, Wang, X & Shen, H-M (2008) Luteolin, a flavonoid with potential for cancer prevention and therapy. *Curr Cancer Drug Targets,* 8, 634-46.
[http://dx.doi.org/10.2174/156800908786241050] [PMID: 18991571]

Liou, GY & Storz, P (2010) Reactive oxygen species in cancer. *Free Radic Res,* 44, 479-96.
[http://dx.doi.org/10.3109/10715761003667554] [PMID: 20370557]

Liu, T, Wang, G, Tao, H, Yang, Z, Wang, Y, Meng, Z, Cao, R, Xiao, Y, Wang, X & Zhou, J (2016) Capsaicin mediates caspases activation and induces apoptosis through P38 and JNK MAPK pathways in human renal carcinoma. *BMC Cancer,* 16, 790.
[http://dx.doi.org/10.1186/s12885-016-2831-y] [PMID: 27729033]

Luo, C & Wu, XG (2011) Lycopene enhances antioxidant enzyme activities and immunity function in N-methyl-N'-nitro-N-nitrosoguanidine-enduced gastric cancer rats. *Int J Mol Sci,* 12, 3340-51.
[http://dx.doi.org/10.3390/ijms12053340] [PMID: 21686188]

Lv, X, Li, J, Zhang, C, Hu, T, Li, S, He, S, Yan, H, Tan, Y, Lei, M, Wen, M & Zuo, J (2016) The role of hypoxia-inducible factors in tumor angiogenesis and cell metabolism. *Genes Dis,* 4, 19-24.
[http://dx.doi.org/10.1016/j.gendis.2016.11.003] [PMID: 30258904]

Manohar, M, Fatima, I, Saxena, R, Chandra, V, Sankhwar, PL & Dwivedi, A (2013) (-)-Epigallocatechi--3-gallate induces apoptosis in human endometrial adenocarcinoma cells *via* ROS generation and p38 MAP kinase activation. *J Nutr Biochem,* 24, 940-7.
[http://dx.doi.org/10.1016/j.jnutbio.2012.06.013] [PMID: 22959059]

Mansour, MMF (2000) Nitrogen containing compounds and adaptation of plants to salinity stress. *Biol Plant,* 43, 491-500.
[http://dx.doi.org/10.1023/A:1002873531707]

Martinez-Outschoorn, UE, Balliet, RM, Rivadeneira, DB, Chiavarina, B, Pavlides, S, Wang, C, Whitaker-Menezes, D, Daumer, KM, Lin, Z, Witkiewicz, AK, Flomenberg, N, Howell, A, Pestell, RG, Knudsen, ES, Sotgia, F & Lisanti, MP (2010) Oxidative stress in cancer associated fibroblasts drives tumor-stroma co-evolution: A new paradigm for understanding tumor metabolism, the field effect and genomic instability in cancer cells. *Cell Cycle,* 9, 3256-76.
[http://dx.doi.org/10.4161/cc.9.16.12553] [PMID: 20814239]

Maurya, BK & Trigun, SK (2016) Fisetin modulates antioxidant enzymes and inflammatory factors to inhibit aflatoxin-B1 induced hepatocellular carcinoma in rats. *Oxid Med Cell Longev,* 20161972793
[http://dx.doi.org/10.1155/2016/1972793] [PMID: 26682000]

Meng, L, Xia, X, Yang, Y, Ye, J, Dong, W, Ma, P, Jin, Y & Liu, Y (2016) Co-encapsulation of paclitaxel and baicalein in nanoemulsions to overcome multidrug resistance *via* oxidative stress augmentation and P-glycoprotein inhibition. *Int J Pharm,* 513, 8-16.
[http://dx.doi.org/10.1016/j.ijpharm.2016.09.001] [PMID: 27596118]

Meybodi, NM, Mortazavian, AM, Monfared, AB, Sohrabvandi, S & Meybodi, FA (2017) Phytochemicals in cancer prevention: A review of the evidence. *Int J Cancer Manag,* 10e7219

Mittler, R (2017) ROS Are Good. *Trends Plant Sci,* 22, 11-9.
[http://dx.doi.org/10.1016/j.tplants.2016.08.002] [PMID: 27666517]

Miyoshi, N, Naniwa, K, Yamada, T, Osawa, T & Nakamura, Y (2007) Dietary flavonoid apigenin is a potential inducer of intracellular oxidative stress: the role in the interruptive apoptotic signal. *Arch Biochem Biophys,* 466, 274-82.
[http://dx.doi.org/10.1016/j.abb.2007.07.026] [PMID: 17870050]

Narayanan, KB, Ali, M, Barclay, BJ, Cheng, QS, D'Abronzo, L, Dornetshuber-Fleiss, R, Ghosh, PM, Gonzalez Guzman, MJ, Lee, TJ, Leung, PS, Li, L, Luanpitpong, S, Ratovitski, E, Rojanasakul, Y, Romano, MF, Romano, S, Sinha, RK, Yedjou, C, Al-Mulla, F, Al-Temaimi, R, Amedei, A, Brown, DG, Ryan, EP, Colacci, A, Hamid, RA, Mondello, C, Raju, J, Salem, HK, Woodrick, J, Scovassi, AI, Singh, N, Vaccari, M, Roy, R, Forte, S, Memeo, L, Kim, SY, Bisson, WH, Lowe, L & Park, HH (2015) Disruptive environmental chemicals and cellular mechanisms that confer resistance to cell death. *Carcinogenesis,* 36 (Suppl. 1), S89-S110.
[http://dx.doi.org/10.1093/carcin/bgv032] [PMID: 26106145]

Naveenkumar, C, Raghunandhakumar, S, Asokkumar, S & Devaki, T (2013) Baicalein abrogates reactive oxygen species (ROS)-mediated mitochondrial dysfunction during experimental pulmonary carcinogenesis *in vivo. Basic Clin Pharmacol Toxicol,* 112, 270-81.

[http://dx.doi.org/10.1111/bcpt.12025] [PMID: 23061789]

Ohnishi, S, Ma, N, Thanan, R, Pinlaor, S, Hammam, O, Murata, M & Kawanishi, S (2013) DNA damage in inflammation-related carcinogenesis and cancer stem cells. *Oxid Med Cell Longev,* 2013387014
[http://dx.doi.org/10.1155/2013/387014] [PMID: 24382987]

Oliveira, MF, Geihs, MA, França, TFA, Moreira, DC & Hermes-Lima, M (2018) Is "preparation for oxidative stress" a case of physiological conditioning hormesis? *Front Physiol,* 9, 945.
[http://dx.doi.org/10.3389/fphys.2018.00945] [PMID: 30116197]

Oyagbemi, AA, Azeez, OI & Saba, AB (2009) Interactions between reactive oxygen species and cancer: the roles of natural dietary antioxidants and their molecular mechanisms of action. *Asian Pac J Cancer Prev,* 10, 535-44.
[PMID: 19827865]

Padma, VV, Kalaiselvi, P, Yuvaraj, R & Rabeeth, M (2015) Mangiferin induces cell death against rhabdomyosarcoma through sustained oxidative stress. *Integr Med Res,* 4, 66-75.
[http://dx.doi.org/10.1016/j.imr.2014.09.006] [PMID: 28664112]

Park, C, Cha, HJ, Lee, H, Hwang-Bo, H, Ji, SY, Kim, MY, Hong, SH, Jeong, JW, Han, MH, Choi, SH, Jin, CY, Kim, GY & Choi, YH (2019) Induction of G2/M cell cycle arrest and apoptosis by genistein in human bladder cancer T24 cells through inhibition of the ROS-dependent PI3k/Akt signal transduction pathway. *Antioxidants,* 8, 1-14.
[http://dx.doi.org/10.3390/antiox8090327] [PMID: 31438633]

Park, CE, Yun, H, Lee, EB, Min, BI, Bae, H, Choe, W, Kang, I, Kim, SS & Ha, J (2010) The antioxidant effects of genistein are associated with AMP-activated protein kinase activation and PTEN induction in prostate cancer cells. *J Med Food,* 13, 815-20.
[http://dx.doi.org/10.1089/jmf.2009.1359] [PMID: 20673057]

Perillo, B, Di Donato, M, Pezone, A, Di Zazzo, E, Giovannelli, P, Galasso, G, Castoria, G & Migliaccio, A (2020) ROS in cancer therapy: the bright side of the moon. *Exp Mol Med,* 52, 192-203.
[http://dx.doi.org/10.1038/s12276-020-0384-2] [PMID: 32060354]

Priya, DKD, Gayathri, R, Gunassekaran, G, Murugan, S & Sakthisekaran, D (2011) Chemopreventive role of sulforaphane by upholding the GSH redox cycle in pre- and post-initiation phases of experimental lung carcinogenesis. *Asian Pac J Cancer Prev,* 12, 103-10.
[PMID: 21517240]

https://pubchem.ncbi.nlm.nih.gov/compound/Ascorbic-acid [Accesssed 11th August 2020]

https://pubchem.ncbi.nlm.nih.gov/compound/Resveratrol [Accesssed 11th August 2020]

https://pubchem.ncbi.nlm.nih.gov/compound/Quercetin [Accesssed 11th August 2020]

https://pubchem.ncbi.nlm.nih.gov/compound/Luteolin [Accesssed 11th August 2020]

https://pubchem.ncbi.nlm.nih.gov/compound/Capsaicin [Accesssed 11th August 2020]

https://pubchem.ncbi.nlm.nih.gov/compound/Curcumin [Accesssed 11th August 2020]

https://pubchem.ncbi.nlm.nih.gov/compound/Epigallocatechin-gallate [Accesssed 11th August 2020]

https://pubchem.ncbi.nlm.nih.gov/compound/Fisetin [Accesssed 11th August 2020]

https://pubchem.ncbi.nlm.nih.gov/compound/Genistein [Accesssed 11th August 2020]

https://pubchem.ncbi.nlm.nih.gov/compound/Apigenin [Accesssed 11th August 2020]

https://pubchem.ncbi.nlm.nih.gov/compound/Piperine [Accesssed 11th August 2020]

https://pubchem.ncbi.nlm.nih.gov/compound/Lycopene [Accesssed 11th August 2020]

https://pubchem.ncbi.nlm.nih.gov/compound/Sulforaphane [Accesssed 11th August 2020]

https://pubchem.ncbi.nlm.nih.gov/compound/Mangiferin [Accesssed 11th August 2020] https://pubchem.ncbi.nlm.nih.gov/compound/Baicalein [Accesssed 11ᵗʰ August 2020]

https://pubchem.ncbi.nlm.nih.gov/compound/Diallyl-sulfide [Accesssed 11ᵗʰ August 2020]

Qian, K, Wang, G, Cao, R, Liu, T, Qian, G, Guan, X, Guo, Z, Xiao, Y & Wang, X (2016) Capsaicin suppresses cell proliferation, induces cell cycle arrest and ROS production in bladder cancer cells through FOXO3a-mediated pathways. *Molecules,* 21, 1-15.
[http://dx.doi.org/10.3390/molecules21101406] [PMID: 27775662]

Rahmani, M, Anderson, A, Habibi, JR, Crabtree, TR, Mayo, M, Harada, H, Ferreira-Gonzalez, A, Dent, P & Grant, S (2009) The BH3-only protein Bim plays a critical role in leukemia cell death triggered by concomitant inhibition of the PI3K/Akt and MEK/ERK1/2 pathways. *Blood,* 114, 4507-16.
[http://dx.doi.org/10.1182/blood-2008-09-177881] [PMID: 19773546]

Rajendran, P, Ekambaram, G & Sakthisekaran, D (2008) Effect of mangiferin on benzo(a)pyrene induced lung carcinogenesis in experimental Swiss albino mice. *Nat Prod Res,* 22, 672-80.
[http://dx.doi.org/10.1080/14786410701824973] [PMID: 18569708]

Rather, RA & Bhagat, M (2018) Cancer chemoprevention and piperine: Molecular mechanisms and therapeutic opportunities. *Front Cell Dev Biol,* 6, 10.
[http://dx.doi.org/10.3389/fcell.2018.00010] [PMID: 29497610]

Ravichandran, N, Suresh, G, Ramesh, B & Siva, GV (2011) Fisetin, a novel flavonol attenuates benzo(a)pyrene-induced lung carcinogenesis in Swiss albino mice. *Food Chem Toxicol,* 49, 1141-7.
[http://dx.doi.org/10.1016/j.fct.2011.02.005] [PMID: 21315788]

Reuter, S, Gupta, SC, Chaturvedi, MM & Aggarwal, BB (2010) Oxidative stress, inflammation, and cancer: how are they linked? *Free Radic Biol Med,* 49, 1603-16.
[http://dx.doi.org/10.1016/j.freeradbiomed.2010.09.006] [PMID: 20840865]

Rigas, B & Sun, Y (2008) Induction of oxidative stress as a mechanism of action of chemopreventive agents against cancer. *Br J Cancer,* 98, 1157-60.
[http://dx.doi.org/10.1038/sj.bjc.6604225] [PMID: 18253125]

Mut-Salud, N, Álvarez, PJ, Garrido, JM, Carrasco, E, Aránega, A & Rodríguez-Serrano, F (2016) Antioxidant intake and antitumor therapy: toward nutritional recommendations for optimal results. *Oxid Med Cell Longev,* 20166719534
[http://dx.doi.org/10.1155/2016/6719534] [PMID: 26682013]

Röhrdanz, E, Bittner, A, Tran-Thi, QH & Kahl, R (2003) The effect of quercetin on the mRNA expression of different antioxidant enzymes in hepatoma cells. *Arch Toxicol,* 77, 506-10.
[http://dx.doi.org/10.1007/s00204-003-0482-7] [PMID: 12756520]

Roy, J, Galano, JM, Durand, T, Le Guennec, JY & Lee, JCY (2017) Physiological role of reactive oxygen species as promoters of natural defenses. *FASEB J,* 31, 3729-45.
[http://dx.doi.org/10.1096/fj.201700170R] [PMID: 28592639]

Russo, GL (2007) Ins and outs of dietary phytochemicals in cancer chemoprevention. *Biochem Pharmacol,* 74, 533-44.
[http://dx.doi.org/10.1016/j.bcp.2007.02.014] [PMID: 17382300]

Sabharwal, SS & Schumacker, PT (2014) Mitochondrial ROS in cancer: initiators, amplifiers or an Achilles' heel? *Nat Rev Cancer,* 14, 709-21.
[http://dx.doi.org/10.1038/nrc3803] [PMID: 25342630]

Saha, SK, Lee, SB, Won, J, Choi, HY, Kim, K, Yang, GM, Dayem, AA & Cho, SG (2017) Correlation between oxidative stress, nutrition, and cancer initiation. *Int J Mol Sci,* 18, 1-30.
[http://dx.doi.org/10.3390/ijms18071544] [PMID: 28714931]

Sahin, K & Kucuk, O (2013) Lycopene in cancer prevention *Natural Products,* 3875-922.Springer, Berlin Heidelberg

Santandreu, FM, Valle, A, Oliver, J & Roca, P (2011) Resveratrol potentiates the cytotoxic oxidative stress

induced by chemotherapy in human colon cancer cells. *Cell Physiol Biochem,* 28, 219-28.
[http://dx.doi.org/10.1159/000331733] [PMID: 21865729]

Schieber, M & Chandel, NS (2014) ROS function in redox signaling and oxidative stress. *Curr Biol,* 24, R453-62.
[http://dx.doi.org/10.1016/j.cub.2014.03.034] [PMID: 24845678]

Sehgal, A, Kumar, M, Jain, M & Dhawan, DK (2012) Synergistic effects of piperine and curcumin in modulating benzo(a)pyrene induced redox imbalance in mice lungs. *Toxicol Mech Methods,* 22, 74-80.
[http://dx.doi.org/10.3109/15376516.2011.603392] [PMID: 21859361]

Selvendiran, K, Senthilnathan, P, Magesh, V & Sakthisekaran, D (2004) Modulatory effect of Piperine on mitochondrial antioxidant system in Benzo(a)pyrene-induced experimental lung carcinogenesis. *Phytomedicine,* 11, 85-9.
[http://dx.doi.org/10.1078/0944-7113-00355] [PMID: 14971727]

Shackelford, RE, Kaufmann, WK & Paules, RS (2000) Oxidative stress and cell cycle checkpoint function. *Free Radic Biol Med,* 28, 1387-404.
[http://dx.doi.org/10.1016/S0891-5849(00)00224-0] [PMID: 10924858]

Sharma, H, Sen, S & Singh, N (2005) Molecular pathways in the chemosensitization of cisplatin by quercetin in human head and neck cancer. *Cancer Biol Ther,* 4, 949-55.
[http://dx.doi.org/10.4161/cbt.4.9.1908] [PMID: 16082193]

Shehzad, A & Lee, YS (2013) Molecular mechanisms of curcumin action: signal transduction. *Biofactors,* 39, 27-36.
[http://dx.doi.org/10.1002/biof.1065] [PMID: 23303697]

Siddiqui, S, Ahamad, MS, Jafri, A, Afzal, M & Arshad, M (2017) Piperine triggers apoptosis of human oral squamous carcinoma through cell cycle arrest and mitochondrial oxidative stress. *Nutr Cancer,* 69, 791-9.
[http://dx.doi.org/10.1080/01635581.2017.1310260] [PMID: 28426244]

Sies, H (2017) Hydrogen peroxide as a central redox signaling molecule in physiological oxidative stress: Oxidative eustress. *Redox Biol,* 11, 613-9.
[http://dx.doi.org/10.1016/j.redox.2016.12.035] [PMID: 28110218]

Silvan, S, Manoharan, S, Baskaran, N, Anusuya, C, Karthikeyan, S & Prabhakar, MM (2011) Chemopreventive potential of apigenin in 7,12-dimethylbenz(a)anthracene induced experimental oral carcinogenesis. *Eur J Pharmacol,* 670, 571-7.
[http://dx.doi.org/10.1016/j.ejphar.2011.09.179] [PMID: 21970806]

Simone, CB, II, Simone, NL, Simone, V & Simone, CB (2007) Antioxidants and other nutrients do not interfere with chemotherapy or radiation therapy and can increase kill and increase survival, Part 2. *Altern Ther Health Med,* 13, 40-7.
[PMID: 17405678]

Singh, K, Bhori, M, Kasu, YA, Bhat, G & Marar, T (2018) Antioxidants as precision weapons in war against cancer chemotherapy induced toxicity - Exploring the armoury of obscurity. *Saudi Pharm J,* 26, 177-90.
[http://dx.doi.org/10.1016/j.jsps.2017.12.013] [PMID: 30166914]

Snezhkina, AV, Kudryavtseva, AV, Kardymon, OL, Savvateeva, MV, Melnikova, NV, Krasnov, GS & Dmitriev, AA (2019) ROS generation and antioxidant defense systems in normal and malignant cells. *Oxid Med Cell Longev,* 20196175804
[http://dx.doi.org/10.1155/2019/6175804] [PMID: 31467634]

Son, TG, Camandola, S & Mattson, MP (2008) Hormetic dietary phytochemicals. *Neuromolecular Med,* 10, 236-46.
[http://dx.doi.org/10.1007/s12017-008-8037-y] [PMID: 18543123]

Sonam, KS & Guleria, S (2017) Synergistic antioxidant activity of natural products. *Ann Pharmacol Pharm,* 2, 1086.

Sriram, N, Kalayarasan, S, Ashokkumar, P, Sureshkumar, A & Sudhandiran, G (2008) Diallyl sulfide induces

apoptosis in Colo 320 DM human colon cancer cells: involvement of caspase-3, NF-kappaB, and ERK-2. *Mol Cell Biochem*, 311, 157-65.
[http://dx.doi.org/10.1007/s11010-008-9706-8] [PMID: 18256791]

Strzelczyk, JK & Wiczkowski, A (2012) Oxidative damage and carcinogenesis. *Contemp Oncol (Pozn)*, 16, 230-3.
[http://dx.doi.org/10.5114/wo.2012.29290] [PMID: 23788885]

Su, C, Zhang, P, Song, X, Shi, Q, Fu, J, Xia, X, Bai, H, Hu, L, Xu, D, Song, E & Song, Y (2015) Tetrachlorobenzoquinone activates Nrf2 signaling by Keap1 cross-linking and ubiquitin translocation but not Keap1-Cullin3 complex dissociation. *Chem Res Toxicol*, 28, 765-74.
[http://dx.doi.org/10.1021/tx500513v] [PMID: 25742418]

Sundarraj, K, Raghunath, A, Panneerselvam, L & Perumal, E (2020) Fisetin, a phytopolyphenol, targets apoptotic and necroptotic cell death in HepG2 cells. *Biofactors*, 46, 118-35.
[http://dx.doi.org/10.1002/biof.1577] [PMID: 31634424]

Sung, H, Ferlay, J, Siegel, RL, Laversanne, M, Soerjomataram, I, Jemal, A & Bray, F (2021) Global Cancer Statistics 2020: GLOBOCAN Estimates of Incidence and Mortality Worldwide for 36 Cancers in 185 Countries. *CA Cancer J Clin*, 71, 209-49.
[http://dx.doi.org/10.3322/caac.21660] [PMID: 33538338]

Surh, YJ (2003) Cancer chemoprevention with dietary phytochemicals. *Nat Rev Cancer*, 3, 768-80.
[http://dx.doi.org/10.1038/nrc1189] [PMID: 14570043]

Tan, BL, Norhaizan, ME, Liew, WPP & Sulaiman Rahman, H (2018) Antioxidant and oxidative stress: A mutual interplay in age-related diseases. *Front Pharmacol*, 9, 1162.
[http://dx.doi.org/10.3389/fphar.2018.01162] [PMID: 30405405]

Tanaka, T, Shnimizu, M & Moriwaki, H (2012) Cancer chemoprevention by carotenoids. *Molecules*, 17, 3202-42.
[http://dx.doi.org/10.3390/molecules17033202] [PMID: 22418926]

Tanaka, T & Sugie, S (2007) Inhibition of colon carcinogenesis by dietary non-nutritive compounds. *J Toxicol Pathol*, 20, 215-35.
[http://dx.doi.org/10.1293/tox.20.215]

Tarumoto, T, Nagai, T, Ohmine, K, Miyoshi, T, Nakamura, M, Kondo, T, Mitsugi, K, Nakano, S, Muroi, K, Komatsu, N & Ozawa, K (2004) Ascorbic acid restores sensitivity to imatinib *via* suppression of Nrf2-dependent gene expression in the imatinib-resistant cell line. *Exp Hematol*, 32, 375-81.
[http://dx.doi.org/10.1016/j.exphem.2004.01.007] [PMID: 15050748]

Tuli, HS, Tuorkey, MJ, Thakral, F, Sak, K, Kumar, M, Sharma, AK, Sharma, U, Jain, A, Aggarwal, V & Bishayee, A (2019) Molecular mechanisms of action of genistein in cancer: Recent advances. *Front Pharmacol*, 10, 1336.
[http://dx.doi.org/10.3389/fphar.2019.01336] [PMID: 31866857]

Ullah, MF, Ahmad, A, Zubair, H, Khan, HY, Wang, Z, Sarkar, FH & Hadi, SM (2011) Soy isoflavone genistein induces cell death in breast cancer cells through mobilization of endogenous copper ions and generation of reactive oxygen species. *Mol Nutr Food Res*, 55, 553-9.
[http://dx.doi.org/10.1002/mnfr.201000329] [PMID: 21462322]

Ulrich, S, Wolter, F & Stein, JM (2005) Molecular mechanisms of the chemopreventive effects of resveratrol and its analogs in carcinogenesis. *Mol Nutr Food Res*, 49, 452-61.
[http://dx.doi.org/10.1002/mnfr.200400081] [PMID: 15830333]

Valadez-Vega, C & Delgado-Olivares, L (2013) https://www.intechopen.com/books/oxidative-stress-a-d-chronic-degenerative-diseases-a-role-for-antioxidants/the-role-of-natural-antioxidants-in-cancer-disease

Vellaichamy, L, Balakrishnan, S, Panjamurthy, K, Manoharan, S & Alias, LM (2009) Chemopreventive potential of piperine in 7,12-dimethylbenz[a]anthracene-induced skin carcinogenesis in Swiss albino mice. *Environ Toxicol Pharmacol*, 28, 11-8.

[http://dx.doi.org/10.1016/j.etap.2009.01.008] [PMID: 21783976]

Visweswara Rao, P, Nallappan, D, Madhavi, K, Rahman, S & Wei, J (2016) L & Hua Gan, S (2016) Phytochemicals and biogenic metallic nanoparticles as anticancer agents. *Oxid Med Cell Longev,* •••, 15.

Vourtsis, D, Lamprou, M, Sadikoglou, E, Giannou, A, Theodorakopoulou, O, Sarrou, E, Magoulas, GE, Bariamis, SE, Athanassopoulos, CM, Drainas, D, Papaioannou, D & Papadimitriou, E (2013) Effect of an all-trans-retinoic acid conjugate with spermine on viability of human prostate cancer and endothelial cells *in vitro* and angiogenesis *in vivo*. *Eur J Pharmacol,* 698, 122-30.
[http://dx.doi.org/10.1016/j.ejphar.2012.11.007] [PMID: 23178525]

Wang, LS & Stoner, GD (2008) Anthocyanins and their role in cancer prevention. *Cancer Lett,* 269, 281-90.
[http://dx.doi.org/10.1016/j.canlet.2008.05.020] [PMID: 18571839]

Wang, Y, Deng, X, Yu, C, Zhao, G, Zhou, J, Zhang, G, Li, M, Jiang, D, Quan, Z & Zhang, Y (2018) Synergistic inhibitory effects of capsaicin combined with cisplatin on human osteosarcoma in culture and in xenografts. *J Exp Clin Cancer Res,* 37, 251.
[http://dx.doi.org/10.1186/s13046-018-0922-0] [PMID: 30326933]

Wang, Z, Li, W, Meng, X & Jia, B (2012) Resveratrol induces gastric cancer cell apoptosis *via* reactive oxygen species, but independent of sirtuin1. *Clin Exp Pharmacol Physiol,* 39, 227-32.
[http://dx.doi.org/10.1111/j.1440-1681.2011.05660.x] [PMID: 22211760]

Watson, J (2013) Oxidants, antioxidants and the current incurability of metastatic cancers. *Open Biol,* 3120144
[http://dx.doi.org/10.1098/rsob.120144] [PMID: 23303309]

Weir, NM, Selvendiran, K, Kutala, VK, Tong, L, Vishwanath, S, Rajaram, M, Tridandapani, S, Anant, S & Kuppusamy, P (2007) Curcumin induces G2/M arrest and apoptosis in cisplatin-resistant human ovarian cancer cells by modulating Akt and p38 MAPK. *Cancer Biol Ther,* 6, 178-84.
[http://dx.doi.org/10.4161/cbt.6.2.3577] [PMID: 17218783]

Wiecek, M, Szymura, J, Maciejczyk, M, Kantorowicz, M & Szygula, Z (2018) Anaerobic exercise-induced activation of antioxidant enzymes in the blood of women and men. *Front Physiol,* 9, 1006.
[http://dx.doi.org/10.3389/fphys.2018.01006] [PMID: 30140236]

Wu, B, Zeng, W, Ouyang, W, Xu, Q, Chen, J, Wang, B & Zhang, X (2020) Quercetin induced NUPR1-dependent autophagic cell death by disturbing reactive oxygen species homeostasis in osteosarcoma cells. *J Clin Biochem Nutr,* 67, 137-45.
[http://dx.doi.org/10.3164/jcbn.19-121] [PMID: 33041510]

Xia, C, Meng, Q, Liu, LZ, Rojanasakul, Y, Wang, XR & Jiang, BH (2007) Reactive oxygen species regulate angiogenesis and tumor growth through vascular endothelial growth factor. *Cancer Res,* 67, 10823-30.
[http://dx.doi.org/10.1158/0008-5472.CAN-07-0783] [PMID: 18006827]

Xu, Y, Xin, Y, Diao, Y, Lu, C, Fu, J, Luo, L & Yin, Z (2011) Synergistic effects of apigenin and paclitaxel on apoptosis of cancer cells. *PLoS One,* 6e29169
[http://dx.doi.org/10.1371/journal.pone.0029169] [PMID: 22216199]

Yang, G, Shang, X, Cui, G, Zhao, L, Zhao, H & Wang, N (2019) Mangiferin attenuated diethynitrosamine-induced hepatocellular carcinoma in sprague-dawley rats *via* alteration of oxidative stress and apoptotic pathway. *Journal of Environmental Pathology, Toxicology, and Oncology Oncol,* 38, 1-12.
[http://dx.doi.org/10.1615/JEnvironPatholToxicolOncol.2018027392] [PMID: 30806285]

Yang, WH, Fong, YC, Lee, CY, Jin, TR, Tzen, JTC, Li, TM & Tang, CH (2011) Epigallocatechin-3-gallate induces cell apoptosis of human chondrosarcoma cells through apoptosis signal-regulating kinase 1 pathway. *J Cell Biochem,* 112, 1601-11.
[http://dx.doi.org/10.1002/jcb.23072] [PMID: 21328612]

Yao, Y & Dai, W (2014) Genomic Instability and Cancer. *J Carcinog Mutagen,* 51000165
[PMID: 25541596]

Zaidieh, T, Smith, JR, Ball, KE & An, Q (2019) ROS as a novel indicator to predict anticancer drug efficacy.

BMC Cancer, 19, 1224.
[http://dx.doi.org/10.1186/s12885-019-6438-y] [PMID: 31842863]

Zimmermann, A, Bauer, MA, Kroemer, G, Madeo, F & Carmona-Gutierrez, D (2014) When less is more: hormesis against stress and disease. *Microb Cell,* 1, 150-3.
[http://dx.doi.org/10.15698/mic2014.05.148] [PMID: 28357237]

CHAPTER 2

Environmental Contaminants and Redox Homeostasis

Zeinab A. Saleh[1,*] and **Khadiga S. Ibrahim**[2]

[1] *Nutrition and Food Science Department -National Research Centre, El-Bohouth St. (Tahrir St.Prev.) Dokki, Cairo, Egypt*

[2] *Environmental & Occupational Medicine Department -National Research Centre, El-Bohouth St. (Tahrir St.Prev.) Dokki, Cairo, Egypt*

Abstract: Contaminants in the environment, such as oxidant fuels, chemical substances, particulate surfaces, cigarette smoke, toxins, metals, medicines, xenobiotics, or radiation, can trigger the generation of the reactive oxygen species (ROS) or the reactive nitrogen species (RNS), which can lead to oxidative stress. Many ROS-mediated mechanisms shield cells from oxidative damage and help them reclaim their redox homeostasis. The activation of metabolic or bioenergetics reaction processes mediated by thiol redox switches is one of the overt or indirect mechanisms of oxidative stress. Furthermore, toxic agents' oxidative stress can be exacerbated through metabolic processes in cells. Excess ROS is regulated by endogenous antioxidant protection mechanisms (both enzymatic and non-enzymatic), which help remove toxic oxygen molecules or scavenge ROS under normal conditions. To sustain redox homeostasis in the presence of environmental stress, the cells are fitted with several complementing energy-dependent structures. The cytochrome (CYP) enzymes are a monooxygenase superfamily that includes several enzymes involved in xenobiotic detoxification. As a result, it seems that the CYP families are the most prominent members. Heavy metal toxicity, such as zinc, arsenic, and cadmium, is believed to be caused by their interaction with sulfhydryl groups in biological systems. Many sulfhydryl residues in antioxidant proteins, including metallothionein and albumin, serve as a sink for heavy metal ions, saving important protein thiols in the process.

Keywords: Antioxidants, Carotenoid, Drugs and Xenobiotics, Environmental Pollutants, GPx, GSH, Ionizing Radiations, Lipoic Acid, Metals, Pesticides, Reactive Oxygen Species, Redox Homeostasis, SOD, Tobacco Smoke, Vitamins.

* **Corresponding author Zeinab A. Saleh**: Nutrition and Food Science Department -National Research Centre, El-Bohouth St. (Tahrir St.Prev.) Dokki, Cairo, Egypt; E-mail: zsaleh_eg@yahoo.com

Pardeep Kaur, Rajendra G. Mehta, Robin, Tarunpreet Singh Thind and Saroj Arora (Eds.)

INTRODUCTION

Humans, wildlife, and household animals are all subject to a diverse combination phase of the mitochondrial respiratory chain produce reactive oxygen species (ROS) as a byproduct of normal metabolism in cells (He *et al.* 2017). The exogenous ROS generation can result from the exposure to various environmental contaminants such as oxidant gases, organic compounds, particulate matter, tobacco smoke, pesticides, metal, drugs, xenobiotics or radiation. Homeostasis is the tendency to maintain a reasonably constant internal condition despite changes in the external environment. ROS development and elimination from the body system are also carefully controlled to ensure redox homeostasis (Kong and Chandel 2018). The human body, for example, controls the internal amounts of charged particles, hydrogen, calcium, potassium, and sodium, on which cells depend for normal operation. Water, oxygen, pH, and blood glucose levels are also maintained through homeostatic cycles and are close to core body temperature. Maintaining "redox homeostasis" in the body requires a daily balance of oxidants and antioxidants. This suggests that, in response to a rise in ROS production, the body would increase the activation of endogenous antioxidant systems through the redox signaling mechanism (Valko *et al.* 2007). "Oxidative stress" is characterised as an accumulation of the reactive oxygen species (ROS) as a consequence of an imbalance between their production and the removal (which is controlled by an antioxidant defense system). On a molecular basis, environmental toxins induce various pathways of toxicity and enhance oxidative stress, causing harm to the cell membrane, lipid, DNA, and protein (Valavanidis *et al.* 2006). Metal ion homeostasis disruption may contribute to oxidative stress, a situation in which the enhanced production of reactive oxygen species (ROS) overwhelms the body's antioxidant defences, resulting in DNA injury, lipid peroxidation, protein alteration, and carcinogenesis (Jomova and Valko 2011). The preference for sulfhydryl groups is believed to underpin the toxicity of heavy metals such as arsenic (As), lead (Pb), and cadmium (Cd). Furthermore, environmental air contaminants (a combination of the particles suspended in the liquid and gaseous phase) may cause redox homeostasis to be disrupted.

Many pesticide groups disturb the cellular redox balance (Čermak *et al.* 2018). Multiple complementary energy-dependent mechanisms exist in the cells to sustain redox homeostasis in the presence of oxidative stress from the environment (Samet and Wages 2018). Several means are available for the treatment of free radical production in the cells that includes the non-enzymatic and enzymatic antioxidants.

FREE RADICALS IN REDOX HOMEOSTASIS

In biology, the importance of free radicals as well as other oxidants have become more valuable due to their predominant role in different physiological environments as well as their impact on a very wide variety of diseases. Reactive oxygen species (ROS) generation are initiated by both endogenous and exogenous sources. They are primarily formed as byproducts of natural cellular metabolism during the oxidative reaction phase of the mitochondrial respiratory chain (Balaban *et al.* 2005, Zorov *et al.* 2014) and exogenous sources or environmental sources (exogenous toxicants). ROS are created, during the conversion of xenobiotics from medications like halothane and paracetamol, *via* exposure to UV irradiation or by the metabolism of the toxic compounds including heavy metals, pesticides, tobacco smoke, and pollution, (Jezek and Hlavatá 2005, Phaniendra *et al.* 2015). Some exogenous toxicants' metabolism may result in formation of the ROS, which are more harmful than their parent compounds. As a consequence, exogenous toxicants could be sources of ROS generated by metabolism.

ROS include hydroxyl radicals, singlet oxygen, as well as hydrogen peroxide. They activate signaling pathways resulting in changes in biochemical, physiological, and molecular processes in the cellular metabolism (Xie *et al.* 2019). Moderate amounts of reactive oxygen species have positive effects on invasive pathogen killing, wounds healing, and repair processes (Bhattacharyya *et al.* 2014). ROS also, serve as a signaling molecule for the regulation of biological and physiological processes (Finkel 2011). ROS may be considered as a signal transduction process to allow the adaptation during changes in the nutrients, and oxidizing environment (Wood *et al.* 2003, Xie *et al.* 2019).

Reactive nitrogen species (RNS), like the nitrogen dioxide (NO_2), dinitrogen trioxide (N_2O_3), nitric oxide (NO), peroxynitrite (OONO), and nitrous acid (HNO_2), contribute to the oxidative stress in addition to ROS (Halliwell 2001, Di Meo *et al.* 2016). When cellular NO interacts with ROS, it produces a large number of RNS, which are involved in oxidative and nitrosative destruction.

ROS and RNS could be divided into two classes, namely the radicals and non-radicals. The radicals are species with at least one unpaired electron within shells around the nucleus and may be independent. Examples of the radicals include the superoxide ($^{\bullet}O_2^{-}$), hydroxyl radical ($^{\bullet}OH$), oxygen radicals (O_2), peroxyl radical ($^{\bullet}ROO^{-}$), nitric monoxide (NO) and nitrogen dioxide (NO_2) (Halliwell 2001). The existence of one unpaired electron around the nucleus, which seeks to donate or receive another electron to achieve equilibrium, results in a higher reaction to certain radicals. The high levels of superoxide anion are more associated with oxidative stress than with cell signaling (Schieber and Chandel 2014). The oxygen derivatives, especially superoxide anion and the OH radicals, are the most effective free radicals in several disease states (Phaniendra *et al.* 2015).

Because it oxidises lipids, proteins, and DNA, the OH radicals are highly reactive of all free radicals, which leads to bimolecular damage or genomic instability (Dizdaroglu and Jaruga 2012).

The non-radical species comprise the hypochlorous acid (HOCl), dinitrogen trioxide (N_2O_3), singlet oxygen ($^1O_2$), dinitrogen tetraoxide (N_2O_4), ozone (O_3), nitrous acid (HNO_2), hydrogen peroxide (H_2O_2), organic peroxides (ROOH), aldehydes (HCOR), and peroxynitrite (ONOOH) (Kohen and Nyska 2002). These non-radical molecules are not free radicals; however certain reactions in living organisms will quickly transform them to free radicals (Genestra 2007, Ahmad 2018). Table **1** illustrates some ROS and RNS in living organisms.

Table 1. Some reactive oxygen and nitrogen species in the living organisms.

Free Radicals		Non Radicals	
Hydroxyl radical	$^.OH$	Hydrogen peroxide	H_2O_2
Superoxide radical	$^.O_2^-$	Hypochlorous acid	HOCl
Nitric oxide radical	$^.NO^-$	Singlet oxygen	$^1O_2$
Lipid peroxyl radical	$^.LOO^-$	Ozone	O_3
Hydroperoxyl radical	$^.HOO^-$	Dinitrogen trioxide	N_2O_3
Peroxyl radicals	$^.ROO^-$	Dinitrogen tetraoxide	N_2O_4

Lipids are the highly susceptible biomolecules to the oxidation from free radicals, especially the polyunsaturated ones. When phospholipids are targeted, they initiate an oxidative chain of events in the other membrane phospholipids, which encourages its propagation and produces a variety of reactive species that may attack proteins and DNA (Gaschler and Stockwell 2017). As a result of the oxidative damage to these phospholipids, cell death can occur not only as a result of changes in the plasma membrane, but also as a consequence of functional changes in proteins and DNA (Trachootham *et al.* 2008).

ROS overproduction disrupts the redox homeostasis and induces oxidative stress leading to the oxidative damage of the cellular macromolecules, such as protein, lipid, and nucleic acids (Jezek and Hlavata 2005).

The term "oxidative stress" refers to a variety of pathological conditions and reactions that occur when a cell or tissue departs from its homeostatic reductive state. The generation of ROS in the cell is a key determinant of cell signalling and oxidative distress (Kaludercic *et al.* 2014).

Pesticides, heavy metals, cigarette smoke, marijuana, and prescription medications are examples of toxins found in the environment that can trigger oxidative stress in cells by direct or indirect pathways, causing metabolic or bioenergetic processes controlled by thiol redox keys to be disrupted (Kovacic and Somanathan 2006, Samet and Wages 2018).

Endogenous ROS Sources

Many cellular components, such as the mitochondria, endoplasmic reticulum, and peroxisomes, are endogenous sources of ROS because oxygen is abundant there. Mitochondria contribute significantly as a source of endogenous ROS because of their primary role in the synthesis of oxidised ATP, in which cellular oxygen (O_2) is converted to water (H_2O) in the mitochondrial electron transport chain. Free radicals as well as non-radicals are the two forms of ROS. Free radicals are molecules, which have one or more unpaired electrons that cause them to interact with another molecule. When the two radicals swap their unpaired electrons, the non-radical molecules are produced. The superoxide anion, hydrogen peroxide as well as hydroxyl radical are the three major ROS of physiological importance.

Superoxide anion is created by adding a single electron to the O_2 (molecular oxygen) (Miller *et al.* 1990). This procedure is intermediated by the nicotine adenine dinucleotide phosphate (NADPH) oxidase or mitochondrial electron transfer system or xanthine oxidase. The mitochondria, the cell's ATP-supplying machinery, are the most critical place for generating superoxide anion. Normally, electrons are relocated *via* the electron transport mechanism in this organelle to transform oxygen to water, but about 1% to 3% of all the electrons leaked out of the cell, resulting in superoxide production (Le Bras *et al.* 2005). The superoxide dismutases (SODs) converts the superoxide to H_2O_2. Further, the H_2O_2 diffuses quickly through the cell wall. Xanthine oxidase, NADPH oxidase, amino acid oxidase, as well as peroxisomes, produce hydrogen peroxide by absorbing molecular oxygen in metabolic processes (Sies 2014).

The peroxyl radicals ($\cdot ROO^-$) are another group of oxygen-derived radicals. Hydroperoxyl radicals are the most basic type of these radicals, and they play a role in lipid peroxidation. By withdrawing a hydrogen (H) atom from the side-chain of methylene carbon, free radicals may initiate lipid peroxidation chain reactions. Peroxyl radicals are generated from the lipid radical in the presence of oxygen. Polyunsaturated fatty acids are converted into lipid hydroperoxides by the peroxyl radical, which starts a chain reaction. Lipid hydroperoxides are extremely unstable and quickly degrade into secondary products like aldehydes and malondialdehydes. Malondialdehyde is a product of lipid peroxidation, which could cause DNA mutations (Marnett 1999) and functional protein alterations

(Breitzig *et al.* 2016). Peroxidation of lipids disrupts cell membrane stability and rearranges membrane composition. Proteins are attacked by reactive species reversibly or irreversibly. All amino acids may oxidize *via* free radicals, with lysine, arginine, histidine, threonine, cysteine, and proline being the most susceptible to metal catalyzed oxidation (Trachootham *et al.* 2008).

Exogenous Sources of ROS (Oxidants)

ROS formation may be facilitated through a variety of factors, including pollutants, exposure to ozone, heavy metals, xenobiotics, tobacco, cigarette smoke, drugs, or ionizing radiation.

Tobacco and Cigarette Smoke (CS)

Tobacco smoke contains many chemical products with harmful health effects. Cigarette smoke is a significant generator for ROS (Halliwell and Cross 1994, Zhao and Hopke 2012). Cigarette smoking is one of the most common social practices in the world today, and it is a leading cause of death that can be avoided. Cigarette smoke is a diverse combination of over 4800 unique components, including high levels of free radicals, the reactive oxygen and nitrogen molecules, superoxide, nitric oxide reactive aldehydes, volatile organic compounds (VOCs), and metals (Church and Pryor 1985, Hoffmann *et al.* 2001). These oxidants have the potential to induce oxidative stress to the biological macromolecules like proteins and lipids, causing harmful effects on tissues (Barreiro *et al.* 2010). The increased production of ROS is linked to antioxidant depletion and the progression of oxidative stress throughout the body (Aycicek *et al.* 2005). The number of cigarettes smoked has a significant impact on the extent of oxidative stress and the antioxidant defences (Kamceva *et al.* 2016). High doses of vitamin C, according to Panta *et al.* (2000), can protect smokers from oxidative damage and the diseases that come with it. Heavy metals, including cadmium, can be transferred to humans by inhaling cigarette smoke, resulting in long-term symptoms and a slew of serious issues such as osteoporosis, kidney failure, and lung injury (Wooten *et al.* 2006).

Ozone Exposure

Ozone is the chief constituent of contaminated air in the major cities of the earth. Exposure to ozone triggers oxidative damage and cell death owing to the increase of the reactive molecules (Pereyra-Muñoz *et al.* 2006). It has the potential to trigger lipid peroxidation and the infiltration of granulocyte into the respiratory epithelium. Inflammatory mediators, as well as lactate dehydrogenase and albumin, are released in response to short-term ozone exposure (Hiltermann *et al.* 1999). Cho *et al.* (2005) demonstrated that fine particles (a suspension of the solid particles or liquid droplets in the atmosphere) stimulate oxygen reduction.

Ionizing Radiations

Ionizing radiations, such as the X-rays and neutrons, and α, β, or γ rays may induce oxidative stress. Ionizing radiation produces, HO radicals by radiolysis of the water and reactive oxygen species *via* secondary reactions (Riley 1994). Ionizing radiations can generate destructive effects by interacting with water, a process called radiolysis. In this event, water (H_2O) loses one electron and converts to its extremely reactive form. Water is successively transformed into hydroxyl radicals, hydrogen peroxide (H_2O_2), $^{\cdot}O_2^{\cdot}$, and in the end O_2 by a three-step chain reactions.

Ionising radiations transform hydroxyl radicals, superoxides, and organic radicals to H2O2 and organic hydroperoxides in the presence of oxygen. Further, these hydroperoxide species may cause oxidative stress by reacting with the redox-active metal ions like Fe and Cu through Fenton's reaction (Biaglow *et al.* 1992, Chiu *et al.* 1993). The amount of intracellular glutathione (GSH) drops for a brief time after being exposed to ionising radiation, but then rises again (Iwanaga 1998).

Heavy Metal Ions

The heavy metals are present naturally in the rocks and soils of vast geographic regions. Lead, cadmium, mercury, and arsenic are also harmful minerals that can be found in large amounts in the atmosphere. The amount of these heavy metals in the atmosphere determine their negative effects (Stankovic *et al.* 2014). These metals enter the human body through a variety of routes, including polluted air, water, dirt, and food. Heavy metals can stimulate ROS formation and cause oxidative damage to macromolecules by depleting enzyme activities *via* lipid peroxidation and react with the nuclear protein and DNA (Valko *et al.* 2005).

Heavy metal ions of zinc (Wu *et al.* 2013), lead (Vaziri 2008), mercury (Mahboob *et al.* 2001) and cadmium (Cuypers *et al.* 2010) are able to coordinate with sulfhydryl groups on the peptides and proteins, leading to their oxidation. Lead, cadmium, mercury, zinc, and nickel, suppress the antioxidative system, by reducing the glutathione and *via* binding to the -SH groups of the antioxidant enzymes (catalases, reductases, and superoxide dismutase) (Fryzova *et al.* 2018).

Some metals, including arsenite, induce ROS production *via* activation of radical generation the cells (Leonard *et al.* 2004). The toxicity of the arsenic compound is attributed to the development of a number of reactive oxygen species (ROS), such as hydrogen peroxide, singlet oxygen, superoxide, peroxyl radicals, nitric oxide, and the dimethylarsinic peroxyl radicals (Shi *et al.* 2004). Antioxidant enzymes, particuarly the GSH-dependent enzymes including glutathione peroxidase, glutathione-S-transferases, and glutathione reductase, can be inhibited by these compounds by reacting with the sulfhydryl (–SH) groups in their structure (Schiller *et al.* 1977).

Lead exposure increases the lipid peroxidation with a significant alterations in the SOD and GPx activities (Monterio *et al.* 1991).

Pesticides

The pesticides use in the agricultural practices has produced severe environmental and health related issues for humans and animals. Plant products, especially fruits and vegetables, are being polluted with pesticide residues due to their intensive treatments on several crops (Keikotlhaile *et al.* 2010). Pesticide exposure has been related to the development of oxidative stress, which causes lipid peroxidation and DNA harm in humans, with agricultural workers becoming particularly vulnerable (Rastogi *et al.* 2009). Pesticide induces the oxidative stress that instigates either by the excess of free radicals or modulation in the detoxification defense mechanisms of enzymatic antioxidants (Mecdad *et al.* 2011).

Drugs and Xenobiotics

The development of the free radicals in the cells is stimulated by a variety of drugs and xenobiotics. Anticancer drugs like anthracyclines and their analogs, actinomycin D, mitoxantrone and quinones, and related chemical compounds could lead to the oxidative stress (Deavall *et al.* 2012). (Fig. **1**) illustrate endogenous and exogenous ROS sources that cause oxidative stress.

ROLE OF ANTIOXIDANTS IN THE METABOLIC REGULATION OF THE REDOX HOMEOSTASIS

Antioxidant molecules turn themselves into reactive species while donating electrons to the free radicals to stabilize the reactive oxygen species. Endogenous antioxidant defense systems are required to recover the ROS welded damage. These systems work by maintaining intracellular ROS activity and redox balance with chelation (Fuchs-Tarlovsky 2013).

Antioxidant enzymes use oxidation-reduction (redox) reactions to reduce reactive species by oxidising another molecule and holding it in a non-reactive state. For cellular homeostasis, the anti/pro-oxidant equilibrium is necessary, and many mechanisms are evolved to control reactive species (Espinosa-Diez *et al.* 2015).

Free Radical Production

The antioxidant defense mechanism includes both enzymatic and the non-enzymatic components for ROS scavenging, and it works at various subcellular compartments. To protect the body's cells and organs from free radical disruption, they function together in a synergistic manner. The peroxiredoxin mechanism, superoxide dismutase, glutathione S-transferases, glutathione reductase, and glutathione peroxidase systems, as well as catalase, comprise the enzymatic antioxidant process (Catalá and Díaz 2016), while Vitamin C and E, carotenoids, thiol antioxidants (thioredoxin, glutathione, and lipoic acid), melatonin, flavonoids, and other molecules are contained in the non-enzymatic antioxidant systems. (Halliwell *et al.* 2005). To control ROS production and maintain physiological levels in the biological processes, the interconnected networks of cellular enzymatic and non-enzymatic antioxidants coordinate with each other.

Enzymatic Antioxidant System

Superoxide Dismutases (SOD)

SOD is a group of cytoplasmic enzymes which facilitate the catalyzed breakdown of the superoxide radicals ($^\cdot O_2^-$) to the less reactive products, molecular oxygen (O_2), and hydrogen peroxide intracellular, providing cellular defense against reactive oxygen species ($2O_2^- + 2H^+ \rightarrow H_2O_2 + O_2$) (Fridovich 1997). Consequently, H_2O_2 is reduced to water and oxygen molecules by enzyme catalase or glutathione peroxidase (Day 2009). The activity of SOD is dependent on the presence of a metal cofactor. Iron (Fe), copper (Cu), zinc (Zn), and manganese (Mn) are the metal ions that are commonly associated with the SOD. The MnSOD (manganese SOD) is produced in the mitochondria, Cu/ZnSOD (copper-zinc SOD) is produced in cytoplasm, and extracellular SOD is produced outside of the cell. SOD is important for cellular health, since it protects body cells from dangerous free radicals, oxygen radicals, and other factors that contribute to ageing and cell death.

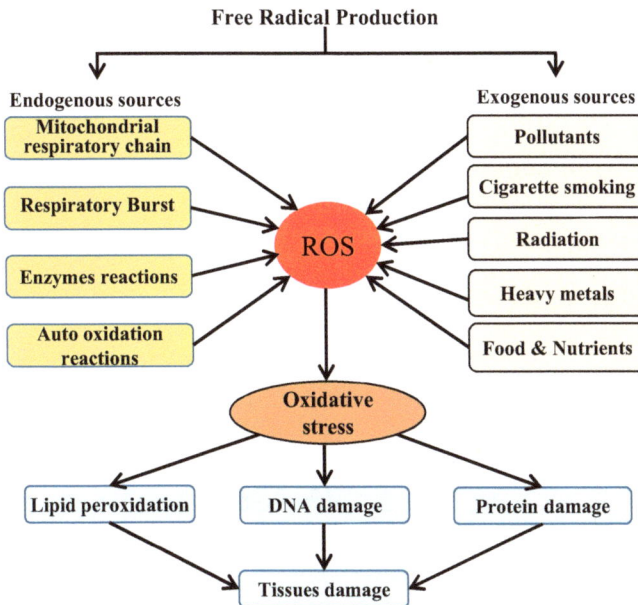

Fig. (1). Endogenous and exogenous ROS sources that cause oxidative stress and tissue damage.

Catalase (CAT)

In cells exposed to environmental stress, catalase has been shown to catalyse H2O2 to water and oxygen inside an energy-efficient manner. It's a common antioxidant enzyme which can be found in nearly all living tissues that use oxygen. In addition, it is a tetrameric heme enzyme present in peroxisomes that provides protection against the ROS-induced cellular impairment (Gasselhuber *et al.* 2015). The enzyme completes the detoxification process started by SOD by catalysing the oxidation or reduction of H_2O_2 to H_2O and O_2 utilising either iron or manganese (Mn) as a cofactor (Chelikani *et al.* 2004). Catalases directly dismutate two H_2O_2 on two H_2O and one O_2 molecule. $2H_2O_2 \rightarrow 2H_2O + O_2$.

The CAT activity is carried out in two stages. The heme is converted to an oxyferryl species by a molecule of hydrogen peroxide. When one oxidation equivalent of iron is extracted and one from the porphyrin ring, the cationic radical of porphyrin is created. To regenerate the resting enzyme, a second H_2O_2 compound acts as a reducing agent, and it produces molecules of oxygen and water (Chelikani *et al.* 2004).

Peroxidases

Peroxidases are oxidoreductases which transform a wide range of substances into oxidised or polymerized products using the free radical mechanism. It is made up of a number of enzymes that suppress H_2O_2 by various catalytic mechanisms. The glutathione and thioredoxin peroxidases are two important peroxidases involved in redox homeostasis. GSH as well as thioredoxin (TRX) are used as cofactors by these enzymes to minimise the amount of energy they consume. Peroxidase catalyses the transition of electrons from these cofactors to reactive species, which are then recovered by reducing enzymes which use electrons from NADPH. Enzymes operate together (peroxidase-reductase) to create an active structure capable of self-recycling (Flohe and Ursini 2008).

Glutathione Peroxidase (GPx)

GPx is an antioxidant enzyme that can scavenge free radicals and prevents lipid peroxidation while still maintaining intracellular homeostasis and redox equilibrium (Lubos *et al.* 2011). GPx is a cytosolic enzyme that reduces hydroperoxides and has a selenocysteine residue that is active at its catalytic core. In erythrocytes, GPx is the most effective antioxidant against oxidant stress and has some significant capacities in phagocytic cells. It catalyses glutathione oxidation at the expense of the hydroperoxide, which can be the H_2O_2 or the other species like lipid hydroperoxide (Takahashi and Cohen 1986).

GPx is the key enzyme accountable for detoxification of H_2O_2 and lipid peroxides by reduced glutathione. Overexpression of this enzyme has been observed to defend cells against lethal oxidative stress (Sies *et al.* 1997). The biochemical role of GPx is to reduce lipid hydroperoxides to their corresponding alcohols and to reduce H2O2 to H2O by using two molecules of GSH as electron donors (Muller *et al.* 2007). This reaction produces oxidised glutathione (GSSG), which could be converted back to the GSH by the glutathione reductase action or transported to the extracellular media (Toppo *et al.* 2009).

Non-Enzymatic Antioxidants

Thiol Antioxidants

1-Glutathione (GSH)

The tripeptide glutathione (GSH) is the multi-functional intra-cellular antioxidant, which is the most effective thiol antioxidant. It's a thiol protein made up of cysteine, glycine, and glutamine that acts as an antioxidant and aids in mitochondrial detoxification (Sies 1999). Many detoxifying enzymes, including GPx and transferase, need GSH as a cofactor. GSH is a very soluble antioxidant found in abundance in the cell. GSH's antioxidant properties express themselves in a variety of forms (Masella *et al.* 2005). GSH is therefore crucial for cellular redox homeostasis to be maintained (Wu *et al.* 2004). It requires the action of GPx to detoxify hydrogen peroxide and lipid peroxides. Vitamin C and E are converted into active forms with the aid of GSH. The dominant redox pair in the cell is GSH and its oxidised form (GSSG) (Van Laer *et al.* 2013). To reduce H_2O_2 to H_2O and O_2, GSH donates one of its electrons to it. GSH reductase, which employs NADPH as electron donor, converts GSSG back to GSH. The membrane lipids are protected from oxidative damage by reduced glutathione, which supplies protons to them (Curello *et al.* 1985). The reduced and oxidised forms of glutathione (GSH and GSSG) regulate and maintain cellular redox state in the presence of other redox-active molecules (Jones *et al.* 2011). GSH inhibits apoptosis in cells by interacting with both proapoptotic and antiapoptotic signalling pathways (Masella *et al.* 2005). GSH levels in cells are maintained and increased, which is an indicator for tumour initiation, growth, and progression (Harris *et al.* 2015, Cramer *et al.* 2017). GSH deficiency, or a drop in the proportion of glutathione and glutathione disulfide (GSH/GSSG), raises the risk of oxidative stress and cancer growth.

2-Thioredoxin

Thioredoxin is also another thiol antioxidant (TRX). These are oxidoreductase-active proteins that are found in mammals and prokaryotic cells as well. A disulfide is also present, as well as two redox-active cysteines inside the conserved active site. As thioredoxin enters redox reactions with many proteins, this comprises two neighbouring –SH groups in reduced state, which are transformed to a disulfide class in oxidised TRX. Many regular and neoplastic cells secrete thioredoxin while they are exposed to oxidative stress and inflammation (Tonissen and Di Trapani 2009). Serum thioredoxin level was significantly higher in disorders linked with oxidative stress in clinical studies (Nakamura *et al.* 1996).

3-α-Lipoic acid

Natural compound *i.e.* α-lipoic acid (ALA), the sulfur-containing antioxidant with the metal-chelating or antiglycation capacities, is the third significant thiol antioxidant (Salehi *et al.* 2019). Lipoic acid works in both the lipid as well as aqueous phases, unlike certain antioxidants that either work in the lipid or aqueous stages. ALA is a cofactor for a number of enzymatic clusters active in the cell's energy metabolism and plays a key function in a variety of chemical reactions. Red meat and organ meats (liver and kidney) are great sources of ALA and it is found in many vegetables like broccoli, potatoes, tomatoes, rice bran, green peas, and spinach. The reduced form of ALA combines with reactive oxygen species and disrupts free radical production (Packer and Cadenas 2010). It acts as metal chelating agent, free radical scavenger, and generator for endogenous antioxidants, like glutathione, vitamins C, E and provide oxidative damage repair (Biewenga *et al.* 1997). Lipoic acid efficiently eradicates heavy metals from the blood, accountable for the oxidative stress (Gorąca *et al.* 2011). ALA also has many other functions, it has a key role in energy transduction in mitochondria as it is a critical cofactor of various oxidative enzymes in metabolism (Keith *et al.* 2012).

Carotenoids

Carotenoids are group of natural organic pigmented compounds of the polyene type. Fungi, several bacteria, and plants synthesize these compounds (Alós et al. 2016). They are lipid-soluble antioxidants that are centered around the isoprenoid carbon skeleton. Further, they are chief precursors of the retinol (vitamin A). The main carotenoids are α-, β- & γ-carotene, neurosporene, lycopene, lutein, phytofluene, zeaxanthin, and phytoene, all of which are found in human plasma (Khachik 2006).

Carotenoids are very powerful natural antioxidants. These are highly effective scavengers of the singlet oxygen and entrap the peroxyl radicals, ROS, and other radicals of various origins (Mortensen *et al.* 1977, Cvetkovic *et al.* 2013).

Carotenoids play a significant part in protecting membranes and lipoproteins against oxidative stress in cells, so they have a protective role against diseases (Sies and Stahl 1995, Mayne 1996). They are relatively non-reactive, but they can also decompose and create non-radical molecules by attaching to them that can stop free radical attacks (Paiva and Russell 1999).

Flavonoids and Phenolic Acids

Fruits, herbs, nuts, tea, flowers, branches, roots, and bark all contain flavonoids, a category of natural products containing complex phenolic structures. Flavonols, flavones, flavanones, anthocyanins, and isoflavonoids are different types of flavonoids. The flavonoids, flavones as well as catechins prove to be the most effective antioxidants in protecting the body from the damage induced by reactive oxygen species (Panche *et al.* 2016). Many flavonoids can actively scavenge superoxides, while others can scavenge peroxynitrite, an extremely reactive oxygen-derived radical (Hanasaki *et al.* 1994). The antioxidant capacity of the flavonoids is estimated by the structural arrangement of functional groups. The mechanism of antioxidant property is strongly influenced by both the structure and total number of OH groups (Rice-Evans *et al.* 1996, Heim *et al.* 2002).

Hydroxycinnamic and hydroxybenzoic acids are two types of phenolic acids. They can be used in a variety of forms in plant products, including esters and glycosides. Further, they have the antioxidant properties, such as chelating power as well as free radical scavenging ability, and have a notable effect on hydroxyl radicals, peroxyl radicals, peroxynitrites, and superoxide anions (Terpinc *et al.* 2011).

Vitamin E (α-Tocopherol)

The key protection against oxidant-induced membrane damage is lipid-soluble vitamin E, which is located in the hydrophobic inner region of the cell membrane. Any of the eight isoforms of vitamin E prevents lipid peroxidation by donating the phenolic hydrogen atom to peroxyl radicals, resulting in tocopheroxyl radicals that are non-reactive and unable to initiate the oxidative chain of events (Niki 2015). The peroxyl radical created during the lipid peroxidation receives an electron from vitamin E. The α-tocopherol is among the main membrane-bound antioxidants within the cell, is the most active source of vitamin E. Vitamin E initiates apoptosis in the cancer cells and inhibit the development of the free radicals (White *et al.* 1997). The α-tocopherol is by far the most effective lipid-soluble antioxidant, which prevents membranes against oxidation by interacting to lipid radicals generated during lipid peroxidation chain of events (Traber and Atkinson 2007). This reaction generates oxidized form of α-tocopheroxyl radicals, which can be decreased through other antioxidants, like ascorbate or retinol, to return to their active antioxidant potential (reduced form) (Wang and Quinn 1999).

Vitamin C (Ascorbic Acid)

Vitamin C is a water-soluble natural antioxidant that has antioxidant properties both intracellularly and extracellularly. It works by scavenging oxygen free radicals including superoxide radicals, hydroxyl radicals, hydrogen peroxide, nitrogen oxide radical, and singlet oxygen (Hacşevki 2009, Barros *et al.* 2011). It is impossible for humans to synthesise it, so it must be ingested by food (Smirnoff 2001). It is held in its reduced state in cells through a reaction with the glutathione, which is catalyzed by the disulfide isomerase as well as glutaredoxins (Meister 1994). It's also a precursor for the antioxidative ascorbate peroxidase, which plays a crucial role in the cell and tissue stress resistance (Shigeoka *et al.* 2002).

Minerals

Several minerals are dietary food ingredients that participate in the antioxidant defense mechanism, and act directly as the antioxidants or support proper functioning of detoxifying enzymes. Antioxidant enzymes like GPx and SOD need selenium (Se), copper (Cu), and zinc (Zn) in the diet (Aziz 2019). The deficiency of minerals increases the activity of cytochrome P450 in the microsomes of liver and lungs, thereby increasing the formation of ROS and NOS expressions (Youdim *et al.* 2000). The main minerals that have an antioxidant function are Se and Zn.

In the human body, selenium can be present in both the organic and the inorganic forms. While it does not specifically interact with free radicals, it is thought to be an essential component of most antioxidant enzymes, since they will not function without it (Tabassum *et al.* 2010). The role of selenium as an antioxidant is due to its occurrence in the essential enzymes like GSH, GPx, and SOD, therefore selenium increases the antioxidant function power of these enzymes (Gupta and Gupta 2016, Zoidis *et al.* 2018).

Zinc is crucial for preventing the formation of free radicals. As NADPH oxidases inhibitor it can stimulate the formation of the singlet oxygen from the oxygen molecule by utilizing NADPH as an electron donor. It is also a constituent of SOD, which is a vital antioxidant enzyme which transforms the singlet oxygen radicals into the hydrogen peroxide. Saad-Hussein *et al.* (2019) reported that Zn supplementation improves the oxidative/antioxidants status in the blood lipids of the pesticide sprayers. Zinc acts by stabilization of protein sulfhydryl groups against oxidation and by replacing redox active metals (copper and iron) (Jarosz *et al.* 2017). Zinc produces the metallothionein, which is the scavenger of hydroxyl radicals. Besides, zinc competes with copper to bind to cell wall, which reduces the formation of OH radicals (Prasad *et al.* 2004).

Uric Acid

Purine nucleotide metabolism produces uric acid as a byproduct in humans.. It can prevent lipid and protein peroxidation and inactivate tetrahydrobiopterin, leading to free radicals scavenging and transitional metal ions chelation (Waring *et al.* 2001). Uric acid is also presumed to defend the central nervous system as an antioxidant (Bowman *et al.* 2010). Uric acid is a strong scavenger of hydroxyl radical ($^{\cdot}$OH), singlet oxygen ($^1O_2$), and peroxyl radical (ROO$^-$) (Álvarez-Lario and Macarron 2010). It also inhibit the excessive production of oxo-heme oxidants resulting from the biochemical reaction of the hemoglobin with the peroxides (Kand'ár *et al.* 2006).

Coenzyme Q10

It works by stopping lipid peroxyl radical development. But once they've formed, it neutralises these radicals. Vitamin E regeneration is an essential function for this coenzyme. This method is more likely to regenerate vitamin E than ascorbate (vitamin C). Further, this coenzyme can be found in all the cells and membranes, and it is vital for the respiratory chain reaction and other cellular metabolic mechanisms (Turunen *et al.* 2004).

Bilirubin (BR)

It is the primary state (unconjugated form) of circulating bilirubin in the healthy individuals, the final product of heme metabolism, and has antioxidant properties (Rizzo *et al.* 2010). Recent studies indicated that bilirubin treatment could increase the accumulation of nuclear factor erythroid 2-related factor (Nrf2) that up-regulate the expression of heme-oxygenase-1 in HepG2 cell line and primary mouse hepatocytes (Kim *et al.* 2013). BR scavenging activity toward $NO^{\cdot}$ is weaker than that of other endogenous substances such as hemoglobin, glutathione or uric acid (Mancuso *et al.* 2006).

Melatonin

Melatonin is generated by the body and can also be absorbed from dietary sources (vegetables, fruits, many herbs, and cereals) (Meng *et al.* 2017). It is a potent antioxidant which can quickly cross the cell membranes. It protects mitochondria from the oxidative damage that reduces oxygen consumption, thereby control the formation of superoxide anion (Reiter *et al.* 1997, López *et al.* 2009). Studies demonstrate that a melatonin molecule can scavenge up to ten molecules of ROS. Melatonin cannot be reduced down to its original state after it has been oxidised because it produces several stable end-products during the reaction with free radicals (Tan *et al.* 2000). Melatonin also recovers the activities of many respiratory chain reaction complexes, thus reduce the leakage of electrons and the production of the free radicals (Solís-Muñoz *et al.* 2011). Melatonin not only scavenges ROS/RNS directly, but it also activates antioxidant enzymes (Barlow-Walden *et al.* 1995).

CONCLUSION

Exposure to different environmental contaminants such as toxic metals, air pollutants, radiation, pesticides, solvents exposure, and tobacco smoke leads to the oxidative stress in cells. This stress affects multiple biological processes by generating excess ROS.

Excessive ROS, a state of the disproportion among the ROS creation and removal of free radicals by the antioxidants, leads to the loss of cellular components and disease development.

Redox homeostasis is accomplished by regulating the formation and removal of the ROS from the body system. The balance amid the ROS generation and its subsequent removal is controlled by a balanced system for surplus ROS neutralization.

Antioxidant systems comprise the enzymatic antioxidants like the superoxide dismutase (SOD), glutathione peroxidase (GPx), and catalase (CAT) as well as the non-enzymatic antioxidants (vitamins, minerals, carotenoids, melatonin, and others), reduce the ROS level maintaining its physiological level in the cell. Therefore, dietary antioxidants are a promising way to avoid and treat varoius health issues caused by the overproduction of ROS.

CONFLICT OF INTEREST

The authors report that there are no conflicts of interest.

ACKNOWLEDGEMENT

We are indebted to our Professor Dr. Laila Hussein for her advice in participating in this valuable Book, deep thanks also to the editorial staff for including us in this work.

CONSENT FOR PUBLICATION

None

REFERENCES

Ahmad, R (2018) Introductory Chapter. *Basics of Free Radicals and Antioxidants,* 1-4
[http://dx.doi.org/10.5772/intechopen.76689]

Alós, E, Rodrigo, MJ & Zacarias, L (2016) Manipulation of carotenoid content in plants to improve human health.*Carotenoids in Nature* Springer, Cham, Switzerland 311-43.
[http://dx.doi.org/10.1007/978-3-319-39126-7_12]

Álvarez-Lario, B & Macarrón-Vicente, J (2010) Uric acid and evolution. *Rheumatology (Oxford),* 49, 2010-5.
[http://dx.doi.org/10.1093/rheumatology/keq204] [PMID: 20627967]

Aycicek, A, Erel, O & Kocyigit, A (2005) Decreased total antioxidant capacity and increased oxidative stress in passive smoker infants and their mothers. *Pediatr Int,* 47, 635-9.
[http://dx.doi.org/10.1111/j.1442-200x.2005.02137.x] [PMID: 16354215]

Aziz, MA, Diab, AS & Mohammed, AA (2019) *Antioxidant Categories and Mode of Action*
[http://dx.doi.org/10.5772/intechopen.83544]

Balaban, RS, Nemoto, S & Finkel, T (2005) Mitochondria, oxidants, and aging. *Cell,* 120, 483-95.
[http://dx.doi.org/10.1016/j.cell.2005.02.001] [PMID: 15734681]

Barlow-Walden, LR, Reiter, RJ, Abe, M, Pablos, M, Menendez-Pelaez, A, Chen, L-D & Poeggeler, B (1995) Melatonin stimulates brain glutathione peroxidase activity. *Neurochem Int,* 26, 497-502.
[http://dx.doi.org/10.1016/0197-0186(94)00154-M] [PMID: 7492947]

Barreiro, E, Peinado, VI, Galdiz, JB, Ferrer, E, Marin-Corral, J, Sánchez, F, Gea, J & Barberà, JA (2010) Cigarette smoke-induced oxidative stress: A role in chronic obstructive pulmonary disease skeletal muscle dysfunction. *Am J Respir Crit Care Med,* 182, 477-88.

[http://dx.doi.org/10.1164/rccm.200908-1220OC] [PMID: 20413628]

Barros, AI, Nunes, FM, Gonçalves, B, Bennett, RN & Silva, AP (2011) Effect of cooking on total vitamin C contents and antioxidant activity of sweet chestnuts (Castanea sativa Mill.). *Food Chem,* 128, 165-72.
[http://dx.doi.org/10.1016/j.foodchem.2011.03.013] [PMID: 25214344]

Bhattacharyya, A, Chattopadhyay, R, Mitra, S & Crowe, SE (2014) Oxidative stress: an essential factor in the pathogenesis of gastrointestinal mucosal diseases. *Physiol Rev,* 94, 329-54.
[http://dx.doi.org/10.1152/physrev.00040.2012] [PMID: 24692350]

Biaglow, JE, Mitchell, JB & Held, K (1992) The importance of peroxide and superoxide in the X-ray response. *Int J Radiat Oncol Biol Phys,* 22, 665-9.
[http://dx.doi.org/10.1016/0360-3016(92)90499-8] [PMID: 1312073]

Biewenga, GP, Haenen, GR & Bast, A (1997) The pharmacology of the antioxidant lipoic acid. *Gen Pharmacol,* 29, 315-31.
[http://dx.doi.org/10.1016/S0306-3623(96)00474-0] [PMID: 9378235]

Bowman, GL, Shannon, J, Frei, B, Kaye, JA & Quinn, JF (2010) Uric acid as a CNS antioxidant. *J Alzheimers Dis,* 19, 1331-6.
[http://dx.doi.org/10.3233/JAD-2010-1330] [PMID: 20061611]

Breitzig, M, Bhimineni, C, Lockey, R & Kolliputi, N (2016) 4-Hydroxy-2-nonenal: a critical target in oxidative stress? *Am J Physiol Cell Physiol,* 311, C537-43.
[http://dx.doi.org/10.1152/ajpcell.00101.2016] [PMID: 27385721]

Catalá, A & Díaz, M (2016) Editorial: impact of lipid peroxidation on the physiology and pathophysiology of cell membranes. *Front Physiol,* 7, 423.
[http://dx.doi.org/10.3389/fphys.2016.00423] [PMID: 27713704]

Čermak, AMM, Pavičić, I & Želježić, D (2018) Redox imbalance caused by pesticides: a review of OPENTOX-related research. *Archives of Industrial Hygiene and Toxicology,* 69, 126-34.
[http://dx.doi.org/10.2478/aiht-2018-69-3105] [PMID: 29990294]

Chelikani, P, Fita, I & Loewen, PC (2004) Diversity of structures and properties among catalases. *Cell Mol Life Sci,* 61, 192-208.
[http://dx.doi.org/10.1007/s00018-003-3206-5] [PMID: 14745498]

Chiu, SM, Xue, LY, Friedman, LR & Oleinick, NL (1993) Copper ion-mediated sensitization of nuclear matrix attachment sites to ionizing radiation. *Biochemistry,* 32, 6214-9.
[http://dx.doi.org/10.1021/bi00075a014] [PMID: 8512931]

Cho, AK, Sioutas, C, Miguel, AH, Kumagai, Y, Schmitz, DA, Singh, M, Eiguren-Fernandez, A & Froines, JR (2005) Redox activity of airborne particulate matter at different sites in the Los Angeles Basin. *Environ Res,* 99, 40-7.
[http://dx.doi.org/10.1016/j.envres.2005.01.003] [PMID: 16053926]

Church, DF & Pryor, WA (1985) Free-radical chemistry of cigarette smoke and its toxicological implications. *Environ Health Perspect,* 64, 111-26.
[http://dx.doi.org/10.1289/ehp.8564111] [PMID: 3007083]

Cramer, SL, Saha, A, Liu, J, Tadi, S, Tiziani, S, Yan, W, Triplett, K, Lamb, C, Alters, SE, Rowlinson, S, Zhang, YJ, Keating, MJ, Huang, P, DiGiovanni, J, Georgiou, G & Stone, E (2017) Systemic depletion of L-cyst(e)ine with cyst(e)inase increases reactive oxygen species and suppresses tumor growth. *Nat Med,* 23, 120-7.
[http://dx.doi.org/10.1038/nm.4232] [PMID: 27869804]

Curello, S, Ceconi, C, Bigoli, C, Ferrari, R, Albertini, A & Guarnieri, C (1985) Changes in the cardiac glutathione status after ischemia and reperfusion. *Experientia,* 41, 42-3.
[http://dx.doi.org/10.1007/BF02005863] [PMID: 3967736]

Cuypers, A, Plusquin, M, Remans, T, Jozefczak, M, Keunen, E, Gielen, H, Opdenakker, K, Nair, AR, Munters, E, Artois, TJ, Nawrot, T, Vangronsveld, J & Smeets, K (2010) Cadmium stress: an oxidative

challenge. *Biometals,* 23, 927-40.
[http://dx.doi.org/10.1007/s10534-010-9329-x] [PMID: 20361350]

Cvetkovic, D, Fiedor, L, Fiedor, J, Wisniewska-Becker, A & Markovic, D (2013) Molecular Base for Carotenoids Antioxidant Activity in Model and Biological Systems: The Health-Related Effects.*Carotenoids: Food Sources, Production and Health Benefits* Nova Science Publishers, Hauppauge, NY, USA 93-126.

Day, BJ (2009) Catalase and glutathione peroxidase mimics. *Biochem Pharmacol,* 77, 285-96.
[http://dx.doi.org/10.1016/j.bcp.2008.09.029] [PMID: 18948086]

Deavall, DG, Martin, EA, Horner, JM & Roberts, R (2012) Drug-induced oxidative stress and toxicity. *J Toxicol,* 2012645460
[http://dx.doi.org/10.1155/2012/645460] [PMID: 22919381]

Di Meo, S, Reed, TT, Venditti, P & Victor, VM (2016) Role of ROS and RNS Sources in Physiological and Pathological Conditions. *Oxid Med Cell Longev,* 20161245049
[http://dx.doi.org/10.1155/2016/1245049] [PMID: 27478531]

Dizdaroglu, M & Jaruga, P (2012) Mechanisms of free radical-induced damage to DNA. *Free Radic Res,* 46, 382-419.
[http://dx.doi.org/10.3109/10715762.2011.653969] [PMID: 22276778]

Espinosa-Diez, C, Miguel, V, Mennerich, D, Kietzmann, T, Sánchez-Pérez, P, Cadenas, S & Lamas, S (2015) Antioxidant responses and cellular adjustments to oxidative stress. *Redox Biol,* 6, 183-97.
[http://dx.doi.org/10.1016/j.redox.2015.07.008] [PMID: 26233704]

Finkel, T (2011) Signal transduction by reactive oxygen species. *J Cell Biol,* 194, 7-15.
[http://dx.doi.org/10.1083/jcb.201102095] [PMID: 21746850]

Flohé, L & Ursini, F (2008) Peroxidase: a term of many meanings. *Antioxid Redox Signal,* 10, 1485-90.
[http://dx.doi.org/10.1089/ars.2008.2059] [PMID: 18479208]

Fridovich, I (1997) Superoxide anion radical (O2-.), superoxide dismutases, and related matters. *J Biol Chem,* 272, 18515-7.
[http://dx.doi.org/10.1074/jbc.272.30.18515] [PMID: 9228011]

Fryzova, R, Pohanka, M, Martinkova, P, Cihlarova, H, Brtnicky, M, Hladky, J & Kynicky, J (2018) Oxidative Stress and Heavy Metals in Plants. *Rev Environ Contam Toxicol,* 245, 129-56.
[http://dx.doi.org/10.1007/398_2017_7] [PMID: 29032515]

Fuchs-Tarlovsky, V (2013) Role of antioxidants in cancer therapy. *Nutrition,* 29, 15-21.
[http://dx.doi.org/10.1016/j.nut.2012.02.014] [PMID: 22784609]

Gaschler, MM & Stockwell, BR (2017) Lipid peroxidation in cell death. *Biochem Biophys Res Commun,* 482, 419-25.
[http://dx.doi.org/10.1016/j.bbrc.2016.10.086] [PMID: 28212725]

Gasselhuber, B, Carpena, X, Graf, MM, Pirker, KF, Nicolussi, A, Sündermann, A, Hofbauer, S, Zamocky, M, Furtmüller, PG, Jakopitsch, C, Oostenbrink, C, Fita, I & Obinger, C (2015) Eukaryotic Catalase-Peroxidase: The Role of the Trp-Tyr-Met Adduct in Protein Stability, Substrate Accessibility, and Catalysis of Hydrogen Peroxide Dismutation. *Biochemistry,* 54, 5425-38.
[http://dx.doi.org/10.1021/acs.biochem.5b00831] [PMID: 26290940]

Genestra, M (2007) Oxyl radicals, redox-sensitive signalling cascades and antioxidants. *Cell Signal,* 19, 1807-19.
[http://dx.doi.org/10.1016/j.cellsig.2007.04.009] [PMID: 17570640]

Gorąca, A, Huk-Kolega, H, Piechota, A, Kleniewska, P, Ciejka, E & Skibska, B (2011) Lipoic acid - biological activity and therapeutic potential. *Pharmacol Rep,* 63, 849-58.
[http://dx.doi.org/10.1016/S1734-1140(11)70600-4] [PMID: 22001972]

Gupta, M & Gupta, S (2017) An Overview of Selenium Uptake, Metabolism, and Toxicity in Plants. *Front Plant Sci,* 7, 2074.

[http://dx.doi.org/10.3389/fpls.2016.02074] [PMID: 28123395]

Halliwell, B & Cross, CE (1994) Oxygen-derived species: their relation to human disease and environmental stress. *Environ Health Perspect,* 102 (Suppl. 10), 5-12.
[PMID: 7705305]

Halliwell, B, Rafter, J & Jenner, A (2005) Health promotion by flavonoids, tocopherols, tocotrienols, and other phenols: direct or indirect effects? Antioxidant or not? *Am J Clin Nutr,* 81 (Suppl.), 268S-76S.
[http://dx.doi.org/10.1093/ajcn/81.1.268S] [PMID: 15640490]

Halliwell, B (2001) *Free Radicals and other reactive species in disease*
[http://dx.doi.org/10.1038/npg.els.0003913]

Hanasaki, Y, Ogawa, S & Fukui, S (1994) The correlation between active oxygens scavenging and antioxidative effects of flavonoids. *Free Radic Biol Med,* 16, 845-50.
[http://dx.doi.org/10.1016/0891-5849(94)90202-X] [PMID: 8070690]

Harris, IS, Treloar, AE, Inoue, S, Sasaki, M, Gorrini, C, Lee, KC, Yung, KY, Brenner, D, Knobbe-Thomsen, CB, Cox, MA, Elia, A, Berger, T, Cescon, DW, Adeoye, A, Brüstle, A, Molyneux, SD, Mason, JM, Li, WY, Yamamoto, K, Wakeham, A, Berman, HK, Khokha, R, Done, SJ, Kavanagh, TJ, Lam, CW, Mak, TW & Mak, TW (2015) Glutathione and thioredoxin antioxidant pathways synergize to drive cancer initiation and progression. *Cancer Cell,* 27, 211-22.
[http://dx.doi.org/10.1016/j.ccell.2014.11.019] [PMID: 25620030]

He, L, He, T, Farrar, S, Ji, L, Liu, T & Ma, X (2017) Antioxidants Maintain Cellular Redox Homeostasis by Elimination of Reactive Oxygen Species. *Cell Physiol Biochem,* 44, 532-53.
[http://dx.doi.org/10.1159/000485089] [PMID: 29145191]

Heim, KE, Tagliaferro, AR & Bobilya, DJ (2002) Flavonoid antioxidants: chemistry, metabolism and structure-activity relationships. *J Nutr Biochem,* 13, 572-84.
[http://dx.doi.org/10.1016/S0955-2863(02)00208-5] [PMID: 12550068]

Hiltermann, JT, Lapperre, TS, van Bree, L, Steerenberg, PA, Brahim, JJ, Sont, JK, Sterk, PJ, Hiemstra, PS & Stolk, J (1999) Ozone-induced inflammation assessed in sputum and bronchial lavage fluid from asthmatics: a new noninvasive tool in epidemiologic studies on air pollution and asthma. *Free Radic Biol Med,* 27, 1448-54.
[http://dx.doi.org/10.1016/S0891-5849(99)00191-4] [PMID: 10641740]

Hoffmann, D, Hoffmann, I & El-Bayoumy, K (2001) The less harmful cigarette: a controversial issue. a tribute to Ernst L. Wynder. *Chem Res Toxicol,* 14, 767-90.
[http://dx.doi.org/10.1021/tx000260u] [PMID: 11453723]

Iwanaga, M, Mori, K, Iida, T, Urata, Y, Matsuo, T, Yasunaga, A, Shibata, S & Kondo, T (1998) Nuclear factor kappa B dependent induction of gamma glutamylcysteine synthetase by ionizing radiation in T98G human glioblastoma cells. *Free Radic Biol Med,* 24, 1256-68.
[http://dx.doi.org/10.1016/S0891-5849(97)00443-7] [PMID: 9626582]

Jarosz, M, Olbert, M, Wyszogrodzka, G, Młyniec, K & Librowski, T (2017) Antioxidant and anti-inflammatory effects of zinc. Zinc-dependent NF-κB signaling. *Inflammopharmacology,* 25, 11-24.
[http://dx.doi.org/10.1007/s10787-017-0309-4] [PMID: 28083748]

Jezek, P & Hlavatá, L (2005) Mitochondria in homeostasis of reactive oxygen species in cell, tissues, and organism. *Int J Biochem Cell Biol,* 37, 2478-503.
[http://dx.doi.org/10.1016/j.biocel.2005.05.013] [PMID: 16103002]

Jomova, K & Valko, M (2011) Advances in metal-induced oxidative stress and human disease. *Toxicology,* 283, 65-87.
[http://dx.doi.org/10.1016/j.tox.2011.03.001] [PMID: 21414382]

Jones, DP, Park, Y, Gletsu-Miller, N, Liang, Y, Yu, T, Accardi, CJ & Ziegler, TR (2011) Dietary sulfur amino acid effects on fasting plasma cysteine/cystine redox potential in humans. *Nutrition,* 27, 199-205.
[http://dx.doi.org/10.1016/j.nut.2010.01.014] [PMID: 20471805]

Kaludercic, N, Deshwal, S & Di Lisa, F (2014) Reactive oxygen species and redox compartmentalization. *Front Physiol,* 5, 285.
[http://dx.doi.org/10.3389/fphys.2014.00285] [PMID: 25161621]

Kamceva, G, Arsova-Sarafinovska, Z, Ruskovska, T, Zdravkovska, M, Kamceva-Panova, L & Stikova, E (2016) Cigarette Smoking and Oxidative Stress in Patients with Coronary Artery Disease. *Open Access Maced J Med Sci,* 4, 636-40.
[http://dx.doi.org/10.3889/oamjms.2016.117] [PMID: 28028404]

Kand'ár, R, Záková, P & Muzáková, V (2006) Monitoring of antioxidant properties of uric acid in humans for a consideration measuring of levels of allantoin in plasma by liquid chromatography. *Clin Chim Acta,* 365, 249-56.
[http://dx.doi.org/10.1016/j.cca.2005.09.002] [PMID: 16194528]

Keikotlhaile, BM, Spanoghe, P & Steurbaut, W (2010) Effects of food processing on pesticide residues in fruits and vegetables: a meta-analysis approach. *Food Chem Toxicol,* 48, 1-6.
[http://dx.doi.org/10.1016/j.fct.2009.10.031] [PMID: 19879312]

Keith, DJ, Butler, JA, Bemer, B, Dixon, B, Johnson, S, Garrard, M, Sudakin, DL, Christensen, JM, Pereira, C & Hagen, TM (2012) Age and gender dependent bioavailability of R- and R,S-α-lipoic acid: a pilot study. *Pharmacol Res,* 66, 199-206.
[http://dx.doi.org/10.1016/j.phrs.2012.05.002] [PMID: 22609537]

Khachik, F (2006) Distribution and metabolism of dietary carotenoids in humans as a criterion for development of nutritional supplements. *Pure Appl Chem,* 78, 1551-7.
[http://dx.doi.org/10.1351/pac200678081551]

Kim, SD, Antenos, M, Squires, EJ & Kirby, GM (2013) Cytochrome P450 2A5 and bilirubin: mechanisms of gene regulation and cytoprotection. *Toxicol Appl Pharmacol,* 270, 129-38.
[http://dx.doi.org/10.1016/j.taap.2013.04.013] [PMID: 23628428]

Kohen, R & Nyska, A (2002) Oxidation of biological systems: oxidative stress phenomena, antioxidants, redox reactions, and methods for their quantification. *Toxicol Pathol,* 30, 620-50.
[http://dx.doi.org/10.1080/01926230290166724] [PMID: 12512863]

Kong, H & Chandel, NS (2018) Regulation of redox balance in cancer and T cells. *J Biol Chem,* 293, 7499-507.
[http://dx.doi.org/10.1074/jbc.TM117.000257] [PMID: 29282291]

Kovacic, P & Somanathan, R (2006) Mechanism of teratogenesis: electron transfer, reactive oxygen species, and antioxidants. *Birth Defects Res C Embryo Today,* 78, 308-25.
[http://dx.doi.org/10.1002/bdrc.20081] [PMID: 17315244]

Le Bras, M, Clément, MV, Pervaiz, S & Brenner, C (2005) Reactive oxygen species and the mitochondrial signaling pathway of cell death. *Histol Histopathol,* 20, 205-19.
[PMID: 15578439]

Leonard, SS, Harris, GK & Shi, X (2004) Metal-induced oxidative stress and signal transduction. *Free Radic Biol Med,* 37, 1921-42.
[http://dx.doi.org/10.1016/j.freeradbiomed.2004.09.010] [PMID: 15544913]

López, A, García, JA, Escames, G, Venegas, C, Ortiz, F, López, LC & Acuña-Castroviejo, D (2009) Melatonin protects the mitochondria from oxidative damage reducing oxygen consumption, membrane potential, and superoxide anion production. *J Pineal Res,* 46, 188-98.
[http://dx.doi.org/10.1111/j.1600-079X.2008.00647.x] [PMID: 19054298]

Lubos, E, Loscalzo, J & Handy, DE (2011) Glutathione peroxidase-1 in health and disease: from molecular mechanisms to therapeutic opportunities. *Antioxid Redox Signal,* 15, 1957-97.
[http://dx.doi.org/10.1089/ars.2010.3586] [PMID: 21087145]

Mahboob, M, Shireen, KF, Atkinson, A & Khan, AT (2001) Lipid peroxidation and antioxidant enzyme activity in different organs of mice exposed to low level of mercury. *J Environ Sci Health B,* 36, 687-97.

[http://dx.doi.org/10.1081/PFC-100106195] [PMID: 11599730]

Mancuso, C, Pani, G & Calabrese, V (2006) Bilirubin: an endogenous scavenger of nitric oxide and reactive nitrogen species. *Redox Rep,* 11, 207-13.
[http://dx.doi.org/10.1179/135100006X154978] [PMID: 17132269]

Marnett, LJ (1999) Lipid peroxidation-DNA damage by malondialdehyde. *Mutat Res,* 424, 83-95.
[http://dx.doi.org/10.1016/S0027-5107(99)00010-X] [PMID: 10064852]

Masella, R, Di Benedetto, R, Varì, R, Filesi, C & Giovannini, C (2005) Novel mechanisms of natural antioxidant compounds in biological systems: involvement of glutathione and glutathione-related enzymes. *J Nutr Biochem,* 16, 577-86.
[http://dx.doi.org/10.1016/j.jnutbio.2005.05.013] [PMID: 16111877]

Mayne, ST (1996) Beta-carotene, carotenoids, and disease prevention in humans. *FASEB J,* 10, 690-701.
[http://dx.doi.org/10.1096/fasebj.10.7.8635686] [PMID: 8635686]

Mecdad, AA, Ahmed, MH, ElHalwagy, MEA & Afify, MMM (2011) A study on oxidative stress biomarkers and immune modulatory effects of pesticides in pesticide-sprayers. *Egypt J Forensic Sci,* 1, 93-8.
[http://dx.doi.org/10.1016/j.ejfs.2011.04.012]

Meister, A (1994) Glutathione-ascorbic acid antioxidant system in animals. *J Biol Chem,* 269, 9397-400.
[http://dx.doi.org/10.1016/S0021-9258(17)36891-6] [PMID: 8144521]

Meng, X, Li, Y, Li, S, Zhou, Y, Gan, R-Y, Xu, D-P & Li, H-B (2017) Dietary Sources and Bioactivities of Melatonin. *Nutrients,* 9E367
[http://dx.doi.org/10.3390/nu9040367] [PMID: 28387721]

Miller, DM, Buettner, GR & Aust, SD (1990) Transition metals as catalysts of "autoxidation" reactions. *Free Radic Biol Med,* 8, 95-108.
[http://dx.doi.org/10.1016/0891-5849(90)90148-C] [PMID: 2182396]

Monteiro, HP, Bechara, EJH & Abdalla, DSP (1991) Free radicals involvement in neurological porphyrias and lead poisoning. *Mol Cell Biochem,* 103, 73-83.
[http://dx.doi.org/10.1007/BF00229595] [PMID: 1857346]

Mortensen, A, Skibsted, LH, Sampson, J, Rice-Evans, C & Everett, SA (1997) Comparative mechanisms and rates of free radical scavenging by carotenoid antioxidants. *FEBS Lett,* 418, 91-7.
[http://dx.doi.org/10.1016/S0014-5793(97)01355-0] [PMID: 9414102]

Muller, FL, Lustgarten, MS, Jang, Y, Richardson, A & Van Remmen, H (2007) Trends in oxidative aging theories. *Free Radic Biol Med,* 43, 477-503.
[http://dx.doi.org/10.1016/j.freeradbiomed.2007.03.034] [PMID: 17640558]

Nakamura, H, De Rosa, S, Roederer, M, Anderson, MT, Dubs, JG, Yodoi, J, Holmgren, A, Herzenberg, LA & Herzenberg, LA (1996) Elevation of plasma thioredoxin levels in HIV-infected individuals. *Int Immunol,* 8, 603-11.
[http://dx.doi.org/10.1093/intimm/8.4.603] [PMID: 8671648]

Niki, E (2015) Evidence for beneficial effects of vitamin E. *Korean J Intern Med (Korean Assoc Intern Med),* 30, 571-9.
[http://dx.doi.org/10.3904/kjim.2015.30.5.571] [PMID: 26354050]

Packer, L & Cadenas, E (2011) Lipoic acid: energy metabolism and redox regulation of transcription and cell signaling. *J Clin Biochem Nutr,* 48, 26-32.
[http://dx.doi.org/10.3164/jcbn.11-005FR] [PMID: 21297908]

Paiva, SA & Russell, RM (1999) β-carotene and other carotenoids as antioxidants. *J Am Coll Nutr,* 18, 426-33.
[http://dx.doi.org/10.1080/07315724.1999.10718880] [PMID: 10511324]

Panche, AN, Diwan, AD & Chandra, SR (2016) Flavonoids: an overview. *J Nutr Sci,* 5e47
[http://dx.doi.org/10.1017/jns.2016.41] [PMID: 28620474]

Panda, K, Chattopadhyay, R, Chattopadhyay, DJ & Chatterjee, IB (2000) Vitamin C prevents cigarette smoke-induced oxidative damage *in vivo*. *Free Radic Biol Med,* 29, 115-24.
[http://dx.doi.org/10.1016/S0891-5849(00)00297-5] [PMID: 10980400]

Pereyra-Muñoz, N, Rugerio-Vargas, C, Angoa-Pérez, M, Borgonio-Pérez, G & Rivas-Arancibia, S (2006) Oxidative damage in substantia nigra and striatum of rats chronically exposed to ozone. *J Chem Neuroanat,* 31, 114-23.
[http://dx.doi.org/10.1016/j.jchemneu.2005.09.006] [PMID: 16236481]

Phaniendra, A, Jestadi, DB & Periyasamy, L (2015) Free radicals: properties, sources, targets, and their implication in various diseases. *Indian J Clin Biochem,* 30, 11-26.
[http://dx.doi.org/10.1007/s12291-014-0446-0] [PMID: 25646037]

Prasad, AS, Bao, B, Beck, FW, Kucuk, O & Sarkar, FH (2004) Antioxidant effect of zinc in humans. *Free Radic Biol Med,* 37, 1182-90.
[http://dx.doi.org/10.1016/j.freeradbiomed.2004.07.007] [PMID: 15451058]

Rastogi, SK, Satyanarayan, PV, Ravishankar, D & Tripathi, S (2009) A study on oxidative stress and antioxidant status of agricultural workers exposed to organophosphorus insecticides during spraying. *Indian J Occup Environ Med,* 13, 131-4.
[http://dx.doi.org/10.4103/0019-5278.58916] [PMID: 20442831]

Reiter, RJ, Carneiro, RC & Oh, CS (1997) Melatonin in relation to cellular antioxidative defense mechanisms. *Horm Metab Res,* 29, 363-72.
[http://dx.doi.org/10.1055/s-2007-979057] [PMID: 9288572]

Reiter, RJ, Tan, DX & Burkhardt, S (2002) Reactive oxygen and nitrogen species and cellular and organismal decline: amelioration with melatonin. *Mech Ageing Dev,* 123, 1007-19.
[http://dx.doi.org/10.1016/S0047-6374(01)00384-0] [PMID: 12044950]

Rice-Evans, CA, Miller, NJ & Paganga, G (1996) Structure-antioxidant activity relationships of flavonoids and phenolic acids. *Free Radic Biol Med,* 20, 933-56.
[http://dx.doi.org/10.1016/0891-5849(95)02227-9] [PMID: 8743980]

Riley, PA (1994) Free radicals in biology: oxidative stress and the effects of ionizing radiation. *Int J Radiat Biol,* 65, 27-33.
[http://dx.doi.org/10.1080/09553009414550041] [PMID: 7905906]

Rizzo, AM, Berselli, P, Zava, S, Montorfano, G, Negroni, M, Corsetto, P & Berra, B (2010) Endogenous antioxidants and radical scavengers. *Adv Exp Med Biol,* 698, 52-67.
[http://dx.doi.org/10.1007/978-1-4419-7347-4_5] [PMID: 21520703]

Saad-Hussein, A, Ibrahim, KS, Abdalla, MSh, El-Mezayen, HA & Osman, NFA (2019) Effects of zinc supplementation on oxidant/antioxidant and lipids status of pesticides sprayers. *J Complement Integr Med,* 17, 1-8.
[http://dx.doi.org/10.1515/jcim-2019-0001] [PMID: 31421040]

Salehi, B, Berkay Yılmaz, Y, Antika, G, Boyunegmez Tumer, T, Fawzi Mahomoodally, M, Lobine, D, Akram, M, Riaz, M, Capanoglu, E, Sharopov, F, Martins, N, Cho, WC & Sharifi-Rad, J (2019) Insights on the Use of α-Lipoic Acid for Therapeutic Purposes. *Biomolecules,* 9, 1-25.
[http://dx.doi.org/10.3390/biom9080356] [PMID: 31405030]

Samet, JM & Wages, PA (2018) Oxidative Stress from Environmental Exposures. *Curr Opin Toxicol,* 7, 60-6.
[http://dx.doi.org/10.1016/j.cotox.2017.10.008] [PMID: 30079382]

Schieber, M & Chandel, NS (2014) ROS function in redox signaling and oxidative stress. *Curr Biol,* 24, R453-62.
[http://dx.doi.org/10.1016/j.cub.2014.03.034] [PMID: 24845678]

Schiller, CM, Fowler, BA & Woods, JS (1977) Effects of arsenic on pyruvate dehydrogenase activation. *Environ Health Perspect,* 19, 205-7.

[http://dx.doi.org/10.1289/ehp.7719205] [PMID: 908299]

Shi, H, Shi, X & Liu, KJ (2004) Oxidative mechanism of arsenic toxicity and carcinogenesis. *Mol Cell Biochem,* 255, 67-78.
[http://dx.doi.org/10.1023/B:MCBI.0000007262.26044.e8] [PMID: 14971647]

Shigeoka, S, Ishikawa, T, Tamoi, M, Miyagawa, Y, Takeda, T, Yabuta, Y & Yoshimura, K (2002) Regulation and function of ascorbate peroxidase isoenzymes. *J Exp Bot,* 53, 1305-19.
[http://dx.doi.org/10.1093/jexbot/53.372.1305] [PMID: 11997377]

Sies, H & Stahl, W (1995) Vitamins E and C, beta-carotene, and other carotenoids as antioxidants. *Am J Clin Nutr,* 62 (Suppl.), 1315S-21S.
[http://dx.doi.org/10.1093/ajcn/62.6.1315S] [PMID: 7495226]

Sies, H (1999) Glutathione and its role in cellular functions. *Free Radic Biol Med,* 27, 916-21.
[http://dx.doi.org/10.1016/S0891-5849(99)00177-X] [PMID: 10569624]

Sies, H (2014) Role of metabolic H_2O_2 generation: redox signaling and oxidative stress. *J Biol Chem,* 289, 8735-41.
[http://dx.doi.org/10.1074/jbc.R113.544635] [PMID: 24515117]

Sies, H, Sharov, VS, Klotz, L-O & Briviba, K (1997) Glutathione peroxidase protects against peroxynitrite-mediated oxidations. A new function for selenoproteins as peroxynitrite reductase. *J Biol Chem,* 272, 27812-7.
[http://dx.doi.org/10.1074/jbc.272.44.27812] [PMID: 9346926]

Smirnoff, N (2001) L-ascorbic acid biosynthesis. *Vitam Horm,* 61, 241-66.
[http://dx.doi.org/10.1016/S0083-6729(01)61008-2] [PMID: 11153268]

Solís-Muñoz, P, Solís-Herruzo, JA, Fernández-Moreira, D, Gómez-Izquierdo, E, García-Consuegra, I, Muñoz-Yagüe, T & García Ruiz, I (2011) Melatonin improves mitochondrial respiratory chain activity and liver morphology in ob/ob mice. *J Pineal Res,* 51, 113-23.
[http://dx.doi.org/10.1111/j.1600-079X.2011.00868.x] [PMID: 21355880]

Stankovic, S, Kalaba, P & Stankovic, AR (2014) Biota as toxic metal indicators. *Environ Chem Lett,* 12, 63-84.
[http://dx.doi.org/10.1007/s10311-013-0430-6]

Tabassum, A, Bristow, RG & Venkateswaran, V (2010) Ingestion of selenium and other antioxidants during prostate cancer radiotherapy: a good thing? *Cancer Treat Rev,* 36, 230-4.
[http://dx.doi.org/10.1016/j.ctrv.2009.12.008] [PMID: 20079573]

Takahashi, K & Cohen, HJ (1986) Selenium-dependent glutathione peroxidase protein and activity: immunological investigations on cellular and plasma enzymes. *Blood,* 68, 640-5.
[http://dx.doi.org/10.1182/blood.V68.3.640.640] [PMID: 3742048]

Tan, DX, Manchester, LC, Reiter, RJ, Qi, WB, Karbownik, M & Calvo, JR (2000) Significance of melatonin in antioxidative defense system: reactions and products. *Biol Signals Recept,* 9, 137-59.
[http://dx.doi.org/10.1159/000014635] [PMID: 10899700]

Terpinc, P, Polak, T, Segatin, N, Hanzlowsky, A, Ulrih, NP & Abramovič, H (2011) Antioxidant properties of 4-vinyl derivatives of hydroxycinnamic acids. *Food Chem,* 128, 62-9.
[http://dx.doi.org/10.1016/j.foodchem.2011.02.077] [PMID: 25214330]

Tonissen, KF & Di Trapani, G (2009) Thioredoxin system inhibitors as mediators of apoptosis for cancer therapy. *Mol Nutr Food Res,* 53, 87-103.
[http://dx.doi.org/10.1002/mnfr.200700492] [PMID: 18979503]

Toppo, S, Flohé, L, Ursini, F, Vanin, S & Maiorino, M (2009) Catalytic mechanisms and specificities of glutathione peroxidases: variations of a basic scheme. *Biochim Biophys Acta,* 1790, 1486-500.
[http://dx.doi.org/10.1016/j.bbagen.2009.04.007] [PMID: 19376195]

Traber, MG & Atkinson, J (2007) Vitamin E, antioxidant and nothing more. *Free Radic Biol Med,* 43, 4-15.

[http://dx.doi.org/10.1016/j.freeradbiomed.2007.03.024] [PMID: 17561088]

Trachootham, D, Lu, W, Ogasawara, MA, Nilsa, R-DV & Huang, P (2008) Redox regulation of cell survival. *Antioxid Redox Signal,* 10, 1343-74.
[http://dx.doi.org/10.1089/ars.2007.1957] [PMID: 18522489]

Turunen, M, Olsson, J & Dallner, G (2004) Metabolism and function of coenzyme Q. *Biochimica et Biophysica Acta (BBA) -. Biomembranes,* 1660, 171-99.
[http://dx.doi.org/10.1016/j.bbamem.2003.11.012]

Valavanidis, A, Vlahogianni, T, Dassenakis, M & Scoullos, M (2006) Molecular biomarkers of oxidative stress in aquatic organisms in relation to toxic environmental pollutants. *Ecotoxicol Environ Saf,* 64, 178-89.
[http://dx.doi.org/10.1016/j.ecoenv.2005.03.013] [PMID: 16406578]

Valko, M, Leibfritz, D, Moncol, J, Cronin, MTD, Mazur, M & Telser, J (2007) Free radicals and antioxidants in normal physiological functions and human disease. *Int J Biochem Cell Biol,* 39, 44-84.
[http://dx.doi.org/10.1016/j.biocel.2006.07.001] [PMID: 16978905]

Valko, M, Morris, H & Cronin, MT (2005) Metals, toxicity and oxidative stress. *Curr Med Chem,* 12, 1161-208.
[http://dx.doi.org/10.2174/0929867053764635] [PMID: 15892631]

Van Laer, K, Hamilton, CJ & Messens, J (2013) Low-molecular-weight thiols in thiol-disulfide exchange. *Antioxid Redox Signal,* 18, 1642-53.
[http://dx.doi.org/10.1089/ars.2012.4964] [PMID: 23075082]

Vaziri, ND (2008) Mechanisms of lead-induced hypertension and cardiovascular disease. *Am J Physiol Heart Circ Physiol,* 295, H454-65.
[http://dx.doi.org/10.1152/ajpheart.00158.2008] [PMID: 18567711]

Wang, X & Quinn, PJ (1999) Vitamin E and its function in membranes. *Prog Lipid Res,* 38, 309-36.
[http://dx.doi.org/10.1016/S0163-7827(99)00008-9] [PMID: 10793887]

Waring, WS, Webb, DJ & Maxwell, SRJ (2001) Systemic uric acid administration increases serum antioxidant capacity in healthy volunteers. *J Cardiovasc Pharmacol,* 38, 365-71.
[http://dx.doi.org/10.1097/00005344-200109000-00005] [PMID: 11486241]

White, E, Shannon, JS & Patterson, RE (1997) Relationship between vitamin and calcium supplement use and colon cancer. *Cancer Epidemiol Biomarkers Prev,* 6, 769-74.
[PMID: 9332757]

Wood, ZA, Poole, LB & Karplus, PA (2003) Peroxiredoxin evolution and the regulation of hydrogen peroxide signaling. *Science,* 300, 650-3.
[http://dx.doi.org/10.1126/science.1080405] [PMID: 12714747]

Wooten, JB, Chouchane, S & McGrath, TE (2006) Tobacco smoke constituents affecting oxidative stress, cigarette smoke and oxidative stress.*Cigarette Smoke and Oxidative Stress* Springer-Verlag, Heidelberg, Berlin, Germany 6-15.
[http://dx.doi.org/10.1007/3-540-32232-9_2]

Wu, G, Fang, YZ, Yang, S, Lupton, JR & Turner, ND (2004) Glutathione metabolism and its implications for health. *J Nutr,* 134, 489-92.
[http://dx.doi.org/10.1093/jn/134.3.489] [PMID: 14988435]

Wu, W, Bromberg, PA & Samet, JM (2013) Zinc ions as effectors of environmental oxidative lung injury. *Free Radic Biol Med,* 65, 57-69.
[http://dx.doi.org/10.1016/j.freeradbiomed.2013.05.048] [PMID: 23747928]

Xie, X, He, Z, Chen, N, Tang, Z, Wang, Q & Cai, Y (2019) The Roles of Environmental Factors in Regulation of Oxidative Stress in Plant. *BioMed Res Int,* 20199732325
[http://dx.doi.org/10.1155/2019/9732325] [PMID: 31205950]

Youdim, KA, Shukitt-Hale, B, MacKinnon, S, Kalt, W & Joseph, JA (2000) Polyphenolics enhance red blood

cell resistance to oxidative stress: *in vitro* and *in vivo*. *Biochim Biophys Acta,* 1523, 117-22.
[http://dx.doi.org/10.1016/S0304-4165(00)00109-4] [PMID: 11099865]

Zhao, JY & Hopke, PK (2012) Concentration of Reactive Oxygen Species (ROS) in Mainstream and Sidestream Cigarette Smoke. *Aerosol Sci Technol,* 46, 191-7.
[http://dx.doi.org/10.1080/02786826.2011.617795]

Zoidis, E, Seremelis, I, Kontopoulos, N & Danezis, GP (2018) Selenium-Dependent Antioxidant Enzymes: Actions and Properties of Selenoproteins. *Antioxidants,* 7E66
[http://dx.doi.org/10.3390/antiox7050066] [PMID: 29758013]

Zorov, DB, Juhaszova, M & Sollott, SJ (2014) Mitochondrial reactive oxygen species (ROS) and ROS-induced ROS release. *Physiol Rev,* 94, 909-50.
[http://dx.doi.org/10.1152/physrev.00026.2013] [PMID: 24987008]

CHAPTER 3

Role of Antioxidants in Redox Homeostasis

Priyanshi S. Desai[1] and **Maushmi S. Kumar**[1,*]

[1] *Shobhaben Pratapbhai Patel School of Pharmacy and Technological Management,SVKM's NMIMS,V. L. Mehta Road, Vile Parle (west), Mumbai- 400056, India*

Abstract: Reactive oxygen species are a result of normal oxygen metabolism, which even possess the ability to damage the cells; and thus, it becomes necessary to eliminate them. Redox homeostasis is a natural mechanism that detoxifies these ROS and involves many cellular processes in the detoxification. However, the production of ROS increases dramatically during environmental stress, which can result in the disruption of redox homeostasis. This disruption can lead to several complications that include the generation of tumour cells, ageing, diabetes and neurodegeneration. Antioxidants can prevent this disruption by reducing the propagation of free radicals and thus, they have an important role to play in the process of redox homeostasis. The chapter highlights the role of enzymatic and non-enzymatic antioxidants in redox homeostasis. Non-enzymatic antioxidants have been further divided into two categories namely, metabolic and nutritional antioxidants. The crucial role played by the antioxidants against ROS can be therefore used in therapeutics to treat the major diseases that are caused due to oxidative stress.

Keywords: Ascorbic Acid, Coenzyme Q10, Ebelsen, Haptoglobin, Lutein, MUA2, Quercetin, Rutin, SOD/CAT-Mimetic Drugs, TLK-199, Tocopherol.

INTRODUCTION

Reactive oxygen species (ROS) are free oxygen radicals that are produced as a result of aerobic metabolism in humans as well as in plants by the cell organelles. ROS, when present in normal amounts, can prove to be helpful in many physiological functions. ROS are important for the excitation-contraction coupling of skeletal muscles as it has been found that antioxidants mediated depletion of ROS lead to a decrease in contractile function (Reid *et al.* 1993).

ROS also act as initiators for apoptosis and it has been observed that an increase in ROS level is one of the starting events in apoptosis (Banki *et al.* 1999). Studies

* **Corresponding author Maushmi S. Kumar:** Shobhaben Pratapbhai Patel School of Pharmacy and Technological Management, SVKM's NMIMS, V. L. Mehta Road, Vile Parle (west), Mumbai- 400056, India;
E-mail: maushmiskumar@gmail.com

Pardeep Kaur, Rajendra G. Mehta, Robin, Tarunpreet Singh Thind and Saroj Arora (Eds.)

show that hydrogen peroxide (H_2O_2) acts as a signalling molecule between the sensor and transcriptional activators, indicating an increase in oxygen levels. NADPH-like oxidase acts as a sensor and the modification in the levels of erythropoietin (Epo) indicates the transcriptional activation (Fandrey *et al.* 1994). H_2O_2 increases the production of inflammatory mediators like interleukin-2, interleukin-2R and transcription factor NF-κB, which shows that ROS plays an important part in T-cell activation and it amplifies the immune response (Los *et al.* 1995). It has also been proved that ROS increases the adherence of leukocytes to endothelial cells by 2-2.5 folds compared to that of control (Sellak *et al.* 1994). Lipid peroxidation is thought to be undesirable, however, the non-enzymatic products generated through this process have been found to be useful. For instance, 15-F_{2t}-isoprostanes obtained from the lipid peroxidation of arachidonic acid assist as the biomarkers and mediators for oxidative injury in many diseases such as ischemia-reperfusion injury, cancer and genetic disorders (Milne *et al.* 2015). Along with these, ROS also plays an important role in stem cell differentiation and regulation of aging.

In spite of the useful nature of ROS at physiological levels, it can cause serious repercussions when its level exceeds the control of defence mechanisms (oxidative stress). In order to maintain the physiological levels of ROS, there is an inbuilt mechanism, which is called redox homeostasis. Redox homeostasis involves several responses, which include signalling, adaption, detoxification and apoptosis. The intensity of the response increases with an increase in the levels of ROS (Ayer *et al.* 2014). However, oxidative stress can be induced in response to environmental chemicals or during the biotransformation of certain drugs (Jezek and Hlavata 2005). The failure of defence mechanisms in oxidative stress results in the disruption of redox homeostasis. This disruption can cause inflammatory and cardiac pathologies as well as other disorders like cancer, diabetes, HIV infection, asthma, obstructive sleep apnoea and cataract (Roy *et al.* 2017). It is proven that the amount of ROS is higher in patients suffering from osteoarthritis than that in healthy individuals. This increase may be due to the increase in lipid peroxidation (Maneesh *et al.* 2005). When there is excess ROS production within the mitochondria of cardiac cells, DNA damage occurs and this results in cell injuries. These cell injuries can serve as one of the causes for major cardiac disorders like arrhythmia, atherosclerosis, hypertension, congestive heart failure and cardiac hypertrophy (Kukreja and Hess 1992). In CNS related disorders like Parkinson's and Alzheimer's disease, moderate levels of ROS have been observed too (Roy *et al.* 2017).

Antioxidants are substances that inhibit oxidation and contribute to limit the damage caused due to ROS. Antioxidants can be endogenous as well as exogenous. Endogenous antioxidants include enzymatic and metabolic ones, whereas exogenous antioxidants are obtained from our diet. Antioxidants are useful therapeutically for diseases in which increased ROS levels are observed. In the following chapter, we bring out the role of antioxidants in redox homeostasis with a therapeutic perspective. This chapter covers enzymatic as well as non-enzymatic antioxidants. The various antioxidants detailed in this chapter are superoxide dismutase (SOD), glutathione peroxidase (GPx), catalase (CAT), glutathione reductase (GR), glutathione-S-transferase (GST), urate, bilirubin, coenzyme Q10, transferrin, haptoglobin, ceruloplasmin, albumin, tocopherol, ascorbic acid, flavonoids, carotenoids, selenium and zinc.

ANTIOXIDANTS - SCAVENGERS OF ROS

Enzymatic Antioxidants

Enzymatic antioxidants (Fig. **1**) are the endogenous antioxidants, which at low concentrations inhibit the oxidation and thus neutralize the harmful effects of free radicals generated in our body due to oxidation (Jeeva *et al.* 2015). The enzymatic antioxidants present in our body include SOD, GPx, catalase, glutathione reductase and glutathione-S-transferase. The different classes, location, structure and mechanism of each enzymatic antioxidant are compiled in Table **1**.

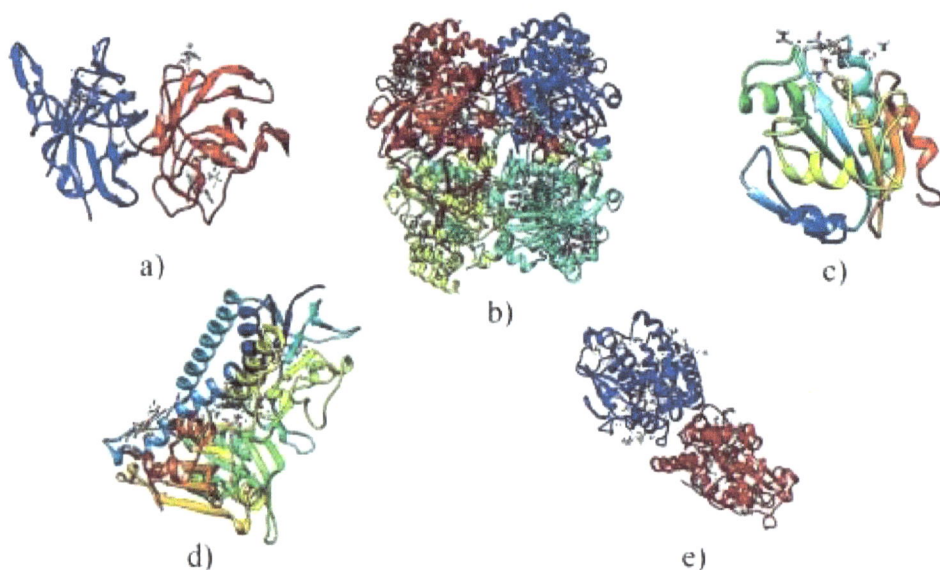

Fig. (1). Enzymatic Antioxidants; a) Superoxide Dismutase (Forest *et al.* 2000); b) Catalase (Foroughi *et al.* 2011); c) Glutathione Peroxidase (Borchert *et al.* 2018); d) Glutathione Reductase (Savvides and Karplus 1996); e) Glutathione-S-Transferase (Meux *et al.* 2011)

Table 1. Enzymatic antioxidants and their mechanism of action.

Enzymatic Antioxidant	Classes	Location	Structure	Mechanism	Reference
Superoxide Dismutase (SOD)	1.Cu/Zn-SOD (SOD1) 2.MnSOD/FeSOD (SOD2) 3. EC-SOD	The 3 classes of SOD are located at different sites. CuSOD- Cytoplasm Fe/MnSOD - Mitochondria EC SOD - Extracellular	The structure of SOD varies according to its type because the folding of the proteins is unique for each type of SOD.	Dismutation of oxygen molecule to hydrogen peroxide is catalysed by SOD. By sequential oxidation and reduction of the transition metal, SOD destroys the free oxygen radicals. $$O_2^- + O_2^- + 2H^+ \xrightarrow{SOD} H_2O_2 + O_2$$	Perry *et al.* 2010, Krishnamurthy and Wadhwani 2012
Catalase (CAT)	1.Monofunctional catalase 2.Catalase peroxidase 3.Pseudocatalase	Predominantly found in the liver in case of mammals and in the cell, it is specifically present in peroxisomes and in cytosol and mitochondria of erythrocytes.	Tetrameric and contains one ferriprotoporphyrin per subunit. The subunits are tetrahedrally arranged	It is a two-step reaction where, initially the heme is oxidised by H_2O_2 to an oxyferryl molecule followed by the generation of porphyrin cation radical. The second H_2O_2 molecule regenerates the enzyme along with production of water and oxygen by acting as a reducing agent. $$2H_2O_2 \xrightarrow{CAT} 2H_2O + O_2$$ $$ROOH + AH_2 \longrightarrow H_2O + ROH + A$$	Krishnamurthy and Wadhwani 2012, Liu and Kokare 2017, Ilyukha 2001
Glutathione peroxidase (GPx)	There are 8 types of GPx namely GPx1, GPx2, GPx3, GPx4, GPx5, GPx6, GPx7 and GPx8.	GPx1- erythrocytes, kidney and liver GPx2- intestines GPx3 - extracellular in kidney GPx4- renal epithelial cells GPx5 - epididymis of the male reproductive system	It consists of four identical subunits, each subunit containing a selenocysteine residue.	Selenium present in each subunit of GPx, reacts with peroxide to give selenic acid. This is followed by the formation of glutathiolated selenol (Se-SG) which is a result of reduction of selenic acid by GSH. After this Se-SG is reduced by another molecule of GSH to restore the active site along with formation of oxidised glutathione. These activities, hence, lead to the detoxification of non-radical H_2O_2. $$ROOH + 2GSH \longrightarrow ROH + GSSG + H_2O$$	Krishnamurthy and Wadhwani 2012, Lubos *et al.* 2011
Glutathione reductase (GR)	-		It is a homodimer and each monomer consist of 3 domains. The domains are NADPH-binding, FAD-binding and dimerization domain	GR catalyses the reduction of glutathione disulphide to glutathione. FAD is reduced to FADH⁻ by NADPH that binds to the oxidised enzyme. The FAD⁻ then helps in reducing the Cys_{58}-Cys_{63} disulphide. This reduced disulphide then binds to the reduced enzyme, which leads to the formation of mixed disulphide and a release of reduced glutathione.	Masella *et al.* 2005, Berkholz *et al.* 2008
Glutathione-S-Transferase	1.Cytosolic 2.Mitochondrial 3.MAPEG (Membrane associated proteins in eicosanoid and glutathione metabolism)	They are majorly present in the cytosol. The binding site for GST is located in the thioredoxin like domain of cytosolic and mitochondrial GSTs.	GST are proteins having N and C terminals. N terminal consists of a mixed helix and beta strand domain. Cytosolic GSTs are dimers and each monomer has a size of about 25kDa.	GST brings the substrate and GSH together, wherein the sulfhydryl group of GSH is activated. This process thus, leads to the nucleophilic attack of GSH on the substrate. As a result of this reaction, the substrate is converted to a less reactive and a more water-soluble product. This facilitates easy elimination of the substrate. $$GSH + RX \xrightarrow{GST} GSR + HX$$	Sheehan *et al.* 2001, Oakley 2011, Eaton and Bammler 1999

Superoxide Dismutase

The therapeutic potential of SOD is explored extensively and it has been found that despite the clinical limitations, SOD can be potentially useful in cancer, ischemia, inflammatory disorders, aging, neurodegenerative disorders and diabetes (Younus 2018). ATN-224, an inhibitor of SOD1 shows remarkable anticancer activity in the case of lung cancer. SOD1 inhibition leads to the death of cancer cells because of the destruction of ROS. Due to the specificity of this inhibitory action, the damage to the normal cells is minimal. Therefore, ATN-224 can be potentially used in lung cancer in combination or as a single agent (Glasauer *et al.* 2014). Analogues of ATN-224 can also be formulated to improve the properties. A study shows that lung injury induced by inhaled nitric oxide and hyperoxia can be reduced by using recombinant human SOD. The lung tissue was kept as a marker for inflammation and SOD act by varying the inflammation as well as oxygen damage (Robbins *et al.* 1997). Transgenic mice became resistant to reperfusion injury when the Cu-SOD was increased by 3-folds. So, exogenously giving supplements of antioxidants increased the cerebral blood flow and thus, improved the conditions of ischemic animals (Yang *et al.* 1994). The role of extracellular-SODs (EC-SODs) has also been studied in aging. EC-SOD has been found to be useful against aging. EC-SOD mimetic drugs have been developed which reduce aging induced cognitive dysfunction. EC-SOD acts by regulating oxidative stress and intercellular signalling. It also reduces the availability of extracellular superoxide (Levin 2005). Patients suffering from rheumatoid arthritis showed high oxidative stress and low antioxidant levels. This could be due to the efforts for reducing lipid peroxidation and hence reducing tissue damage (Karatas *et al.* 2003). Since the levels of antioxidants are low, the administration of SOD could prove to be helpful. Studies show that experimentally induced arthritis can be treated by liposomal administration of SOD (Ugur *et al.* 2004). Alzheimer's disease (AD) has been associated with increased oxidative stress. Studies show that SOD and S-Adenosylmethionine (SAM) supplementation show a synergistic effect. Patients having dementia showed oxidative damage. High levels of homocysteine (Hcy) were induced in transgenic CRND8 mice by giving them a vitamin B deficient diet, followed by SAM and SOD supplements administration. It was observed that SAM did not show any significant effect on the increased Hcy levels. In contrast, SOD exhibited a corrective effect in vitamin B deficiency and contributed to the reduction of Hcy levels. Thiol levels which increased in AD were reduced in the case of SOD supplementation (Persichilli *et al.* 2015). In a study conducted on streptozotocin (STZ) induced diabetic rats, modified SOD proved to be successful in reducing the effects of diabetes. SOD was modified with two polymers to make carboxymethylcellulose-SOD (CMC-SOD) and poly(methyl vinyl ether-co-maleic anhydride)-SOD   (PMVE/MA-SOD).   PMVE/MA-SOD   reduced   the malondialdehyde (MA) levels compared to the control and CMC-SOD as well as PMVE/MA-SOD increased the activity of glutathione and SOD enzymes. It was observed during histopathological examinations that the SOD polymers had a protective effect on the degenerative changes (Mansuroğlu *et al.* 2015).

Due to the numerous applications of SOD, drugs called SOD mimetics have been developed. Manganese pyridoxyl ethyl diamine (Mn-PLED) derivatives have been developed which show effective results in preclinical trials against cancer, acute myocardial infarction and paracetamol intoxication. These derivatives are small and lipophilic due to which intracellular penetration improves. The penetration of these drugs then lead to the dismutation of free radicals and this target omits the underlying causes for many disorders (Karlsson *et al.* 2015). However, clinical limitations still exist which mainly include instability, high immunogenicity, low cellular uptake as well as low half-life. These limitations can be overcome by developing SOD-mimetic drugs, which are formulated as high loaded or long circulating liposomes (Younus 2018).

Catalase

Catalase (CAT) is an enzymatic antioxidant found in almost all aerobic organisms. It is one such enzyme that has industrial as well as therapeutic application. Different neurological and metabolic disorders caused due to catalase deficiency include Alzheimer's disease, Parkinson's disease, bipolar diseases, schizophrenia, diabetes, hypertension and osteoporosis. Other serious catalase-related diseases comprise of acatalasemia, vitiligo, anaemia, cancer, asthma and Wilson disease (Nandi *et al.* 2019). Due to the wide applications, SOD/catalase mimetic drugs like EUK-8 and EUK-134 have been developed. These are salen-manganese complexes and have been found to possess potential therapeutic uses. EUK-8 was administered in lipopolysaccharide (LPS) induced lung injury and it was observed that high doses of EUK-8 reduced the effects of lung injury. LPS increased malondialdehyde which get treated in EUK-8 treated groups (Gonzalez *et al.* 1995). Further, it was also observed that EUK-8 administration resulted in protection of pressure-overload induced heart failure in harlequin mice. This, therefore, throws light upon its potential use in human heart failure (van Empel *et al.* 2006). EUK-134 was administered in a rat ischemic brain injury model and exhibited higher catalase and cytoprotective activity compared to EUK-8, which was protective but less effective (Baker *et al.* 1998). In one of the studies, EUK-134 was used in rats for pneumo toxicity of lungs and the broncho alveolar lavage (BAL) fluid was examined. As a result, EUK-134 increased the activity of lactate dehydrogenase (LDH) and alkaline phosphatase (ALP) in the BAL fluid. Increased SOD activity was also observed upon the examination of lung homogenates (Shopova *et al.* 2009). Pulmonary hypertension (PH) was induced by monocrotaline in male wistar rats. PH results in decline in tetanic contraction force in diaphragm and also leads to hyper nitration and aggregation of actin. These effects due to PH were prevented when EUK-134 was administered (Himori *et al.* 2017).

However, clinical limitations related to the catalase administration exist. These clinical limitations are mainly associated with the delivery of the catalase in adequate amounts to the accurate site (Nandi *et al.* 2019). To overcome this limitation, the drug can be delivered using nanoparticles. Poly (lactic co-glycolic acid) (PLGA) has been used as a polymer to carry the drug. Catalase loaded-PLGA nanoparticles can deliver antioxidant therapy to neurons and this PLGA encapsulation provides sustainable release. The administration of these particles leads to neuroprotection and neuronal recovery. Additionally, it was observed that nano-catalase protected human neurons from H_2O_2 induced cellular injury, DNA damage and loss of neuronal cytoskeleton structure and plasma membrane integrity (Singhal *et al.* 2013). Hence, this nanotechnology approach to deliver catalase can serve in the treatment of various brain pathological processes.

Glutathione Peroxidase

Glutathione peroxidase (GPx), similar to SOD and CAT, is related to many serious disorders like cancer and aging. GPx mimetic drugs like ebselen, diselenide and peptide compounds have been developed (Day 2009). Ebselen, which is also known as PZ-51, has been studied by many researchers. In a study, ebselen was administered to rats on a Se-deficient diet and it was observed that ebselen was able to replace GPx to a great extent (Muller *et al.* 1984). Ebselen has also been found to decrease the levels of leukotriene B_4 (LB$_4$) and 5-hydroxyeicosatetraenoic acid (5-HETE) which in turn reduces the formation of H_2O_2 (Safayhi *et al.* 1985). It also interacts with components like protein kinase C (PKc) and NADPH oxidase to inhibit the oxidative burst in human granulocytes and also plays a role in protecting the uptake of oxygen by cells. However, these actions are shown by ebselen at high doses and at low doses it does not interact with PKc and 5-HETE (Cotgreave *et al.* 1989). GPx mimics like BXT-51072 have exhibited potential therapeutic value to pathologies of TNF-α and interleukin-1 (Moutet *et al.* 1998). Another GPx mimetic, ovothiol, has also been identified but it has lesser GPx activity than that exerted by ebselen (Bailly *et al.* 2000). However, GPx mimetic drugs are not as efficient and therapeutically active as SOD/CAT mimetics.

Glutathione Reductase

Glutathione reductase (GR) seems to be an important potential target for the treatment of malaria. Low cytosolic levels of GR provide protection against malarial parasites without having significant effect on the function of erythrocytes. However, in order to exploit this potential target successfully, the drugs need to be specific towards the *Plasmodium falciparum*'s GR (PfGR). Studying the differences between GR and PfGR will help to a great extent in achieving this target. The other advantage of targeting GR that has been pointed out is the prevention of resistance. In the long term, PfGR inactivators might also become important (Sarma *et al.* 2003).

Glutathione-S-Transferase

Like other enzymatic antioxidants, glutathione-S-transferase (GST) is also being investigated for its therapeutic potential. GST targeting drugs are of mainly two types namely GST inhibitors and GST activated prodrugs. It has been observed that the resistance to anticancer drugs is associated with increased cytosolic GST levels. In a study conducted using indomethacin as an inhibitor of GST, the results indicated an increase in the activity of chlorambucil (Hall *et al.* 1989). Ethacrynic acid (EA) is one of the inhibitors of GST, which again resulted in an increase in cytotoxic activity of chlorambucil and melphalan (Clapper *et al.* 1990). However, EA was found to have certain limitations due to its diuretic properties and the lack of isoenzyme specificity (Townsend and Tew 2003). Hence, in order to get a better inhibitor with a greater isoenzyme specificity TLK-199 was developed which inhibit GST P1-1 expression. TLK 199 gets converted into the active form which is TLK 117 with the help of esterase. This TLK-117 was found to enhance the activity of melphalan in xenografts (Morgan *et al.* 1996). TLK-199 also inhibits the multidrug resistant protein-1 (MRP-1). A study show that accumulation of daunorubicin in MRP-1 transfected NIH3T3 was reversed and its intracellular concentrations were maintained due to TLK-199. It is also revealed through the cytotoxic assays that the resistance of MRP-1 transfected NIH3T3 cells towards drugs like vincristine, doxorubicin, mitoxantrone and etoposide was reversed by TLK-199 (O'Brien *et al.* 1999). Another study was conducted to test TLK-199 for the treatment of myelodysplastic syndrome. The results of this study indicated that TLK-199 tablets were safe, tolerable and also showed hematologic improvement in myelodysplastic syndrome (MDS) patients, which points towards the further development of this drug (Raza *et al.* 2009). GST is also being targeted for diseases not related to cancer. Vaccines like Sm28GST and Sh28GST have been developed to prevent schistosomiasis. Sh28GST was found to block the transmission of the disease and was well tolerated in phase I and phase II clinical trials (Townsend and Tew 2003).

Non-Enzymatic Antioxidants

Metabolic Antioxidants

Metabolic antioxidants are produced as metabolites in the biochemical reactions of the body. The metabolic antioxidants include urate, bilirubin, coenzyme Q10, ceruloplasmin, transferrin, albumin and haptoglobin.

Uric Acid

Uric acid is the final product of purine metabolism and is majorly produced in the liver. Uric acid reduces the free radicals and neutralises them to molecular products. During this process of reduction and neutralization it gets converted to allantoin (Sautin and Johnson 2008). Due to the ability of uric acid to form a complex with iron, the ascorbic acid oxidation is inhibited which is usually catalysed by Fe^{3+} (Davies *et al.* 1986). Uric acid also inhibits the lipid peroxidation that is initiated by singlet oxygen (Ames *et al.* 1981).

A study was conducted for treating ischemic stroke with a dual therapy of uric acid and recombinant tissue plasminogen activator (rt-PA). It was observed that lipid peroxidation reduced in patients those who were given a high dose of uric acid and no adverse effects were observed when uric acid was administered with rt-PA (Amaro *et al.* 2007). 1,7-Dimethyluric acid (mUA2) and 6,8-dithiouric acid (sUA2) were identified as the two analogues of uric acid, which when administered in mice intravenously resulted in decreased brain damage. It was also observed that the damage to the cerebral cortex was also reduced (Haberman *et al.* 2007). A study shows that levels of uric acid go down in patients suffering from myasthenia gravis. So, in such cases, the administration of uric acid analogues or their precursors can prove to be useful (Fuhua *et al.* 2012).

Bilirubin

Bilirubin is produced by the degradation of heme carried out by heme oxygenase (HO). It gets converted to biliverdin on reaction with free radicals. Due to the solubility of bilirubin in lipids, it lowers the lipid peroxidation. This is followed by the neutralization and detoxification of soluble oxidants with the help of glutathione. Hence, bilirubin and glutathione act as complementary antioxidants (Otero Regino *et al.* 2009). Due to the antioxidant property of bilirubin, it is being targeted for many diseases that involve ROS to some extent. It has been observed that the levels of bilirubin reduce during multiple sclerosis. This decrease in the levels of bilirubin is hypothesized to be due to the higher rates of ROS generation. Hence, administration of bilirubin supplements can be considered as one of the treatment options for multiple sclerosis (Peng *et al.* 2011). Bilirubin is also found to be associated with diabetes. The results from some studies show the low levels of diabetes markers such as fasting blood glucose and HbA1c in the Gunn rats with hyperbilirubinemia, as compared to the normal rats (Vítek 2012). The responsiveness of bilirubin towards ROS has been exploited for the development of bilirubin nanoparticles (BRNPs). These nanoparticles can rapidly release drugs in response to ROS. However, this is not only useful as a drug delivery method but the anticancer properties of bilirubin also makes it a potential therapeutic agent for cancer (Lee *et al.* 2016).

Coenzyme Q10

CoQ_{10} is produced as a final product in the mevalonate cycle in the mitochondria. CoQ_{10} is the only endogenously synthesized liposoluble antioxidant. Due to the redox properties of CoQ_{10}, it can neutralize the free radicals and by sequestering these free radicals, it can inhibit lipid peroxidation (Casagrande *et al.* 2018). CoQ_{10} protects the mitochondria from oxidative damage. When the cells were exposed to UVB-irradiation it led to the death of astrocytes due to accumulation of ROS. However, CoQ_{10} was able to stabilize the mitochondrial membrane, reduce the ROS accumulation and contributed in improving the respiration of mitochondria (Jing *et al.* 2015). CoQ_{10} has also been investigated for its anti-cancer properties. Studies show that CoQ_{10} can inhibit the inflammatory cascade that is activated by the ROS due to its antioxidant property. A clinical study shows that CoQ_{10} is well tolerated in patients with hepatocellular carcinoma after surgery. CoQ_{10} acts by increasing the antioxidant capacity and reducing the markers of inflammation (Liu *et al.* 2015). CoQ_{10} can prove to be a potential therapeutic target for retinal degeneration, which majorly involves oxidative stress in its process (Zhang *et al.* 2017).

Ceruloplasmin

Ferrous (Fe^{2+}) ion is very harmful as it produces free radicals. Ceruloplasmin acts as an antioxidant by converting Fe^{2+} to Fe^{3+}, thus inhibiting the generation of free radicals. Ceruloplasmin also helps in catalysing the destruction of free oxygen radicals (Wiggins *et al.* 2006). The antioxidant property of ceruloplasmin makes it a potential target for neurodegenerative diseases like Parkinson and Alzheimer's disease. Parkinson disease exhibits a decrease in the levels of ceruloplasmin, which results in the loss of the activity of substantia nigra. However, the administration of ceruloplasmin peripherally resulted in decreased nigral damage (Ayton *et al.* 2013). It has been found that Alzheimer's disease (AD) is related to oxidative stress and the levels of ceruloplasmin decrease in the hippocampus. This results in an increase in the iron concentration, which in turn leads to free radical generation and thus, causes neuronal damage. Due to the involvement of ceruloplasmin in AD, it can be targeted for developing new therapies for AD (Zhao *et al.* 2018).

Transferrin

Similar to ceruloplasmin, transferrin also exhibits its antioxidant property with the help of iron. However, it cannot convert Fe^{2+} to Fe^{3+}, but it can reduce the amount of free ferrous (Fe^{2+}) ions, which are responsible for the generation of ROS (Mirończuk-Chodakowska *et al.* 2018). It has been observed that, in diseases like diabetes, transferrin is downregulated, which further affects the lipid peroxidation, and the pro-oxidant ability of iron is enhanced due to the decreased binding with transferrin (Campenhout *et al.* 2003). Autism, another neurodegenerative disease, is associated with oxidative stress. It was found that the levels of transferrin as well as ceruloplasmin were lower in children suffering from autism compared to the non-autistic children (Chauhan *et al.* 2004). Along with ceruloplasmin, even transferrin can be a potential target in neurodegenerative diseases like Parkinson and AD.

Albumin

The antioxidant property of albumin can be attributed to its structure, which confers it the ability of trapping free radicals and binding with ligands. Free transition metals like iron and copper have the ability to give rise to ROS. However, this can be controlled when they bind to proteins like albumin, thus limiting their reactivity. This ligand binding property of albumin also results in its binding with bilirubin. This albumin-bound bilirubin accounts for the indirect antioxidant activity of albumin by inhibiting the lipid peroxidation. The free radical trapping of albumin is because it exists as a disulphide with cysteine, glutathione or homocysteine and the Cys34 residue has the ability to trap multiple ROS such as H_2O_2 and superoxide (Taverna *et al.* 2013). A study showed that the administration of albumin could increase the antioxidant capacity in patients with acute lung injury (Quinlan *et al.* 2004). However, the therapeutic potentials of albumin as an antioxidant are not as extensive as the other metabolic antioxidants.

Haptoglobin

Studies show that haptoglobin is a very potent antioxidant that strengthens cellular resistance against oxidative stress. Due to the antioxidant activity of haptoglobin, it can be useful in diseases like atherosclerosis and myocardial infarction (Tseng *et al.* 2004). It has been found that the amount of haptoglobin increases initially during myocardial infarction but later on, due to an altered glycosylation of haptoglobin and limited haemolysis, the levels of haptoglobin go down (Bernard *et al.* 1997). It has also been found that the levels of haptoglobin were higher in post-acute myocardial infarction. These high levels accounted for the severity of inflammation and reduced the chances of overall survival of patients suffering from myocardial infarction (Chiang *et al.* 2017). Similar to albumin, the therapeutic potential of haptoglobin as an antioxidant is also not as extensive as the other metabolic antioxidants.

Nutritional Antioxidants

Nutritional antioxidants are not synthesized in our body and are obtained from diet; therefore, these are also called exogenous antioxidants. The dietary source of the nutritional antioxidants has been mentioned in Table **2**.

Table 2. Major dietary sources for nutritional antioxidants (Rizvi *et al.* 2014, Barros *et al.* 2018, Pietta 2000).

Nutritional Antioxidants	Source
Tocopherol (Vitamin E)	Nuts, seeds and green leafy vegetables
Ascorbic acid (Vitamin C)	Citrus fruits (*e.g.* orange), vegetables like tomato, potato, broccoli, Brussels sprouts, red and green bell peppers
Carotenoids	Carrot, grapefruit, apricots, oranges, lettuce, spinach and green pepper
Flavonoids	Tea, citrus fruits, apples, legumes, red wine and soy products
Selenium	Brazil nuts, fish, beef, chicken and ham
Zinc	Milk products, whole grains, oysters, cereals, red meat and chickpeas

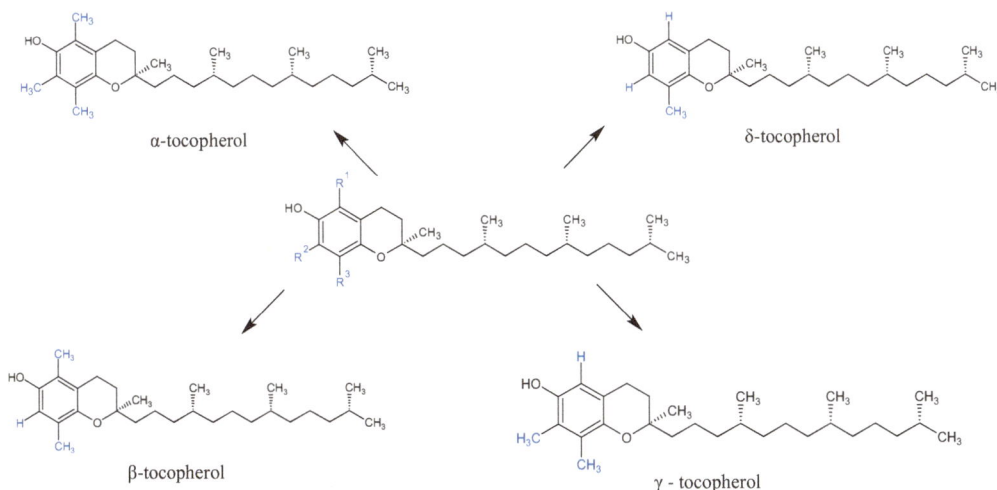

Fig. (2). Different forms of tocopherols.

Tocopherol

Tocopherol, also known as Vitamin E is obtained from nuts, seeds and green leafy vegetables. Vitamin E is usually the first line of defence in case of lipid peroxidation. It can act by four ways which includes, getting oxidized to produce tocopherol quinones, oxidizes other lipids, itself gets reduced by other antioxidants and reacts with other tocopheryl radicals to form non-reactive tocopherol dimers. Tocopherol exists in four different forms namely alpha (α), beta (β), gamma (γ) and delta (δ) (Fig. **2**).

It has been observed that formation of new radicals is inhibited by α-tocopherol whereas the existing radicals are trapped and neutralized by the γ-tocopherol (Rizvi *et al.* 2014). The therapeutic potential of vitamin E has been studied and vitamin E has turned out to be of potential use in many diseases. It has been found that vitamin E prevents atherosclerosis by reducing the oxidation of lipoproteins, which in turn reduces the risk of non-fatal myocardial infarction in patients suffering from angina or coronary atherosclerosis (Shklar and Oh 2000). γ-tocopherol traps the free radicals that can induce mutations in the DNA and cause malignant transformation in the cells, as a result of which the growth of cancer cells is inhibited (Stone *et al.* 2004). Vitamin E supplementation can also slow down the progression of cataracts, which are a result of accumulation of proteins damaged by free radicals (Rizvi *et al.* 2014). It was observed in a study that the administration of alpha-tocopherol in patients with AD slowed the disease progression (Sano *et al.* 1997). In leprosy, there is an imbalance observed between the amount of ROS produced and availability of antioxidants. The co-supplementation of vitamin E along with the ongoing multi-drug therapy provides a greater protection against oxidative stress. The benefits of using vitamin E are its ability to inhibit lipid peroxidation and membrane stabilizing property (Vijayaraghavan *et al.* 2005). A study was conducted in which 6---propylthiouracil (PTU) induced hypothyroid rats were used. The PTU-induced hypothyroidism increased the oxidative stress and to treat this, vitamin E was administered, which resulted in a decrease in oxidative stress (Hedayati *et al.* 2017).

Ascorbic Acid

Ascorbic acid (Vitamin C) (Fig. **3**) is derived from glucose, and acts as a scavenger of ROS. Vitamin C is a water-soluble molecule due to which it can act inside as well as outside the cell, resulting in the neutralization of free radicals and prevention of oxidative damage.

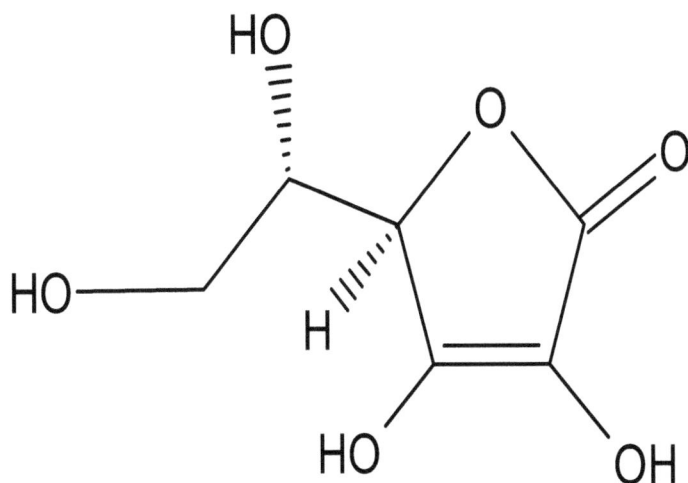

Fig. (3). Ascorbic acid (Vitamin C).

Ascorbic acid is a good electron donor and using this property ascorbate peroxidase reduces H_2O_2 to water. The antioxidant form of vitamin E can be regenerated by vitamin C through the reduction of tocopheryl radicals. In this process of neutralization of free radicals, ascorbic acid is oxidized to dehydroascorbic acid, which is further reduced to ascorbic acid for reuse or gets metabolised. Vitamin C attenuates the free radical induced lipid peroxidation and converts these free radicals into their unreactive forms (Pehlivan 2017).

It has been suggested in various studies that the diseases like hypertension and diabetes mellitus involves oxidative stress, which can be protected to some extent by intake of natural antioxidants like vitamin C and vitamin E (Maxwell 2000). Vitamin C can increase the synthesis of nitric oxide in the endothelial cells by stabilizing tetrahydropterin which is a cofactor, this in turn, facilitates the dilation of the endothelial cells (Heller *et al.* 2001). Hyperglycaemia can contribute in impaired vascular function. However, a studies show that the administration vitamin C restores the impairment of vasodilation. This can be attributed to its ability to increase the NO by removing the free radicals (Beckman *et al.* 2001). Some studies also suggest that the higher levels of vitamin C in the body can provide a protective effect against cancer due to its antioxidant properties (Byers and Guerrero 1995).

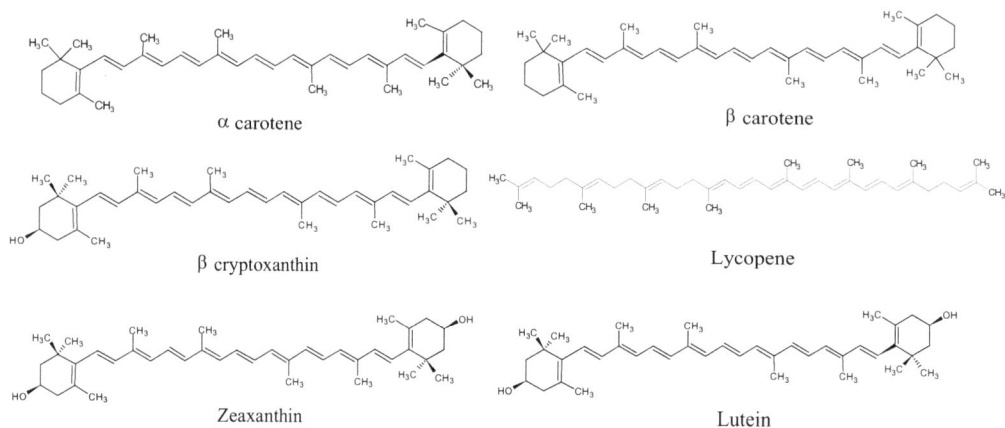

Fig. (4). Carotenoids.

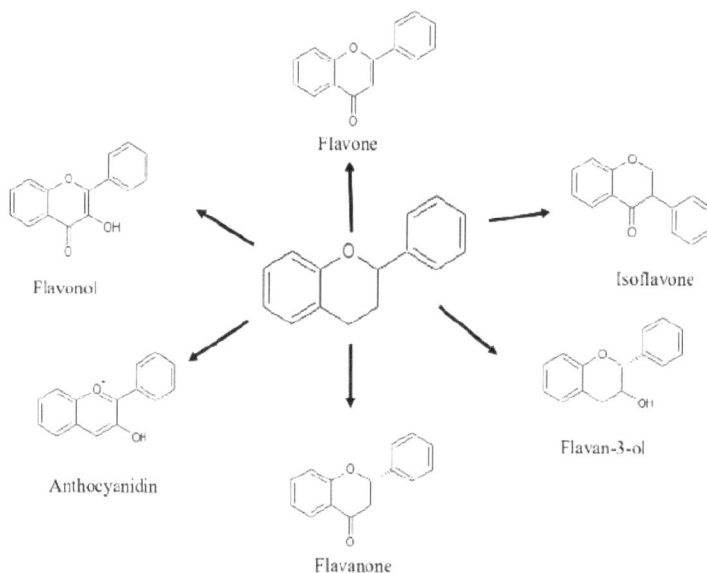

Fig. (5). Different types of flavonoids.

Carotenoids

Carotenoids (Fig. **4**) can be classified as two major classes namely, carotenes and xanthophylls. α-carotene, β-carotene, γ-carotene and β-cryptoxanthin are the four different forms of carotenoids and these can be converted into retinol. Other carotenoids include lutein, lycopene and zeaxanthin, which are not converted into retinol. Carotenoids show their antioxidant property by three mechanisms that include electron transfer, radical addition or adduct formation and allylic hydrogen abstraction (Barros *et al.* 2018).

Oxidative stress appears to be involved in liver dysfunction and it has been observed that nutritional intake of carotenoids can inhibit the development of liver dysfunction by participating in antioxidant defence systems (Sugiura 2012). Like the other antioxidants, carotenoids have also been found to be useful in neurodegenerative diseases. Carotenoids act by various mechanisms in these diseases. For instance, the administration of lycopene, in the rat model of AD resulted in a decrease in the mitochondrial dysfunction and cytokine mediators (Sachdeva and Chopra 2015).

Flavonoids

Flavonoids are formed in the plants from phenylalanine and tyrosine. Flavonoids are mainly divided into six broad classes, which include flavanols, flavanones, isoflavones, flavones, flavan-3-ols and anthocyanins (Fig. **5**). The antioxidant properties of flavonoids can be exhibited in three ways, which include chelation with iron or copper, scavenging free radicals and increasing the antioxidant defenses. In the body, the flavonoids that are ingested are initially hydrolyzed to their respective aglycone. Some flavonoids can also be converted into phenolic compounds, which possess radical scavenging properties (Pietta 2000).

Quercetin and rutin, which belong to the flavanols class, exhibited a protective effect in sickle cell anaemia which is characterised by oxidative stress. Hence, flavonoids showed a remarkable antioxidant effect against ROS that caused cellular damage in case of sickle cell anaemia (Henneberg *et al.* 2013). Other flavonoids like genistein and catechin also possess antioxidant properties. Genistein exhibits anticancer activity and analogues of genistein like B43-genistein and EGF-genistein have been developed to treat leukemia and breast cancer (Wang 2000).

Metals (Selenium and Zinc)

Selenium obtained from diet is converted into selenoproteins in the body. Vertebrates obtain Se in the form of selenomethionine and the conversion of selenium into selenoproteins requires a special mechanism for decoding the UGA codon in the mRNA (Zoidis *et al.* 2018). SeIM, SeIW and SeIR are some of the selenoproteins involved in maintaining redox homeostasis by scavenging the free radicals. Se and selenoproteins play an important role in the physiologic regulation of neurons, hence the downregulation of selenium can cause dysfunction in the brain. Various studies show that Se is important for reducing the oxidative stress in diseases like Parkinson's disease and AD. A study on humans confirmed that Se can be useful in the prevention and treatment of brain-related disorders, but it is not yet clear whether high selenium levels are safe for the body (Dominiak *et al.* 2016).

Another metal that exhibits antioxidant property is zinc. The antioxidant property of zinc is exhibited by various mechanisms some of which include the regulation of oxidant levels and oxidative damage by metals in cells, free radical scavenging action of zinc-binding metalloprotein (metallothionein) *via* release of metal in response to oxidative stress and the regulation of glutathione metabolism (Oteiza 2012). A study was conducted in which toxicity was induced in male albino rats using dimethylmercury (DMM), which caused oxidative damage. Combination of selenium, zinc and N-acetyl cysteine was administered and this resulted in the decrease in the levels of oxidative damage induced by DMM (Joshi *et al.* 2012).

CONCLUSION

Various studies discussed here draw our attention towards a very significant role played by the antioxidants in regulating the process of redox homeostasis. However, this role is not only limited to the physiological process but also extends to the therapeutic area. As described in the chapter, various studies and clinical trials have been conducted in order to exploit this therapeutic potential of the antioxidants. Enzymatic antioxidants seem to be the most useful targets in many diseases because the analogues of these antioxidants can be well tolerated. SOD/CAT-mimetic drugs emerge out to be the most successful ones as compared to the other antioxidant analogues. Among the metabolic antioxidants, uric acid and bilirubin appear to have better therapeutic potentials and can be targeted for many other diseases that shows the involvement of oxidative stress. Nutritional antioxidants also play an important role in redox homeostasis but since they are exogenous, the extent of contribution becomes limited in contrast to those present endogenously. The therapeutic potential of selenium and zinc restricts due to the possible adverse effects that can be caused by these metals. Due to the significance of antioxidants in redox homeostasis, the antioxidant therapy can be investigated in depth in order to come out with newer and more potent drugs.

CONFLICT OF INTEREST

The authors declare no conflict of interest.

ACKNOWLEDGEMENT

We thank SVKM's NMIMS for all the necessary support to carry out this work.

CONSENT FOR PUBLICATION

None

REFERENCES

Amaro, S, Soy, D, Obach, V, Cervera, A, Planas, AM & Chamorro, A (2007) A pilot study of dual treatment with recombinant tissue plasminogen activator and uric acid in acute ischemic stroke. *Stroke,* 38, 2173-5.
[http://dx.doi.org/10.1161/STROKEAHA.106.480699] [PMID: 17525395]

Ames, BN, Cathcart, R, Schwiers, E & Hochstein, P (1981) Uric acid provides an antioxidant defense in humans against oxidant- and radical-caused aging and cancer: a hypothesis. *Proc Natl Acad Sci USA,* 78, 6858-62.
[http://dx.doi.org/10.1073/pnas.78.11.6858] [PMID: 6947260]

Ayer, A, Gourlay, CW & Dawes, IW (2014) Cellular redox homeostasis, reactive oxygen species and replicative ageing in Saccharomyces cerevisiae. *FEMS Yeast Res,* 14, 60-72.
[http://dx.doi.org/10.1111/1567-1364.12114] [PMID: 24164795]

Ayton, S, Lei, P, Duce, JA, Wong, BX, Sedjahtera, A, Adlard, PA, Bush, AI & Finkelstein, DI (2013) Ceruloplasmin dysfunction and therapeutic potential for Parkinson disease. *Ann Neurol,* 73, 554-9.
[http://dx.doi.org/10.1002/ana.23817] [PMID: 23424051]

Bailly, F, Zoete, V, Vamecq, J, Catteau, JP & Bernier, JL (2000) Antioxidant actions of ovothiol-derived 4-mercaptoimidazoles: glutathione peroxidase activity and protection against peroxynitrite-induced damage. *FEBS Lett,* 486, 19-22.
[http://dx.doi.org/10.1016/S0014-5793(00)02234-1] [PMID: 11108835]

Baker, K, Marcus, CB, Huffman, K, Kruk, H, Malfroy, B & Doctrow, SR (1998) Synthetic combined superoxide dismutase/catalase mimetics are protective as a delayed treatment in a rat stroke model: a key role for reactive oxygen species in ischemic brain injury. *J Pharmacol Exp Ther,* 284, 215-21.
[PMID: 9435181]

Banki, K, Hutter, E, Gonchoroff, NJ & Perl, A (1999) Elevation of mitochondrial transmembrane potential and reactive oxygen intermediate levels are early events and occur independently from activation of caspases in Fas signaling. *J Immunol,* 162, 1466-79.
[PMID: 9973403]

Barros, MP, Rodrigo, MJ & Zacarias, L (2018) Dietary carotenoid roles in redox homeostasis and human health. *J Agric Food Chem,* 66, 5733-40.
[http://dx.doi.org/10.1021/acs.jafc.8b00866] [PMID: 29785849]

Beckman, JA, Goldfine, AB, Gordon, MB & Creager, MA (2001) Ascorbate restores endothelium-dependent vasodilation impaired by acute hyperglycemia in humans. *Circulation,* 103, 1618-23.
[http://dx.doi.org/10.1161/01.CIR.103.12.1618] [PMID: 11273987]

Berkholz, DS, Faber, HR, Savvides, SN & Karplus, PA (2008) Catalytic cycle of human glutathione reductase near 1 A resolution. *J Mol Biol,* 382, 371-84.
[http://dx.doi.org/10.1016/j.jmb.2008.06.083] [PMID: 18638483]

Bernard, DR, Langlois, MR, Delanghe, JR & De Buyzere, ML (1997) Evolution of haptoglobin concentration in serum during the early phase of acute myocardial infarction. *Eur J Clin Chem Clin Biochem,* 35, 85-8.
[http://dx.doi.org/10.1515/cclm.1997.35.2.85] [PMID: 9056748]

Borchert, A, Kalms, J, Roth, SR, Rademacher, M, Schmidt, A, Holzhutter, HG, Kuhn, H & Scheerer, P (2018) Crystal structure and functional characterization of selenocysteine-containing glutathione peroxidase 4 suggests an alternative mechanism of peroxide reduction. *Biochim Biophys Acta Mol Cell Biol Lipids,* 1863, 1095-107.
[http://dx.doi.org/10.1016/j.bbalip.2018.06.006] [PMID: 29883798]

Byers, T & Guerrero, N (1995) Epidemiologic evidence for vitamin C and vitamin E in cancer prevention.

Am J Clin Nutr, 62 (Suppl.), 1385S-92S.
[http://dx.doi.org/10.1093/ajcn/62.6.1385S] [PMID: 7495236]

van Campenhout, A, van Campenhout, CM, Lagrou, AR & Manuel-y-Keenoy, B (2003) Transferrin modifications and lipid peroxidation: implications in diabetes mellitus. *Free Radic Res,* 37, 1069-77.
[http://dx.doi.org/10.1080/10715760310001600390] [PMID: 14703796]

Casagrande, D, Waib, PH & Júnior, AAJ (2018) Mechanisms of action and effects of the administration of Coenzyme Q10 on metabolic syndrome. *J Nutr Intermed Metab,* 13, 26-32.
[http://dx.doi.org/10.1016/j.jnim.2018.08.002]

Chauhan, A, Chauhan, V, Brown, WT & Cohen, I (2004) Oxidative stress in autism: increased lipid peroxidation and reduced serum levels of ceruloplasmin and transferrin--the antioxidant proteins. *Life Sci,* 75, 2539-49.
[http://dx.doi.org/10.1016/j.lfs.2004.04.038] [PMID: 15363659]

Chiang, KH, Kao, YT, Leu, HB, Huang, PH, Huang, SS, Cheng, TM & Pan, JP (2017) Higher post-acute myocardial infarction plasma haptoglobin level is associated with poor long-term overall survival. *Int J Cardiol,* 229, 102-7.
[http://dx.doi.org/10.1016/j.ijcard.2016.11.220] [PMID: 27913007]

Clapper, ML, Hoffman, SJ & Tew, KD (1990) Sensitization of human colon tumor xenografts to L-phenylalanine mustard using ethacrynic acid. *Journal of Cellular and Molecular Pharmacology,* 1, 71-8.

Cotgreave, IA, Duddy, SK, Kass, GE, Thompson, D & Moldéus, P (1989) Studies on the anti-inflammatory activity of ebselen. Ebselen interferes with granulocyte oxidative burst by dual inhibition of NADPH oxidase and protein kinase C? *Biochem Pharmacol,* 38, 649-56.
[http://dx.doi.org/10.1016/0006-2952(89)90211-6] [PMID: 2537084]

Davies, KJA, Sevanian, A, Muakkassah-Kelly, SF & Hochstein, P (1986) Uric acid-iron ion complexes. A new aspect of the antioxidant functions of uric acid. *Biochem J,* 235, 747-54.
[http://dx.doi.org/10.1042/bj2350747] [PMID: 3753442]

Day, BJ (2009) Catalase and glutathione peroxidase mimics. *Biochem Pharmacol,* 77, 285-96.
[http://dx.doi.org/10.1016/j.bcp.2008.09.029] [PMID: 18948086]

Dominiak, A, Wilkaniec, A, Wroczyński, P & Adamczyk, A (2016) Selenium in the therapy of neurological diseases. Where is it going? *Curr Neuropharmacol,* 14, 282-99.
[http://dx.doi.org/10.2174/1570159X14666151223100011] [PMID: 26549649]

Eaton, DL & Bammler, TK (1999) Concise review of the glutathione S-transferases and their significance to toxicology. *Toxicol Sci,* 49, 156-64.
[http://dx.doi.org/10.1093/toxsci/49.2.156] [PMID: 10416260]

Fandrey, J, Frede, S & Jelkmann, W (1994) Role of hydrogen peroxide in hypoxia-induced erythropoietin production. *Biochem J,* 303, 507-10.
[http://dx.doi.org/10.1042/bj3030507] [PMID: 7980410]

Forest, KT, Langford, PR, Kroll, JS & Getzoff, ED (2000) Cu,Zn superoxide dismutase structure from a microbial pathogen establishes a class with a conserved dimer interface. *J Mol Biol,* 296, 145-53.
[http://dx.doi.org/10.1006/jmbi.1999.3448] [PMID: 10656823]

Foroughi, LM, Kang, YN & Matzger, AJ (2011) Polymer-induced heteronucleation for protein single crystal growth: structural elucidation of bovine liver catalase and concanavalin a forms. *Cryst Growth Des,* 11, 1294-8.
[http://dx.doi.org/10.1021/cg101518f]

Fuhua, P, Xuhui, D, Zhiyang, Z, Ying, J, Yu, Y, Feng, T, Jia, L, Lijia, G & Xueqiang, H (2012) Antioxidant status of bilirubin and uric acid in patients with myasthenia gravis. *Neuroimmunomodulation,* 19, 43-9.
[http://dx.doi.org/10.1159/000327727] [PMID: 22067621]

Glasauer, A, Sena, LA, Diebold, LP, Mazar, AP & Chandel, NS (2014) Targeting SOD1 reduces experimental non–small-cell lung cancer. *J Clin Invest,* 124, 117-28.

[http://dx.doi.org/10.1172/JCI71714] [PMID: 24292713]

Gonzalez, PK, Zhuang, J, Doctrow, SR, Malfroy, B, Benson, PF, Menconi, MJ & Fink, MP (1995) EUK-8, a synthetic superoxide dismutase and catalase mimetic, ameliorates acute lung injury in endotoxemic swine. *J Pharmacol Exp Ther,* 275, 798-806.
[PMID: 7473169]

Haberman, F, Tang, SC, Arumugam, TV, Hyun, DH, Yu, QS, Cutler, RG, Guo, Z, Holloway, HW, Greig, NH & Mattson, MP (2007) Soluble neuroprotective antioxidant uric acid analogs ameliorate ischemic brain injury in mice. *Neuromolecular Med,* 9, 315-23.
[http://dx.doi.org/10.1007/s12017-007-8010-1] [PMID: 17999205]

Hall, A, Robson, CN, Hickson, ID, Harris, AL, Proctor, SJ & Cattan, AR (1989) Possible role of inhibition of glutathione S-transferase in the partial reversal of chlorambucil resistance by indomethacin in a Chinese hamster ovary cell line. *Cancer Res,* 49, 6265-8.
[PMID: 2804972]

Hedayati, M, Niazmand, S, Hosseini, M, Baghcheghi, Y, Beheshti, F & Niazmand, S (2017) Vitamin E improved redox homeostasis in heart and aorta of hypothyroid rats. *Endocr Regul,* 51, 205-12.
[http://dx.doi.org/10.1515/enr-2017-0021] [PMID: 29232192]

Heller, R, Unbehaun, A, Schellenberg, B, Mayer, B, Werner-Felmayer, G & Werner, ER (2001) L-ascorbic acid potentiates endothelial nitric oxide synthesis *via* a chemical stabilization of tetrahydrobiopterin. *J Biol Chem,* 276, 40-7.
[http://dx.doi.org/10.1074/jbc.M004392200] [PMID: 11022034]

Henneberg, R, Otuki, MF, Furman, AEF, Hermann, P, do Nascimento, AJ & Leonart, MSS (2013) Protective effect of flavonoids against reactive oxygen species production in sickle cell anemia patients treated with hydroxyurea. *Rev Bras Hematol Hemoter,* 35, 52-5.
[http://dx.doi.org/10.5581/1516-8484.20130015] [PMID: 23580885]

Himori, K, Abe, M, Tatebayashi, D, Lee, J, Westerblad, H, Lanner, JT & Yamada, T (2017) Superoxide dismutase/catalase mimetic EUK-134 prevents diaphragm muscle weakness in monocrotalin-induced pulmonary hypertension. *PLoS One,* 12e0169146
[http://dx.doi.org/10.1371/journal.pone.0169146] [PMID: 28152009]

Ilyukha, VA (2001) Superoxide dismutase and catalase in the organs of mammals of different ecogenesis. *J Evol Biochem Physiol,* 37, 241-5.
[http://dx.doi.org/10.1023/A:1012663105999]

Jeeva, JS, Sunitha, J, Ananthalakshmi, R, Rajkumari, S, Ramesh, M & Krishnan, R (2015) Enzymatic antioxidants and its role in oral diseases. *J Pharm Bioallied Sci,* 7 (Suppl. 2), S331-3.
[http://dx.doi.org/10.4103/0975-7406.163438] [PMID: 26538872]

Jezek, P & Hlavatá, L (2005) Mitochondria in homeostasis of reactive oxygen species in cell, tissues, and organism. *Int J Biochem Cell Biol,* 37, 2478-503.
[http://dx.doi.org/10.1016/j.biocel.2005.05.013] [PMID: 16103002]

Jing, L, He, MT, Chang, Y, Mehta, SL, He, QP, Zhang, JZ & Li, PA (2015) Coenzyme Q10 protects astrocytes from ROS-induced damage through inhibition of mitochondria-mediated cell death pathway. *Int J Biol Sci,* 11, 59-66.
[http://dx.doi.org/10.7150/ijbs.10174] [PMID: 25552930]

Joshi, D, Mittal, DK, Shukla, S & Srivastav, AK (2012) Therapeutic potential of N-acetyl cysteine with antioxidants (Zn and Se) supplementation against dimethylmercury toxicity in male albino rats. *Exp Toxicol Pathol,* 64, 103-8.
[http://dx.doi.org/10.1016/j.etp.2010.07.001] [PMID: 20688495]

Karatas, F, Ozates, I, Canatan, H, Halifeoglu, I, Karatepe, M & Colakt, R (2003) Antioxidant status & lipid peroxidation in patients with rheumatoid arthritis. *Indian J Med Res,* 118, 178-81.
[PMID: 14700353]

Karlsson, JOG, Ignarro, LJ, Lundström, I, Jynge, P & Almén, T (2015) Calmangafodipir [Ca4Mn(DPDP)5], mangafodipir (MnDPDP) and MnPLED with special reference to their SOD mimetic and therapeutic properties. *Drug Discov Today,* 20, 411-21.
[http://dx.doi.org/10.1016/j.drudis.2014.11.008] [PMID: 25463039]

Krishnamurthy, P & Wadhwani, A (2012)

Kukreja, RC & Hess, ML (1992) The oxygen free radical system: from equations through membrane-protein interactions to cardiovascular injury and protection. *Cardiovasc Res,* 26, 641-55.
[http://dx.doi.org/10.1093/cvr/26.7.641] [PMID: 1423428]

Lee, Y, Lee, S, Lee, DY, Yu, B, Miao, W & Jon, S (2016) Multistimuli-Responsive Bilirubin Nanoparticles for Anticancer Therapy. *Angew Chem Int Ed Engl,* 55, 10676-80.
[http://dx.doi.org/10.1002/anie.201604858] [PMID: 27485478]

Levin, ED (2005) Extracellular superoxide dismutase (EC-SOD) quenches free radicals and attenuates age-related cognitive decline: opportunities for novel drug development in aging. *Curr Alzheimer Res,* 2, 191-6.
[http://dx.doi.org/10.2174/1567205053585710] [PMID: 15974918]

Liu, HT, Huang, YC, Cheng, SB, Huang, YT & Lin, PT (2016) Effects of coenzyme Q10 supplementation on antioxidant capacity and inflammation in hepatocellular carcinoma patients after surgery: a randomized, placebo-controlled trial. *Nutr J,* 15, 85.
[http://dx.doi.org/10.1186/s12937-016-0205-6] [PMID: 27716246]

Liu, X & Kokare, C (2017) *Biotechnology of Microbial Enzymes, Microbial enzymes of use in industry* Academic Press 267-98.
[http://dx.doi.org/10.1016/B978-0-12-803725-6.00011-X]

Los, M, Dröge, W, Stricker, K, Baeuerle, PA & Schulze-Osthoff, K (1995) Hydrogen peroxide as a potent activator of T lymphocyte functions. *Eur J Immunol,* 25, 159-65.
[http://dx.doi.org/10.1002/eji.1830250127] [PMID: 7843227]

Lubos, E, Loscalzo, J & Handy, DE (2011) Glutathione peroxidase-1 in health and disease: from molecular mechanisms to therapeutic opportunities. *Antioxid Redox Signal,* 15, 1957-97.
[http://dx.doi.org/10.1089/ars.2010.3586] [PMID: 21087145]

Maneesh, M, Jayalekshmi, H, Suma, T, Chatterjee, S, Chakrabarti, A & Singh, TA (2005) Evidence for oxidative stress in osteoarthritis. *Indian J Clin Biochem,* 20, 129-30.
[http://dx.doi.org/10.1007/BF02893057] [PMID: 23105509]

Mansuroğlu, B, Derman, S, Yaba, A & Kızılbey, K (2015) Protective effect of chemically modified SOD on lipid peroxidation and antioxidant status in diabetic rats. *Int J Biol Macromol,* 72, 79-87.
[http://dx.doi.org/10.1016/j.ijbiomac.2014.07.039] [PMID: 25124383]

Masella, R, Di Benedetto, R, Varì, R, Filesi, C & Giovannini, C (2005) Novel mechanisms of natural antioxidant compounds in biological systems: involvement of glutathione and glutathione-related enzymes. *J Nutr Biochem,* 16, 577-86.
[http://dx.doi.org/10.1016/j.jnutbio.2005.05.013] [PMID: 16111877]

Maxwell, SRJ (2000) Coronary artery disease--free radical damage, antioxidant protection and the role of homocysteine. *Basic Res Cardiol,* 95 (Suppl. 1), I65-71.
[http://dx.doi.org/10.1007/s003950070012] [PMID: 11192356]

Meux, E, Prosper, P, Ngadin, A, Didierjean, C, Morel, M, Dumarçay, S, Lamant, T, Jacquot, JP, Favier, F & Gelhaye, E (2011) Glutathione transferases of Phanerochaete chrysosporium: S-glutathionyl-p-hydroquinone reductase belongs to a new structural class. *J Biol Chem,* 286, 9162-73.
[http://dx.doi.org/10.1074/jbc.M110.194548] [PMID: 21177852]

Milne, GL, Dai, Q & Roberts, LJ, II (2015) The isoprostanes—25 years later. *Biochimica et Biophysica Acta (BBA)-. Molecular and Cell Biology of Lipids,* 1851, 433-45.
[http://dx.doi.org/10.1016/j.bbalip.2014.10.007]

Mirończuk-Chodakowska, I, Witkowska, AM & Zujko, ME (2018) Endogenous non-enzymatic antioxidants in the human body. *Adv Med Sci,* 63, 68-78.
[http://dx.doi.org/10.1016/j.advms.2017.05.005] [PMID: 28822266]

Morgan, AS, Ciaccio, PJ, Tew, KD, Kauvar, LM & Ciaccio, FJ (1996) Isozyme-specific glutathione S-transferase inhibitors potentiate drug sensitivity in cultured human tumor cell lines. *Cancer Chemother Pharmacol,* 37, 363-70.
[http://dx.doi.org/10.1007/s002800050398] [PMID: 8548883]

Moutet, M, d'Alessio, P, Malette, P, Devaux, V & Chaudière, J (1998) Glutathione peroxidase mimics prevent TNFalpha- and neutrophil-induced endothelial alterations. *Free Radic Biol Med,* 25, 270-81.
[http://dx.doi.org/10.1016/S0891-5849(98)00038-0] [PMID: 9680172]

Müller, A, Cadenas, E, Graf, P & Sies, H (1984) A novel biologically active seleno-organic compound--I. Glutathione peroxidase-like activity *in vitro* and antioxidant capacity of PZ 51 (Ebselen). *Biochem Pharmacol,* 33, 3235-9.
[PMID: 6487370]

Nandi, A, Yan, LJ, Jana, CK & Das, N (2019) Role of Catalase in Oxidative Stress- and Age-Associated Degenerative Diseases. *Oxid Med Cell Longev,* 20199613090
[http://dx.doi.org/10.1155/2019/9613090] [PMID: 31827713]

Oakley, A (2011) Glutathione transferases: a structural perspective. *Drug Metab Rev,* 43, 138-51.
[http://dx.doi.org/10.3109/03602532.2011.558093] [PMID: 21428697]

O'Brien, ML, Vulevic, B, Freer, S, Boyd, J, Shen, H & Tew, KD (1999) Glutathione peptidomimetic drug modulator of multidrug resistance-associated protein. *J Pharmacol Exp Ther,* 291, 1348-55.
[PMID: 10565860]

Oteiza, PI (2012) Zinc and the modulation of redox homeostasis. *Free Radic Biol Med,* 53, 1748-59.
[http://dx.doi.org/10.1016/j.freeradbiomed.2012.08.568] [PMID: 22960578]

Otero Regino, W, Velasco, H & Sandoval, H (2009) The protective role of bilirubin in human beings. *Rev Colomb Gastroenterol,* 24, 293-301.

Pehlivan, FE (2017) Vitamin C: An antioxidant agent.*Vitamin C.*IntechOpen.
[http://dx.doi.org/10.5772/intechopen.69660]

Peng, F, Deng, X, Yu, Y, Chen, X, Shen, L, Zhong, X, Qiu, W, Jiang, Y, Zhang, J & Hu, X (2011) Serum bilirubin concentrations and multiple sclerosis. *J Clin Neurosci,* 18, 1355-9.
[http://dx.doi.org/10.1016/j.jocn.2011.02.023] [PMID: 21782448]

Perry, JJP, Shin, DS, Getzoff, ED & Tainer, JA (2010) The structural biochemistry of the superoxide dismutases. *Biochimica et Biophysica Acta (BBA)-. Proteins and Proteomics,* 1804, 245-62.
[http://dx.doi.org/10.1016/j.bbapap.2009.11.004]

Persichilli, S, Gervasoni, J, Di Napoli, A, Fuso, A, Nicolia, V, Giardina, B, Scarpa, S, Desiderio, C & Cavallaro, RA (2015) Plasma thiols levels in Alzheimer's disease mice under diet-induced hyperhomocysteinemia: effect of S-adenosylmethionine and superoxide-dismutase supplementation. *J Alzheimers Dis,* 44, 1323-31.
[http://dx.doi.org/10.3233/JAD-142391] [PMID: 25672765]

Pietta, PG (2000) Flavonoids as antioxidants. *J Nat Prod,* 63, 1035-42.
[http://dx.doi.org/10.1021/np9904509] [PMID: 10924197]

Quinlan, GJ, Mumby, S, Martin, GS, Bernard, GR, Gutteridge, JM & Evans, TW (2004) Albumin influences total plasma antioxidant capacity favorably in patients with acute lung injury. *Crit Care Med,* 32, 755-9.
[http://dx.doi.org/10.1097/01.CCM.0000114574.18641.5D] [PMID: 15090958]

Raza, A, Galili, N, Smith, S, Godwin, J, Lancet, J, Melchert, M, Jones, M, Keck, JG, Meng, L, Brown, GL & List, A (2009) Phase 1 multicenter dose-escalation study of ezatiostat hydrochloride (TLK199 tablets), a novel glutathione analog prodrug, in patients with myelodysplastic syndrome. *Blood,* 113, 6533-40.

[http://dx.doi.org/10.1182/blood-2009-01-176032] [PMID: 19398716]

Reid, MB, Khawli, FA & Moody, MR (1993) Reactive oxygen in skeletal muscle. III. Contractility of unfatigued muscle. *J Appl Physiol,* 75, 1081-7.
[http://dx.doi.org/10.1152/jappl.1993.75.3.1081] [PMID: 8226515]

Rizvi, S, Raza, ST, Ahmed, F, Ahmad, A, Abbas, S & Mahdi, F (2014) The role of vitamin e in human health and some diseases. *Sultan Qaboos Univ Med J,* 14, e157-65.
[PMID: 24790736]

Robbins, CG, Horowitz, S, Merritt, TA, Kheiter, A, Tierney, J, Narula, P & Davis, JM (1997) Recombinant human superoxide dismutase reduces lung injury caused by inhaled nitric oxide and hyperoxia. *Am J Physiol,* 272, L903-7.
[PMID: 9176255]

Roy, J, Galano, JM, Durand, T, Le Guennec, JY & Lee, JCY (2017) Physiological role of reactive oxygen species as promoters of natural defenses. *FASEB J,* 31, 3729-45.
[http://dx.doi.org/10.1096/fj.201700170R] [PMID: 28592639]

Sachdeva, AK & Chopra, K (2015) Lycopene abrogates Aβ(1-42)-mediated neuroinflammatory cascade in an experimental model of Alzheimer's disease. *J Nutr Biochem,* 26, 736-44.
[http://dx.doi.org/10.1016/j.jnutbio.2015.01.012] [PMID: 25869595]

Safayhi, H, Tiegs, G & Wendel, A (1985) A novel biologically active seleno-organic compound--V. Inhibition by ebselen (PZ 51) of rat peritoneal neutrophil lipoxygenase. *Biochem Pharmacol,* 34, 2691-4.
[http://dx.doi.org/10.1016/0006-2952(85)90569-6] [PMID: 2990494]

Sano, M, Ernesto, C, Thomas, RG, Klauber, MR, Schafer, K, Grundman, M, Woodbury, P, Growdon, J, Cotman, CW, Pfeiffer, E, Schneider, LS & Thal, LJ (1997) A controlled trial of selegiline, alpha-tocopherol, or both as treatment for Alzheimer's disease. The Alzheimer's Disease Cooperative Study. *N Engl J Med,* 336, 1216-22.
[http://dx.doi.org/10.1056/NEJM199704243361704] [PMID: 9110909]

Sarma, GN, Savvides, SN, Becker, K, Schirmer, M, Schirmer, RH & Karplus, PA (2003) Glutathione reductase of the malarial parasite Plasmodium falciparum: crystal structure and inhibitor development. *J Mol Biol,* 328, 893-907.
[http://dx.doi.org/10.1016/S0022-2836(03)00347-4] [PMID: 12729762]

Sautin, YY & Johnson, RJ (2008) Uric acid: the oxidant-antioxidant paradox. *Nucleosides Nucleotides Nucleic Acids,* 27, 608-19.
[http://dx.doi.org/10.1080/15257770802138558] [PMID: 18600514]

Savvides, SN & Karplus, PA (1996) Kinetics and crystallographic analysis of human glutathione reductase in complex with a xanthene inhibitor. *J Biol Chem,* 271, 8101-7.
[http://dx.doi.org/10.1074/jbc.271.14.8101] [PMID: 8626496]

Sellak, H, Franzini, E, Hakim, J & Pasquier, C (1994) Reactive oxygen species rapidly increase endothelial ICAM-1 ability to bind neutrophils without detectable upregulation. *Blood,* 83, 2669-77.
[http://dx.doi.org/10.1182/blood.V83.9.2669.2669] [PMID: 7513210]

Sheehan, D, Meade, G, Foley, VM & Dowd, CA (2001) Structure, function and evolution of glutathione transferases: implications for classification of non-mammalian members of an ancient enzyme superfamily. *Biochem J,* 360, 1-16.
[http://dx.doi.org/10.1042/bj3600001] [PMID: 11695986]

Shklar, G & Oh, SK (2000) Experimental basis for cancer prevention by vitamin E. *Cancer Invest,* 18, 214-22.
[http://dx.doi.org/10.3109/07357900009031826] [PMID: 10754990]

Shopova, VL, Dancheva, VY, Salovsky, PT & Stoyanova, AM (2009) Protective effects of a superoxide dismutase/catalase mimetic compound against paraquat pneumotoxicity in rat lung. *Respirology,* 14, 504-10.
[http://dx.doi.org/10.1111/j.1440-1843.2009.01531.x] [PMID: 19645869]

Singhal, A, Morris, VB, Labhasetwar, V & Ghorpade, A (2013) Nanoparticle-mediated catalase delivery protects human neurons from oxidative stress. *Cell Death Dis,* 4, e903-3.
[http://dx.doi.org/10.1038/cddis.2013.362] [PMID: 24201802]

Stone, WL, Krishnan, K, Campbell, SE, Qui, M, Whaley, SG & Yang, H (2004) Tocopherols and the treatment of colon cancer. *Ann N Y Acad Sci,* 1031, 223-33.
[http://dx.doi.org/10.1196/annals.1331.022] [PMID: 15753148]

Sugiura, M (2012)

Taverna, M, Marie, AL, Mira, JP & Guidet, B (2013) Specific antioxidant properties of human serum albumin. *Ann Intensive Care,* 3, 4.
[http://dx.doi.org/10.1186/2110-5820-3-4] [PMID: 23414610]

Townsend, DM & Tew, KD (2003) The role of glutathione-S-transferase in anti-cancer drug resistance. *Oncogene,* 22, 7369-75.
[http://dx.doi.org/10.1038/sj.onc.1206940] [PMID: 14576844]

Tseng, CF, Lin, CC, Huang, HY, Liu, HC & Mao, SJ (2004) Antioxidant role of human haptoglobin. *Proteomics,* 4, 2221-8.
[http://dx.doi.org/10.1002/pmic.200300787] [PMID: 15274115]

Ugur, M, Yildirim, K, Kiziltunc, A, Erdal, A, Karatay, S & Senel, K (2004) Correlation between soluble intercellular adhesion molecule 1 level and extracellular superoxide dismutase activity in rheumatoid arthritis: a possible association with disease activity. *Scand J Rheumatol,* 33, 239-43.
[http://dx.doi.org/10.1080/03009740310004054] [PMID: 15370719]

van Empel, VP, Bertrand, AT, van Oort, RJ, van der Nagel, R, Engelen, M, van Rijen, HV, Doevendans, PA, Crijns, HJ, Ackerman, SL, Sluiter, W & De Windt, LJ (2006) EUK-8, a superoxide dismutase and catalase mimetic, reduces cardiac oxidative stress and ameliorates pressure overload-induced heart failure in the harlequin mouse mutant. *J Am Coll Cardiol,* 48, 824-32.
[http://dx.doi.org/10.1016/j.jacc.2006.02.075] [PMID: 16904556]

Vijayaraghavan, R, Suribabu, CS, Sekar, B, Oommen, PK, Kavithalakshmi, SN, Madhusudhanan, N & Panneerselvam, C (2005) Protective role of vitamin E on the oxidative stress in Hansen's disease (Leprosy) patients. *Eur J Clin Nutr,* 59, 1121-8.
[http://dx.doi.org/10.1038/sj.ejcn.1602221] [PMID: 16015260]

Vítek, L (2012) The role of bilirubin in diabetes, metabolic syndrome, and cardiovascular diseases. *Front Pharmacol,* 3, 55.
[http://dx.doi.org/10.3389/fphar.2012.00055] [PMID: 22493581]

Wang, HK (2000) The therapeutic potential of flavonoids. *Expert Opin Investig Drugs,* 9, 2103-19.
[http://dx.doi.org/10.1517/13543784.9.9.2103] [PMID: 11060796]

Wiggins, JE, Goyal, M, Wharram, BL & Wiggins, RC (2006) Antioxidant ceruloplasmin is expressed by glomerular parietal epithelial cells and secreted into urine in association with glomerular aging and high-calorie diet. *J Am Soc Nephrol,* 17, 1382-7.
[http://dx.doi.org/10.1681/ASN.2005111239] [PMID: 16597684]

Yang, G, Chan, PH, Chen, J, Carlson, E, Chen, SF, Weinstein, P, Epstein, CJ & Kamii, H (1994) Human copper-zinc superoxide dismutase transgenic mice are highly resistant to reperfusion injury after focal cerebral ischemia. *Stroke,* 25, 165-70.
[http://dx.doi.org/10.1161/01.STR.25.1.165] [PMID: 8266365]

Younus, H (2018) Therapeutic potentials of superoxide dismutase. *Int J Health Sci (Qassim),* 12, 88-93.
[PMID: 29896077]

Zhang, X, Tohari, AM, Marcheggiani, F, Zhou, X, Reilly, J, Tiano, L & Shu, X (2017) Therapeutic potential of co-enzyme Q10 in retinal diseases. *Curr Med Chem,* 24, 4329-39.
[http://dx.doi.org/10.2174/0929867324666170801100516] [PMID: 28762311]

Zhao, YS, Zhang, LH, Yu, PP, Gou, YJ, Zhao, J, You, LH, Wang, ZY, Zheng, X, Yan, LJ, Yu, P & Chang, YZ (2018) Ceruloplasmin, a potential therapeutic agent for Alzheimer's disease. *Antioxid Redox Signal,* 28, 1323-37.
[http://dx.doi.org/10.1089/ars.2016.6883] [PMID: 28874056]

Zoidis, E, Seremelis, I, Kontopoulos, N & Danezis, GP (2018) Selenium-dependent antioxidant enzymes: Actions and properties of selenoproteins. *Antioxidants,* 7, 66.
[http://dx.doi.org/10.3390/antiox7050066] [PMID: 29758013]

CHAPTER 4

Antioxidants (Natural and Synthetic) Screening Assays: An Overview

Basharat Ahmad Bhat[1], **Safura Nisar**[1], **Bashir Ahmad Sheikh**[1], **Wajahat Rashid Mir**[1] and **Manzoor Ahmad Mir**[1,*]

[1] *Department of Bioresources, School of Biological Sciences, University of Kashmir, Srinagar-190006, India*

Abstract: Antioxidants are used to inhibit the deterioration of a molecule and are used at a low concentration to slow or avoid the degradation of a molecule. They have the ability to chelate transition metals and work through a variety of synthetic processes like hydrogen atom transfer (HAT) and single electron transfer (SET). Understanding the biology of antioxidants, their possible applications, and their synthesis using different biotechnological methods are important aspects of antioxidant mechanisms. Antioxidant molecules can react in one of two ways: through multiple mechanisms or through a single mechanism. Understanding the antioxidant reaction process is possible due to the molecular structure of the antioxidant material. This chapter presents an overview of various antioxidants, their reaction mechanism against free radicals as well as the most utilized techniques to assess their different activities.

Keywords: Antioxidant activity, Antioxidant screening assays, Antioxidant, Free radicals, Hydrogen atom transfer (HAT), Reactive oxygen species, Single electron transfer (SET).

INTRODUCTION

In biological systems, oxidative stress is comprised of multiple and diverse mechanisms, which is considered to be a disproportion amid the creation of the free radicals and capability of our body to remove these species by the utilization of intrinsic and extrinsic antioxidants. Free radicals are extremely reactive species or molecular compound with an odd number of electrons which are considered to be very active with other atoms or molecules in a chemical reaction. Due to their unstable nature within the cell, they can oxidize numerous biomolecules, cause tissue injury and lead to cell death. When our body uses oxygen molecule, free

---

[*] **Corresponding author Manzoor Ahmad Mir:** Department of Bioresources, School of Biological Sciences, University of Kashmir, Srinagar-190006, J&K India. E-mails: drmanzoor@kashmiruniversity.ac.in and mirmanzoor110@gmail.com

Pardeep Kaur, Rajendra G. Mehta, Robin, Tarunpreet Singh Thind and Saroj Arora (Eds.)

radicals are generated due to cell death. When our body uses oxygen molecule, free radicals are generated due to loss or gain of electrons and these reactive molecules damage the internal environment of the cell called oxidative stress. This free radical reaction depends on the existence of oxygen, nitrogen, and sulphur radicals. Superoxide ($\cdot O_2^-$), alkoxyl (RO·), hydroxyl (HO·), peroxyl (ROO·), and nitric oxide (NO·) are examples of O_2 dependent free radicals and reactive oxygen species (ROS). There are other non-radical ROS in the body, including hydrogen peroxide (H_2O_2), and singlet oxygen ($^1O_2$) and hypochlorous acid (HOCl) (Pietta 2000).

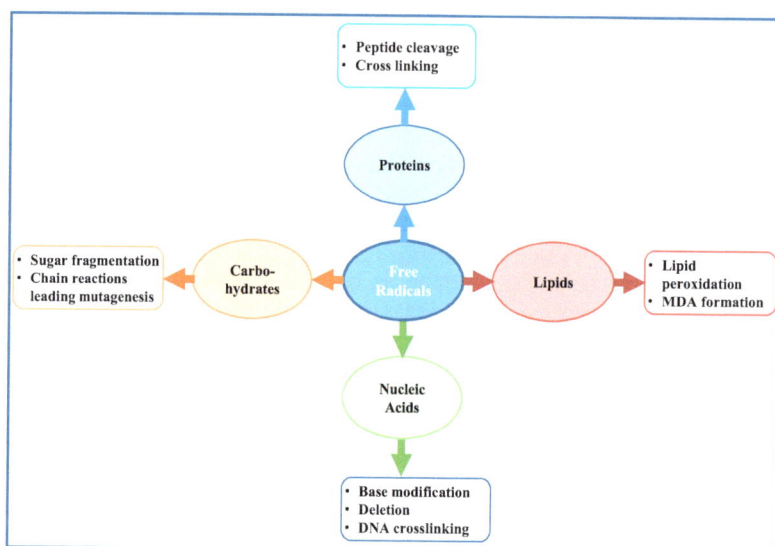

Fig. (1). Biological targets of free radicals.

ROS could be produced throughout the metabolism of biomolecules, respiration, and therefore autoxidation of the xenobiotics as a function of this cause various diseases in the living organisms (Cakmak and Gülçin 2019, Anraku *et al.* 2018). Moreover, there are more reactive nitrogen species (RNS), like, peroxynitrite (ONOO−), nitric oxide (NO•), nitrosoperoxycarbonate ($ONOOCO_2^-$), nitrogen dioxide (NO_2•), and nitronium particles (NO_2^+), dinitrogen trioxide (N_2O_3), and peroxynitrous acid (ONOOH). These reactive species are produced in lesser quantities in the cellular functions including cell flagging, neurotransmission, the unwinding of muscle, peristalsis, accumulation of platelet, pulse adjustment, blood pressure inflection, phagocytosis and cell development (Limón-Pacheco and Gonsebatt 2009). In the biological, environmental conditions, they are generally known as the pro-oxidants or antioxidant agents, and in chemical terms, they are referred to as oxidants and reductants, respectively (Cao and Prior 1998).

The pro-oxidants are agents that cause oxidative harm to the biological targets including sugars, nucleic acids, proteins, and lipids (Fig. **1**).

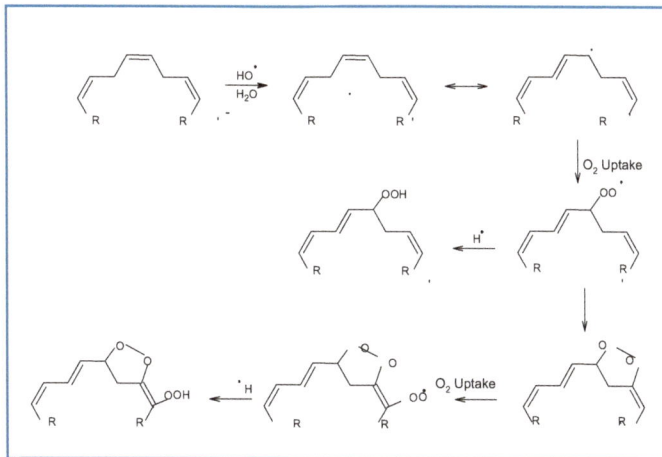

Fig. (2). The hydroxyl (OH) radical reaction with the polyunsaturated fatty acids.

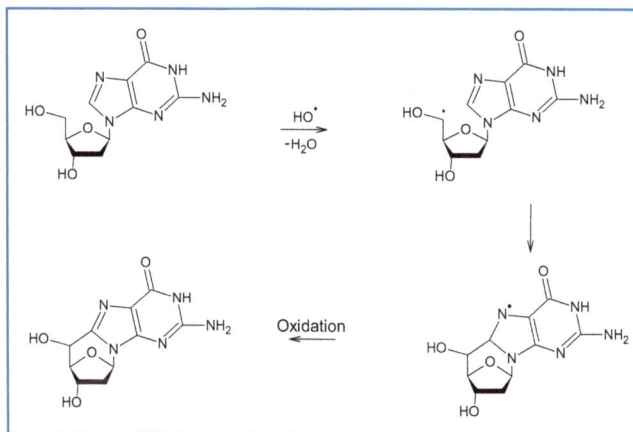

Fig. (3). The hydroxyl radical reaction with the sugar.

Free radicals create assorted activities on the metabolism, which can be the basis of cell injury (Nakamura *et al.* 1997).

1. In the polyunsaturated lipids, lipid peroxidation occurs due to ROS molecules causing cell lysis (Fig. **2**)
2. Altering cellular processes correlated with interleukin involvement and the production of prostaglandins, neurotransmitters, and hormones in the

glycosides (Fig. **3**) (Nimse and Pal 2015).

3. In the proteins, causing denaturation and inactivation (Fig. **4**) (Dean *et al.* 1997).

4. In the nucleic acids, causes carcinogenesis via altering bases (Fig. **5**) (Carocho and Ferreira 2013).

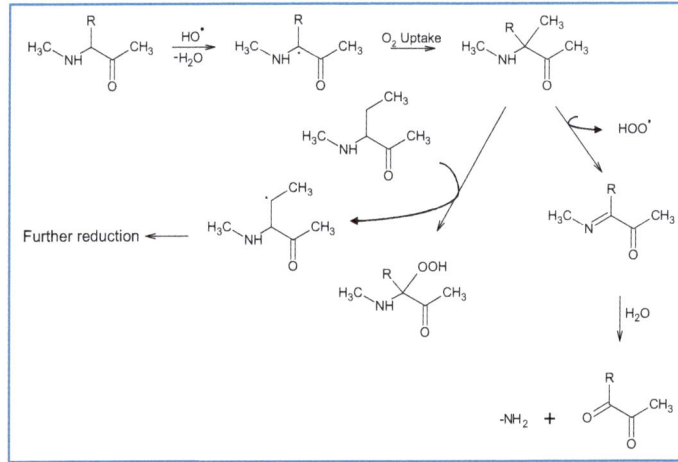

Fig. (4). The hydroxyl radical reaction with α-amino acids.

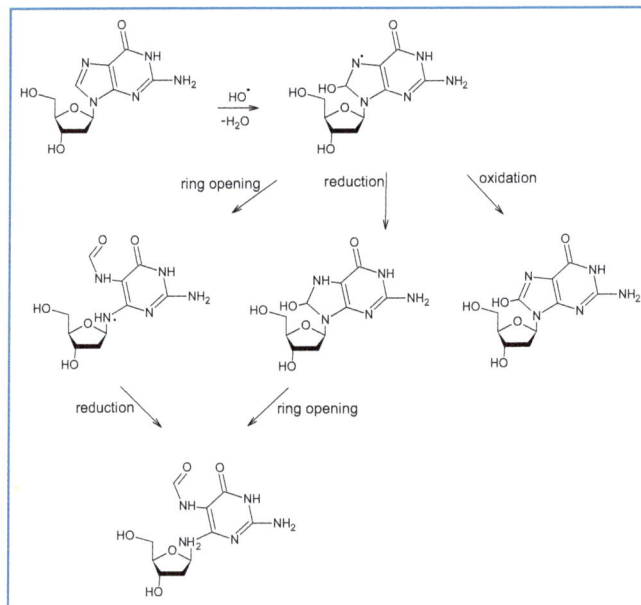

Fig. (5). The hydroxyl (OH) radical reaction with base pair of the DNA guanosine.

There are completely different reaction mechanisms in free radical molecules. They interact with the molecules around them by donating electrons, accepting electrons, oxidising radicals, and eliminating radicals (Carocho and Ferreira 2013).

a. hydrogen abstraction $OH^{\bullet} + RS^{-} \rightarrow OH^{-} + RS^{\bullet}$
b. addition reactions $CCl_3^{\bullet} + RH \rightarrow CHCl_3 + R^{\bullet}$
c. self-annihilation $CCl_3^{\bullet} + CCl_3^{\bullet} \rightarrow C_2Cl_6$
d. disproportionation $CCl_3 + CH_2 = CH_2 \rightarrow CH_2 (CCl_3) - CH_2$

ROS molecules cause injury to cells by harming DNA, proteins, RNA, and lipids and eventually disrupt cell functions (Işık *et al.* 2017, Krawczyk 2019). ROS molecules have capability of injuring important biological molecules like carbohydrates and polyunsaturated fatty acids (Tohma *et al.* 2017, Köksal *et al.* 2017). The harmful impacts of ROS molecules on mitochondria in the cell are to cause stress and eventually death (Koksal *et al.* 2011, Krawczyk 2019). Living organisms can defend themselves by scavenging ROS and manufacturing inhibitor molecules that are free radicals scavengers (Hamad *et al.* 2017, Anraku *et al.* 2018, Alam *et al.* 2013, Ekinci Akdemir *et al.* 2016). Table **1** depicts the most prominent free radicals generated during the energy production phase in aerobic biological processes.

Table 1. Free radicals and their biological function.

Species	Source	Function
$O_2^{\bullet-}$	Enzymatic reactions, nonenzymatic electron transfer reactions and autoxidation reaction	Act as a reducing agent for complexes of iron including cytochrome-c or an oxidising agent for ascorbate and α-tocopherol oxidation
$HO^{\bullet}$	H_2O_2 generates HO• via Fenton's reaction catalyzed by metal	HO• enters into intermolecular reactions within the cell membranes with both inorganic and organic molecules like proteins, DNA, lipids, and carbohydrates
$HO_2^{\bullet}$	Protonation of $O_2^{\bullet-}$	HO$_2$• causes fatty acid peroxidation
$NO^{\bullet}$	NADPH as electron source and arginine as a base for nitric oxide-synthase	NO• is a cellular secondary messenger that tends to relax smooth muscle in blood vessels by stimulating guanylate cyclase and protein kinases.
$ONOO^{\bullet}$	Reaction of O_2 with NO•	ONOO• oxidises DNA to form nitroguanine and is a potent oxidising and nitrating agent of tyrosine and methionine residue in the proteins.
$NO^{\bullet}_2$	ONOO− protonation or ONOOCO$_2$− hemolytic fragmentation	This radical inhibits the antioxidative mechanisms, lowering plasma levels of ascorbate as well as α-tocopherol.

ANTIOXIDANTS

Antioxidants play an important role in the body to decrease oxidative damage and damaging action of the ROS as well as in the food systems (Çakmakçı *et al.* 2015, Göçer *et al.* 2013). In the food industry, utilization of nutritional antioxidants molecules help to preserve the flavor, texture, and colour of the food products at the time of storage by retarding the lipid peroxidation (Bursal and Gülçin 2011, Çakmakçı *et al.* 2015). Moreover, antioxidants also help to prevent the alteration of protein function by reducing amino acids, protein degradation, and lipid-derived carbonyl interactions with proteins (Kalra 2019). Antioxidant molecules inhibit the oxidation of products that are readily oxidised, like fats. Antioxidant is characterised as any molecule present in smaller amounts in comparison to that of the oxidizable substrate that substantially slows or inhibits the oxidation of that substrate or eliminates oxidative stress to a target molecule in the context of food (Halliwell and Gutteridge 1989, Halliwell 1995, Sies 1993).

Antioxidants are added to the food items in order to avert the activation and proliferation of the oxidation mechanism and cause a reaction to come to a halt (Ahmad *et al.* 2020, Gülçin *et al.* 2006). Antioxidants have exclusive properties of prolonging the storage lifespan of the food products without affecting the other secondary nutritional qualities of the food products. The antioxidants which are utilized in food systems should be effective. They are nontoxic at small doses; they are extremely stable and can withstand processing; they have no colour, taste, and odour of their own. They're simple to use, cheap, and have a high level of product solubility (Shahidi and Ambigaipalan 2015). A number of scientific studies showed that antioxidant defences protect the body from oxidative damage. The antioxidants have beneficial health effects in various metabolic processes in stress, pathogen incursion, ageing, apoptosis, and neurological disorders. Currently, it has been shown that numerous diseases are developed with the creation of these radicals like DNA mutagenesis, transformation of cell, cancers, myocardial infarction, diabetes, arteriosclerosis, inflammatory disorders, central nervous system ailments, as well as aging (Rice-Evans and Bruckdorfer 1995, Halliwell 1996).

Antioxidants help to avoid or lower the rate of these illnesses by suppressing the development of free radicals. A wide variety against disease through offering an abundant supply of flavonoid antioxidants through fresh or dried fruits and veggies, which is rich in antioxidants, offers a broad-spectrum protection against disease (Anjana *et al.* 2020).

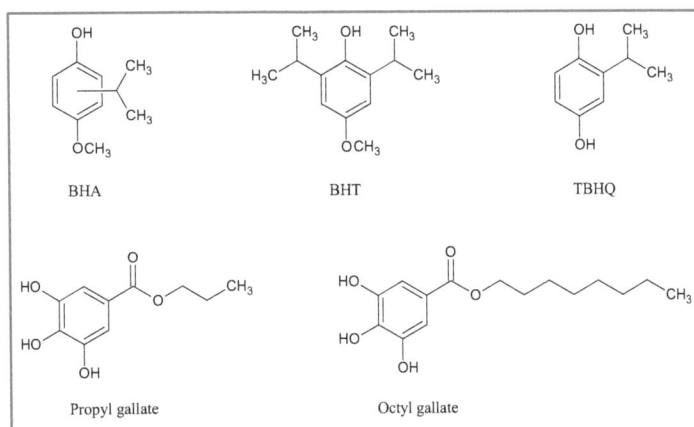

Fig. (6). The molecular structures of the most likely and well-known synthetic antioxidants.

Synthetic Antioxidants

Natural and synthetic or artificial antioxidants are commonly utilized in food and drug products being measured today using the commonly established measuring device in the food and drug industry. Food additives can be applied to different items to extend shelf life or serve other purposes, such as protecting them from various treatments and keeping them fresh. Synthetic antioxidants are incorporated in all processed food materials that have been reported to be safe, despite the fact that a few research studies indicate otherwise (Fig. **6**) (Carocho and Ferreira 2013). The most regularly utilized synthetic form of antioxidants are the phenolic molecules like butylated hydroxyanisole (BHA), dibutylhydroxytoluene (BHT) *tertiary*-butylhydroquinone (TBHQ), octyl gallate (OG), and propyl gallate (PG) (Gülcin 2012). The short-chain fatty acids oxidation is particularly controlled by BHA synthetic antioxidants. However, because of the inclusion of two *tertiary*-butyl groups, which induce a higher steric hindrance to a molecule than the BHA, BHT antioxidant is not more successful than BHA (Nanditha and Prabhasankar 2008).

TBHQ is another active synthetic antioxidant, which is used in plenty of food materials like edible fats from animals, unsaturated forms of vegetable oils, and other products from meat. TBHQ does not cause any discoloration or change the flavor or color even in the iron containing foods and it also stabilizes animal food items' freshness, nutritive benefit, colour, and taste (Kashanian and Dolatabadi 2009). TBHQ is more powerful than BHA and BHT synthetic antioxidants and it is the most potent antioxidant in beverages and herbaceous plant oil. The antioxidant function of TBHQ is because of the availability of two *para*-OH groups (Nanditha and Prabhasankar 2008, Shahidi and Ambigaipalan 2015). Another important secure synthetic antioxidant is propyl gallate, which is a useful antioxidant to shield oils, foods, and fats comprising fats from rancidification effect and formation of peroxides. It was demonstrated that the continuous use of propyl gallate can cause hepatotoxicity and enhance cancer development (Shahidi and Ambigaipalan 2015). The OG consists of octan-1-ol and the gallic acid esters and utilized as an antioxidative agent and preservative of food products. BHT and BHA, on the other hand, are widely utilized synthetic antioxidants in food processing industry as well as for pharmacological uses, and have been approved as food ingredients by a number of national authorities (Koudelka *et al.* 2015). It has been demonstrated that synthetic antioxidants can cause hepatic damage and cancers if utilized at greater levels in the laboratory animals. It's also been noted that BHA, TBHQ, and PG, among other food additives, have the capacity to shape the complexes of molecules with the structure of nucleic acids and harm DNA's double helical structural form (Dolatabadi and Kashanian 2010). The suitability of these synthetic compounds is diminished in consumers because they may be antioxidants but raise concerns about their associated protective ability, metabolism and accumulation in the cell, tissue, organ and body (Kulawik *et al.* 2013, Anraku *et al.* 2018).

Natural Antioxidants

Plant phenolics can be found in every portion of the plant, such as fruits, berries, seeds, nuts, stems, leaves, bulbs, and barks. The plants yield a large number of the secondary metabolite which includes flavonoids, important oils, some alkaloids, terpenes, lignans, terpenoids, organic acids, tocopherols, phenolics, polyfunctional organic acids, peptides, in their regular metabolic mechanisms. Plant phenolics, which may be found in all areas of plants, are the most common sources of herbal antioxidants (Shahidi and Ambigaipalan 2015). This metabolite play a key function in shielding plants against harmful consequences. The normal human diet includes a variety of molecules and compounds with antioxidative properties and scavenge the reactive oxygen species (ROS). The ascorbic acid, tocopherols, carotenoids, and flavonoids are the most common nutritional antioxidants found in the form of human diet (Sies and Stahl 1995, Rice-Evans and Miller 1994).

Phenolics

Phenolics include a wide group of the various secondary metabolites encompassing greater than 8000 compounds with a expanded range of different chemical properties and the biological processes and present at substantial quantities in human and animal diet (Martínez-Valverde *et al.* 2000). The phenolic molecules are very essential to protect vegetation from various diseases and in plant signalling pathways. They help in the regulation of plant growth and defence against various diseases. Phenolic compounds behave as donors of hydrogen or metallic ions chelator together with iron and copper, with the aid of preventing the oxidation of the low-density lipoproteins. These features of phenolic molecules help in the control and management of the neurodegenerative illnesses, such as cardiovascular ailments (Paran *et al.* 2009), gastrointestinal cancers (Yoshida *et al.* 1990), colon (Ranelletti *et al.* 1992), breast and ovarian cancers (Scambia *et al.* 1990), and leukemia (Yoshida *et al.* 1992, Teofili *et al.* 1992, Ren *et al.* 2001). Phenolics also have anti-allergenic and vasorelaxant properties, as well as the ability to suppress the oxidation of the low-density lipoproteins *in vitro* (Riemersma *et al.* 2001, Sakakibara *et al.* 2003).

Flavonoids

Flavonoids are cyclic diphenylpropane compounds present particularly in plants and foods. Flavonoids are polyphenolic compounds with powerful antioxidant activity. These chemicals are used to cure a variety of serious illnesses. About 4000 flavonoids have been found in different plant types, out of over 8000 polyphenolic compounds, and their numbers are still increasing (Baxter *et al.* 1999, Ghosh *et al.* 2015). They've been found in nearly any section of the plant, including the leaves, branches, roots, fruits, and seeds. Plants make flavonoids from aromatic form of amino acids including phenylalanine, malonate, and tyrosine (Cody *et al.* 1986). Higher plant tissues include flavonoids such as flavones, chalcones, isoflavones, flavanones, and, flavanols.

Flavonoids can provide protection against the cardiovascular disease by lowering the oxidation of the low-density lipoproteins, according to one theory. In addition, antioxidant flavonoids are one of our diet's most important components. Flavonoids are present in various kinds of foods, like fruits, nuts, and plant-based beverages, as well as tea. Consumption of flavonoids in the dietary supplements form is a few hundred milligrammes per day It has been demonstrated that flavonoids offer defense against the oxidative stress induced diseases via modulation of the enzymatic activities and interactions with the unique receptors (Williams *et al.* 2004).

Carotenoids

Carotenoids are present in the living things, including plants, animals, as well as bacteria. The vast majority of carotenoids have been detected and more than 700 have been reported (Mercadante *et al.* 2004). These compounds give pigmentation to biological systems. The most current research efforts have been designed to ascertain the potential use of these substances as an antioxidants. The molecular structure base forms of these carotenoids represent the conjugated form of polyunsaturated chain. Further, this form of carotenoid has the potential to constrain free radicals formation. There are differences in the forms of polyunsaturated chain from individual carotenoid to the next and the collective presence of OH groups extensively regulates the reactions of the carotenoids. Environmental factors have an effect on the reactivity of these substances. For example, it has been shown that as a function of oxygen concentration, carotenoids transform from antioxidant to prooxidant activity (Edge and Truscott 2018). Carotenoids are considered as exquisite scavengers of peroxyl radical and possess lipophilic character. They also play an essential part in cell membrane and lipoprotein defence in opposition to peroxyl radicals.

Ascorbic Acid (Vitamin C)

At physiological pH, vitamin C is a ketolactone with the two ionizable OH groups, and ascorbate monoanion is the major type. It has been reported as the most powerful natural antioxidant and is very effective against free radicals like O_2^-, H_2O_2, OH, $^1O_2$ as well as reactive $NO_2^{\cdot}$ (Barros *et al.* 2011). This is a water-soluble vitamin that can be present in high amounts in a variety of plants. It normally interacts with oxidants. By transferring electrons, ascorbic acid may end chain radical reactions. Vitamin C has the molecular ability to react with the majority of the physiologically important ROS molecules. The HAT towards peroxyl radicals, the inhibition of the singlet oxygen, as well as the reduction of the molecular oxygen are the antioxidant reaction pathways of the vitamin C (Sisein 2014). Moreover, it has been demonstrated that SET allows ascorbate to generate reactions with oxidising agents (Williams and Yandell 1985) or a coordinated electron/proton (SET/HAT) transfer (Marcus and Sutin 1985). *In vivo* and *in vitro*, vitamin C was used to revive α-tocopherol out from its tocopheroxyl radical form, revamping its antioxidative function (Kamal-Eldin and Budilarto 2015). Fruits, particularly citrus fruits, kiwi fruit, melons, cherries, and vegetables, like leafy greens, brussels sprouts, broccoli, tomatoes, cabbage, and cauliflower are the vital sources of ascorbate in the diet. In a recent study by Bursal and Gülçin (2011) documented roughly 1000 mg ascorbic acid per kg in the lyophilized extract of kiwifruit (*Actinidia deliciosa*). Bioavailability of vitamin C from the foods and synthetic products is almost identical at low doses (100 mg) (Mangels *et al.* 1993).

Methods to Detrmine the Antioxidant Activity

The antioxidative action of various compounds such as foods, prescription drugs, pharmaceuticals and biological samples can be determined both *in vitro* and *in vivo* by various procedures. The determination of antioxidant capability of compounds instigated from the molecular chemistry and later on it was tailored to the biology, pharmaceutics, epidemiology as well as diet (Floegel *et al.* 2011). There is an increased interest in antioxidant research studies of the foods and nutrition, owing to the recognized consequences of oxygen free radicals which cause the development of cardiovascular and neurodegenerative sickness, aging and cancers (Maltos *et al.* 2010). Many alternative procedures are established to assess the overall antioxidant potential of food products (Pérez-Jiménez and Saura-Calixto 2005). A reliable and consistent methodology is needed to estimate the antioxidant effect of food elements (Prior *et al.* 2005, Magalhães *et al.* 2008). Moreover, antioxidant action cannot be determined only on the basis of a single antioxidative testing model. Many *in vitro* procedures of antioxidant must to be evaluated for the specimens of interest antioxidant (Alam *et al.* 2013). There are variety of antioxidant tests that vary in several oxidation steps and procedure of almost every method is different. However, the best methodology for estimation of antioxidant potential ought to measure the impact of the food complexes in reaction environments that impersonate the oxidative stress elicited *in vivo* through ROS and RNS. Antioxidant assays are classified as the hydrogen atom transport (HAT) or single electron transmission (SET) approaches based on reaction mechanisms. The procedures for estimating the antioxidant activity of food elements are based on SET or HAT reaction assays. In both, the end result remains the same, in spite of different reaction mechanisms and kinetics. The power of a possible antioxidant to pass one electron to minimise every molecule, like metals, carbonyls, and radicals, is detected using SET-based protocols. SET methods display results via the colour change as the oxidant diminished. (Apak *et al.* 2016, Huang *et al.* 2005). HAT-based procedures are focused on an antioxidant's conventional capacity to remove the free radicals via hydrogen/electron donation. The HAT reactions are not affected by the presence of a solvent or the pH of the environment with the usual completion time in moments to minutes. The reducing agents' presence, together with metals, maybe a problem in HAT analyses that might cause highly inaccurate raections (Prior *et al.* 2005).

The following are some of HAT reaction-based procedures (Huang *et al.* 2005).

- Oxygen radical absorbance capacity (ORAC)
- Total radical trapping antioxidant parameter (TRAP)
- Total radical scavenging capacity assay (TOSCA)
      The following assays use SET-based approaches.
- Total phenolics via Folin–Ciocalteu reagent.
- Ferric ion reducing antioxidant power (FRAP) assay.
- 2, 2-Diphenyl-1-picrylhydrazyl radical (DPPH˙) scavenging assay.
- 2, 2-Azinobis 3-ethylbenzthiazoline-6-sulfonic acid radical (ABTS˙⁺) scavenging assay.

HAT and SET processes were used in ABTS methods, according to reports (Prior *et al.* 2005). Further, there are some assays which assess a sample's capacity to scavenge oxidants that interfere with and disrupt large macromolecules in the biological systems and foodstuffs (Huang *et al.* 2005) (MacDonald-Wicks *et al.* 2006, Miguel 2010).

- Superoxide anion radical (O_2-) scavenging assays
- Hydroxyl radical (HO·) scavenging assays
- Hydrogen peroxide (H_2O_2) scavenging assays
- Total peroxyl radical-trapping antioxidant potential (TRAP)

In Vitro Evaluation of Antioxidant Capacity/Activity

The methods to estimate the antioxidant potential require just a limited quantity of the chemical substances to be examined and must be very fast, reproducible, and, furthermore, physical properties of said molecules had little impact on them. (Marco 1968). *In vitro* assay findings could be utilized to predict antioxidant function *in vivo*; a drug which is inefficient *in vitro* would not be more effective *in vivo* (Aruoma 1996). Since several variables may influence the oxidation stage, the antioxidant ability can differ based on the oxidative conditions used in antioxidant assay, which includes temperature, the oxygen concentration level of the reaction media, and metals as catalysts. Based on their precision, tests that quantify substrates or products may provide varying results (Fukumoto and Mazza 2000). Table **2** displays the procedures of estimation of antioxidant action *in vitro*.

Table 2. The most common methods for evaluating antioxidant properties *in vitro*.

Method	Reaction mechanism	Characteristics	Reference
Total radical-trapping antioxidant parameter (TRAP)	HAT	TRAP method includes the start of the lipid peroxidation via producing water-soluble ROO• and it is extremely sensitive to every antioxidant that weaken chains	(Wayner *et al.* 1985)
Oxygen radical absorbance capacity (ORAC)	HAT	This assay is focused on the production of the free radicals with AAPH and the calculation of the decline in fluorescence when free radical scavengers are present	(Cao *et al.* 1997)

(Table 2) cont.....

Method	Reaction mechanism	Characteristics	Reference
Inhibition of 2,2-diphenyl-1-picrylhydrazyl radical (DPPH•)	SET or HAT	Colorimetric technique used to measure the scavenging capacity of antioxidants towards DPPH•	(Brand-Williams *et al.* 1995)
Ferric-reducing antioxidant power (FRAP)	SET	Colorimetric method used to evaluate the Fe_3^+-tripyridyltriazine complex (Fe_3^+-TPTZ) reduction by converting it to the ferrous form (Fe_2^+-TPTZ)	(Benzie and Strain 1996)
Inhibition of 2,2'-azino-bis- (3-ethylbenzothiazoline-6- sulphonic acid) (ABTS•+) cation radical	SET or HAT	Colorimetric technique to calculate the ABTS•$^+$ decay in the antioxidant agent presence	(Re *et al.* 1999)
Total antioxidant capacity (TAC)	SET	Use of this assay is to determine the amount of peroxide in the early stages of lipid oxidation. While continouos oxidation of the linoleic acid, peroxides are produced, which combine with Fe_2^+ to create Fe_3^+, and these metal ions later form thiocyanate complex	(Roginsky and Lissi 2005)

Total Radical-Trapping Antioxidant Parameter (TRAP)

TRAP method is utilized to estimate the prominence of an antioxidant level in the plasma. Outcomes (TRAP values) are evaluated as the µmol concentration of ROO• caught per liter of the plasma (Wayner *et al.* 1985). The test depends on estimation of oxygen take-up for the duration of a controlled peroxidation response, advanced by the 2,2'-azobis-(2-amidopropane) (ABAP) deterioration by heat, which generates ROO• at a consistent rate. Further, this begins through the expansion of the ABAP to the plasma and the parameter assessed is the "defer time" of the oxygen assimilation in the plasma initiated through antioxidant availablility in the medium. This defer time estimated from oxygen concentration in the plasma maintained in the buffer solution is examined by the electrode. Among the fundamental demerits of TRAP technique is chance of an inaccuracy in the discovery of the endpoint brought about through the weakness of the oxygen cathode since this stage could take up to 2 hours to achieve. Further, to limit this issue, the identification of O_2 electrochemically could be done with the chemiluminescence recognition dependent on utilization of the luminol and the horseradish peroxidase (HRP) (Bastos *et al.* 2003).

Total Oxyradical Scavenging Capacity Assay (TOSCA)

This strategy depends on assessment of the antioxidant action in gaseous phase, which comprises uncovering of the α-keto-γ-methylthiobutyric acid (KMBA) with incredible oxidizing ability against •OH, ROO•, as well as ONOO− (Silvester *et al.* 1998, Seeram *et al.* 2008). These oxidizing substances actuate a change of the KMBA to the ethylene. Further, to assess impact of the antioxidants, ethylene arrangement is assessed and contrasted with the controlled response via the utilization of the head-space gas chromatography (HS-GC). Moreover, the TOSCA analysis depends on hindrance of the ethylene development with the addition of the antioxidant sample, which compete with the KMBA for the ROS. This technique is not reasonable for an elite investigation on the grounds that separate injections of each specimen are needed to calculate ethylene output (Prior *et al.* 2005). The kinetics of this reaction technique doesn't permit the linear or direct relationship in between the level of reticence of the KMBA oxidation and the antioxidants concentration, which is a severe impediment (Lichtenthäler and Marx 2005).

Oxygen Radical Absorbance Capacity (ORAC) Method

ORAC stands for Oxygen Radical Absorbance Ability and is a novel tool for determining the antioxidant function of foods and other pharmaceuticals. By controlling the inhibition of ROO•- induced oxidation by HAT, this approach assesses antioxidants' capacity to break radical chains (Ou *et al.* 2001). In the ORAC process, beta-phycoerythrin serves as the oxidizable protein substrate, with 2, 2'-azobis (2-amidinopropane) dihydrochloride (AAPH) serving as the peroxyl radical producer and Cu^{2+}-H_2O_2 mechanism serving as a OH radical generator. This approach completes the free radical reaction and quantifies it using the area-under-the-curve (AUC) procedure, integrating a percentage of inhibition and the time or duration of the free radical's prevention period into the single quantity (Miller *et al.* 1993, Whitehead *et al.* 1992).

2,2-Diphenyl-1-picrylhydrazyl Radical (DPPH•) Method

It is the most frequently utilized antioxidant assays for plant samples described first by Blois (1958) and it was then modified slightly by many researchers later. The DPPH is a stable long lived nitrogen centred free radical species in aqueous or ethanol solution (Gulcin *et al.* 2002). This process is performed by the inclusion of a reactive species and an antioxidant which decolorizes a DPPH solution. The antioxidant capacity is tested at a wavelength of 515 nm and monitored to see whether it decreases (Alam *et al.* 2013). In this step, 0.1 mM DPPH prepared in methanol is formulated, and 4 ml of DPPH solution is applied to 1 ml of antioxidant/sample solution prepared in a methanol at various concentrations. Further, the absorbance using spectrophotometer was estimated at 517 nm after 30 minutes. A substantial reduction in the spectrophotometric absorbance of a reaction medium means that the compound has strong free radical scavenging activity.

2,2'-Azino-bis(3-ethylbenzothiazoline-6-sulfonic acid (ABTS) Method

It is the most widely utilized technique to asses the antioxidative potential of the food products and other chemicals developed by the Rice Evans and Miller in 1994 and were then later improved by Re *et al.* (1999). The ABTS radical cation is formed using one of the spectrophotometric criteria for estimating total antioxidant capacity of the pure substances, water-soluble mixtures as well as the beverages (Gülçin *et al.* 2009). The alteration is dependent on the production of a radical cation by activating metmyoglobin with H_2O_2 in the vicinity of ABTS•+ (Miller *et al.* 1993). Further, the mixture of ABTS and potassium persulfate produces a blue/green ABTS•+ chromophore in this improved method. Moreover, the ABTS radical scavenging procedure, together with the DPPH, is one of the extensively employed antioxidant assay methods for the plant species. The ABTS radical cation is formed when ABTS is oxidised with potassium persulfate $(K_2S_2O_8)$, and its reduction is determined spectrophotometrically at 734 nm in the hydrogen-donating antioxidants' presence. The overall antioxidant potential of lipophilic and hydrophilic compounds is measured in this decolorization assay (Awika *et al.* 2003). When determining antioxidant function, the influence of antioxidant level and the extent of the prevention of radical cation absorption are taken into account. As a positive control, Trolox, a water-soluble vitamin E analogue, is used. The activity is measured in the Trolox-equivalent antioxidative potential per milligramme of extract (TEAC/mg).

Photochemiluminescence (PCL) Assay

In both lipid and aqueous phases, the PCL assay tests a compound's antioxidant potential against the superoxide radical. This approach may be used to determine the antioxidant ability of hydrophilic and lipophilic compounds as the pure compounds or as a part in the complex matrix derived from synthetic/artificial, animal, vegetable, or human sources. The PCL system is a simple and accurate calculation method. Researchers used the PCL assay to determine the antioxidant potential of marigold flowers (Wang *et al.* 2006).

Carotene Linoleic Acid Bleaching Assay

Miller (1971) was the first to characterise the carotene linoleic acid bleaching assay and is an antioxidant assay that could be used for the plant samples. The antioxidant potential is measured in this assay by recording the prevention of volatile organic compounds as well as conjugated diene hydroperoxides produced during oxidation of linoleic acid, which causes carotene to discolour. Further, 25 litres of linoleic acid with 200 mg of a Tween 40 emulsifier solution are mixed with carotene (0.5 mg) in 1 ml chloroform. Following the vacuum evaporation of the chloroform, 100 mL of oxygen (O_2)-saturated distilled water is applied with the intense shaking. The mixture (4 ml) is then taken into the test tubes comprising various proportions of the specimen. A spectrophotometer is used to calculate the zero time point absorbance at 470 nm as quickly as the emulsifying agent is added to each tube. The emulsion is incubated for 2 h at 50 °C. Further, at 50 °C, 2 hours incubation of emulsion is achieved. For background subtraction, a blank solution devoid of the carotene is prepared. Standards include quercetin, tocopherol, and BHT. However, the main limitations of this technique are the inaqurate quantification, little reproducibility, difficulty of reagent formulation, and definite interfering parameters like pH, solvents, and temperature (Alam *et al.* 2013, Apak *et al.* 2016).

CONCLUSION

The ability of electrons to neutralise free radicals is expected by theory of antioxidant action. Phenolic compounds or molecules are a diverse category of the phytochemicals found in the plants like apples, onions, tea, olive oil, tobacco, and many others. Antioxidant agents, which are provided to human bodies as dietary ingredients or as specialised protective pharmaceutical medications, are gaining popularity these days. As a result, antioxidants have been an essential aspect of food safety and current health treatment. It is well established that the existence of the phenolic compounds, particularly phenolic acids and the flavonoids, is correlated with plants that have antioxidative and pharmacological properties. Antioxidant activity analysis techniques that are accurate are needed for successful research study for naturally occurring antioxidant compounds. In the current research, however, a wide range of bioanalytical criteria for estimating the antioxidant ability of food components are possible, as described here. In terms of the antioxidant kinetics, substrate form, oxidant and the target organisms, process conditions and the oxidation originator, outcome expression, and ease of activity, these bioanalytical assays vary from one another. The mechanism and execution of these approaches differ. In this case, after a strategy has been chosen, the first thing to consider is the reaction process. For a reliable evaluation of antioxidative potential and, finally, for the ability of antioxidants as the food preservatives, medicines, or health-promoting agents, choosing the right approach or combination of techniques is critical.

CONFLICT OF INTEREST

The authors have no conflict of interest to declare and are responsible for the content and writing of the manuscript

ACKNOWLEDGEMENTS

This chapter was designed and initiated by MAM. It has been written by BAB, SN and edited and compiled by Dr. MAM. The Authors are thankful to Dr MAM for his assistance in the preparation of this manuscript.

CONSENT FOR PUBLICATION

None

REFERENCES

Ahmad, S, Jafarzadeh, S, Ariffin, F & Abidin, SZ (2020) Evaluation of physicochemical, antioxidant and antimicrobial properties of chicken sausage incorporated with different vegetables. *Ital J Food Sci,* 32.

Alam, MN, Bristi, NJ & Rafiquzzaman, M (2013) Review on *in vivo* and *in vitro* methods evaluation of antioxidant activity. *Saudi Pharm J,* 21, 143-52.
[http://dx.doi.org/10.1016/j.jsps.2012.05.002] [PMID: 24936134]

Anjana, A, Rajagopal, P, Kumar, PS, Arthi, I, Nair, MB & Aneeshia, S (2020) Antioxidant activity of the leaves of Sphagneticola trilobata (L.). *International Journal of Modern Pharmaceutical Research,* 4, 138-42.

Anraku, M, Gebicki, JM, Iohara, D, Tomida, H, Uekama, K, Maruyama, T, Hirayama, F & Otagiri, M (2018) Antioxidant activities of chitosans and its derivatives in *in vitro* and *in vivo* studies. *Carbohydr Polym,* 199, 141-9.
[http://dx.doi.org/10.1016/j.carbpol.2018.07.016] [PMID: 30143114]

Apak, R, Özyürek, M, Güçlü, K & Çapanoğlu, E (2016) Antioxidant activity/capacity measurement. 1. Classification, physicochemical principles, mechanisms, and electron transfer (ET)-based assays. *J Agric Food Chem,* 64, 997-1027.
[http://dx.doi.org/10.1021/acs.jafc.5b04739] [PMID: 26728425]

Aruoma, OI (1996) Assessment of potential prooxidant and antioxidant actions. *J Am Oil Chem Soc,* 73, 1617-25.
[http://dx.doi.org/10.1007/BF02517962]

Awika, JM, Rooney, LW, Wu, X, Prior, RL & Cisneros-Zevallos, L (2003) Screening methods to measure antioxidant activity of sorghum (sorghum bicolor) and sorghum products. *J Agric Food Chem,* 51, 6657-62.
[http://dx.doi.org/10.1021/jf034790i] [PMID: 14582956]

Barros, AI, Nunes, FM, Gonçalves, B, Bennett, RN & Silva, AP (2011) Effect of cooking on total vitamin C contents and antioxidant activity of sweet chestnuts (Castanea sativa Mill.). *Food Chem,* 128, 165-72.
[http://dx.doi.org/10.1016/j.foodchem.2011.03.013] [PMID: 25214344]

Bastos, EL, Romoff, P, Eckert, CR & Baader, WJ (2003) Evaluation of antiradical capacity by H2O2-hemi--induced luminol chemiluminescence. *J Agric Food Chem,* 51, 7481-8.
[http://dx.doi.org/10.1021/jf0345189] [PMID: 14640603]

Baxter, H, Harborne, J & Moss, G (1999) *Phytochemical dictionary A Handbook of Bioactive Compounds from Plants* Taylor and Francis LTD, London, UK.

Benzie, IF & Strain, JJ (1996) The ferric reducing ability of plasma (FRAP) as a measure of "antioxidant

power": the FRAP assay. *Anal Biochem,* 239, 70-6.
[http://dx.doi.org/10.1006/abio.1996.0292] [PMID: 8660627]

Blois, MS (1958) Antioxidant determinations by the use of a stable free radical. *Nature,* 181, 1199-200.
[http://dx.doi.org/10.1038/1811199a0]

Brand-Williams, W, Cuvelier, M-E & Berset, C (1995) Use of a free radical method to evaluate antioxidant activity. *Lebensm Wiss Technol,* 28, 25-30.
[http://dx.doi.org/10.1016/S0023-6438(95)80008-5]

Bursal, E & Gülçin, İ (2011) Polyphenol contents and *in vitro* antioxidant activities of lyophilised aqueous extract of kiwifruit (*Actinidia deliciosa*). *Food Res Int,* 44, 1482-9.
[http://dx.doi.org/10.1016/j.foodres.2011.03.031]

Cetin Cakmak, K & Gülçin, İ (2019) Anticholinergic and antioxidant activities of usnic acid-an activity-structure insight. *Toxicol Rep,* 6, 1273-80.
[http://dx.doi.org/10.1016/j.toxrep.2019.11.003] [PMID: 31832335]

Çakmakçı, S, Topdaş, EF, Kalın, P, Han, H, Şekerci, P & Köse, P (2015) Antioxidant capacity and functionality of oleaster (E laeagnus angustifolia L.) flour and crust in a new kind of fruity ice cream. *Int J Food Sci Technol,* 50, 472-81.
[http://dx.doi.org/10.1111/ijfs.12637]

Cao, G, Sofic, E & Prior, RL (1997) Antioxidant and prooxidant behavior of flavonoids: structure-activity relationships. *Free Radic Biol Med,* 22, 749-60.
[http://dx.doi.org/10.1016/S0891-5849(96)00351-6] [PMID: 9119242]

Carocho, M & Ferreira, IC (2013) A review on antioxidants, prooxidants and related controversy: natural and synthetic compounds, screening and analysis methodologies and future perspectives. *Food Chem Toxicol,* 51, 15-25.
[http://dx.doi.org/10.1016/j.fct.2012.09.021] [PMID: 23017782]

Cody, V, Middleton, E & Harborne, JB (1986) Plant flavonoids in biology and medicine: biochemical, pharmacological, and structure-activity relationships

Dean, RT, Fu, S, Stocker, R & Davies, MJ (1997) Biochemistry and pathology of radical-mediated protein oxidation. *Biochem J,* 324, 1-18.
[http://dx.doi.org/10.1042/bj3240001] [PMID: 9164834]

Dolatabadi, JEN & Kashanian, S (2010) A review on DNA interaction with synthetic phenolic food additives. *Food Res Int,* 43, 1223-30.
[http://dx.doi.org/10.1016/j.foodres.2010.03.026]

Edge, R & Truscott, TG (2018) Singlet oxygen and free radical reactions of retinoids and carotenoids—a review. *Antioxidants,* 7, 5.
[http://dx.doi.org/10.3390/antiox7010005] [PMID: 29301252]

Ekinci Akdemir, FN, Gülçin, İ, Karagöz, B, Soslu, R & Alwasel, SH (2016) A comparative study on the antioxidant effects of hesperidin and ellagic acid against skeletal muscle ischemia/reperfusion injury. *J Enzyme Inhib Med Chem,* 31, 114-8.
[http://dx.doi.org/10.1080/14756366.2016.1220378] [PMID: 27555116]

Floegel, A, Kim, D-O, Chung, S-J, Koo, SI & Chun, OK (2011) Comparison of ABTS/DPPH assays to measure antioxidant capacity in popular antioxidant-rich US foods. *J Food Compos Anal,* 24, 1043-8.
[http://dx.doi.org/10.1016/j.jfca.2011.01.008]

Fukumoto, LR & Mazza, G (2000) Assessing antioxidant and prooxidant activities of phenolic compounds. *J Agric Food Chem,* 48, 3597-604.
[http://dx.doi.org/10.1021/jf000220w] [PMID: 10956156]

Ghosh, N, Chakraborty, T, Mallick, S, Mana, S, Singha, D, Ghosh, B & Roy, S (2015) Synthesis, characterization and study of antioxidant activity of quercetin-magnesium complex. *Spectrochim Acta A Mol Biomol Spectrosc,* 151, 807-13.

[http://dx.doi.org/10.1016/j.saa.2015.07.050] [PMID: 26172468]

Göçer, H, Akıncıoğlu, A, Öztaşkın, N, Göksu, S & Gülçin, İ (2013) Synthesis, antioxidant, and antiacetylcholinesterase activities of sulfonamide derivatives of dopamine-related compounds. *Arch Pharm (Weinheim)*, 346, 783-92.
[http://dx.doi.org/10.1002/ardp.201300228] [PMID: 24591156]

Gülçin, İ (2012) Antioxidant activity of food constituents: an overview. *Arch Toxicol*, 86, 345-91.
[http://dx.doi.org/10.1007/s00204-011-0774-2] [PMID: 22102161]

Gulcin, I, Buyukokuroglu, ME, Oktay, M & Kufrevioglu, OI (2002) On the *in vitro* antioxidative properties of melatonin. *J Pineal Res*, 33, 167-71.
[http://dx.doi.org/10.1034/j.1600-079X.2002.20920.x] [PMID: 12220332]

Gülçin, İ, Elias, R, Gepdiremen, A & Boyer, L (2006) Antioxidant activity of lignans from fringe tree (*Chionanthus virginicus* L.). *Eur Food Res Technol*, 223, 759.
[http://dx.doi.org/10.1007/s00217-006-0265-5]

Gülçin, İ, Elias, R, Gepdiremen, A, Taoubi, K & Köksal, E (2009) Antioxidant secoiridoids from fringe tree (*Chionanthus virginicus* L.). *Wood Sci Technol*, 43, 195.
[http://dx.doi.org/10.1007/s00226-008-0234-1]

Halliwell, B (1996) Antioxidants in human health and disease. *Annu Rev Nutr*, 16, 33-50.
[http://dx.doi.org/10.1146/annurev.nu.16.070196.000341] [PMID: 8839918]

Halliwell, B (1995) Antioxidant characterization. Methodology and mechanism. *Biochem Pharmacol*, 49, 1341-8.
[http://dx.doi.org/10.1016/0006-2952(95)00088-H] [PMID: 7763275]

Halliwell, B & Gutteridge, J (1989) *Free radicals in biology and medicine* Clarendon, Oxford.

Hamad, HO, Alma, MH, Gulcin, İ, Yılmaz, MA & Karaoğul, E (2017) Evaluation of phenolic contents and bioactivity of root and nutgall extracts from Iraqian Quercus infectoria Olivier. *Rec Nat Prod*, 11, 205-10.

Huang, D, Ou, B & Prior, RL (2005) The chemistry behind antioxidant capacity assays. *J Agric Food Chem*, 53, 1841-56.
[http://dx.doi.org/10.1021/jf030723c] [PMID: 15769103]

Işık, M, Beydemir, Ş, Yılmaz, A, Naldan, ME, Aslan, HE & Gülçin, İ (2017) Oxidative stress and mRNA expression of acetylcholinesterase in the leukocytes of ischemic patients. *Biomed Pharmacother*, 87, 561-7.
[http://dx.doi.org/10.1016/j.biopha.2017.01.003] [PMID: 28081467]

Kalra, BS (2019) Supplemental Antioxidants: A Hype in Disease Prevention. *J Assoc Physicians India*, 67, 66-8.
[PMID: 31562721]

Kamal-Eldin, A & Budilarto, E (2015) *Tocopherols and tocotrienols as antioxidants for food preservation Handbook of antioxidants for food preservation.* Elsevier.

Kashanian, S & Dolatabadi, JEN (2009) DNA binding studies of 2-tert-butylhydroquinone (TBHQ) food additive. *Food Chem*, 116, 743-7.
[http://dx.doi.org/10.1016/j.foodchem.2009.03.027]

Koksal, E, Bursal, E, Dikici, E, Tozoglu, F & Gulcin, I (2011) Antioxidant activity of Melissa officinalis leaves. *J Med Plants Res*, 5, 217-22.

Köksal, E, Tohma, H, Kılıç, Ö, Alan, Y, Aras, A, Gülçin, İ & Bursal, E (2017) Assessment of antimicrobial and antioxidant activities of Nepeta trachonitica: analysis of its phenolic compounds using HPLC-MS/MS. *Sci Pharm*, 85, 24.
[http://dx.doi.org/10.3390/scipharm85020024] [PMID: 28505129]

Koudelka, S, Turanek Knotigova, P, Masek, J, Prochazka, L, Lukac, R, Miller, AD, Neuzil, J & Turanek, J (2015) Liposomal delivery systems for anti-cancer analogues of vitamin E. *J Control Release*, 207, 59-69.

[http://dx.doi.org/10.1016/j.jconrel.2015.04.003] [PMID: 25861728]

Krawczyk, H (2019) The stilbene derivatives, nucleosides, and nucleosides modified by stilbene derivatives. *Bioorg Chem,* 90103073
[http://dx.doi.org/10.1016/j.bioorg.2019.103073] [PMID: 31234131]

Kulawik, P, Özogul, F, Glew, R & Özogul, Y (2013) Significance of antioxidants for seafood safety and human health. *J Agric Food Chem,* 61, 475-91.
[http://dx.doi.org/10.1021/jf304266s] [PMID: 23256644]

Lichtenthäler, R & Marx, F (2005) Total oxidant scavenging capacities of common European fruit and vegetable juices. *J Agric Food Chem,* 53, 103-10.
[http://dx.doi.org/10.1021/jf0307550] [PMID: 15631516]

Limón-Pacheco, J & Gonsebatt, ME (2009) The role of antioxidants and antioxidant-related enzymes in protective responses to environmentally induced oxidative stress. *Mutat Res,* 674, 137-47.
[http://dx.doi.org/10.1016/j.mrgentox.2008.09.015] [PMID: 18955158]

Macdonald-Wicks, LK, Wood, LG & Garg, ML (2006) Methodology for the determination of biological antioxidant capacity *in vitro*: a review. *J Sci Food Agric,* 86, 2046-56.
[http://dx.doi.org/10.1002/jsfa.2603]

Magalhães, LM, Segundo, MA, Reis, S & Lima, JL (2008) Methodological aspects about *in vitro* evaluation of antioxidant properties. *Anal Chim Acta,* 613, 1-19.
[http://dx.doi.org/10.1016/j.aca.2008.02.047] [PMID: 18374697]

Maltos, DAF, Cortés, JS, Urdiales, BV & González, CNA (2010) Uso de técnicas electroquímicas para evaluar el poder antioxidante en alimentos. *Investig Cienc,* 18, 20-5.

Mangels, AR, Block, G, Frey, CM, Patterson, BH, Taylor, PR, Norkus, EP & Levander, OA (1993) The bioavailability to humans of ascorbic acid from oranges, orange juice and cooked broccoli is similar to that of synthetic ascorbic acid. *J Nutr,* 123, 1054-61.
[PMID: 8505665]

Marco, GJ (1968) A rapid method for evaluation of antioxidants. *J Am Oil Chem Soc,* 45, 594-8.
[http://dx.doi.org/10.1007/BF02668958]

Marcus, RA & Sutin, N (1985) Electron transfers in chemistry and biology. *Biochimica et Biophysica Acta (BBA)-. Reviews on Bioenergetics,* 811, 265-322.

Martínez-Valverde, I, Periago, MJ & Ros, G (2000) Significado nutricional de los compuestos fenólicos de la dieta. *Arch Latinoam Nutr,* 50, 5-18.
[PMID: 11048566]

Mercadante, A, Egeland, E, Britton, G, Liaaen-Jensen, S & Pfander, H (2004) Carotenoids handbook.*Britton, G, Liaaen-Jensen, S*

Miguel, MG (2010) Antioxidant activity of medicinal and aromatic plants. A review. *Flavour Fragrance J,* 25, 291-312.
[http://dx.doi.org/10.1002/ffj.1961]

Miller, H (1971) A simplified method for the evaluation of antioxidants. *J Am Oil Chem Soc,* 48, 91-1.
[http://dx.doi.org/10.1007/BF02635693]

Miller, NJ, Rice-Evans, C, Davies, MJ, Gopinathan, V & Milner, A (1993) A novel method for measuring antioxidant capacity and its application to monitoring the antioxidant status in premature neonates. *Clin Sci (Lond),* 84, 407-12.
[http://dx.doi.org/10.1042/cs0840407] [PMID: 8482045]

Nakamura, H, Nakamura, K & Yodoi, J (1997) Redox regulation of cellular activation. *Annu Rev Immunol,* 15, 351-69.
[http://dx.doi.org/10.1146/annurev.immunol.15.1.351] [PMID: 9143692]

Nanditha, B & Prabhasankar, P (2009) Antioxidants in bakery products: a review. *Crit Rev Food Sci Nutr,* 49,

1-27.
[http://dx.doi.org/10.1080/10408390701764104] [PMID: 18949596]

Nimse, SB & Pal, D (2015) Free radicals, natural antioxidants, and their reaction mechanisms. *RSC Advances*, 5, 27986-8006.
[http://dx.doi.org/10.1039/C4RA13315C]

Ou, B, Hampsch-Woodill, M & Prior, RL (2001) Development and validation of an improved oxygen radical absorbance capacity assay using fluorescein as the fluorescent probe. *J Agric Food Chem*, 49, 4619-26.
[http://dx.doi.org/10.1021/jf010586o] [PMID: 11599998]

Paran, E, Novack, V, Engelhard, YN & Hazan-Halevy, I (2009) The effects of natural antioxidants from tomato extract in treated but uncontrolled hypertensive patients. *Cardiovasc Drugs Ther*, 23, 145-51.
[http://dx.doi.org/10.1007/s10557-008-6155-2] [PMID: 19052855]

Pérez-Jiménez, J & Saura-Calixto, F (2005) Literature data may underestimate the actual antioxidant capacity of cereals. *J Agric Food Chem*, 53, 5036-40.
[http://dx.doi.org/10.1021/jf050049u] [PMID: 15941353]

Pietta, P-G (2000) Flavonoids as antioxidants. *J Nat Prod*, 63, 1035-42.
[http://dx.doi.org/10.1021/np9904509] [PMID: 10924197]

Prior, RL, Wu, X & Schaich, K (2005) Standardized methods for the determination of antioxidant capacity and phenolics in foods and dietary supplements. *J Agric Food Chem*, 53, 4290-302.
[http://dx.doi.org/10.1021/jf0502698] [PMID: 15884874]

Ranelletti, FO, Ricci, R, Larocca, LM, Maggiano, N, Capelli, A, Scambia, G, Benedetti-Panici, P, Mancuso, S, Rumi, C & Piantelli, M (1992) Growth-inhibitory effect of quercetin and presence of type-II estrogen-binding sites in human colon-cancer cell lines and primary colorectal tumors. *Int J Cancer*, 50, 486-92.
[http://dx.doi.org/10.1002/ijc.2910500326] [PMID: 1735617]

Re, R, Pellegrini, N, Proteggente, A, Pannala, A, Yang, M & Rice-Evans, C (1999) Antioxidant activity applying an improved ABTS radical cation decolorization assay. *Free Radic Biol Med*, 26, 1231-7.
[http://dx.doi.org/10.1016/S0891-5849(98)00315-3] [PMID: 10381194]

Ren, W, Qiao, Z, Wang, H, Zhu, L, Zhang, L, Lu, Y, Cui, Y, Zhang, Z & Wang, Z (2001) Tartary buckwheat flavonoid activates caspase 3 and induces HL-60 cell apoptosis. *Methods Find Exp Clin Pharmacol*, 23, 427-32.
[http://dx.doi.org/10.1358/mf.2001.23.8.662129] [PMID: 11838316]

Rice-Evans, C & Bruckdorfer, KR (1995) *Oxidative stress, lipoproteins and cardiovascular dysfunction.* Ashgate Publishing.

Rice-Evans, C & Miller, NJ (1994) [241 Total antioxidant status in plasma and body fluids. *Methods in enzymology*. Elsevier. Riemersma, R, Rice-Evans, C, Tyrrell, R, Clifford, M & Lean, M (2001) Tea flavonoids and cardiovascular health. *QJM*, 94, 277-82.

Roginsky, V & Lissi, EA (2005) Review of methods to determine chain-breaking antioxidant activity in food. *Food Chem*, 92, 235-54.
[http://dx.doi.org/10.1016/j.foodchem.2004.08.004]

Sakakibara, H, Honda, Y, Nakagawa, S, Ashida, H & Kanazawa, K (2003) Simultaneous determination of all polyphenols in vegetables, fruits, and teas. *J Agric Food Chem*, 51, 571-81.
[http://dx.doi.org/10.1021/jf020926l] [PMID: 12537425]

Scambia, G, Ranelletti, FO, Panici, PB, Piantelli, M, Bonanno, G, De Vincenzo, R, Ferrandina, G, Rumi, C, Larocca, LM & Mancuso, S (1990) Inhibitory effect of quercetin on OVCA 433 cells and presence of type II oestrogen binding sites in primary ovarian tumours and cultured cells. *Br J Cancer*, 62, 942-6.
[http://dx.doi.org/10.1038/bjc.1990.414] [PMID: 2257224]

Seeram, NP, Aviram, M, Zhang, Y, Henning, SM, Feng, L, Dreher, M & Heber, D (2008) Comparison of antioxidant potency of commonly consumed polyphenol-rich beverages in the United States. *J Agric Food Chem*, 56, 1415-22.

[http://dx.doi.org/10.1021/jf073035s] [PMID: 18220345]

Shahidi, F & Ambigaipalan, P (2015) Phenolics and polyphenolics in foods, beverages and spices: Antioxidant activity and health effects–A review. *J Funct Foods,* 18, 820-97.
[http://dx.doi.org/10.1016/j.jff.2015.06.018]

Sies, H (1993) Strategies of antioxidant defense. *Eur J Biochem,* 215, 213-9.
[http://dx.doi.org/10.1111/j.1432-1033.1993.tb18025.x] [PMID: 7688300]

Sies, H & Stahl, W (1995) Vitamins E and C, beta-carotene, and other carotenoids as antioxidants. *Am J Clin Nutr,* 62 (Suppl.), 1315S-21S.
[http://dx.doi.org/10.1093/ajcn/62.6.1315S] [PMID: 7495226]

Silvester, JA, Timmins, GS & Davies, MJ (1998) Photodynamically generated bovine serum albumin radicals: evidence for damage transfer and oxidation at cysteine and tryptophan residues. *Free Radic Biol Med,* 24, 754-66.
[http://dx.doi.org/10.1016/S0891-5849(97)00327-4] [PMID: 9586806]

Sisein, EA (2014) Biochemistry of free radicals and antioxidants. *Scholars Acad J Biosci,* 2, 110-8.

Teofili, L, Pierelli, L, Iovino, MS, Leone, G, Scambia, G, De Vincenzo, R, Benedetti-Panici, P, Menichella, G, Macrì, E & Piantelli, M (1992) The combination of quercetin and cytosine arabinoside synergistically inhibits leukemic cell growth. *Leuk Res,* 16, 497-503.
[http://dx.doi.org/10.1016/0145-2126(92)90176-8] [PMID: 1625476]

Tohma, H, Gülçin, İ, Bursal, E, Gören, AC, Alwasel, SH & Köksal, E (2017) Antioxidant activity and phenolic compounds of ginger (*Zingiber officinale* Rosc.) determined by HPLC-MS/MS. *J Food Meas Charact,* 11, 556-66.
[http://dx.doi.org/10.1007/s11694-016-9423-z]

Wang, M, Tsao, R, Zhang, S, Dong, Z, Yang, R, Gong, J & Pei, Y (2006) Antioxidant activity, mutagenicity/anti-mutagenicity, and clastogenicity/anti-clastogenicity of lutein from marigold flowers. *Food Chem Toxicol,* 44, 1522-9.
[http://dx.doi.org/10.1016/j.fct.2006.04.005] [PMID: 16757077]

Wayner, DD, Burton, GW, Ingold, KU & Locke, S (1985) Quantitative measurement of the total, peroxyl radical-trapping antioxidant capability of human blood plasma by controlled peroxidation. The important contribution made by plasma proteins. *FEBS Lett,* 187, 33-7.
[http://dx.doi.org/10.1016/0014-5793(85)81208-4] [PMID: 4018255]

Whitehead, T, Thorpe, G & Maxwell, S (1992) Enhanced chemiluminescent assay for antioxidant capacity in biological fluids. *Anal Chim Acta,* 266, 265-77.
[http://dx.doi.org/10.1016/0003-2670(92)85052-8]

Williams, NH & Yandell, JK (1985) Reduction of oxidized cytochrome c by ascorbate ion. *Biochimica et Biophysica Acta (BBA)-. Bioenergetics,* 810, 274-7.
[http://dx.doi.org/10.1016/0005-2728(85)90142-2]

Williams, RJ, Spencer, JP & Rice-Evans, C (2004) Flavonoids: antioxidants or signalling molecules? *Free Radic Biol Med,* 36, 838-49.
[http://dx.doi.org/10.1016/j.freeradbiomed.2004.01.001] [PMID: 15019969]

Yoshida, M, Sakai, T, Hosokawa, N, Marui, N, Matsumoto, K, Fujioka, A, Nishino, H & Aoike, A (1990) The effect of quercetin on cell cycle progression and growth of human gastric cancer cells. *FEBS Lett,* 260, 10-3.
[http://dx.doi.org/10.1016/0014-5793(90)80053-L] [PMID: 2298289]

Yoshida, M, Yamamoto, M & Nikaido, T (1992) Quercetin arrests human leukemic T-cells in late G1 phase of the cell cycle. *Cancer Res,* 52, 6676-81.
[PMID: 1423313]

CHAPTER 5

Oxidative Stress and Biochemical Approaches of Antioxidant Analysis

Samiksha [1], **Sandeep Kaur**[2], **Drishtant Singh**[3], **Ajay Kumar**[2], **Satwinderjeet Kaur**[2] and **Satwinder Kaur Sohal**[*, 1]

[1] *Department of Zoology, Guru Nanak Dev University Amritsar, Punjab, 143005, India*

[2] *Department of Botanical and Environmental Sciences, Guru Nanak Dev University Amritsar, Punjab, 143005, India*

[3] *Department of Molecular Biology and Biochemistry, Guru Nanak Dev University Amritsar, Punjab, 143005, India*

Abstract: Abiotic stresses have contributed to the generation of reactive oxygen species called as free radicals which are highly toxic to the organism. Free radicals may be evaluated either explicitly or inadvertently after the production of oxidative by-products of nucleic acids, proteins or lipids, a method also known as fingerprinting. Though the approaches for analyzing such reactive intermediates have been thoroughly studied; we concentrated primarily on recent implementations of these techniques to quantify free radicals and different candidate biomarkers of oxidative stress such as nitrotyrosine, isoprostane, *etc*. Further, the various biochemical approaches along with the conventional methods are also discussed for the evaluation of antioxidant activity of natural products.

Keywords: Antioxidants, Biochemical approaches, Biomarkers, Oxidative stress.

INTRODUCTION

Oxidative stress is associated with a delayed release of free radicals or with a reduction in antioxidant concentration. The disruption in the stability of prooxidants and antioxidants is the result of oxidative stress (Husain and Kumar 2012). Free radicals or prooxidants produce fewer electrons that respond strongly to certain kinds of radicals in an unstable manner. Continuous metabolic pathways in humans generate ROS/free radicals that especially target fats, proteins and DNA. There are few endogenous causes for the production of ROS such as certain organelles (mitochondria, peroxisomes), xanthine oxidase (Sisein 2014), phagocytosis, arachidonic acid pathway (Husain and Kumar 2012), respiratory

---

* **Corresponding author Satwinder Kaur Sohal:** Department of Zoology, Guru Nanak Dev University Amritsar, Punjab, 143005, India. E-mail: satudhillon63@gmail.com

Pardeep Kaur, Rajendra G. Mehta, Robin, Tarunpreet Singh Thind and Saroj Arora (Eds.)

explosion (Takashima *et al.* 2012), whereas exogenous sources include UV radiation, industrial solvents and atmospheric pollutants. In addition, the reactive oxygen species (ROS) are produced as a result of partial reduction by non-reactive dioxygen (Kumar 2014). ROS usually involves nitric oxide (NO), superoxide anion (O_2), H_2O_2, radical hydroxyl (OH), single oxygen *etc.* The importance of free radicals in pathogenesis is increasingly being recognized in past years amongst people for the prevention of various diseases. Oxygen is an important aspect of life however, the regular use of oxygen by the body continually creates free radicals (Shinde *et al.* 2012). The development of chronic and degenerative diseases including cancer, diabetes, aging, cardiovascular and neuropathic disease that has a significant role to play when it comes to oxidative stress (Shinde *et al.* 2012).

The human body offers many mechanisms to combat oxidative stress by providing antioxidants that are produced naturally or delivered externally *via* food and/or supplementation. Antioxidants from external as well as internal sources function as free radical scavengers that can enhance the immune response and reduce the risk of various diseases (Valko *et al.* 2006). The previous reports suggested that disparities in free radicals and saliva antioxidants could be a contributing factor in the development of periodontal diseases, thus it is necessary to evaluate oxidation stress in saliva to provide a more precise account of oral surroundings (Shinde *et al.* 2012).

There are two kinds of biological free radicals: nitrogen-based radicals, also known as RNS and oxygen dependent radicals, also known as ROS. Free radicals may trigger lipid peroxidation (LPO), breakdown in DNA strands and oxidation of proteins and other essential molecules that can cause injury (Phaniendra *et al.* 2015). Some of the RNS and ROS are given in Table **1**.

Table 1. Some of the common reactive oxygen and nitrogen species.

S. NO.	Reactive oxygen species	
1.	Alkoxy radical	RO·
2.	Hydrogen peroxide	H_2O_2
3.	Hydroperoxyl radical	HOO·
4.	Hydroxyl radical	·OH
5.	Hypochlorous acid	HOCl
6.	Ozone	O_3
7.	Perhydroxyl radical	HO_2·
8.	Peroxyl radical	ROO·
9.	Singlet oxygen	O_2

S. NO.	Reactive oxygen species	
10.	Superoxide	$O_2^{\cdot-}$
	Reactive nitrogen species	
1.	Nitric oxide	NO
2.	Nitric dioxide	NO_2
3.	Peroxynitrite	ONO_2^{-}

BIOMARKERS OF OXIDATIVE STRESS

The cellular ROS rates and ROS mediated protein and membrane lipid products, thiobarbituric acid reactive substances (TBARS), reactive carbonyls and malondialdehyde (MDA) are known to be the main biomarkers of oxidative stress (Anjum *et al.* 2019).

Malondialdehyde (MDA)

MDA is a small, reactive organic molecule omnipresent throughout eukaryotes, which is formed by 3 carbon molecules at C1 and C3 positions containing dual aldehyde groups. Because of its pH-dependent tautomeric chemical activity MDA occurs in aqueous solutions in various types. The dominant form at a pH higher than pKa of 4.46 is the enolic anion which demonstrates weak chemical reactivity. During conditions of oxidative stress, MDA occurs in a balance amongst its protonated enol aldehyde and the dialdehyde form at lower pH (Morales and Munné-Bosch 2019). Numerous approaches for evaluating MDA content have already been introduced through derivatization combined with specific isolation methods, which took advantage of the MDA molecule's electrophilic character. Such approaches include liquid chromatography (LC); gas chromatography (GC) and mass spectrometry (MS) (Morales and Munne-Bosch 2019).

Thiobarbituric Acid Reactive Substances (TBARS)

TBARS is known to be the primary biomarker of oxidative stress (Anjum *et al.* 2019). The technique involves the reaction of lipid peroxidation products, especially thiobarbituric acid (TBA), with MDA which leads to the formation of MDA-TBA2 product, TBARS. TBARS generates a red-pink colour that can be evaluated at 532nm spectrophotometrically. The TBARS test is conducted at 95 °C in acidic conditions (pH = 4). Pure MDA is unstable, but these conditions allow MDA to be released from MDA bis(dimethyl acetal), which is used as an analytical standard. This approach is not very precise, as 2, 4-alkadienals, 4-hydroxyalkenals, and nucleic acids can also react with TBA, resulting in the formation of a chromophore (Miguel 2010).

8-Hydroxy-2-deoxyguanosine (8-OHdG)

Different kinds of DNA products occur during oxidative DNA damage based on modulation of the nucleobase, particularly on 8-OHdG lesions. They are produced *in vivo* which can be measured following DNA hydrolysis in cells (Valavanidis *et al.* 2009). Direct 8-OHdG detection is mostly achieved with high performance liquid chromatography (HPLC) (Utari and Auerkari 2020). Some of the biomarkers of oxidative stress are listed in Table **2**.

Table 2. Some of the biomarkers of the oxidative stress.

Molecule	Biomarker	Evaluation format	References
Antioxidant	Glutathione	High Performance Liquid Chromatography (HPLC), Spectrophotometric	Appala *et al.* (2016), Yilmaz *et al.* (2009)
	Oxygen radical absorbance capacity	Fluorometric	Naguib (2000)
	Glutathione peroxidase	Spectrophotometric	Shekhar *et al.* (2019)
	Glutathione reductase	Spectrophotometric	Elavarthi and Martin (2010), Kertulis-Tartar *et al.* (2009)
	Superoxide dismutase	Spectrophotometric	Elavarthi and Martin (2010), Magnani *et al.* (2000)
	Catalase	Spectrophotometric	Slaughter and O'Brien (2000), Hadwan, (2018)
	Ascorbate (vitamin C)	Spectrophotometric	Miller and Rice-Evans (1996), Khan *et al.* (2006)
	Tocopherol (vitamin E)	HPLC	Katsanidis and Addis (1999), Mendoza *et al.* (2003)
Protein	Protein carbonyls	Spectrophotometric, Enzyme Linked Immunosorbent Assay (ELISA), Western blot	Pazos *et al.* (2011), Mohanty *et al.* (2010), Shacter *et al.* (1994), Augustyniak *et al.* (2015), Buss and Winterbourn (2002)
	Individual oxidized amino acids	GC–MS, Western blot	Shacter (2000)
	Nitrotyrosine	ELISA	Shacter (2000)

(Table 2) cont.....

Molecule	Biomarker	Evaluation format	References
Lipid	Isoprostane	Gas Chromatography–Mass Spectroscopy (GC–MS), ELISA	Il'yasova *et al.* (2004), Soffler *et al.* (2010)
	Lipid hydroperoxides	Spectrophotometric, ELISA	Hicks and Gebicki (1979), Mottaran *et al.* (2002)
	Malondialdehyde	HPLC, Spectrophotometric	Lykkesfeldt (2001), Mendes et al (2009)
	Thiobarbituric acid reactive substances	HPLC, Fluorometric, Spectrophotometric	Dani *et al.* (2008), Vinson and Zhang (2005), Feoli *et al.* (2006)
	Conjugated dienes	Spectrophotometric	Recknagel *et al.* (1991), Faas *et al.* (2020)
DNA	8-Hydroxydeoxyguanosine	HPLC, ELISA	Kayamba *et al.* (2020), Chiou *et al.* (2003)
	Oxidized DNA bases	HPLC	Kawai *et al.* (2018), Gackowski *et al.* (2016)
	Strand breaks	Comet assay	Lightbourn and Thomas (2019), Park et al (2016)

Free Radical Measurement by Electron Paramagnetic Resonance (EPR)

ROS can be specifically monitored by EPR, which can be employed to track alterations in the chemical structures of the oxidizable ions (transition metal) involved in reactive oxygen species production (Jackson *et al.* 2004). Due to the poor sensitivity of EPR the analysis of strongly reactive radicals directly *in vivo* remains exceptionally difficult. A method called spin trapping is sometimes used to address the sensitivity problem (Shulaev and Oliver 2006). The recent development in the EPR approach is its integration with spin traps (Venkidasamy *et al.* 2019). EPR reacts with selected trap molecules in spin-trapping studies to create less reactive and stable products that can be easily monitored (Khan *et al.* 2003). EPR's greatest benefit is its ability to calculate and localize reactive oxygen species *in vivo*. The major drawback to using EPR is the need for the infiltration of spin trap molecules to be penetrated into the cells.

Superoxide

Superoxide detection can be accomplished by EPR using superoxide-specific spin samples (*i.e.,* 5-diethoxyphosphoryl-5-methyl-1-pyrroline-N-oxide or 5,5-dimethylpyrroline-N-oxide), employing superoxide-based assays to reduce nitroblue tetrazolium (NBT), cytochrome c (Shulaev and Oliver 2006). The NBT analysis could also be utilized for superoxide histochemical localisation. Infiltration of leaves with NBT contributes to the formation of a dark blue insoluble forming molecule which can be microscopically identified to standardize the production of superoxides in plant tissues (Flohe and Otting 1984). Poor accuracy and sensitivity are serious inconveniences in both *in vitro* and histochemical assays. Including superoxide, other compounds may reduce cytochrome c or NBT, skewing the amounts of superoxide determined with such approaches. But on the other side, lucigenin oxidation by certain compounds can cause the production of artificial superoxide. EPR with nitrone spin trap may be used to evaluate the free radicals production and can be utilized to measure alterations in the generation of free radicals (superoxide and hydroxyl) at room temperature. Superoxide assessment must be carried out with several controls and should also be checked by alternative methods. Dudylina *et al.* (2018) also used EPR spectroscopy with a combination of TIRON probe to study the potential of phenols to scavenge superoxide radicals.

Hydrogen Peroxide

A variety of methods for evaluating hydrogen peroxide (H_2O_2) in biological tissues have already been identified. Assays utilize a range of substrates like scopoletin, 4-aminoantipyrine, amplex red, homovanillic acid and dichlorofluorescence diacetate (DCFDA). The simplicity of utilization and accessibility of industrial kits have made peroxidase assays a common methodology in separated subcellular fractions for measuring H_2O_2 levels. Histochemical approaches of staining have a benefit above other tests as they enable for subcellular differentiation of H_2O_2, even though these tests are semi-quantitative in several cases. In general, ROS histochemical identification samples have specific permeability and can concentrate in a specific cellular compartment, exacerbating the analysis of the findings. A popular method for locating H_2O_2 in plants is leaf infiltration with 3,3-diaminobenzidine (DAB) (Shulaev and Oliver 2006). In the presence of peroxidase, DAB reacts with H_2O_2, forming a brown coloured polymerized product. Some other commonly used cytochemical methods are dependent on the cerium chloride H_2O_2 reaction for the production of electron dense cerium perhydroxide precipitates (Shulaev and Oliver 2006).

Nucleic Acid Oxidation

The chemistry of DNA damage caused by ROS has been widely studied both *in vitro* and *in vivo* (Beckman and Ames 1997). ROS may cause the deoxyribose sugar and bases to change/split DNA strands. Different DNA adducts were classified which occurred due to oxidative damage (Gedik *et al.* 2002). Some other distinctive attributes of DNA oxidation include the formation of DNA-MDA adducts, 8-hydroxyguanine, and 8-hydroxy2-deoxyguanosine (Bruskov *et al.* 2002). Such metabolic markers are the basis for most of the assays designed to assess oxidative damage to DNA. Although evaluating oxidative DNA damage is among the most commonly used methods for quantifying oxidative stress in animals and humans, implementation of this method is very restricted in plants.

Measuring Protein Oxidation

Protein oxidation is characterized mostly as covalent binding that is a special group of post-translational alterations, stimulated either through direct ROS responses or by explicit binding with fatty acid peroxidation degrading enzymes. Specific modification entails stimulation of protein expression *via* disulphide bonding, nitrosylation, glutathione and carbonylation (Soares *et al.* 2019). Implicit protein modulation is aimed primarily at metabolites like amino acids lysine, arginine, threonine, histidine, and tryptophan resulting in greater sensitivity of enzymes to oxidative damage (Soares *et al.* 2019). The permanently inactivated proteins could not be reversed and must be identified and damaged by cell proteolytic mechanisms, since their effective deterioration and deletion are exceptionally crucial for the sustainability of metabolic processes. It's been known that oxidized proteins are also considered as good substrates for enzymatic degradation for ubiquitination. Protein carbonyls are the much investigated hallmark of protein oxidation by free radicals as their reaction with DNPH makes them readily detectable. Absolute oxidation levels of proteins in whole organ extracts can be evaluated spectrophotometrically. This method is simple and easily versatile for high-throughput studies. Bulk protein oxidation measurements include a clear, unbiased oxidative stress assessment that can validate findings based upon the analyses of lipid oxidation product formation.

ESR Spectroscopy and Oxidative Stress

Free radicals could be seen accurately and quickly using ESR, as it identifies the involvement of unpaired electrons. Spin traps could be used to interact with reactive radicals to produce stable ones that can be detected through ESR spectroscopy (Iravani and Soofi 2019). ESR is beneficial for non-invasive measurement of the redox state of living organisms. It has been shown that *in vivo* ESR / nitroxyl spin probe approaches could be an important strategy for selectively becoming aware of free radicals and tracking free radical *in vivo* reactions (Iravani and Soofi 2019). Oxidative stress contributes to extreme over activity of cell metabolism and homeostasis of the cells that plays a major role in insulin resistance pathogenesis and β-cell dysfunction.

METHODS FOR DETERMINING ANTIOXIDANT ACTIVITY

Besides the methods for determining the chain-breaking antioxidant activity, the methods for assessing the ability to scavenge certain free radicals, like superoxide, nitric oxide, peroxynitrite, hydroxyl or chelating metals are also accessible. Several approaches were formulated with the advantages and drawbacks of these methods also recorded in some of them (Huang *et al.* 2005, Frankel and Meyer 2000, Antolovich *et al.* 2002, Sánchez-Moreno *et al.* 2003, Becker *et al.* 2004, Decker *et al.* 2005, Frankel 1993, Prior *et al.* 2005, MacDonalds *et al.* 2006). Furthermore, the antioxidant potential of the different substances was assessed using certain biochemical approaches. Analysis of the variety of measures used by various authors to assess the antioxidant efficacy of different substances is discussed below.

Assays Associated with Lipid Peroxidation

An example of role and action of antioxidants is lipid peroxidation. The suppressed chain initiation, propagation and the enhanced chain termination inhibit lipid peroxidation. The physiological function of active oxygen and associated organisms are of significance, which cause toxic effects. There are three different reactions that are linked with complex lipid peroxidation viz. 1. Free radical induced chain reactions (non enzymatic); 2. Non-radical photooxidation (non enzymatic) 3. Enzymatic reactions (Miguel 2010). The first path catalyses advanced, damaging chains mechanisms, which produce hydroperoxide and other compounds *via* induction, progression and completion process. These species are extremely unstable and are stabilized by reacting rapidly to O_2 which lead to the formation of peroxyl radicals (propagation phase). The generated peroxyl radicals can further oxidize the lipid and produce hydroperoxides in the proliferation process. The antioxidant activity can be monitored by evaluating the substrate and oxidant intake, and the composition of the intermediate or finishing product (Miguel 2010).

Peroxidation Level Evaluation Using the Ferric Thiocyanate

Peroxides (primary oxidative products), which oxidize Fe^{2+} to Fe^{3+}, are formed during linoleum acid oxidation. This forms a complex with thiocyanate whose peak absorption is at 500 nm. High absorption therefore, suggests strong oxidation of linoleic acid (Yang *et al.* 2010).

Conjugated Diene Assay

The antioxidant activity of the sample materials can be assessed in the preliminary stage of lipid peroxidation by measuring the conjugated diene formation. The hydroperoxides produced by oxidation at 40 °C from methyl linoleate were analyzed spectrophotometrically (for conjugated diene absorption) at 234 nm (Miguel 2010).

β-Carotene Bleaching Test

The β-carotene bleaching test assesses the capacity of antioxidants to slow down the decoloration of β-carotene triggered by conjugated diene hydroperoxides due to oxidative deterioration of linoleic acid (Djenidi *et al.* 2020). In this method, linoleic acid and tween 40 are introduced to β-carotene suspended in chloroform. Upon evapo-transpiration of chloroform, oxygen-saturated distilled water is added with continuous stirring. Some amount of this emulsion is added to the tubes and BHT is applied as a comparison antioxidant. The kinetics of discoloration (in the presence and absence of antioxidant) is evaluated at a time interval of 24 hours at a wavelength of 490 nm (Bouaziz *et al.* 2015). In the absence of an antioxdant, β-carotene develops fast de-coloration, even though free linoleic acid substantially targets β-carotene that also keeps losing its double bond and thus its orange color (Miguel 2010).

Aldehyde/Carboxylic Acid Assay

This technique is important for assessing the effect of antioxidants on delayed oxidation processes that occur over prolonged periods of time (Moon and Shibamoto 2009). Wei and Shibamoto (2010) using this approach demonstrated that the essential oils extracted from different plants like *Eugenia caryophyllus, Thymus vulgaris, Cinnamomum zeylanicum* Blume, *Illicium verum* and *Ocimum basilicum* prevented the oxidation of hexanal to hexanoic acid. The hexanal decrease was accompanied by gas chromatography coupled with a detector for flame ionisation.

Formic Acid Evaluation

The rancimat approach is an automation assay which determines the conductance of formic acid produced at or above 100 °C during auto-oxidation of lipids (Miguel 2010). The antioxidant potential of oils from different spice plants being utilized in the Mediterranean food was assessed using the TBARS method (Viuda-Martos *et al.* 2010) and was also analyzed using the rancimat approach. The machine was heated at 120 °C and the mixture was continuously blown in with an air flow of 20 l/h. Due to the dissociation of volatile carboxylic acids the end of the induction cycle was marked by the unexpected incline in water conductivity.

Free Radical Scavenging Potential

To determine free radical scavenging efficiency, the approaches are divided into 2 classes: reaction-based methods for the transfer of hydrogen atoms and reaction-based methods for single electron transfer (Miguel 2010).

DPPH Assay

1,1-Diphenyl-2-picrylhydrazyl (DPPH) radical scavenging is the most widely used method which provides an early evaluation of antioxidant properties. Due to its stability DPPH is manufactured in a radical form. This radical displays a strong maximum absorption at 517 nm (violet). It has a dark blue color and could be a nitrogen radical species owing to its failure to endure dimerization (Gulcin 2020). Its color changes from pale pink to yellow in the presence of antioxidants. Hence a UV-Vis spectrophotometer is the only equipment required for the assay. Whenever the DPPH radical approach is combined with an antioxidant molecule that can provide a hydrogen atom, the degradation of this violet color results in a reduced form (Gulcin 2020). The DPPH process is based on a reduction of purple DPPH· to 1,1-diphenyl2-picryl hydrazine. This approach is based on the evaluation of reduction of antioxidant capacity towards DPPH (Gulcin 2020). Capacity can be assessed by ESR or by assessing the reduction of its absorbance. Furthermore, several new research has shown that there is a rapid transfer of electrons from the test sample to DPPH radical (Miguel 2010). Due to its efficiency and sensitivity, some scientists only utilize the DPPH approach to assess the antioxidant activity of essential oils.

ABTS·$^+$ Assay

In this method, ABTS is metabolized by oxidizing agents to some of its radical cations ABTS·$^+$ which are a strong colored radicals. The antioxidant potential is evaluated as the tendency of the test samples to reduce the color effectively reacting to its ABTS radical. ABTS·$^+$ applies to both hydrophilic and lipophilic substances. The effective tool for the approach is a color removal strategy wherein the radical produced converts to its stable form after reacting with antioxidants. The initial ABTS·$^+$ scavenging method was conducted by Miller *et al.* (1993). This method was associated with activation of metmyoglobin, functioning as peroxidase, with H_2O_2 for the production of radical ferrylmyoglobin. This approach is based on reducing blue-green cation radicals (ABTS·$^+$) and calculating radical cation reduction as the percent inhibition at 734 nm.

FRAP Assay

FRAP assay is a standard ET-based technique in which under acidic conditions, a Fe^{3+} and 2,4,6-tripyridyl-s-triazine (TPTZ) complex undergoes reduction by an antioxidant to the form Fe^{2+} ions and intense blue color develops with a maximum absorption at a wavelength of 593 nm. The antioxidant effect can be assessed by observing the formation of a Fe^{2+}-TPTZ complex using a spectrophotometer (Moon and Shibamoto 2009). With regard to its drawbacks, any substance with a redox potential less than that of redox pair may cause the reduction of Fe^{3+} to Fe^{2+}, which contribute to the FRAP value and produce falsely negative results. But from the other side, not all antioxidants are capable of reducing Fe^{3+} quickly enough to enable it to be assessed within in the time of measurement. The FRAP assay evolves from an assay based on the assumption that the redox reaction starts so quickly that certain reactions are completed in less than 4 and 6 minutes, respectively, but that's not always accurate. The outcomes of FRAP can vary considerably depending on the timeframe of the evaluation.

Reducing Power

The theory of this approach is based on a rise in absorbance which implies an incline in antioxidant properties. Substances with reduction potential are electron donors and thus exhibit the potential to reduce the oxidized transitional mechanism of lipid peroxidation. Its reaction comprises test solution, sodium phosphate buffer (0.2 M, pH 6.6) and potassium ferric cyanide (1.0%) which is then incubated at 50 °C for 20 min and trichloroacetic acid (10% w/v) is added followed by centrifugation for 10 min at 1,000 xg. Then top layer (supernatant) is obtained and distilled water and ferric chloride are added to solution which is then analyzed at a wavelength of 700 nm (Haida and Hakiman 2019). One such approach for testing antioxidant potential is based on the reduction of Fe^{3+} to Fe^{2+} wherein the yellowish color of the test sample shifts to varying spectra of green and blue, depending on the reduction power of each sample. The existence of reducing factors contributes to the conversion of the Fe^{3+}/ferricyanide complex to the ferrous form, which can be observed at 700 nm due to the production of the prussian blue $Fe^4[Fe(CN)_6]3$ (Miguel 2010).

Chelating Activity

Transitional metal chelation is among the proposed pathways of antioxidant functions. Transition of metal ions can activate lipid peroxidation by speeding up peroxidation, removing lipid hydroperoxides into certain products capable of absorbing hydrogen, perpetuating the lipid peroxidation chain (Viuda-Martos *et al.* 2010). Generally one tool used to assess chelating behavior involves ferrozine that quantitatively come from Fe^{2+} structures. The activation of chelates with Fe^{2+}, ferrozine, may create a structure of red colour. The complex formation is disturbed in the presence of other chelating agents, resulting in a decrease in the complex ferrozine-Fe^{2+} red colour. Consequently, analysis of the colour reduction rate enables evaluation of the coexisting chelating activity (Wannes *et al.* 2010).

Hydroxyl Radical Scavenging

Hydroxyl is highly reactive among the oxygen radicals, causing serious losses to the contingent biological molecules. There have been many approaches to determine how hydroxyl radicals can be formed. Deoxyribose is uitilized for the evaluation of radical scavenging activity. This process involves a combination of ethylenediaminetetraacetic acid (EDTA) and ferric chloride ($FeCl_3$) which form Fe^{2+}-EDTA in the presence of ascorbic acid (oxidized ascorbic acid). HO• and Fe^{3+} EDTA are formed after introduction of the hydrogen peroxide (H_2O_2). It is the Fenton's reaction that creates extremely reactive hydroxyl radicals. Deoxyribose is attacked by hydroxyl radicals which are not diminish by either component of the reaction and degraded into many small fragments. Most of these molecules are prepared in response to heating at an acidic pH with thiobarbituric acid, resulting in a pink pigment that can be measured by spectrophotometer (Miguel 2010).

Superoxide Anion Scavenging Activity

Since this superoxide anion is a poor oxidant, it might eventually induce strong and hazardous hydroxyl radicals and singlet oxygen, which make a significant contribution to oxidative damage (Haida and Hakiman 2019). Adenine dinucleotide nicotinamide (NAD^+) after accepting electron from xanthine oxidase (dehydrogenase) is reduced to NADH. Xanthine oxidase also oxidises hypoxanthine/xanthine. However, the dehydrogenase is modified to an oxidase during stress conditions, and the oxidase enzyme absorbs oxygen rather than NAD^+ in these conditions (Miguel 2010). That way, dioxygen is reduced to superoxide anion and hydrogen peroxide. The superoxide anion is produced in the presence of NADH and dioxygen by the reaction of phenazine methosulphate (Miguel 2010).

One Dimensional Polyacrylamide Gel Electrophoresis

It is dependent on the transfer of denatured proteins to polyacrylamide gels as affected by molecular weight (Smith 1994). In accordance with Western blot, conventional 1D PAGE-based proteomic techniques are mostly conducted out where protein-specific antibodies are being used to classify and quantify proteins. While postranslational modification research is currently controlled by MS-based proteomics, the proteomic methodology dependent on 1D PAGE/WB is still a key pillar, particularly for identifying covalent NP-protein interactions. Unique protein binding sites like cysteine residues cannot be identified by 1D polyacrylamide gel electrophoresis/Western blot. The introduction of mutations to these residues *via* SDM allows SDM/1D PAGE/WB an effective strategy to study the covalent NP-protein interactions with reactive cysteine residues. Cells harbouring mutations are subjected to NPs in a standard workflow that involves SDM and cell lysates are exposed to 1D PAGE and WBBE. The C288 residue of

Keap1 was identified as the target of DATS for covalent modification using this method.

Electrophoretic Mobility Shift Assay

Using electrophoretic mobility shift assays, interactions between proteins and DNA are studied. A double-stranded oligonucleotide fragment containing the sequence of response elements is synthesised in this method (Jiang *et al.* 2009). Instead, with a hapten or fluoro-labelled dNTP, the target duplex DNA fragment can be synthesized. The labelled DNA fragment is incubated with a nuclear protein fraction in a typical EMSA experiment, allowing the development of a protein-response element complex. By non-denaturing (native) PAGE, this protein-response element complex is then resolved to allow differential migration of protein-response element complex and free DNA molecules, with protein-response element migrating slower than free DNA (Tocmo *et al.* 2020).

2D GE Coupled MS

The 2D GE is a method of protein separation based on two different protein properties: first-dimensional isoelectric point (pI) and second-dimensional relative molecular weight (Tocmo *et al.* 2020). The 2D GE separation of proteins is no longer the only method used in modern proteomics, but its use has become a keystone in bottom-up proteomics (BUP) workflows. Cell lysates or tissue extracts from cell cultures or animals exposed to the natural products (or from unexposed controls) are subjected to 2D GE followed by LC-MS/MS analysis in a standard 2D GE coupled MS approach that aims to detect covalent alteration by an electrophilic natural products (Issaq and Veenstra 2008). In an immobilised pH gradient (IPG) strip, modern 2D GE experiments proceed with protein separation and allow first dimension protein separation through isoelectric focusing (IEF). This is accompanied by the SDS-PAGE separation of the second dimension (Issaq and Veenstra 2008). Proteins are stained with MS-compatible dyes, visualised, and proteins of interest are sliced for digestion in gel after 2D GE.

Ability to Localize Oxidative Stress

One of the specific benefits of combining research on protein oxidative stress is that it preserves some spatial knowledge on stress localization. Although H_2O_2 does not cross cell membranes, superoxides and radicals of hydroxide, such data is helpful in locating where ROS is generated and oxidative stress is encountered. It is possible to obtain this sort of spatial information in many ways. Classic biochemical approaches may isolate organelles and then evaluate oxidised proteins inside certain preparations, or if proteomics approaches are utilized and unique oxidised proteins are found, bioinformatics methods may be employed to evaluate the subcellular location of a protein in a whole cell extract. Intact organs can also be derivatized with DNPH and immunological labelling.

CONCLUSION

Free radical generation is a continuous mechanism where ample proofs are available for its presence in several pathological conditions, in which antioxidant counteracts the harmful impact of free radicals. As studies shows less antioxidant consumption and lower rates of antioxidants cause disease, natural antioxidants in food may compensate for this. The advantages of antioxidants can be recommended to the public and should therefore be advised to consume food containing seeds, fruits and vegetables that are fabulously wealthy high in antioxidants. The conventional methods along certain biochemical approaches are used for evaluation of the antioxidant potential of the different substances. The proteomics approaches can be applied for better understanding of the antioxidant biomolecules and oxidative stress biomarkers (MDA, TBARS and 8-OHdG).

CONFLICT OF INTEREST

All authors declared that they have no conflict of interest. There is no financial or other dependency between authors and any of the companies considered.

ACKNOWLEDGEMENTS

The grant received from UGC New Delhi under the scheme "University with Potential for Excellence (UPE)" for conducting the research work is gratefully acknowledged.

CONSENT FOR PUBLICATION

None

REFERENCES

Anjum, NA, Gill, SS, Duarte, AC & Pereira, E (2019) Oxidative stress biomarkers and antioxidant defense in plants exposed to metallic nanoparticles.*Nanomaterials and Plant Potential* Springer 427-39.
[http://dx.doi.org/10.1007/978-3-030-05569-1_17]

Antolovich, M, Prenzler, PD, Patsalides, E, McDonald, S & Robards, K (2002) Methods for testing antioxidant activity. *Analyst (Lond),* 127, 183-98.
[http://dx.doi.org/10.1039/b009171p] [PMID: 11827390]

Appala, RN, Chigurupati, S, Appala, RV, Krishnan Selvarajan, K & Islam Mohammad, J (2016) A simple HPLC-UV method for the determination of glutathione in PC-12 cells. *Scientifica (Cairo),* 20166897890
[http://dx.doi.org/10.1155/2016/6897890] [PMID: 27127683]

Augustyniak, E, Adam, A, Wojdyla, K, Rogowska-Wrzesinska, A, Willetts, R, Korkmaz, A, Atalay, M, Weber, D, Grune, T, Borsa, C, Gradinaru, D, Chand Bollineni, R, Fedorova, M & Griffiths, HR (2015) Validation of protein carbonyl measurement: a multi-centre study. *Redox Biol,* 4, 149-57.

[http://dx.doi.org/10.1016/j.redox.2014.12.014] [PMID: 25560243]

Bandyopadhyay, U, Das, D & Banerjee, RK (1999) Reactive oxygen species: oxidative damage and pathogenesis. *Curr Sci,* 77, 658-66.

Becker, EM, Nissen, LR & Skibsted, LH (2004) Antioxidant evaluation protocols: Food quality or health effects. *Eur Food Res Technol,* 219, 561-71.
[http://dx.doi.org/10.1007/s00217-004-1012-4]

Beckman, KB & Ames, BN (1997) Oxidative decay of DNA. *J Biol Chem,* 272, 19633-6.
[http://dx.doi.org/10.1074/jbc.272.32.19633] [PMID: 9289489]

Bloomer, RJ (2008) Effect of exercise on oxidative stress biomarkers. *Adv Clin Chem,* 46, 1-50.
[http://dx.doi.org/10.1016/S0065-2423(08)00401-0] [PMID: 19004186]

Bouaziz, A, Abdalla, S, Baghiani, A & Charef, N (2015) Phytochemical analysis, hypotensive effect and antioxidant properties of Myrtus communis L. growing in Algeria. *Asian Pac J Trop Biomed,* 5, 19-28.
[http://dx.doi.org/10.1016/S2221-1691(15)30165-9]

Bruskov, VI, Malakhova, LV, Masalimov, ZK & Chernikov, AV (2002) Heat-induced formation of reactive oxygen species and 8-oxoguanine, a biomarker of damage to DNA. *Nucleic Acids Res,* 30, 1354-63.
[http://dx.doi.org/10.1093/nar/30.6.1354] [PMID: 11884633]

Buss, IH & Winterbourn, CC (2002) Protein carbonyl measurement by ELISA.*Oxidative Stress Biomarkers and Antioxidant Protocols* Humana Press 123-8.
[http://dx.doi.org/10.1385/1-59259-173-6:123]

Cao, G, Alessio, HM & Cutler, RG (1993) Oxygen-radical absorbance capacity assay for antioxidants. *Free Radic Biol Med,* 14, 303-11.
[http://dx.doi.org/10.1016/0891-5849(93)90027-R] [PMID: 8458588]

Chen, J, Lindmark-Månsson, H, Gorton, L & Åkesson, B (2003) Antioxidant capacity of bovine milk as assayed by spectrophotometric and amperometric methods. *Int Dairy J,* 13, 927-35.
[http://dx.doi.org/10.1016/S0958-6946(03)00139-0]

Chiou, CC, Chang, PY, Chan, EC, Wu, TL, Tsao, KC & Wu, JT (2003) Urinary 8-hydroxydeoxyguanosine and its analogs as DNA marker of oxidative stress: development of an ELISA and measurement in both bladder and prostate cancers. *Clin Chim Acta,* 334, 87-94.
[http://dx.doi.org/10.1016/S0009-8981(03)00191-8] [PMID: 12867278]

Dani, C, Pasquali, MA, Oliveira, MR, Umezu, FM, Salvador, M, Henriques, JA & Moreira, JC (2008) Protective effects of purple grape juice on carbon tetrachloride-induced oxidative stress in brains of adult Wistar rats. *J Med Food,* 11, 55-61.
[http://dx.doi.org/10.1089/jmf.2007.505] [PMID: 18361738]

Decker, EA, Warner, K, Richards, MP & Shahidi, F (2005) Measuring antioxidant effectiveness in food. *J Agric Food Chem,* 53, 4303-10.
[http://dx.doi.org/10.1021/jf058012x] [PMID: 15884875]

Djenidi, H, Khennouf, S & Bouaziz, A (2020) Antioxidant activity and phenolic content of commonly consumed fruits and vegetables in Algeria. *Prog Nutr,* 22, 224-35.

Dudylina, AL, Ivanova, MV, Shumaev, KB & Ruuge, EK (2019) Superoxide formation in cardiac mitochondria and effect of phenolic antioxidants. *Cell Biochem Biophys,* 77, 99-107.
[http://dx.doi.org/10.1007/s12013-018-0857-2] [PMID: 30218405]

Duthie, G, Campbell, F, Bestwick, C, Stephen, S & Russell, W (2013) Antioxidant effectiveness of vegetable powders on the lipid and protein oxidative stability of cooked Turkey meat patties: implications for health. *Nutrients,* 5, 1241-52.
[http://dx.doi.org/10.3390/nu5041241] [PMID: 23595133]

Elavarthi, S & Martin, B (2010) Spectrophotometric assays for antioxidant enzymes in plants.*Plant Stress Tolerance* Humana Press 273-80.

[http://dx.doi.org/10.1007/978-1-60761-702-0_16]

Faas, N, Röcker, B, Smrke, S, Yeretzian, C & Yildirim, S (2020) Prevention of lipid oxidation in linseed oil using a palladium-based oxygen scavenging film. *Food Packag Shelf Life,* 24100488
[http://dx.doi.org/10.1016/j.fpsl.2020.100488]

Feoli, AM, Siqueira, IR, Almeida, L, Tramontina, AC, Vanzella, C, Sbaraini, S, Schweigert, ID, Netto, CA, Perry, ML & Gonçalves, CA (2006) Effects of protein malnutrition on oxidative status in rat brain. *Nutrition,* 22, 160-5.
[http://dx.doi.org/10.1016/j.nut.2005.06.007] [PMID: 16459228]

Flohe, L (1984) Superoxide dismutase assays.*Methods in enzymology* Academic Press 93-104. [10]

Frankel, EN (1993) In search of better methods to evaluate natural antioxidants and oxidative stability in food lipids. *Trends Food Sci Technol,* 4, 220-5.
[http://dx.doi.org/10.1016/0924-2244(93)90155-4]

Frankel, EN & Meyer, AS (2000) The problems of using one-dimensional methods to evaluate multifunctional food and biological antioxidants. *J Sci Food Agric,* 80, 1925-41.
[http://dx.doi.org/10.1002/1097-0010(200010)80:13<1925::AID-JSFA714>3.0.CO;2-4]

Gackowski, D, Starczak, M, Zarakowska, E, Modrzejewska, M, Szpila, A, Banaszkiewicz, Z & Olinski, R (2016) Accurate, direct, and high-throughput analyses of a broad spectrum of endogenously generated DNA base modifications with isotope-dilution two-dimensional ultraperformance liquid chromatography with tandem mass spectrometry: possible clinical implication. *Anal Chem,* 88, 12128-36.
[http://dx.doi.org/10.1021/acs.analchem.6b02900] [PMID: 28193047]

Gedik, CM, Boyle, SP, Wood, SG, Vaughan, NJ & Collins, AR (2002) Oxidative stress in humans: validation of biomarkers of DNA damage. *Carcinogenesis,* 23, 1441-6.
[http://dx.doi.org/10.1093/carcin/23.9.1441] [PMID: 12189185]

Hadwan, MH (2018) Simple spectrophotometric assay for measuring catalase activity in biological tissues. *BMC Biochem,* 19, 7.
[http://dx.doi.org/10.1186/s12858-018-0097-5] [PMID: 30075706]

Haida, Z & Hakiman, M (2019) A comprehensive review on the determination of enzymatic assay and nonenzymatic antioxidant activities. *Food Sci Nutr,* 7, 1555-63.
[http://dx.doi.org/10.1002/fsn3.1012] [PMID: 31139368]

Halliwell, B & Gutteridge, JM (2015) *Free radicals in biology and medicine.*Oxford University Press, USA.
[http://dx.doi.org/10.1093/acprof:oso/9780198717478.001.0001]

Hicks, M & Gebicki, JM (1979) A spectrophotometric method for the determination of lipid hydroperoxides. *Anal Biochem,* 99, 249-53.
[http://dx.doi.org/10.1016/S0003-2697(79)80003-2] [PMID: 517738]

Huang, D, Ou, B & Prior, RL (2005) The chemistry behind antioxidant capacity assays. *J Agric Food Chem,* 53, 1841-56.
[http://dx.doi.org/10.1021/jf030723c] [PMID: 15769103]

Husain, N & Kumar, A (2012) Reactive oxygen species and natural antioxidants: a review. *Adv Biores,* 3, 164-75.

Il'yasova, D, Morrow, JD, Ivanova, A & Wagenknecht, LE (2004) Epidemiological marker for oxidant status: comparison of the ELISA and the gas chromatography/mass spectrometry assay for urine 2,3-dino--5,6-dihydro-15-F2t-isoprostane. *Ann Epidemiol,* 14, 793-7.
[http://dx.doi.org/10.1016/j.annepidem.2004.03.003] [PMID: 15519902]

Iravani, S & Soofi, GJ (2019) Measurement of oxidative stress using ESR spectroscopy.*Electron Spin Resonance Spectroscopy in Medicine* Springer, Singapore 73-81.
[http://dx.doi.org/10.1007/978-981-13-2230-3_4]

Issaq, H & Veenstra, T (2008) Two-dimensional polyacrylamide gel electrophoresis (2D-PAGE): advances

and perspectives. *Biotechniques,* 44, 697-698, 700.
[http://dx.doi.org/10.2144/000112823] [PMID: 18474047]

Jackson, SK, Thomas, MP, Smith, S, Madhani, M, Rogers, SC & James, PE (2004) *in vivo* EPR spectroscopy: biomedical and potential diagnostic applications. *Faraday Discuss,* 126, 103-17.
[http://dx.doi.org/10.1039/b307162f] [PMID: 14992402]

Jiang, D, Jarrett, HW & Haskins, WE (2009) Methods for proteomic analysis of transcription factors. *J Chromatogr A,* 1216, 6881-9.
[http://dx.doi.org/10.1016/j.chroma.2009.08.044] [PMID: 19726046]

Katsanidis, E & Addis, PB (1999) Novel HPLC analysis of tocopherols, tocotrienols, and cholesterol in tissue. *Free Radic Biol Med,* 27, 1137-40.
[http://dx.doi.org/10.1016/S0891-5849(99)00205-1] [PMID: 10641704]

Kawai, K, Kasai, H, Li, YS, Kawasaki, Y, Watanabe, S, Ohta, M, Honda, T & Yamato, H (2018) Measurement of 8-hydroxyguanine as an oxidative stress biomarker in saliva by HPLC-ECD. *Genes Environ,* 40, 5.
[http://dx.doi.org/10.1186/s41021-018-0095-2] [PMID: 29632621]

Kayamba, V, Zyambo, K, Mulenga, C, Mwakamui, S, Tembo, MJ, Shibemba, A, Heimburger, DC, Atadzhanov, M & Kelly, P (2020) Biomass Smoke Exposure Is Associated With Gastric Cancer and Probably Mediated *via* Oxidative Stress and DNA Damage: A Case-Control Study. *JCO Global Oncology,* 6, 532-41.
[http://dx.doi.org/10.1200/GO.20.00002] [PMID: 32228314]

Kertulis-Tartar, GM, Rathinasabapathi, B & Ma, LQ (2009) Characterization of glutathione reductase and catalase in the fronds of two Pteris ferns upon arsenic exposure. *Plant Physiol Biochem,* 47, 960-5.
[http://dx.doi.org/10.1016/j.plaphy.2009.05.009] [PMID: 19574057]

Khan, N, Wilmot, CM, Rosen, GM, Demidenko, E, Sun, J, Joseph, J, O'Hara, J, Kalyanaraman, B & Swartz, HM (2003) Spin traps: *in vitro* toxicity and stability of radical adducts. *Free Radic Biol Med,* 34, 1473-81.
[http://dx.doi.org/10.1016/S0891-5849(03)00182-5] [PMID: 12757857]

Khan, MR, Rahman, MM, Islam, MS & Begum, SA (2006) A simple UV-spectrophotometric method for the determination of vitamin C content in various fruits and vegetables at Sylhet area in Bangladesh. *J Biol Sci,* 6, 388-92.
[http://dx.doi.org/10.3923/jbs.2006.388.392]

Kumar, S (2014) The importance of antioxidant and their role in pharmaceutical science-a review. *Asian Journal of Research in Chemistry and Pharmaceutical Sciences,* 1, 27-44.

Landry, LG, Chapple, CC & Last, RL (1995) Arabidopsis mutants lacking phenolic sunscreens exhibit enhanced ultraviolet-B injury and oxidative damage. *Plant Physiol,* 109, 1159-66.
[http://dx.doi.org/10.1104/pp.109.4.1159] [PMID: 8539286]

Levine, RL, Williams, JA, Stadtman, EP & Shacter, E (1994) Carbonyl assays for determination of oxidatively modified proteins.*Methods in enzymology* Academic Press 346-57. [37]

Lightbourn, AV & Thomas, RD (2019) Crude Edible Fig (*Ficus carica*) Leaf Extract Prevents Diethylstilbestrol (DES)-Induced DNA Strand Breaks in Single-Cell Gel Electrophoresis (SCGE)/Comet Assay: Literature Review and Pilot Study. *J Bioequivalence Bioavailab,* 11, 19-28.
[PMID: 31814674]

Lykkesfeldt, J (2001) Determination of malondialdehyde as dithiobarbituric acid adduct in biological samples by HPLC with fluorescence detection: comparison with ultraviolet-visible spectrophotometry. *Clin Chem,* 47, 1725-7.
[http://dx.doi.org/10.1093/clinchem/47.9.1725] [PMID: 11514418]

MacDonald-Wicks, LK, Wood, LG & Garg, ML (2006) Methodology for the determination of biological antioxidant capacity *in vitro*: a review. *J Sci Food Agric,* 86, 2046-56.
[http://dx.doi.org/10.1002/jsfa.2603]

Machac, N, Kaya Karasu, G, Sahin, N, Orhan, C, Sahin, K & Iben, C (2019) Effects of supplementation of chromium histidinate on glucose, lipid metabolism and oxidative stress in cats. *J Anim Physiol Anim Nutr (Berl),* 103, 331-8.
[http://dx.doi.org/10.1111/jpn.13023] [PMID: 30467904]

Magnani, L, Gaydou, EM & Hubaud, JC (2000) Spectrophotometric measurement of antioxidant properties of flavones and flavonols against superoxide anion. *Anal Chim Acta,* 411, 209-16.
[http://dx.doi.org/10.1016/S0003-2670(00)00717-0]

Mendes, R, Cardoso, C & Pestana, C (2009) Measurement of malondialdehyde in fish: A comparison study between HPLC methods and the traditional spectrophotometric test. *Food Chem,* 112, 1038-45.
[http://dx.doi.org/10.1016/j.foodchem.2008.06.052]

Rodas Mendoza, B, Morera Pons, S, Castellote Bargalló, AI & López-Sabater, MC (2003) Rapid determination by reversed-phase high-performance liquid chromatography of Vitamins A and E in infant formulas. *J Chromatogr A,* 1018, 197-202.
[http://dx.doi.org/10.1016/j.chroma.2003.08.018] [PMID: 14620570]

Miguel, MG (2010) Antioxidant and anti-inflammatory activities of essential oils: a short review. *Molecules,* 15, 9252-87.
[http://dx.doi.org/10.3390/molecules15129252] [PMID: 21160452]

Miguel, MG (2010) Antioxidant activity of medicinal and aromatic plants. *Flavour Fragrance J,* 25, 291-312.
[http://dx.doi.org/10.1002/ffj.1961]

Miller, NJ & Rice-Evans, CA (1996) Spectrophotometric determination of antioxidant activity. *Redox Rep,* 2, 161-71.
[http://dx.doi.org/10.1080/13510002.1996.11747044] [PMID: 27406072]

Mohanty, JG, Bhamidipaty, S, Evans, MK & Rifkind, JM (2010) A fluorimetric semi-microplate format assay of protein carbonyls in blood plasma. *Anal Biochem,* 400, 289-94.
[http://dx.doi.org/10.1016/j.ab.2010.01.032] [PMID: 20122892]

Moon, JK & Shibamoto, T (2009) Antioxidant assays for plant and food components. *J Agric Food Chem,* 57, 1655-66.
[http://dx.doi.org/10.1021/jf803537k] [PMID: 19182948]

Morales, M & Munné-Bosch, S (2019) Malondialdehyde: Facts and Artifacts. *Plant Physiol,* 180, 1246-50.
[http://dx.doi.org/10.1104/pp.19.00405] [PMID: 31253746]

Mottaran, E, Stewart, SF, Rolla, R, Vay, D, Cipriani, V, Moretti, M, Vidali, M, Sartori, M, Rigamonti, C, Day, CP & Albano, E (2002) Lipid peroxidation contributes to immune reactions associated with alcoholic liver disease. *Free Radic Biol Med,* 32, 38-45.
[http://dx.doi.org/10.1016/S0891-5849(01)00757-2] [PMID: 11755315]

Murphy, TM, Vu, H & Nguyen, T (1998) The superoxide synthases of rose cells. Comparison Of assays. *Plant Physiol,* 117, 1301-5.
[http://dx.doi.org/10.1104/pp.117.4.1301] [PMID: 9701585]

Naguib, YM (2000) A fluorometric method for measurement of oxygen radical-scavenging activity of water-soluble antioxidants. *Anal Biochem,* 284, 93-8.
[http://dx.doi.org/10.1006/abio.2000.4691] [PMID: 10933861]

Niki, E (2010) Assessment of antioxidant capacity *in vitro* and *in vivo. Free Radic Biol Med,* 49, 503-15.
[http://dx.doi.org/10.1016/j.freeradbiomed.2010.04.016] [PMID: 20416370]

Park, S, Choi, S & Ahn, B (2016) DNA strand breaks in mitotic germ cells of Caenorhabditis elegans evaluated by comet assay. *Mol Cells,* 39, 204-10.
[http://dx.doi.org/10.14348/molcells.2016.2206] [PMID: 26903030]

Pazos, M, da Rocha, AP, Roepstorff, P & Rogowska-Wrzesinska, A (2011) Fish proteins as targets of

ferrous-catalyzed oxidation: identification of protein carbonyls by fluorescent labeling on two-dimensional gels and MALDI-TOF/TOF mass spectrometry. *J Agric Food Chem,* 59, 7962-77.
[http://dx.doi.org/10.1021/jf201080t] [PMID: 21630660]

Phaniendra, A, Jestadi, DB & Periyasamy, L (2015) Free radicals: properties, sources, targets, and their implication in various diseases. *Indian J Clin Biochem,* 30, 11-26.
[http://dx.doi.org/10.1007/s12291-014-0446-0] [PMID: 25646037]

Prasad, TK (1996) Mechanisms of chilling-induced oxidative stress injury and tolerance in developing maize seedlings: changes in antioxidant system, oxidation of proteins and lipids, and protease activities. *Plant J,* 10, 1017-26.
[http://dx.doi.org/10.1046/j.1365-313X.1996.10061017.x]

Prior, RL, Wu, X & Schaich, K (2005) Standardized methods for the determination of antioxidant capacity and phenolics in foods and dietary supplements. *J Agric Food Chem,* 53, 4290-302.
[http://dx.doi.org/10.1021/jf0502698] [PMID: 15884874]

Recknagel, RO, Glende, EA & Britton, RS (1991) Free radical damage and lipid peroxidation. *Hepatotoxicology,* 401, 436.

Sánchez-Moreno, C, Cao, G, Ou, B & Prior, RL (2003) Anthocyanin and proanthocyanidin content in selected white and red wines. Oxygen radical absorbance capacity comparison with nontraditional wines obtained from highbush blueberry. *J Agric Food Chem,* 51, 4889-96.
[http://dx.doi.org/10.1021/jf030081t] [PMID: 12903941]

Shacter, E (2000) Quantification and significance of protein oxidation in biological samples. *Drug Metab Rev,* 32, 307-26.
[http://dx.doi.org/10.1081/DMR-100102336] [PMID: 11139131]

Shacter, E, Williams, JA, Lim, M & Levine, RL (1994) Differential susceptibility of plasma proteins to oxidative modification: examination by western blot immunoassay. *Free Radic Biol Med,* 17, 429-37.
[http://dx.doi.org/10.1016/0891-5849(94)90169-4] [PMID: 7835749]

Shekhar, S, Jain, S & Priya, P (2019) Assessment of serum antioxidant enzymes superoxide dismutase (SOD) and glutathione peroxidase in oral submucous fibrosis. *Journal of Advanced Medical and Dental Sciences Research,* 7, 1-5.

Shinde, A, Ganu, J & Naik, P (2012) Effect of free radicals & antioxidants on oxidative stress: a review. *Journal of Dental and Allied Sciences,* 1, 63.
[http://dx.doi.org/10.4103/2277-4696.159144]

Shulaev, V & Oliver, DJ (2006) Metabolic and proteomic markers for oxidative stress. New tools for reactive oxygen species research. *Plant Physiol,* 141, 367-72.
[http://dx.doi.org/10.1104/pp.106.077925] [PMID: 16760489]

Sisein, EA (2014) Biochemistry of free radicals and antioxidants. *Scholars Acad J Biosci,* 2, 110-8.

Slaughter, MR & O'Brien, PJ (2000) Fully-automated spectrophotometric method for measurement of antioxidant activity of catalase. *Clin Biochem,* 33, 525-34.
[http://dx.doi.org/10.1016/S0009-9120(00)00158-2] [PMID: 11124337]

Smith, BJ (1994) SDS Polyacrylamide Gel Electrophoresis of Proteins.*Basic Protein and Peptide Protocols Methods in Molecular Biology*™ Humana Press 23-34.
[http://dx.doi.org/10.1385/0-89603-268-X:23]

Soares, C, Carvalho, ME, Azevedo, RA & Fidalgo, F (2019) Plants facing oxidative challenges—A little help from the antioxidant networks. *Environ Exp Bot,* 161, 4-25.
[http://dx.doi.org/10.1016/j.envexpbot.2018.12.009]

Soffler, C, Campbell, VL & Hassel, DM (2010) Measurement of urinary F2-isoprostanes as markers of *in vivo* lipid peroxidation: a comparison of enzyme immunoassays with gas chromatography-mass spectrometry in domestic animal species. *J Vet Diagn Invest,* 22, 200-9.

[http://dx.doi.org/10.1177/104063871002200205] [PMID: 20224077]

Takashima, M, Horie, M, Shichiri, M, Hagihara, Y, Yoshida, Y & Niki, E (2012) Assessment of antioxidant capacity for scavenging free radicals *in vitro*: a rational basis and practical application. *Free Radic Biol Med,* 52, 1242-52.
[http://dx.doi.org/10.1016/j.freeradbiomed.2012.01.010] [PMID: 22306582]

Tocmo, R, Veenstra, JP, Huang, Y & Johnson, JJ (2021) Covalent Modification of Proteins by Plant-Derived Natural Products: Proteomic Approaches and Biological Impacts. *Proteomics,* 21e1900386
[http://dx.doi.org/10.1002/pmic.201900386] [PMID: 32949481]

Utari, DR, Budiawan, & Auerkari, EI (2020) Detection of DNA *adduct 8-hydroxy-2'-deoxyguanosine* (8-OHdG) as a toxicity bioindicator to the effects of nickel on Ni-Cr alloy prosthesis users. *Saudi J Biol Sci,* 27, 1643-8.
[http://dx.doi.org/10.1016/j.sjbs.2020.03.006] [PMID: 32489306]

Valavanidis, A, Vlachogianni, T & Fiotakis, C (2009) 8-hydroxy-2' -deoxyguanosine (8-OHdG): A critical biomarker of oxidative stress and carcinogenesis. *J Environ Sci Health Part C Environ Carcinog Ecotoxicol Rev,* 27, 120-39.
[http://dx.doi.org/10.1080/10590500902885684] [PMID: 19412858]

Valko, M, Rhodes, CJ, Moncol, J, Izakovic, M & Mazur, M (2006) Free radicals, metals and antioxidants in oxidative stress-induced cancer. *Chem Biol Interact,* 160, 1-40.
[http://dx.doi.org/10.1016/j.cbi.2005.12.009] [PMID: 16430879]

Venkidasamy, B, Karthikeyan, M & Ramalingam, S (2019)

Vinson, JA & Zhang, J (2005) Black and green teas equally inhibit diabetic cataracts in a streptozotocin-induced rat model of diabetes. *J Agric Food Chem,* 53, 3710-3.
[http://dx.doi.org/10.1021/jf048052l] [PMID: 15853424]

Viuda-Martos, M, Ruiz Navajas, Y, Sánchez Zapata, E, Fernández-López, J & Pérez-Álvarez, JA (2010) Antioxidant activity of essential oils of five spice plants widely used in a Mediterranean diet. *Flavour Fragrance J,* 25, 13-9.
[http://dx.doi.org/10.1002/ffj.1951]

Aidi Wannes, W, Mhamdi, B, Sriti, J, Ben Jemia, M, Ouchikh, O, Hamdaoui, G, Kchouk, ME & Marzouk, B (2010) Antioxidant activities of the essential oils and methanol extracts from myrtle (*Myrtus communis* var. italica L.) leaf, stem and flower. *Food Chem Toxicol,* 48, 1362-70.
[http://dx.doi.org/10.1016/j.fct.2010.03.002] [PMID: 20211674]

Wei, A & Shibamoto, T (2010) Antioxidant/lipoxygenase inhibitory activities and chemical compositions of selected essential oils. *J Agric Food Chem,* 58, 7218-25.
[http://dx.doi.org/10.1021/jf101077s] [PMID: 20499917]

Yang, SA, Jeon, SK, Lee, EJ, Shim, CH & Lee, IS (2010) Comparative study of the chemical composition and antioxidant activity of six essential oils and their components. *Nat Prod Res,* 24, 140-51.
[http://dx.doi.org/10.1080/14786410802496598] [PMID: 20077307]

Yilmaz, Ö, Keser, S, Tuzcu, M, Güvenc, M, Cetintas, B, Irtegün, S, Tastan, H & Sahin, K (2009) A practical HPLC method to measure reduced (GSH) and oxidized (GSSG) glutathione concentrations in animal tissues. *J Anim Vet Adv,* 8, 343-7.

CHAPTER 6

Advances in Extraction and Profiling of Antioxidants

Gülşen Kaya[1] and **Merve Keskin[2,*]**

[1] *Scientific and Technology Research Centre, Inonu University, Turkey*

[2] *Vocational School of Health Services, Bilecik Seyh Edebali University, Turkey*

Abstract: The natural antioxidants are plant secondary metabolites that play a key role in preventing the development of various oxidative stress-induced degenerative and age-related disorders such as cardiovascular disease, cancer, *etc*. As a result, interest in these antioxidant compounds from natural sources has increased in recent years. For this reason, antioxidant substances in plants are extracted and presented to the market as a standardized solution. The first method of antioxidant extraction from plant sources is classical solvent extraction. Conventional solvent extraction takes place in two ways: liquid-liquid extraction and solid-liquid extraction. However, there are some disadvantages of using the classical extraction method to obtain antioxidants from plant sources. These methods use high amounts of solvents and require more time for extraction. Low selectivity, less efficiency, and environmental effects are some of the disadvantages. Therefore, the trend towards new extraction techniques has increased. Ultrasound-assisted, microwave-assisted, supercritical fluid, and accelerated extraction systems are very effective methods compared to conventional solvent extraction. These extraction procedures can be used in low temperatures and prevent the thermal degradation of antioxidants. In this study, the efficiency of new extraction methods and classical extraction methods are compared and the effect of extraction on antioxidant components has been compiled.

Keywords: Antioxidants, Catalase, Enzymatic antioxidants, Glutathione reductase, Microwave-assisted extraction, Natural antioxidants, Solid-liquid extraction, Soxhlet extraction, Supercritical fluid extraction, Ultrasound-assisted extraction.

INTRODUCTION

Sample preparation is a process that decides the qualitative and quantitative analysis of antioxidants. One of the indispensable steps of analytical processes is extraction. F. Soxhlet developed soxhlet extraction in 1879 with massive

* **Corresponding author Merve Keskin:** Vocational School of Health Services, Bilecik Seyh Edebali University, Turkey. E-mail: merveozdemirkeskin@gmail.com

Pardeep Kaur, Rajendra G. Mehta, Robin, Tarunpreet Singh Thind and Saroj Arora (Eds.)

popularity until mid-1980s and is still most routinely used procedure in laboratories. Demand for advanced extraction techniques has been increasing in recent years. As it is suitable for automation with reduced extraction time and consumption of organic solvents, thereby preventing pollution in analytical laboratories with reduced sample cost (Wan and Wong 1996, Eskilson *et al.* 2000).

The basic understanding of extraction principles has progressed in parallel with the development of new technologies. This progress led to new trends in sample preparation. These are the integration of sampling, separation and quantitation steps used in micro extraction, miniaturization and analytical processes (Pawliszyn *et al.* 2003). The required sample preparation depends on the nature of the sample and the analytical method used. Sample matrices can be classified as organic or inorganic and subdivided into solids, liquids or gases. For example, homogenization and drying are usually the first steps of the process. The next sample pretreatment step is usually extraction. For this purpose, the need for new extraction techniques that shorten the extraction time, reduce organic solvent consumption and prevent environmental pollution is increasing. Ultrasound-assisted, microwave-assisted, supercritical and accelerated extraction systems, which are used in the extraction of antioxidant substances from plants, are very fast and effective. In these techniques, the possibility of working at high pressure and / or high temperatures greatly reduces the extraction time.

ANTIOXIDANTS

Antioxidants are molecules that prevent the formation of free radicals or prevent damage to the cell by sweeping existing radicals and generally carry phenolic groups in its structure (Kahkönen *et al.* 1999). Antioxidants, at lower concentrations than oxidizable substrates severely hamper or delay the oxidation-induced stress. Pro-oxidants (reactive oxygen and nitrogen types, free radicals) are toxic substances that cause oxidative damage in lipids, proteins and nucleic acids, resulting in various pathological events and/or diseases. The presence of these dangerous compounds makes antioxidants important for a healthy life because antioxidants effectively reduce pro-oxidants into low-toxic or non-toxic products (Cao and Prior 1999). The most important factors that determine the place of antioxidants in human health are their chemical structure, solubility, structure/activity relationships and their availability from natural sources (Güçlü *et al.* 2009).

Antioxidants are produced by body cells and can be taken through foods as well. The main natural antioxidants present in foods that protect the human body from harmful free radicals are mainly vitamins (C, E and A), flavonoids, carotenoids and polyphenols. Studies show an inverse relationship between the consumption of fruits/vegetables and the occurrence of certain cancers and heart diseases (Kaur and Kapoor 2001). The most important antioxidants are polyphenols and their derivatives. These compounds can behave in different ways in the oxidative system. For example, they can reduce oxygen concentration by absorbing singlet oxygen, prevent the initiation of chain reactions using their ability to scavenge primary radicals, such as hydroxyl radicals and prevent the catalytic synthesis of pro-oxidants *via* metal ions (Shahidi *et al.* 1996). Antioxidants are oxidizable substances and can protect the biological macromolecules for a limited time only, and after a certain point, the biomolecule continues to oxidize as if there were no antioxidants in the environment. The reduction potential of antioxidants as hydrogen or electron donor is usually expressed as free radical scavenging (Kaur and Kapoor 2001). In an evaluation of chain-breaking antioxidant activity, both the number of electrons that the antioxidant can give per molecule or the number of free radicals it can remove (reaction stoichiometry) and the reaction rate (kinetics) are important (Rice-Evans *et al.* 1997).

Classification of Antioxidants

Cells are protected by antioxidants against oxidative damage caused by free radicals and peroxides under normal physiological conditions (Rice-Evans *et al.* 1997). Antioxidants are divided into two groups, natural and synthetic:

a. Natural Antioxidants: Natural antioxidants are classified as enzymatic and non-enzymatic.
  1. Enzymatic antioxidants are present in all plants, microorganisms and animals. These enzymes are as follows:
     i. Superoxide Dismutase (SOD): Superoxide dismutase (E.C.1.15.1.1) catalyzes single-electron dismutation of superoxide to hydrogen peroxide and oxygen (Chaudiere *et al.* 1999).
     ii. Catalase (CAT): Catalase (E.C.1.11.1.6) is a protein with a tetrameric structure of 240,000 daltons molecular weight, consisting of four subunits, each having a group of [Fe (III) -protoporphirin] in each subunit (Özkan *et al.* 2000). Catalase enzyme neutralizes hydrogen peroxide by converting it into water and oxygen. Although H_2O_2 formed as a result of SOD activity is not a radical, it can cause oxidative damage because it is the precursor of the most reactive species, ˙OH radical. Therefore, catalase facilitates the reduction of the hydrogen peroxide concentration by catalyzing the dismutation of two electrons of hydrogen peroxide into water and oxygen.
     iii. Glutathione Peroxidase (GPx): Glutathione peroxidase (E.C.1.11.1.4),

which is a class of selenoenzymes, is responsible for the protection against H_2O_2 induced oxidative stress. In this reaction, hydrogen peroxide is reduced to water and alcohol, while glutathione (GSH) is converted to oxidized glutathione (GSSG) (Chaudiere *et al.* 1999).

    iv. Glutathione Reductase (GR): Glutathione reductase (E.C.1.8.1.7) catalyzes the conversion of oxidized glutathione (GSSG) to reduced glutathione (GSH), which is formed by the reduction of hydroperoxides *via* GPx (Pektaş 2009).

    v. Glutathione-S-Transferase (GST): Glutathione-S-transferases (E.C. 2.5.1.18) form an antioxidant defense mechanism by showing selenium-independent GSH-Px activity against lipid peroxides, primarily arachidonic acid and lineolate hydroperoxides (Pektaş 2009).

2. Non-Enzymatic Antioxidants: Non-enzymatic natural antioxidants are found in almost all plants, microorganisms and animal tissues (Görünmezoğlu 2008). Natural antioxidants include phenolic compounds, and the most important are ascorbic acid, tocopherols, carotenoids, and flavonoids (Antmen 2005).

    i. Tocopherols (Vitamin E): It exists in nature in four different forms *i.e.,* α, β, γ, and δ. The most biologically common and active form of vitamin E is α-tocopherol. These oil-soluble but water-insoluble compounds are resistant to acid and temperature in oxygen-free environments. They contain a hydroxyl group that donates hydrogen atoms to free radicals and provides protection against oxidative stress (Antmen 2005).

    ii. Carotenoids: Red-yellow pigments found in plants and animal tissues. Carotenoids are highly complex C_{40} tetraterpenoids molecules formed by the combination of eight C_5 isoprenoid units. Most of the carotenoids in nature show antioxidant activity (Çöllü 2007).

    iii. Polyphenols: It is among the widest categories of phytochemicals in the plant kingdom. Dietary phenolic compounds include phenolic acids, phenolic polymers (commonly known as tannins) and flavonoids. The classification of these compounds is shown below (Fig. **1**).

b. Synthetic Antioxidants: Many researchers are in search of synthetic compounds with high antioxidant activity and no harm to the organism. Identical forms or derivatives of natural antioxidants, as well as artificial antioxidants, have been synthesized in the laboratory. Although hundreds of artificial antioxidant substances have been synthesized since the 1940s, only a few of them are used today (Eken 2007).

Antioxidants have become one of the most important subject in human nutrition.

The main properties that antioxidants should have are the following:

- It should be harmless to human health,
- It should be used in very small amounts so that it does not increase the cost,
- It must be dissolved or mixed well in the substance it will protect,
- It should not lose its effect during normal production (especially in high temperature applications (Sezgin 2006).

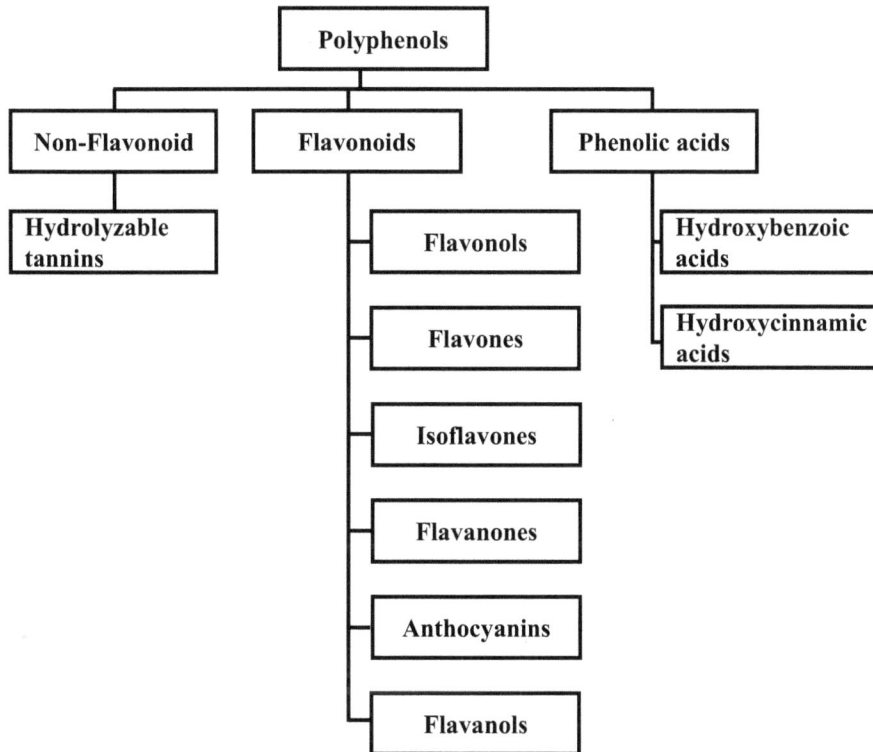

Fig. (1). Classification of polyphenolic compounds.

The amount of lipid free radicals increases as a result of storage, heating and digestion. Antioxidants prevent or delay lipid peroxidation. However, recent findings have shown that synthetic antioxidants can show toxicity, require high costs, and have less effect than natural antioxidants. For this reason, the search for natural antioxidants has increased considerably. Today, the use of stabilizing synthetic antioxidant compounds added to food and drugs is legally limited due to their harmful effects and natural antioxidant compounds are preferred instead. In addition, synthetic antioxidants have been observed to cause liver, lung and intestinal damage (Wanasundara and Shahidi 1998) and have a carcinogenic effect. The increasing interest in using natural products instead of synthetic compounds has led to an increase in the number of studies on plants.

CLASSICAL EXTRACTION METHOD (SOXHLET EXTRACTION)

Soxhlet extraction, performed in a special device, consists of a solvent bottle, a liquid flow tube (siphon) in the middle, condenser and a heating system (Fig. **2**). Solid samples are placed in the extraction chamber inside the middle circle. The solvent is put into the solvent bottle under it. The solvent is heated above the boiling temperature and the vapors from the boiling solvent are carried to the condensate where condensation occurs, condense and drip to the sample. As soon as the solvent level reaches the top of the siphon, the solvent begins to drip back into the solvent bottle and empties the entire sample container. Thus, the hot solvent circulates several times in the sample. While the analytes remain in the solvent bottle, the fresh solvent is evaporated. Solvents used in extraction are mostly pure organic solvents or mixtures thereof. Soxhlet extraction is generally used to remove organic compounds from solid samples. Solvents with boiling temperatures at which the compounds can be thermally stable are preferred. The cleaning of the sample chamber is one of the many problems encountered during this extraction method. It is recommended to use a clean solvent before each use (Kellner and Otto 2004).

Soxhlet extraction has some attractive advantages. The sample is in constant contact with the fresh solvent. Thus, it is easier to remove the component from the solid matrix. In addition, filtration is not required after extraction, and the amount of substance obtained can be increased by performing several simultaneous extractions. The major disadvantages of Soxhlet extraction compared to other solid sample preparation techniques are the use of large amounts of organic solvent and its long duration. Although it is expensive to dispose of the large amount of solvent used, it also constitutes the source of environmental problems. The extraction at the boiling temperature of the solvent may lead to the thermal degradation of some antioxidants. Since a large amount of solvent is used, the evaporation/concentration step is required for the preparation of extract. Modern extraction methods and green technologies have been developed as an alternative, due to the limited selectivity of solvent and difficult automation (de Castro and Garcia-Ayuso 1998, de Castro and Priego-Capote 2010). More sample mass can be extracted from other extraction methods (microwave-assisted extraction, supercritical liquid extraction, *etc.*) (Luque-Garcia and Castro 2004, de Castro and Priego-Capote 2010).

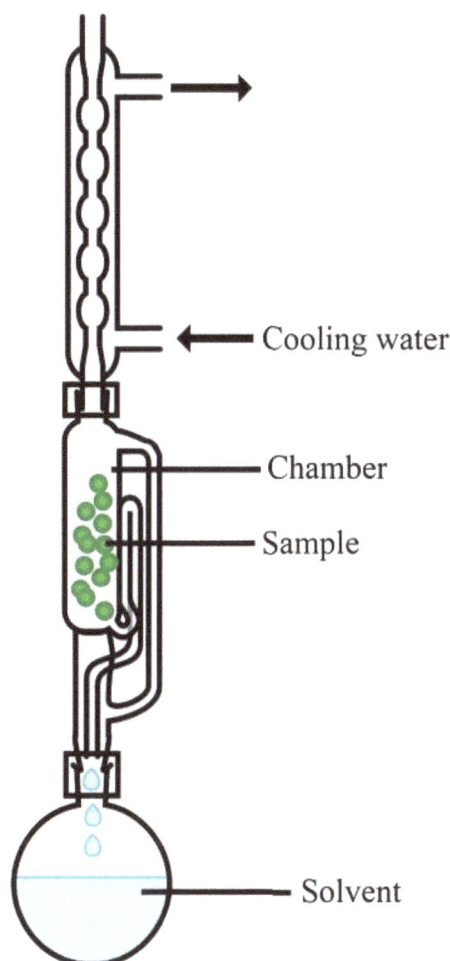

Fig. (2). Soxhlet extraction method.

MODERN EXTRACTION METHODS AND GREEN TECHNOLOGIES

Extraction is very important for industrial applications and analytical purposes. Studies in this field are mostly concentrated in the production of compounds such as anthocyanins and phenolic derivatives that enrich the functional properties of foods. The problems in classical extraction methods are long extraction time, high cost, high purity solvent requirement, the necessity of evaporation of large amounts of solvent, low extraction selectivity and thermal degradation of temperature sensitive components that have led to the development of new extraction techniques (Chemat *et al.* 2017). Green extraction methods developed as an alternative to traditional extraction methods are aimed to reduce solvent use and extraction time, as well as to increase efficiency. Green extraction techniques used for this purpose are microwave, ultrasound, high pressure, accent electric field, ohmic and supercritical fluid extraction techniques.

Pulsed Electric Field Assisted Extraction

The pulsed electric field (PEF) has been recognized as a useful method in the improvement of pressing, drying, extraction and diffusion processes over the past decade (Barsotti and Cheftel 1998, Angerbach *et al.* 2000, Vorobiev *et al.* 2005, Vorobiev and Lebovka 2006). The basic principle of PEF is to break the structure of the cell membrane and increase the effectiveness of the extraction by applying high electric field to the product placed between a series of electrodes for 1-100 μs. In the cell exposed to PEF, the molecules accumulate on both sides of the membrane surface according to their loads based on their dipole properties. Accumulating surface charges increase transmembrane potential and electromechanical stress. When the transmembrane potential exceeds a critical value of approximately 1 volt, repulsion occurs between the load-bearing molecules in the weak regions of the membrane and pore is formed. This causes an increase in the permeability intensity (Azmir *et al.* 2013).

In general, simple circuits with exponentially decaying pulses are used in the extraction of plants. The system has a processing chamber consisting of two electrodes where plant material is placed. Depending on the design and application of the processing chamber, PEF operates continuously or intermittently (Puértolas *et al.* 2010). PEF efficiency depends on various factors such as energy input, strength of electric field, temperature and properties of the material to be extracted (Heinz *et al.* 2003). Extraction time can be shortened and mass transfer can be increased by destroying the membrane structure of plant material by PEF application (Toepfl *et al.* 2006). PEF increases the cell membrane permeability and facilitates the release of intracellular compounds from plant tissue. It has been determined that PEF application in a moderate electrical field of 500 to 1000 V/cm for 102-104 seconds does not damage the cell membrane and increase temperature (Fincan and Dejmek 2002, Lebovka *et al.* 2002). Therefore, the degradation of heat-sensitive components can be minimized by PEF application (Ade-Omowaye *et al.* 2001). In addition, this application can be applied as a pre-treatment before classical extraction to reduce the energy and time consumed (López *et al.* 2009).

Fincan *et al.* (2004) suggests that PEF used for the extraction of betanin from beet roots performs a more effective extraction compared to processes such as freezing and mechanical pressing. Guderjan *et al.* (2005) applied PEF as a pretreatment and reported that the recovery of corn phytosterols increased by 32.4% and the recovery of genistein and daidzein isoflavonoids from soybean by 20-21%. PEF application increases the extraction of polyphenols and anthocyanins (Singh *et al.* 1999, Delsart *et al.* 2012). Corralesa *et al.* (2012) stated that they found the best result with the help of PEF among many methods used to extract the anthocyanins from grape wastes (stalks, kernels and bark).

Enzyme-assisted Extraction

Some phytochemicals in the plant matrix are dispersed in the cell cytoplasm, and some compounds are kept in the polysaccharide-lignin network with hydrogen bonds or hydrophobic bonds that cannot be accessed with a solvent in a routine extraction process (Azmir *et al.* 2013). Enzymatic pretreatment is seen as an effective way to release bound compounds or increase overall yield (Singh *et al.* 1999). The addition of specific enzymes such as cellulase, α-amylase and pectinase during extraction facilitate the cell wall breakdown and increases the hydrolysis of polysaccharides and lipid components (Singh *et al.* 1999, Latif and Anwar 2009). For enzyme-assisted extraction, there are two different applications: enzyme-assisted aqueous extraction and enzyme-assisted cold pressing. Enzyme-assisted aqueous extraction has been developed for the extraction of oils from various seeds (Singh *et al.* 1999, Rosenthal *et al.* 1996, Sharma *et al.* 2002). Since there is no polysaccharide-protein colloid system in the cold pressing rose-hip oil extraction from seeds, the enzyme-assisted extraction facilitates the hydrolysis of the cell wall enabling improved yield of oil (Concha *et al.* 2004). Besides the moisture content of the plant (Dominguez *et al.* 1995), parameters such as enzyme composition and concentration, particle size of plant material, solid to liquid ratio and hydrolysis time are key factors for enzyme-assisted extraction (Niranjan *et al.* 2004). Bhattacharjee *et al.* (2006) reported that this extraction method is an ideal alternative for the extraction of bioactive components from oilseeds as the enzymes are non-toxic and non-flammable. Enzyme-assisted extraction is an environmentally friendly technology as this method uses water as a solvent instead of organic chemicals (Puri *et al.* 2012).

Gómez-García *et al.* (2012) stated that the use of enzymes is an effective technology in the extraction of bioactive components from agricultural and industrial by-products. Maier *et al.* (2008) extracted phenolic acids, non-anthocyanin flavonoids and anthocyanins using a mixture of pectinolytic and cellulolytic enzymes in a 2:1 ratio and obtained higher yields than sulfite-assisted extraction. In a study for the recovery of phenolic antioxidants from raspberry pulp, it has been reported that adding enzymes to hydro-alcoholic extraction works better than non-enzymatic control (Lazore *et al.* 2010).

Microwave-assisted Extraction

Microwave-assisted extraction (Fig. **3**) is considered as a new method that can be used to extract components dissolved in liquid from the material using microwave energy (Azmir *et al.* 2013). Microwaves are electromagnetic fields in the range of 300 MHz to 300 GHz. Microwave-assisted extraction is mainly based on the effect of microwaves on polar molecules (Letellier *et al.* 1999). Electromagnetic energy is converted into heat by ionic conduction and dipole rotation mechanisms (Jain 2009). During ionic conduction, heat is formed as a result of the medium's resistance to the flow of ions. As the ions continue to migrate, they alter their directions according to the changing fields that cause intermolecular collisions and lead to heat generation (Azmir *et al.* 2013).

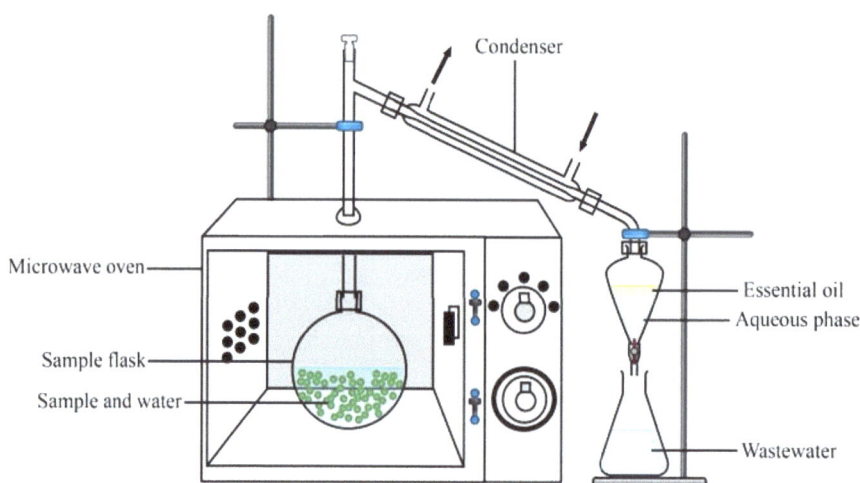

Fig. (3). Microwave-assisted extraction method (Kusuma and Mahfud 2016).

The microwave-assisted extraction mechanism includes three consecutive steps, as noted by Alupului (2012). The first step includes the separation of the components from the material matrix by increasing temperature and pressure. The second and third steps involve diffusion of the solvent through the sample matrix and the release of components from the material matrix dissolved in the solvent. Instant heating with increased extraction efficiency and smaller equipment are the advantages of the system for extraction of bioactive components from plant material (Cravottoa *et al.* 2008). In addition, because it reduces the use of organic solvent, microwave-assisted extraction method is described as an environmental friendly technology (Alupului 2012). Pan *et al.* (2003) stated that they obtained higher yields with microwave-assisted extraction process for extraction of polyphenols and caffeine from green tea leaves than other extraction methods applied at room temperature for 20 hours. Dhobi *et al.* (2009) achieved the highest efficiency with microwave-assisted extraction of flavolignin and silybin from *Silybum marianum*, as compared to the classical extraction techniques such as soxhlet and maceration. Asghari *et al.* (2011) reported that some bioactive components including cinnamaldehyde and guggulsterone from various plants were extracted faster and easier using the microwave-assisted extraction method than conventional methods. Wei *et al.* (2019) evaluated the *in vitro* and *in vivo* antioxidant activities of polysaccharides obtained from the false spindle (*Hippophae rhamnoides* L.) by microwave-assisted extraction. The researchers reported that the optimum polysaccharide extraction was obtained at 85 °C with 600 W microwave power for 6 minutes with a 10:1 liquid to solid ratio and revealed that 600 W microwave power provides high efficiency in the extraction of polysaccharides. In a study comparing microwave-assisted extraction and ultrasound-assisted extraction methods, natural phenolic compounds were extracted from lime (*Citrus aurantiifolia*) shells. It has been demonstrated that ultrasound-assisted extraction is more effective in obtaining natural antioxidant extracts than microwave-assisted extraction (Rodsamrana and Sothornvita 2019).

Pressurized Liquid Extraction

The method discovered by Richter *et al.* (1996) is known today by names such as accelerated fluid extraction, advanced solvent extraction or high pressure solvent extraction (Nieto *et al.* 2010). Pressurized liquid extraction is the application of high pressure to keep the solvent in the environment well above its boiling point (Azmir *et al.* 2013). Applied high pressure and temperature facilitate quick extraction with minimal use of solvents. The high extraction temperature increases the solubility and mass transfer while reducing the viscosities and surface tensions of the solvents, resulting in higher analyte solubility and thus increasing the extraction efficiency (Ibañez *et al.* 2012).

The method has been found to significantly reduce solvent and time as compared to conventional soxhlet extraction (Richter *et al.* 1996). According to Wang and Weller (2006), the pressurized liquid extraction technique can also be used effectively for removing organic pollutants from the environmental matrices at high temperatures. Ibañez *et al.* (2012) used the pressurized liquid extraction method for the extraction of bioactive components from sea sponges and reported effective results. In addition, the same researchers stated that the method is an environment-friendly extraction technique since the use of organic solvents is very low. Extraction of isoflavones from soybean was performed with this method without its degradation under optimized conditions (Rostagno *et al.* 2004).

Shen and Shao (2005) performed the pressurized fluid extraction of terpenoids and sterols from tobacco along with soxhlet extraction and ultrasound-assisted extraction as well. Researchers reported that, considering the yield, repeatability, extraction time and solvent use, pressure liquid extraction is less effective than the ultrasound-assisted extraction method, but it may be a good alternative to classical extraction methods. Unlike this research, Mroczek and Mazurek (2009) have optimized the pressurized liquid extraction conditions for the extraction of lycorine and galanthamine alkaloids and emphasized that the results are more efficient than hot solvent extraction, microwave-assisted extraction and ultrasound-assisted extraction. Luthria (2008) determined that parameters such as temperature, pressure, particle size, duration and sample to solvent ratio were highly effective on the pressurized liquid extraction of phenolic compounds from the parsley plant. Pressurized liquid extraction is also used in extraction of phenolic compounds such as catechin, gallocatechin, myricetin, epicatechin gallate, caffeic acid and chlorogenic acid from Anatolia propolis (Erdogan *et al.* 2011).

Supercritical Fluid Extraction

In nature, substances exist in solid, liquid or gaseous form. The supercritical state is distinctive, but it can only be achieved by keeping a substance under temperature and pressure above the critical point. The temperature and pressure values of the substance above the critical point are the characteristic of supercritical fluid where its distinctive gas and liquid phases do not exist (Inczedy *et al.* 1998). Since the specific properties of gas and liquid disappear in the supercritical state, the supercritical fluid can never be liquefied by changing the temperature and pressure (Azmir *et al.* 2013). Supercritical fluid is a gas-like compressible fluid with liquid-like density and solvating power. Supercritical fluid has low viscosity and high diffusivity. These properties enable the extraction of compounds with higher efficiency (Sihvonen *et al.* 1999).

A simple supercritical fluid extraction system has a mobile phase tank with CO_2, pump, solvent, solvent container, oven in which the extraction vessel is placed, a control device for measuring and maintaining the high pressure, and a capture unit. Generally, different types of meters, such as dry and wet gas meters can also be connected to the system (Azmir *et al.* 2013).

Carbon dioxide is the ideal solvent used in supercritical fluid extraction. The critical temperature and pressure of CO_2 are 31 °C (close to room temperature) and 74 bar, respectively. In general, the systems offer extractions to operate at moderate pressures between 100-450 bar (Temelli and Güçlü-Üstündag *et al.* 2005). The only disadvantage of carbon dioxide is that it is ideal for non-polar substances such as lipids and oils, but due to its low polarity, it is not suitable for most pharmaceuticals and medicinal samples. This negative situation is overcome by the use of chemical modifiers (Lang and Wai 2001, Ghafoor *et al.* 2010).

The main variables of supercritical fluid that affect the yield of bioactive components from plants are temperature, pressure, particle size, moisture content of the sample, extraction time, CO_2 flow rate and solvent to sample ratio (Ibañez *et al.* 2012, Temelli and Güçlü-Üstündag 2005).

Supercritical fluid extraction, which has become popular in the last 10 years, is frequently used in the extraction of active ingredients from materials such as leaves, flowers, seeds, and fruits. Supercritical fluid extraction has many advantages over conventional extraction methods. Since supercritical fluid has higher diffusion coefficient with lower viscosity and surface tension than other liquid solutions, it penetrates more into the sample matrix and significantly reduces the extraction time as compared to the conventional methods. A complete extraction is achieved by repeatedly returning the supercritical fluid to the sample. In conventional extraction methods, it is quite a time consuming effort to separate the solute from the solvent. The separation process in supercritical fluid extraction can be shortened easily by lowering the fluid pressure. It is an ideal method for the extraction of temperature sensitive components since it works at room temperature. Compared to conventional extraction methods, a small amount of samples can be studied with this method. Since a small amount of organic solvent is used with minimal waste generation, the method can be described as environment-friendly (Lang and Wai 2001).

The most important disadvantage of supercritical fluid extraction is the high investment cost for the system, as it works at high pressure above 80 atm (standard atmosphere). Another disadvantage is that 1-2% oxygen, even in the CO_2 tubes, which are considered pure, reacts with components such as antioxidants sensitive to oxidation, and causes their degradation, albeit in small amounts (Cocero *et al.* 2000).

One of the studies using supercritical fluid extraction is on the extraction of caffeine from the stems and fiber wastes of the tea by İçen and Gürü (2010). The researchers reported the maximum caffeine yield as 14.95 mg/g tea stem waste and 18.92 mg/g tea fiber waste. In a study of oil extraction from yarrow, supercritical fluid extraction was carried out at 10 MPa pressure and 40-60 °C temperature using CO_2. The essential oil obtained was found to contain camphor, 1,8-cineole, bornyl acetate, terpinen and terpinolen (Bocevska and Sovov 2007). Kavoura *et al.* (2019) reported that, in supercritical carbon dioxide extraction from greek sage (*Salvia fruticosa*) with the pressure between 100 bar and 280 bar at 60 °C, the extraction efficiency increased as the pressure increased. In a different study, Xu *et al.* (2011) extracted oil, carotenoid, squalene and sterols (campesterol, stigmasterol, β-sitosterol and β-amyrin) from the pollen by supercritical carbon dioxide extraction and determined the maximum yield at 38.2 MPa pressure and 49.7 °C.

Ultrasound-assisted Extraction

Ultrasound-assisted extraction method is a technique that enables the degradation of the plant cell wall by using ultrasonic waves. The mechanical waves propagate in an elastic environment and accelerate the mass transfer, obtaining the desired bioactive components in a shorter time with higher efficiency as compared to the conventional techniques (Fig. **4**). In addition, it is an environment-friendly technology with lower energy consumption and less solvent usage (Vilkhu *et al.* 2008, Jadhav *et al.* 2009). The ultrasound-assisted extraction method, which has gained popularity since 2010, is still used today (Poongothai *et al.* 2010, Dabre *et al.* 2011, Márquez-Sillero *et al.* 2013, Gliszczy´nska-Swigło *et al.* 2015, Benkerrou *et al.* 2018, Kurek *et al.* 2018).

EFFECTS OF EXTRACTION ON ANTIOXIDANTS

Antioxidant compounds, especially in the food industry, are added as additives to fat-containing products in order to eliminate the bitterness caused by lipid oxidation, prevent or reduce the formation of toxic compounds, maintain nutritional quality and prolong the shelf life of food. For this purpose, synthetic antioxidants such as butylated hydroxytoluene (BHT), butylated hydroxyanisole (BHA), propyl gallate (PG), tert-butyl hydroxyquinone (TBHQ) have been used as food additives for many years. However, toxic effects of synthetic antioxidants and therefore restrictions on their use, high production costs and increased consumer awareness have accelerated the research on the efforts to use natural antioxidants instead of synthetic antioxidants (Moure *et al.* 2001, Martínez 2007, Balasundram *et al.* 2006). Among the phenolic antioxidant sources, fruits and vegetables, seeds, cereals and tea leaves are the most studied one. Agricultural and industrial wastes are renewable, cheap and easy to access phenolic antioxidant sources. In obtaining these cheap and alternative natural antioxidants, the classical extraction methods require a long extraction time. Also, it has low selectivity and low extraction efficiency with large usage of toxic solvents. The obtained extract contains solvent residues in the extraction process (Kaur *et al.* 2019). The compounds sensitive to light, oxygen and heat may cause their autooxidation. These problems of classical extraction methods may lead to the degradation of antioxidants (Herrero *et al.* 2006). Therefore, in recent years, there has been a growing interest in the development of alternative energy-efficient technological processes that have minimal environmental impacts with efficient use of by-products for high-quality and safe end-products with less toxic residues and meet the legal requirements for CO_2 emissions. It is important to investigate the effects of these technological processes on antioxidants and the parameters that affect them.

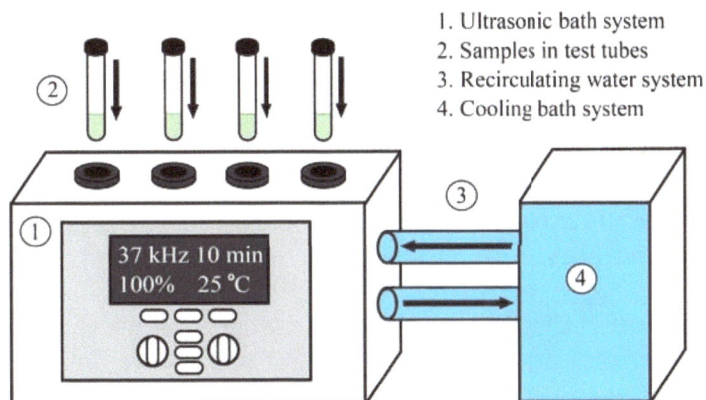

1. Ultrasonic bath system
2. Samples in test tubes
3. Recirculating water system
4. Cooling bath system

37 kHz 10 min
100%   25 °C

Fig. (4). Ultrasound-assisted extraction method (Che-Galicia *et al.* 2020).

In a study by Wang *et al.* (2014), subcritical water extraction of pectin from citrus peels and apple pulp was investigated. Antioxidant activities with physicochemical, rheological, and gelling properties of pectin extract were also investigated along with the effects of extraction temperature on these properties. The pectin obtained in the process was extracted without adding any acid or alkali. The maximum pectin yield extracted from citrus peel and apple pulp was determined as 21.95% and 16.68%, respectively. While no clear differences were observed in the FTIR spectra, differential scanning calorimetric (DSC) analysis showed that the endothermic properties of the pectin were affected by the extraction temperature and the exothermic properties were influenced by its structure and raw material. In addition, pectin produced from citrus peel and apple pulp reduced more than 60% of the DPPH radicals and 80% of the ABTS radicals *in vitro* and showed an extremely high growth inhibition rate of 76.4% and 45.23% against HT-29 (colon cancer cell), respectively.

Using the supercritical-carbon dioxide (SC-CO_2) and 10% (w/w) ethanol as the solvent, Farías-Campomanes *et al.* (2013) determined the economic feasibility required to perform large-scale operation in the recovery of phenolic compounds from grape pulp by supercritical fluid extraction at 313 K temperature and 20-35 MPa pressure. With the SC-CO_2 / ethanol extraction process, they obtained a higher concentration of phenolic extracts than conventional extraction methods. Qualitative analysis of the extracted compounds was clarified by thin layer chromatography (TLC) and HPLC analysis revealing syringic, vanillic, gallic, p-hydroxybenzoic, protocatechuic, p-coumaric acids and quercetin as the main components in extract. An economic evaluation of the process showed that the industrial supercritical fluid extraction (SFE) plant with a capacity of 0.5 m^3 would have a production cost of \$ 133.16/kg, where the targeted phenolic concentration is about 23 g/kg of extract.

In a study conducted by Yılmaz and Gökmen (2013), the chemical composition of cherry seeds was examined and it was emphasized that it could be a potentially valuable by-product in the food industry as a source of fat, protein and nutritional fiber. The study stated that sour cherry seeds obtained by traditional hexane extraction and SC-CO$_2$ extraction methods consist of 17.0% fat, 29.3% protein and 30.3% nutritional fiber. It was found that cherry kernel contains palmitic acid (6.4%), stearic acid (1.2%), oleic acid (46.3%), linoleic acid (41.5%) and linolenic acid (4.6%). It reported that the extraction technique used in the study did not have a significant effect on the composition of fatty acids. It was determined that the total amount of tocopherol and beta carotene extracted during the extraction process, where hexane was used as solvent, was more recovered by the SC-CO$_2$ extraction system. In both extraction techniques ethanol use as a co-solvent increases the total phenolic content, antioxidant capacity and beta carotene amount.

Juntachote *et al.* (2006) extracted the phenolic components from lemon grass (*Cymbopogon citratus*), galangal (*Alpinia galanga*), holy basil (*Ocimum sanctum*) and rosemary (*Rosmarinus officinalis*). The extraction efficiency and antioxidant properties of phenolic components were optimized using response surface methodology using three variables, ethanol to water ratio, temperature, and time. For extraction, ethanol to water ratio between 3:1-1:3 v/v, extraction temperature between 25-75 °C, and extraction time between 30-90 minutes was used. They found the optimum extraction conditions as 3:1 ethanol to water ratio at 25 °C for 30 minutes for lemongrass, 3:1 ethanol to water ratio for galangal and holy basil at 75 °C for 90 minutes, and 3:1 ethanol to water ratio for rosemary at 75 °C for 30 minutes. They found that the ethanol to water ratio was the independent variable that had the greatest effect on extraction efficiency, reducing power and total amount of phenolic substances. Temperature had significant effect on extraction efficiency of lemongrass and reducing power of galangal. A significant effect of temperature was observed on reducing power and total phenolic constituents of holy basil and rosemary. The extraction time only showed an effect on the reducing power of holy basil.

In another study, anthocyanin production from *Aronia melanocarpa* wastes was investigated with the ultrasound-assisted extraction method. D'Alessandro *et al.* (2014) examined the effects of temperature, ethanol concentration and ultrasound power on extraction efficiency at different times and found that the increase in temperature and ethanol concentration had a positive effect on 17 polyphenolic extracts. Ultrasound assistance was found to be more effective at the beginning of extracts and at low temperature in extraction of polyphenols. However, it was found that the extraction conditions performed at high temperatures decreased the efficiency of anthocyanin production.

Corbin *et al.* (2015) performed the extraction of lignan and other phenolic materials supported by ultrasound from flax seeds. This method reduced the formation of mucilage and increased the extraction efficiency. Optimum extraction conditions were achieved with the addition of 0.2 N sodium hydroxide solvent at 25 °C temperation and 30 kHz ultrasonic frequency for 60 minutes extraction. It has been determined that ultrasound-assisted method provides the highest phenolic content compared to other methods.

In the study, Virot *et al.* (2010) extracted phenolic substances from apple pulp. It was determined that ultrasound-assisted extraction achieved more than 20% efficiency as compared to classical extraction.

In a study by İnce *et al.* (2012), a microwave-assisted, ultrasound-assisted, conventional and maceration extraction of phenolic components from balm plant were compared. The extraction was carried out using a laboratory type microwave oven and water was used as a solvent. Microwave power kept constant at 400 W with different extraction times (5, 10, 15 and 20 minutes). Different solid to solvent ratios of 1:10, 1:20, and 1:30 g/ml were compared. The highest total phenolic amount was obtained at a solid to solvent ratio of 1:30 g/ml with 5 minutes extraction time. The highest phenolic content and antioxidant activity were observed in the microwave-assisted extraction. Also, it was revealed that extraction time was reduced by 83% with this procedure.

Bampouli *et al.* (2014) made a comparison of yield and antioxidant activity by using four different extraction methods (soxhlet, microwave-assisted, ultrasound-assisted and supercritical CO_2 extraction) from gum tree leaves. Samples were analyzed both fresh and lyophilized. The results show that extraction method and drying process have an important effect on extraction efficiency and antioxidant activity. While the highest yield is obtained from microwave-assisted extraction from fresh leaves, the highest antioxidant activity is provided by ultrasound-assisted extraction from fresh leaves. It has been reported that the high efficiency was obtained by performing supercritical fluid extraction at ambient pressure and low flow rate.

CONCLUSION

Using antioxidants from natural sources has increased. Therefore, antioxidant substances in plants are extracted and presented to the market as a standardized solution. To obtain these solutions, antioxidants should be extracted. The first method of antioxidant extraction from plant sources is classical solvent extraction. It has disadvantages like high amounts of solvent usage, time cosuming, low selectivity, low efficiency with environmental impacts. Therefore, the trend towards new extraction techniques (green extraction) has increased. Compared to conventional solvent extraction, microwave-assisted, ultrasound-assisted, supercritical fluid and accelerated extraction systems are very effective methods and can be used at low temperatures to prevent thermal degradation.

CONFLICT OF INTEREST

None declared.

ACKNOWLEDGEMENTS

None declared.

CONSENT FOR PUBLICATION

None

REFERENCES

Ade-Omowaye, BIO, Angersbach, A, Taiwo, KA & Knorr, D (2001) Use of Pulsed Electric Field Pre-Treatment to İmprove Dehydration Characteristics of Plant Based Foods. *Trends Food Sci Technol,* 12, 285-95.
[http://dx.doi.org/10.1016/S0924-2244(01)00095-4]

Alupului, A (2012) Microwave Extraction of Active Principles From Medicinal Plants. *UPB Science Bulletin, Series B,* 74

Antmen, E (2005) *Oxidative Stress in Beta Thalassemia.*

Angersbach, A, Heinz, V & Knorr, D (2000) Effects of Pulsed Electric Fields on Cell Membranes in Real Food Systems. *Innov Food Sci Emerg Technol,* 1, 135-49.
[http://dx.doi.org/10.1016/S1466-8564(00)00010-2]

Asghari, J, Ondruschka, B & Mazaheritehrani, M (2011) Extraction of Bioactive Chemical Compounds From the Medicinal Asian Plants by Microwave Irradiation. *J Med Plants Res,* 5, 495-506.

Azmir, J, Zaidul, ISM, Rahman, MM, Sharif, KM, Mohamed, A, Sahena, F, Jahurul, MHA, Ghafoor, K, Norulaini, NAN & Omar, AKM (2013) Techniques for Extraction of Bioactive Compounds From Plant Materials: A Review. *J Food Eng,* 117, 426-36.
[http://dx.doi.org/10.1016/j.jfoodeng.2013.01.014]

Balasundram, N, Sundram, K & Samman, S (2006) Phenolic compounds in plants and agri industrial by-products: Antioxidant activity, occurrence, and potentialuses. *Food Chem,* 99, 191-203.
[http://dx.doi.org/10.1016/j.foodchem.2005.07.042]

Bampouli, A, Kyriakopoulou, K, Papaefstathiou, G, Louli, V, Krokida, M & Magoulas, K (2014) Comparison of different extraction methods of Pistacia lentiscus var. chia leaves: Yield, antioxidant activity and essential oil chemical composition. *J Appl Res Med Aromat Plants,* 1, 81-91.
[http://dx.doi.org/10.1016/j.jarmap.2014.07.001]

Barsotti, L & Cheftel, JC (1998) Traitement Des Aliments Par Champs Electriques Pulses. *Sci Aliments,* 18, 584-601.

Benkerrou, F, Bey, MB, Amrane, M & Louaileche, H (2018) Ultrasonic-Assisted Extraction of Total Phenolic Contents from *Phoenix dactylifera* and Evaluation of Antioxidant Activity: Statistical Optimization of Extraction Process Parameters. *J Food Meas Charact,* 12, 1910-6.
[http://dx.doi.org/10.1007/s11694-018-9805-5]

Bhattacharjee, P, Singhal, RS & Tiwari, SR (2006) Supercritical Carbon Dioxide Extraction of Cottonseed Oil. *J Food Eng,* 79, 892-989.
[http://dx.doi.org/10.1016/j.jfoodeng.2006.03.009]

Bocevska, M & Sovov´, AH (2007) Supercritical CO2 Extraction of Essential Oil from Yarrow. *J Supercrit Fluids,* 40, 360-7.
[http://dx.doi.org/10.1016/j.supflu.2006.07.014]

Prior, RL & Cao, G (1999) *In vivo* total antioxidant capacity: comparison of different analytical methods. *Free Radic Biol Med,* 27, 1173-81.
[http://dx.doi.org/10.1016/S0891-5849(99)00203-8] [PMID: 10641708]

Chaudière, J & Ferrari-Iliou, R (1999) Intracellular antioxidants: from chemical to biochemical mechanisms. *Food Chem Toxicol,* 37, 949-62.
[http://dx.doi.org/10.1016/S0278-6915(99)00090-3] [PMID: 10541450]

Che-Galicia, G, Váquiro-Herrera, HA, Sampieri, Á & Corona-Jiménez, E (2020) Ultrasound-assisted extraction of phenolic compounds from avocado leaves (*Persea americana* Mill. var. Drymifolia): optimization and modeling. *Int J Chem React Eng,* 18
[http://dx.doi.org/10.1515/ijcre-2020-0023]

Chemat, F, Rombaut, N, Sicaire, AG, Meullemiestre, A, Fabiano-Tixier, AS & Abert-Vian, M (2017) Ultrasound assisted extraction of food and natural products. Mechanisms, techniques, combinations, protocols and applications. A review. *Ultrason Sonochem,* 34, 540-60.
[http://dx.doi.org/10.1016/j.ultsonch.2016.06.035] [PMID: 27773280]

Cocero, MJ, Gonzalez, S, Perez, S & Alonso, E (2000) Supercritical Extraction of Unsaturated Products: Degradation of Beta Carotene Supercritical Extraction Processes. *J Supercrit Fluids,* 19, 39-44.
[http://dx.doi.org/10.1016/S0896-8446(00)00077-2]

Concha, J, Soto, C, Chamy, R & Zuniga, ME (2004) Enzymatic Pretreatment on Rosehip Oil Extraction: Hydrolysis and Pressing Conditions. *J Am Oil Chem Soc,* 81, 549-52.
[http://dx.doi.org/10.1007/s11746-006-0939-y]

Corbin, C, Fidel, T, Leclerc, EA, Barakzoy, E, Sagot, N, Falguiéres, A, Renouard, S, Blondeau, JP, Ferroud, C, Doussot, J, Lainé, E & Hano, C (2015) Development and validation of an efficient ultrasound assisted extraction of phenolic compounds from flax (*Linum usitatissimum* L.) seeds. *Ultrason Sonochem,* 26, 176-85.
[http://dx.doi.org/10.1016/j.ultsonch.2015.02.008] [PMID: 25753491]

Corralesa, M, Toepflb, S, Butza, P, Knorrc, D & Tauschera, B (2008) Extraction of Anthocyanins From Grape By-Products Assisted by Ultrasonics, High Hydrostatic Pressure or Pulsed Electric Fields: A Comparison. *Innov Food Sci Emerg Technol,* 9, 85-91.
[http://dx.doi.org/10.1016/j.ifset.2007.06.002]

Cravotto, G, Boffa, L, Mantegna, S, Perego, P, Avogadro, M & Cintas, P (2008) Improved extraction of vegetable oils under high-intensity ultrasound and/or microwaves. *Ultrason Sonochem,* 15, 898-902.
[http://dx.doi.org/10.1016/j.ultsonch.2007.10.009] [PMID: 18093864]

Çöllü, Z (2007)

D'Alessandro, LG & Dimitrov, K (2014) Kinetics of ultrasound assisted extraction of anthocyanins from Aronia melanocarpa (black chokeberry) wastes. *Chem Eng Res Des,* 92, 1818-26.
[http://dx.doi.org/10.1016/j.cherd.2013.11.020]

Dabre, R, Azad, N, Schwämmle, A, Lämmerhofer, M & Lindner, W (2011) Simultaneous separation and analysis of water- and fat-soluble vitamins on multi-modal reversed-phase weak anion exchange material by HPLC-UV. *J Sep Sci,* 34, 761-72.
[http://dx.doi.org/10.1002/jssc.201000793] [PMID: 21384549]

Luque de Castro, MD & Priego-Capote, F (2010) Soxhlet extraction: Past and present panacea. *J Chromatogr A,* 1217, 2383-9.
[http://dx.doi.org/10.1016/j.chroma.2009.11.027] [PMID: 19945707]

de Castro, MDL & Garcia-Ayuso, LE (1998) Soxhlet extraction of solid materials: an out-dated technique with a promising innovative future. *Anal Chim Acta,* 369, 1-10.
[http://dx.doi.org/10.1016/S0003-2670(98)00233-5]

Delsart, C, Ghidossi, R, Poupot, C, Cholet, C, Grimi, N, Vorobiev, E, Milisic, V & Peuchot, MM (2012) Enhanced Extraction of Phenolic Compounds From Merlot Grapes By Pulsed Electric Field Treatment. *Am J Enol Vitic,* 63, 205-11.
[http://dx.doi.org/10.5344/ajev.2012.11088]

Dhobi, M, Mandal, V & Hemalatha, S (2009) Optimization of Microwave Assisted Extraction of Bioactive Flavolignan–Silybinin. *J Chem Metrol,* 3, 13-23.

Dominguez, H, Ntiiiez, MJ & Lema, JM (1995) Enzyme-Assisted Hexane Extraction of Soybean Oil. *Food Chem,* 54, 223-31.
[http://dx.doi.org/10.1016/0308-8146(95)00018-E]

Eken, S (2007) *Antioxidant Determinations in Some Materials.*

Erdogan, S, Ates, B, Durmaz, G, Yilmaz, I & Seckin, T (2011) Pressurized liquid extraction of phenolic compounds from Anatolia propolis and their radical scavenging capacities. *Food Chem Toxicol,* 49, 1592-7.
[http://dx.doi.org/10.1016/j.fct.2011.04.006] [PMID: 21530603]

Eskilsson, CS & Björklund, E (2000) Analytical-scale microwave-assisted extraction. *J Chromatogr A,* 902, 227-50.
[http://dx.doi.org/10.1016/S0021-9673(00)00921-3] [PMID: 11192157]

Farías-Campomanes, AM, Rostagno, MAA & Meireles, MA (2013) Production of polyphenol extracts from grape bagasse using supercritical fluids: Yield, extract composition and economic evaluation. *J Supercrit Fluids,* 77, 70-8.
[http://dx.doi.org/10.1016/j.supflu.2013.02.006]

Fincan, M, De Vito, F & Dejmek, P (2004) Pulsed Electric Field Treatment for Solid– Liquid Katı-Sıvı Extraction of Red Beetroot Pigment. *J Food Eng,* 64, 381-8.
[http://dx.doi.org/10.1016/j.jfoodeng.2003.11.006]

Fincan, M & Dejmek, P (2002) *In Situ* Visualization of the Effect of A Pulsed Electric Field on Plant Tissue. *J Food Eng,* 55, 223-30.
[http://dx.doi.org/10.1016/S0260-8774(02)00079-1]

Ghafoor, K, Park, J & Choi, YH (2010) Optimization of Supercritical Carbon Dioxide Extraction of Bioactive Compounds From Grape Peel (*Vitis labrusca* B.) by Using Response Surface Methodology. *Innov Food Sci Emerg Technol,* 11, 485-90.
[http://dx.doi.org/10.1016/j.ifset.2010.01.013]

Gliszczy'nska-Swigło, A & Rybicka, I (2015) Simultaneous Determination of Caffeine and Water-Soluble Vitamins ´ In Energy Drinks by HPLC With Photodiode Array and Fluorescence Detection. *Food Anal Methods,* 8, 139-46.
[http://dx.doi.org/10.1007/s12161-014-9880-0]

Görünmezoğlu, Ö (2008) *Comparison of Antioxidant Capacity of Apricot and Fig Fruit.*

Gómez-García, R, Martínez-Ávila, GCG & Aguilar, CN (2012) Enzyme-Assisted Extraction of Antioxidative Phenolics From Grape (Vitis vinifera L.) Residues. *3 Biotech,* 2, 297-300.

Guderjan, M, Töpfl, S, Angersbach, A & Knorr, D (2005) Impact of Pulsed Electric Field Treatment on the Recovery and Quality of Plant Oils. *J Food Eng,* 67, 281-7.
[http://dx.doi.org/10.1016/j.jfoodeng.2004.04.029]

Güçlü, K, Apak, R & Özyürek, M (2009) *Development of New Antioxidant Activity Determination Methods Based on the Sweep of Hydroxyl and Superoxide Radicals*

Hanmoungjai, P, Pyle, DL & Niranjan, K (2001) Enzymatic Process for Extracting Oil and Protein From Rice Bran. *J Am Oil Chem Soc,* 78, 817-21.
[http://dx.doi.org/10.1007/s11746-001-0348-2]

Heinz, V, Toepfl, S & Knorr, D (2003) Impact of Temperature on Lethality and Energy Efficiency of Apple Juice Pasteurization by Pulsed Electric Fields Treatment. *Innov Food Sci Emerg Technol,* 4, 167-75.
[http://dx.doi.org/10.1016/S1466-8564(03)00017-1]

Herrero, M, Alejandro, C & Elena, I (2006) Sub-and supercritical fluid extraction of functional ingredients from different natural sources: Plants, food-byproducts, algae and microalgae: A review. *Food Chem,* 98, 1136-48.
[http://dx.doi.org/10.1016/j.foodchem.2005.05.058]

Ibañez, E, Herrero, M, Mendiola, JA & Castro-Puyana, M (2012) Extraction and Characterization of Bioactive Compounds With Health Benefits From Marine Resources: Macro and Micro Algae, Cyanobacteria, and İnvertebrates.*Marine Bioactive Compounds: Sources, Characterization and Applications* Springer 55-98.
[http://dx.doi.org/10.1007/978-1-4614-1247-2_2]

İçen, H & Gürü, M (2010) Effect of Ethanol Content on Supercritical Carbon Dioxide Extraction of Caffeine From Tea Stalk and Fiber Wastes. *J Supercrit Fluids,* 55, 156-60.
[http://dx.doi.org/10.1016/j.supflu.2010.07.009]

İnce, AE, Şahin, S & Şümnü, SG (2012) Extraction of phenolic compounds from melissa using microwave and ultrasound. *Turk J Agric For,* 37, 6-75.

Inczedy, J, Lengyel, T & Ure, AM (1998) *Supercritical Fluid Chromatography and Extraction*

Jadhav, D, Rekha, BN, Parag, RG & Virendra, KR (2009) Extraction of Vanillin From Vanilla Pods: A Comparison Study of Conventional Soxhlet and Ultrasound Assisted Extraction. *J Food Eng,* 93, 421-6.
[http://dx.doi.org/10.1016/j.jfoodeng.2009.02.007]

Jain, T (2009) Microwave Assisted Extraction for Phytoconstituents – An Overview. *Asian J Res Chem,* 2, 19-25.

Juntachote, T, Berghofer, E, Bauer, F & Siebenhandl, S (2006) The application of response surface methodology to the production of phenolic extracts of lemon grass, galangal, holy basil and rosemary. *Int J Food Sci Technol,* 41, 121-33.
[http://dx.doi.org/10.1111/j.1365-2621.2005.00987.x]

Kähkönen, MP, Hopia, AI, Vuorela, HJ, Rauha, JP, Pihlaja, K, Kujala, TS & Heinonen, M (1999) Antioxidant activity of plant extracts containing phenolic compounds. *J Agric Food Chem,* 47, 3954-62.
[http://dx.doi.org/10.1021/jf990146l] [PMID: 10552749]

Kaur, P, Robin, , Mehta, RG, Singh, B & Arora, S (2019) Development of aqueous-based multi-herbal combination using principal component analysis and its functional significance in HepG2 cells. *BMC Complement Altern Med,* 19, 18.
[http://dx.doi.org/10.1186/s12906-019-2432-9] [PMID: 30646883]

Kaur, C & Kapoor, HC (2001) *Antioxidants in fruits and vegetables–theMillennium's health*

Kavoura, D, Kyriakopoulou, K, Papaefstathiou, G, Spanidi, E, Gardikis, K, Loulia, V, Aligiannis, N, Krokida, M & Magoulasa, K (2019) Supercritical CO2 extraction of Salvia fruticosa. *J Supercrit Fluids,* 146, 159-64.
[http://dx.doi.org/10.1016/j.supflu.2019.01.010]

Kellner, RMM, Otto, M, Valcarcel, M & Widmer, HM (2004) Sample Preparation.*AnalyticalChemistry: Modern Approach to Analytical Science* Wiley, Weinheim 506-8.

Kurek, MA, Karp, S, Wyrwisz, J & Niu, YG (2018) Physicochemical Properties of Dietary Fibers Extracted From Gluten-Free Sources: Quinoa (*Chenopodium quinoa*), Amaranth (*Amaranthus caudatus*) and Millet (*Panicum miliaceum*). *Food Hydrocoll,* 85, 321-30.
[http://dx.doi.org/10.1016/j.foodhyd.2018.07.021]

Kusuma, HS & Mahfud, M (2016) Preliminary study: Kinetics of oil extraction from sandalwood by microwave-assisted hydrodistillation. *IOP Conf Series Mater Sci Eng,* 128012009
[http://dx.doi.org/10.1088/1757-899X/128/1/012009]

Lang, Q & Wai, CM (2001) Supercritical fluid extraction in herbal and natural product studies - a practical review. *Talanta,* 53, 771-82.
[http://dx.doi.org/10.1016/S0039-9140(00)00557-9] [PMID: 18968166]

Laroze, L, Soto, C & Zúñiga, ME (2010) Phenolic Antioxidants Extraction From Raspberry Wastes Assisted by-Enzymes. *Electron J Biotechnol,* 13, 1-11.
[http://dx.doi.org/10.2225/vol13-issue6-fulltext-12]

Latif, S & Anwar, F (2009) Physicochemical Studies of Hemp (*Cannabis sativa*) Seed Oil Using Enzyme-Assisted Cold-Pressing. *Eur J Lipid Sci Technol,* 111, 1042-8.
[http://dx.doi.org/10.1002/ejlt.200900008]

Letellier, M & Budzinski, H (1999) Microwave Assisted Extraction of Organic Compounds. *Analusis,* 27, 259-70.
[http://dx.doi.org/10.1051/analusis:1999116]

Lebovka, NI, Bazhal, MI & Vorobiev, E (2002) Estimation of Characteristic Damage Time of Food Materials in Pulsed-Electric Fields. *J Food Eng,* 54, 337-46.
[http://dx.doi.org/10.1016/S0260-8774(01)00220-5]

López, N, Puértolas, E, Condón, S, Raso, J & Álvarez, I (2009) Enhancement of the Extraction of Betanine From Red Beet Root by Pulsed Electric Fields. *J Food Eng,* 90, 60-6.
[http://dx.doi.org/10.1016/j.jfoodeng.2008.06.002]

Luque-García, JL & Luque de Castro, MD (2004) Focused microwave-assisted Soxhlet extraction: devices and applications. *Talanta,* 64, 571-7.
[http://dx.doi.org/10.1016/j.talanta.2004.03.054] [PMID: 18969643]

Luthria, DL (2008) Influence of Experimental Conditions on the Extraction of Phenolic Compounds From Parsley (*Petroselinum crispum*) Flakes Using a Pressurized Liquid Extractor. *Food Chem,* 107, 745-52.
[http://dx.doi.org/10.1016/j.foodchem.2007.08.074]

Maier, T, Göppert, A, Kammerer, DR, Schieber, A & Carle, R (2008) Optimization of a Process for Enzyme-Assisted Pigment Extraction From Grape (*Vitis vinifera* L.) pomace. *Eur Food Res Technol,* 227, 267-75.
[http://dx.doi.org/10.1007/s00217-007-0720-y]

Márquez-Sillero, I, Cárdenas, S & Valcárcel, M (2013) Determination of water-soluble vitamins in infant milk and dietary supplement using a liquid chromatography on-line coupled to a corona-charged aerosol detector. *J Chromatogr A,* 1313, 253-8.
[http://dx.doi.org/10.1016/j.chroma.2013.05.015] [PMID: 23726354]

Martínez, JL (2007) *Supercritical Fluid Extraction of Nutraceuticals and Bioactive Compounds* CRC Press, United States Of America 402.
[http://dx.doi.org/10.1201/9781420006513]

Mroczek, T & Mazurek, J (2009) Pressurized liquid extraction and anticholinesterase activity-based thin-layer chromatography with bioautography of Amaryllidaceae alkaloids. *Anal Chim Acta,* 633, 188-96.
[http://dx.doi.org/10.1016/j.aca.2008.11.053] [PMID: 19166722]

Moure, A, Cruz, JM, Franco, D, Domınguez, JM, Sineiro, J, Domınguez, H & Parajó, JC (2001) Natural antioxidants from residual sources. *Food Chem,* 72, 145-71.
[http://dx.doi.org/10.1016/S0308-8146(00)00223-5]

Nieto, A, Borrull, F, Pocurull, E & Marcé, RM (2010) Pressurized Liquid Extraction: A Useful Technique to Extract Pharmaceuticals and Personal-Care Products From Sewage Sludge. *Trends Analyt Chem,* 29, 752-64.
[http://dx.doi.org/10.1016/j.trac.2010.03.014]

Niranjan, K & Hanmoungjai, P (2004) Enzyme-aided aquous extraction.

Pan, X, Niu, G & Liu, H (2003) Microwave-Assisted Extraction of Tea Polyphenols and Tea Caffeine From Green Tea Leaves. *Chem Eng Process,* 42, 129-33.
[http://dx.doi.org/10.1016/S0255-2701(02)00037-5]

Pawliszyn, J (2003) Sample preparation: quo vadis? *Anal Chem,* 75, 2543-58.
[http://dx.doi.org/10.1021/ac034094h] [PMID: 12948120]

Pektaş, İ (2009) *Investigation of the Effect of Plant Growth Regulators on Antioxidant Enzymes.*

Poongothai, S, Ilavarasan, R & Karrunakaran, CM (2010) Simultaneous and Accurate Determination of Vitamins B1, B6, B12 and Alpha-Lipoic Acid in Multivitamin Capsule by Reverse-Phase High Performance Liquid Chromatographic Method. *Int J Pharm Pharm Sci,* 2, 133-9.

Puri, M, Sharma, D & Barrow, CJ (2012) Enzyme-assisted extraction of bioactives from plants. *Trends Biotechnol,* 30, 37-44.
[http://dx.doi.org/10.1016/j.tibtech.2011.06.014] [PMID: 21816495]

Puértolas, E, López, N, Saldaña, G, Álvarez, I & Raso, J (2010) Evaluation of Phenolic Extraction During Fermentation of Red Grapes Treated by A Continuous Pulsed Electric Fields Process at Pilot-Plant Scale. *J Food Eng,* 119, 1063-70.
[http://dx.doi.org/10.1016/j.jfoodeng.2009.12.017]

Rice-Evans, CA, Miller, NJ & Paganga, G (1997) Antioxidant properties of phenolic compounds. *Trends Plant Sci,* 2, 152-9.
[http://dx.doi.org/10.1016/S1360-1385(97)01018-2]

Richter, BE, Jones, BA, Ezzell, JL, Porter, NL, Avdalovic, N & Pohl, C (1996) Accelerated Solvent Extraction: A Technology for Sample Preparation. *Anal Chem,* 68, 1033-9.
[http://dx.doi.org/10.1021/ac9508199]

Rodsamrana, P & Sothornvita, R (2019) Extraction of Phenolic Compounds from Lime Peel Waste Using Ultrasonicassisted and Microwave-Assisted Extractions. *Food Biosci,* 28, 66-73.
[http://dx.doi.org/10.1016/j.fbio.2019.01.017]

Rosenthal, A, Pyle, DL & Niranjan, K (1996) Aqueous and Enzymatic Processes for Edible Oil Extraction. *Enzyme Microb Technol,* 19, 402-20.
[http://dx.doi.org/10.1016/S0141-0229(96)80004-F]

Rostagno, MA, Palma, M & Barroso, CG (2004) Pressurized Liquid Extraction of İsoflavones From Soybeans. *Anal Chim Acta,* 522, 169-77.
[http://dx.doi.org/10.1016/j.aca.2004.05.078]

Sezgin, N (2006)

Shahidi, F (1996) *Natural antioxidants: chemistry, health effects, and applications AOCS Press, Champaign-Illinois 1-11* AOCS Press, Champaign, Illinois, USA 209.

Sharma, A, Khare, SK & Gupta, MN (2002) Enzyme-Assisted Aqueous Extraction of Peanut Oil. *J Am Oil Chem Soc,* 79, 215-8.

[http://dx.doi.org/10.1007/s11746-002-0463-0]

Shen, J & Shao, X (2005) A comparison of accelerated solvent extraction, Soxhlet extraction, and ultrasonic-assisted extraction for analysis of terpenoids and sterols in tobacco. *Anal Bioanal Chem,* 383, 1003-8.
[http://dx.doi.org/10.1007/s00216-005-0078-6] [PMID: 16231136]

Sihvonen, M, Järvenpää, E, Hietaniemi, V & Huopalahti, R (1999) Advances in Supercritical Carbon Dioxide Technologies. *Trends Food Sci Technol,* 10, 217-22.
[http://dx.doi.org/10.1016/S0924-2244(99)00049-7]

Singh, RK, Sarker, BC, Kumbhar, BK, Agrawal, YC & Kulshreshtha, MK (1999) Response Surface Analysis of Enzyme-Assisted Oil Extraction Factors for Sesame, Groundnut, and Sunflower Seeds. *J Food Sci Technol,* 36, 511-4.

Temelli, F & Güçlü-Üstündag, Ö (2005) *Supercritical Technologies for Further Processing of Edible Oils Bailey's Industrial Oil and Fat Products.*John Wiley & Sons, Inc.

Toepfl, S, Mathys, A, Heinz, V & Knorr, D (2006) Review: Potential of High Hydrostatic Pressure and Pulsed Electric Fields for Energy Efficiency and Environmentally Friendly Food Processing. *Food Rev Int,* 22, 405-23.
[http://dx.doi.org/10.1080/87559120600865164]

Wan, HB & Wong, MK (1996) Minimization of solvent consumption in pesticide residue analysis. *J Chromatogr A,* 754, 43-7.
[http://dx.doi.org/10.1016/S0021-9673(96)00537-7] [PMID: 10839139]

Wang, L & Weller, CL (2006) Recent advances in extraction of nutraceuticals from plants. *Trends Food Sci Technol,* 17, 300-12.
[http://dx.doi.org/10.1016/j.tifs.2005.12.004]

Wang, X, Chen, Q & Lü, X (2014) Pectin extracted from apple pomace and citrus peel by subcritical water. *Food Hydrocoll,* 38, 129-37.
[http://dx.doi.org/10.1016/j.foodhyd.2013.12.003]

Wanasundara, UN & Shahidi, F (1998) Antioxidant and pro-oxidant activity ofgreen tea extracts in marine oils. *Food Chem,* 63, 335-42.
[http://dx.doi.org/10.1016/S0308-8146(98)00025-9]

Wei, E, Yang, R, Zhao, H, Wang, P, Zhao, S, Zhai, W, Zhang, Y & Zhou, H (2019) Microwave-assisted extraction releases the antioxidant polysaccharides from seabuckthorn (*Hippophae rhamnoides* L.) berries. *Int J Biol Macromol,* 123, 280-90.
[http://dx.doi.org/10.1016/j.ijbiomac.2018.11.074] [PMID: 30445071]

Xu, X, Dong, J, Mu, X & Sun, L (2011) Supercritical CO_2 Extraction of Oil, Carotenoids, Squalene and Sterols From Lotus (*Nelumbo nucifera* Gaertn) Bee Pollen. *Food Bioprod Process,* 89, 47-52.
[http://dx.doi.org/10.1016/j.fbp.2010.03.003]

Vilkhu, K, Mawson, R, Simons, L & Bates, D (2008) Applications and Opportunities for Ultrasound Assisted Extraction in the Food Industry-A Review. *Innov Food Sci Emerg Technol,* 9, 161-9.
[http://dx.doi.org/10.1016/j.ifset.2007.04.014]

Vorobiev, E, Jemai, AB, Bouzrara, H, Lebovka, NI & Bazhal, MI (2005) *Pulsed Electric Field Assisted Extraction of Juice from Food Plants In Novel Food Processing Technologies* Crc Press, New York 105-30.

Vorobiev, E & Lebovka, NI (2006) Extraction of intercellular components by pulsed electric fields.
[http://dx.doi.org/10.1007/978-0-387-31122-7_6]

Virot, M, Tomao, V, Le Bourvellec, C, Renard, CMCG & Chemat, F (2010) Towards the industrial production of antioxidants from food processing by-products with ultrasound-assisted extraction. *Ultrason Sonochem,* 17, 1066-74.
[http://dx.doi.org/10.1016/j.ultsonch.2009.10.015] [PMID: 19945900]

Yılmaz, C & Gökmen, V (2013) Compositional characteristics of sour cherry kernel and its oil as influenced

by different extraction and roasting conditions‖. *Ind Crops Prod,* 49, 130-5.
[http://dx.doi.org/10.1016/j.indcrop.2013.04.048]

CHAPTER 7

Advances in the Profiling and Characterization of Antioxidants

Poonam Jaglan[1], Vikas Kumar[2], Priyanka Suthar[1], Anna Aleena Paul[1] and Satish Kumar[1,3,*]

[1] *Food Technology and Nutrition, School of Agriculture, Lovely Professional University, Phagwara, Punjab-144411, India*

[2] *Department of Food Science and Technology, Punjab Agricultural University, Ludhiana, Punjab-141004, India*

[3] *College of Horticulture and Forestry, Thunag- Mandi, Dr. Y. S. Parmar University of Horticulture and Forestry, Nauni, Solan (HP)-173230, India*

Abstract: The growing interest in plant foods as a source of phytochemicals in general and antioxidants like polyphenols in particular continues to receive a great deal of attention of nutritionists, food scientists and consumers as well. Food is no more regarded as just a source of energy and nutrition but is gaining importance as a functional or nutraceutical diet ingredient. The functional compounds are the secondary metabolites (PSM), produced by the plants as a natural defense against insect pest damage or adverse environmental conditions and represents a large and diverse group of bioactive compounds. PSMs are strong antioxidants that complement or improve the functions of antioxidant vitamins and enzymes which have a protective role to play in the bodily system against reactive oxygen and nitrogen species, UV light exposure, attack of pathogens, parasites and predators. Antioxidants are prophylactic compounds that can possibly even be used to cure several prevailing human diseases by traditional medicinal and health care system. Antioxidants are very sensitive compounds and their bioavailability in food is subject to their occurrence in food and the food processing conditions. The complexity in structure, function and expression of different antioxidants coupled with their frequent occurrence in different herbals from negligible to significant amounts, extraction, identification and their analysis remain a challenging task as ever for the scientists and technologists, despite the recent advances in the analytical and the instrumentation procedures. Keeping in view the high health potential and the related concerns, the current contribution is focussed on extraction, profiling, characterization, biological activity and implications of antioxidant consumption on human health to diversify food applications.

[*] **Corresponding author Satish Kumar:** Food Technology and Nutrition, School of Agriculture, Lovely Professional University, Phagwara, Punjab-144411, India; College of Horticulture and Forestry, Thunag-Mandi, Dr. Y. S. Parmar University of Horticulture and Forestry, Nauni, Solan (HP)-173230, India; E-mail: satishsharma1666@gmail.com

Keywords: Antioxidant activity, Biological activity, Characterization, Extraction, Plant secondary metabolites, Profiling.

INTRODUCTION

In the past decades, research conducted and publications dealing with antioxidants, their stability, bioavailability and potential application in human health and disease management reflected tremendous growth. Free radicals can harm DNA, lipids, proteins and negatively affect the aging process and diseases. Antioxidants are substances that neutralize the free radical chain reactions. Plants undergo various environmental stresses like nutrient deficiency, salinity, drought, UV radiation, temperature variations (heat shock, chilling, and frost), heavy metals, pathogen attacks and air pollution, from which they cannot escape. During these oxidative stress, reactive oxygen species (ROS) are formed such as superoxide radicals ($O_2{}^-$), singlet oxygen ($^1O_2$), hydroxyl radicals ($^\cdot OH$), and hydrogen peroxide (H_2O_2). The imbalance in the ROS equilibrium determines its toxic response in a stressed condition. These ROS molecules can attack high molecular mass compounds like DNA. Hence, ROS are capable of causing damage at the cellular levels and antioxidants are essential to scavenge these toxic molecules. Antioxidants act on the ROS and other free radicals to restrict or prevent various cellular damages from free radicals that are responsible for a variety of diseases. The recent research in plant sciences and nutrition has shifted its focus around various practices to protect crucial tissues and organs from damage induced by free these radicals. Mainly, four defence mechanisms of antioxidants suggested by McDowell *et al.* (2007) include (a) quenching active oxygen species, (b) preventive antioxidants, (c) sequestration of elements by chelation, and (d) free radical scavengers. The first mechanism explains the conversion of active oxygen species into a more stable form. For example, vitamin E and carotenoids are helpful in stabilizing singlet oxygen radicals. The second mechanism involves the suppression of free radical generation. The catalase enzymes inhibit hydrogen peroxide and prevent oxygen radical formation. The third mechanism of antioxidant activity suggests their strong bonding with trace minerals like Fe and Cu during protein transportation. These trace elements facilitate the formation of radicals. The fourth mechanism reflects the role of antioxidants in stabilizing free radicals as they donate electrons and oxidize themselves. This process is also referred to as "free radical scavenging." Vitamin E scavenges the peroxyl radical in a similar manner (McDowell *et al.* 2007). The effective action of antioxidants may vary with their activation energy, oxidation-reduction potential, rate constant, their susceptibility towards heat and their stability in various environmental conditions.

Plant tissues are under constant stress (oxidative) and continuously generate the free radicals. As a result, they develop an antioxidant system to protect themselves from free radicals attack. Various drought stressed plants are reported to synthesize low molecular-weight antioxidants, like α-tocopherol. Two types of antioxidants have been reported in the literature, including synthetic and natural antioxidants. Structurally, antioxidants have at least one aromatic ring and their activity greatly depends on a number of –OH groups present on these aromatic rings whereas, the arrangement of this functional group on aromatic rings is helpful in chelating peroxidative metals. The examples of synthetic antioxidants are BHT, BHA and propyl gallate that possess one aromatic ring. Natural antioxidants, ascorbic acid and vitamin E also possess one aromatic ring. However, phenols and other antioxidants possess more than one aromatic ring. Natural antioxidants have great diversity and generally, they include all bioactive compounds (Brewer 2011).

Naturally, each and every cell of the body has a defence mechanism against harmful effects of free radicals which involve various enzymes like superoxide dismutase, glutathione reductase, glutathione peroxidase, thiols and di-sulfide bonding. The theory of free radicals accelerates the broad interest in the bioactivity of antioxidants in preventing chronic disease like stroke, cancer, diabetes, arthritis and neurodegeneration in past few decades. The utilization of dietary antioxidants showed positive evidence especially in preventing fatal disorders like cancer and cardiovascular disease (CV). The traditional medicinal systems like Ayurveda, Siddha, Chinese medicinal system, *etc.*, include a wide range of plants for the treatment of many chronic diseases. These plant materials have therapeutic activity and are widely incorporated in the foods through which they enter the body system and interact with the living tissue (Biesalski *et al.* 2009). A vast range of diversity is available in plant compounds, including alcohols, aldehydes, alkyls, benzyl rings, and steroids, and all of them possess different characteristic features (Roessner and Beckles 2009). Further, the concept of nutraceutical and functional foods are trending in developed countries. These functional and nutraceutical foods claim their therapeutic effects due to the presence of bioactive compounds in high concentrations. The bioactive compounds are broadly classified as phenols, terpenes, saponins, alkaloids, vitamins, lipids and carbohydrates. In industries, antioxidants are required for wide spectrum applications *i.e.*, they restrict the deterioration of oxidative products in pharmaceuticals and cosmetics. In plants, the antioxidants are distributed in all parts like leaves, roots, stem/bark, fruits and fruit shells/peels, flowers and seeds. This is the reason behind the extensive study on whole plants for their therapeutic effects in the past few years. In traditional Indian diet, medicinal plants and spices are used which possess a high amount of natural antioxidants. Spices are rich in essential oils that have strong antioxidant properties. In view of the wide range of the applications of the antioxidants in both the food and non-food industries, the present chapter has been compiled to provide the readers with in-hand information about their distribution, functional importance, classification, characterisation, profiling and health apprehensions.

CLASSIFICATION

Antioxidants are classified into two broad classes- enzymatic and non- enzymatic antioxidants. A brief classification of antioxidants is depicted in Fig. (**1**).

Enzymatic Antioxidants

Enzymes play a significant role in eliminating toxic ROS in each cellular compartment. Superoxide dismutase (SOD), ascorbate peroxidase (APX), catalase (CAT), glutathione peroxidases (GPX) and glutathione reductase (GR) are well established as enzymatic antioxidants. The action mechanism behind the antioxidant activity of SOD is in scavenging superoxide radicals. Whereas, the combined effect of CAT and SOD effectively converts hazardous radicals $\cdot O_2^-$ and H_2O_2 to water molecules and thus minimizes the cellular damage. Also, many studies reported the increased activity of SOD under various stress conditions in plants. CAT is well known for converting $2H_2O_2$ molecules into $2H_2O$ and O_2. CAT is grouped into 3 classes, where class 1 CAT is involved in eliminating hydrogen peroxides from photosynthetic tissues. Class 2 and class 3 CAT are produced in vascular tissues and seeds. CAT is directly involved in the detoxification of ROS induced by hydrogen peroxide during a stress environment. Similarly, GPX and APX are reported with their effective involvement in the elimination of hydroperoxides radicals and convert them into non-toxic water molecules. The activity of GR is in increasing the ratio of NADP+/NADPH which ensures NADP+ bioavailability to accept the electrons and minimize the formation of O_2^- (Ahmad *et al.* 2010). These enzymes (SOD, CAT and GPX) effectively remove superoxide and peroxides radicals and restrict their further metal catalyzed reactions which in turn generate ROS. The chain breaking antioxidants like vitamin E terminates the chain reaction propagation (Matés *et al.* 1999).

Non Enzymatic Antioxidants

Non-enzymatic antioxidants are categorized into 3 important classes *i.e.*, plant secondary metabolites (PSM), minerals and vitamins.

Plant Secondary Metabolites

As discussed above, under stress conditions plants produce some defensive compounds and express them. Plant secondary metabolites are among such compounds and hence are majorly used during oxidative stress conditions. These metabolites are further divided into 6 broad categories *i.e.*, phenols, alkaloids, terpenoids, lipids, saponins and plant sugar (carbohydrates). All plant secondary metabolites are termed "bioactive compounds." All these compounds are discussed hereunder for their potential antioxidant activities.

Polyphenols

Polyphenols are secondary metabolites which are produced by the plants to prevent themselves from various stress conditions. These are important for human beings as well, as they are linked to lower risk of chronic diseases like cardiovascular diseases, degenerative diseases, arthritis, asthma, cancer, chronic obstructive pulmonary disease, diabetes and some viral diseases such as hepatitis C and acquired immunodeficiency syndrome (Duthie and Brown 1994, Milner 1994). Polyphenols are regarded as the oxidation chain-breakers which donate the extra electron from their configuration to the free radical to neutralize it and themselves becoming stable (less reactive) radicals, thus stopping the chain reactions (Guo *et al.* 2009, Pietta 2000, Rice-Evans *et al.* 1996). Other than free radical scavengers, polyphenols are also called chelators. Chelation of transition metals directly reduces the rate of reaction by preventing oxidation reaction. Polyphenols are not supposed to act alone but they function as co-antioxidants and are also involved in the regeneration of the essential vitamins (McHugh and Krukonis 1986).

Polyphenols are broadly classified as flavonoids and non flavonoids. Flavonoids account for around 60% of all polyphenols. Examples include quercetin, kaempferol, catechins, and anthocyanins, which are found in foods like apples, onions, dark chocolate and red cabbage. The basic structure of flavonoids is aglycone; however, in plants, most of these compounds exist as glycosides. The biological activities of these compounds depend on both the structural difference and the glycosylation patterns. Anthocyanins are reported in different colored fruits and vegetables and are responsible for the characteristic red, purple or blue color. The example of anthocyanin rich fruits are grapes and cranberries. Initially, anthocyanins were known for their colored pigments but now the interest has shifted towards their potential role in preventing fatal diseases such as CVD, cancer, inflammation, diabetes and many more. Also, the stability of these antioxidant compounds is challenging and various improvements have been tried for ensuring their bioavailability such as encapsulation (Yousuf *et al.* 2016).

Quercetin is the most common and abundant flavonol widely distributed among various plant organs. This compound received great attention due to its strong free radical quenching activity and its bonding with transition metal ions. The processing of food significantly affects the bioavailability of quercetin due to its thermal degradability (Bentz 2017).

Phenolic acids are another popular group of flavonoids which accounts for around 30% of all polyphenols. Examples include stilbenes and lignans, which are mostly found in fruits, vegetables, whole grains, and seeds particularly in the bran or hull in which the phenolic acids are often in the bound form. These phenolic acids can only be freed or hydrolyzed upon acid or alkaline hydrolysis, or by enzymes. Tannins are classified under simple phenols with molecular weight between 500 to 3000 D. As reported, tannins in legumes play significant role in plant defense system when introduced under oxidative stress environment. Tannins are present in condensed form in various seed coats and beans (Singh *et al.* 2017). Coumarins are another example of simple phenols which are involved in health promoting activities. Coumarins and their derivatives are strong free radical scavengers and thereby, act as antioxidants. These are thermally stable hence possess wide applicability in food, cosmetic or pharmaceutical industries (Al-Majedy *et al.* 2017). Resveratrol, a polyphenol found in red wine plays a critical role in inhibiting LDL oxidation. Raspberries are rich in ellagic acid and are present in 3 most common forms *i.e.*, free ellagic acid, ellagic acid glycosides and ellagitannins. The curcumin from turmeric is extensively reported in past 2 decades and is used widely in pharmaceutical industries. It is a yellow phenolic compound which possesses antioxidant activity both *in vivo* and *in vitro* experiments. Polyphenolic amides include capsaicinoids in chilli peppers and avenanthramides in oats. The hotness of chilli powder is because of the presence of the capsaicinoids only. It is a strong antioxidant and anti-inflammatory substance.

Terpenoids

Terpenoids are plant secondary metabolites and are further subdivided as monoterpene, diterpene, and so on based on the number of isoprene units present. In general, terpenoids are versatile in their bioactivity and possess potential effect against cancer and brain related disorders. The terpenoids from mushrooms are well established as antitumor agents (Dasgupta and Acharya 2019). Sometimes, they are classified as carotenoids and non-carotenoids. In carotenoid class, lycopene and β-carotene are most popular. Mostly carotenoids are coloured molecules. Dietary sources of lycopene are tomato, watermelon, guava, *etc.* Lycopene is a heat stable and potent antioxidant which reduces the risk associated with ischemic stroke. Other carotenoids like zeaxanthin and lutein also showed protective effects against oxidative damages and contributed in lowering the risk related with stroke and CVD in humans (Bahonar *et al.* 2017). The non-carotenoid class includes limonene which is monocyclic monoterpene and is colorless. It is present abundantly in citrus family plants like lemon, grape, orange and mandarin. It acts as a gastroprotective, antioxidant, anti-diabetic, antitumour and anti-inflammatory agent (Ashrafizadeh *et al.* 2020).

Alkaloids

Another class of secondary metabolites of plants are alkaloids. They possess bioactivity majorly in plants related to *Solanaceae* family. They are N-containing compounds and generally heat stable. They can be very toxic in nature and can be fatal even at low doses. More than 12,000 alkaloids are already reported. *Solanaceae*, *Convolvulaceae*, *Erythroxylaceae*, *Euphorbiaceae*, *Proteaceae*, *Brassicaceae* and *Rhizophoraceae* are common representative families of various alkaloids. Alkaloid berberine is reported with its significant role in treating diabetes, tumor, inflammation, hyperlipidemia, hepatotoxicity and mental diseases (Imenshahidi and Hosseinzadeh 2016). Alkaloid mahanimbine is extracted from roots and stem bark of *Murraya koenigii* and is utilized in treating cancer, inflammation and diabetes (Ng *et al.* 2018).

Saponins

Previously, saponins were classified as antinutrients due to their fungitoxic, hemolytic and membranolytic activity. In past few years, studies reported their active role in promoting human health. They are non-volatile compounds with polar sugar and non-polar algycone molecules. Major dietary sources of saponins are pulses. They are concentrated mainly in seed coat, hypocotyl, plumule and radicle of plants. Many studies claim their potential antioxidant, anticancerous, antimutagenic, hepatoprotective and neuroprotective effects. Saponins showed strong scavenging activity against superoxide radicals, which are initiator of various chronic diseases. The bioavailability of saponins is reduced during the soaking, sprouting and cooking. Though this processing results in great loss in saponin content, leftover saponins are sufficient to exert their therapeutic effects in human health (Singh *et al.* 2017). Saponins like astragaloside IV, glycyrrhizic acid, elatoside C, asperosaponin VI, trillin, tribulosin, protodioscin and platycodin D play critical role in enhancing activity of enzymatic antioxidants like SOD, CAT and GPX, thereby, promoting antioxidant defence mechanism against reactive oxygen species (Singh and Chaudhuri 2018).

Lipids

Steroids, phytosterols, phytoestrogens, polyacetylesnes, waxes, *etc.*, are lipid-based plant secondary metabolites. Due to their structural similarity with cholesterol, phytosterols and stanols can be replaced with cholesterol in human diet. This led to the low cholesterol absorption in intestine. Also, plant seeds have squalene which acts as an antioxidant. The lipid secondary metabolites stanols (sterol) are involved in diet as sistostanol, sitosterol, campesterol, campestanol and stigmasterol. They are reported with their positive activities which include low CVD risk and reduced hepatic inflammation. The common physterols enriched food products are milk, chocolates, cheese and spreads. Flaxseeds are important source of phytosterol, majorly β-sitosterol. These compounds reported their positive role against diabetes and CVD. The rice bran oil has avenasterols, which is a well-established potential antioxidant at high temperature.

Carbohydrates

Carbohydrates are important source of energy in plants and humans. Carbohydrates have ketone and aldehydes as their functional group and they can be hydrolysed to form polyhydroxy ketones and aldehydes. Various studies have reported anti-tumour, antiviral and immunomodulatory effects of polysaccharides. Polysaccharides are novel source of antioxidant (Hu *et al.* 2016). Very few studies are available on the antioxidant activity of highly purified polysaccharides. Fructans are defined as non-reducing sugars or carbohydrates with fructosyl unit and one glucose molecule as a terminator. The soluble dietary fibre, fructans are recently studied for their antioxidant activities in rats. The high oligofructose diet given to rats showed pro-oxidative effects. The representatives of fructans rich plants are garlic, onion, leek, asparagus and chicory roots (Franco-Robles and López 2015).

Minerals

Minerals are inorganic molecules required by the body in small amount and act as co-factors for antioxidant enzymes. Zinc is one such example, which possess active role in SOD, responsible for expression of metallothionein and manage the glutathione metabolism. Zinc also competes with other minerals like Fe and Cu in cell for binding with NADPH-oxidase enzyme. A study reported that diabetic mice

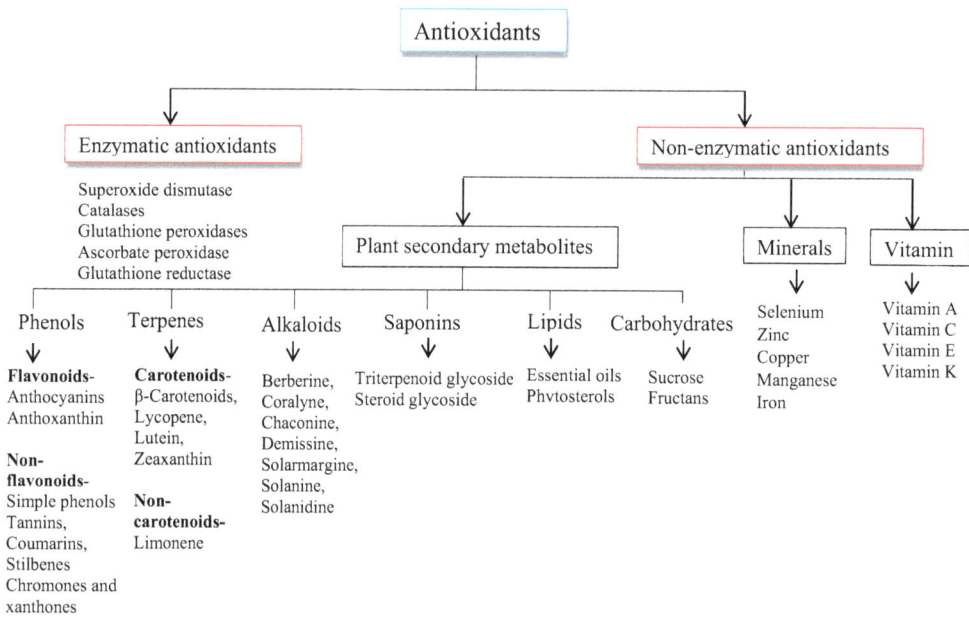

Fig. (1). Classification of antioxidants in plants.

supplemented with zinc showed elevated SOD activity in pancreas and blood serum (Cruz *et al.* 2015). Also, selenium or selenoprotein P showed defensive action against LDL oxidation due to free radicals in blood serum (Tinggi 2008). Iron is reported with its active role in CAT and helps in conversion of hydrogen peroxide to water.

Vitamins

Vitamins are the essential organic molecules, which play a significant role in metabolism activity. Vitamin A, B-complex, C, D, E and K are existing types of vitamin. Among them, A, C, E and K are recognized for their antioxidant activities. The carotenoids are the precursor for Vitamin A synthesis. Vitamin C and E restrict peroxyl radicals efficiently thereby, protecting lipids in tissues from the reactive oxygen species. Major sources of vitamin E are vegetable oils, nuts (peanuts, almonds) and seeds. Another vitamin K is mostly present in leafy vegetables and is available in diet in two forms phyllquinone and menaquinones. The special compound Vitamin K- hydroquinone could act as potent antioxidant.

EXTRACTION, PROFILING AND CHARACTERIZATION OF ANTIOXIDANTS

Prehistorically, food has been given prime importance and records states that during 2000 BC, philosophers advised that food is a medicine, even though the components consumed through herbs, fruits, vegetables, spices, milk, wine, *etc.*, were unknown to humans. Studies were conducted by truth-seekers to verify the facts of their therapeutic potential. This gave ascend in folk-medicines, where people started consuming concentrated and diluted forms of herbs and different parts of plants. Later, concentration pills and now concepts of functional compounds and nutraceutical came into existence. This sum-up history itself is a proof that from medieval period different types of extraction techniques were developed for extracting various bioactive compounds from the plants for various therapeutic applications. With the increase in knowledge on biologically active components, scientists and researchers started characterization and profiling of each molecule. Application of these bioactive components in food, nutraceutical, pharmaceutical and cosmetic industries affected the extraction techniques directly and indirectly from conventional methods (maceration, distillation, reflux extraction methods, *etc.*) to advanced technologies (chromatographic techniques, hyphenated systems).

The traditional and the conventional methods of isolation of polyphenols are now being replaced by the modern techniques (Kenz 2016). The technique to be used for isolation of specific compounds depends on the nature, sample size and the presence of the substances which can interfere in the isolation. The yield of the extraction is affected by the parameters like temperature, extraction time, number of repeated extractions of the sample, solvent-to feed ratio, and the choice of extraction solvents. Solubility depends on the temperature and extraction time. High temperature lowers the viscosity and surface tension of the solvents and increases solubility and mass transfer velocities (Brunner 1994 2005). Prior to extraction of the polyphenols, the sample materials are subjected to homogenisation, grinding, milling and drying. The different kinds of drying techniques are responsible for the phenolic content during extraction. However, freeze drying technique retains the higher amount of phenolic content in plant samples relatively (Abascal *et al.* 2005). Some commonly practiced extraction methods used for characterization and profiling of antioxidants are illustrated in Fig. (**2**). Precise information on various extraction protocols has been presented hereunder.

Conventional Methods of Extraction

Extraction techniques have been using for centuries when some are modified and developed to new and economical level, whilst very few are applied in a similar pattern. Though, the technologies are developed, yet the conventional methods play a vital role in the utilization of bioactive compounds, especially in small-scale. For instance, house-hold and primary laboratory procedures for extracting polyphenolic and other active biological compounds are mostly through conventional methods such as decoction, digestion, distillation, solvent extraction, soxhlet extraction, *etc*. Key factor for efficient extraction is the solvent used for the procedure (Azmir *et al.* 2013). For small scale purposes, simple extraction procedures were adopted. Therefore, according to its easiness to carry out, process conditions like temperature, pressure, solvents, *etc.*, available instruments and sample, we can classify them into various methods. That is, oils can be easily extracted through pressing methods; based on the boiling point of desired component, distillation process can be suggested; and for better result achievement, solvent extraction techniques are advised. Even though there are several disadvantages of conventional extraction methods over modern methods; liquid-liquid and solid- liquid are commonly used because of the ease to handle and use, high efficiency and wide range of applicability (Qiu *et al.* 2010, Stalikas 2007). In both the processes, conventional solvents are used, for instance acetone, methanol, ethanol, diethyl ether and acetate along with the mixture of water with different dilutions.

The demand for foods, spices and herbs is increasing day-to-day, which indirectly gives rise to related industries and allied sectors. Now, we know, most of the components that are antioxidant in nature are lost during various processing operations in the form of waste/ residues generated from the processing industries. In this stage, cold pressing (CP) extraction, which is considered one of the best conventional methods for oil extraction, can be utilized at room temperature. Also, this technique is easy, simple, convenient and easy to handle for achieving product within short period of time, produces a protein-rich cake as by-product. Also, oil obtained using pressing method can be consumed directly. Use of mechanical extraction technique has therefore benefit over methods that require temperature (can cause degradation of antioxidant compounds), solvents (can be toxic or expensive during disposal), and complex procedures (Çakaloğlu *et al.* 2018). However, limitations like difficulty in separation and quantification of components, incapability for extracting other antioxidant components and selectivity are some of the drawbacks faced by mechanical conventional extraction methods.

Distillation is another method used for extraction of essential oils. Working of this technique utilizes the property of volatility of many antioxidants at given temperature conditions. Thus, transferring required antioxidant molecule to its vapour phase and then combining with steam produced during distillation process is an effective extraction method (*e.g.* in steam distillation, essential oils that have boiling point lower than 100 °C are appropriate) (Çakaloğlu *et al.* 2018). Similar to mechanical cold-press extraction method, distillation has some limitations, except, separation of a limited number of components is possible. The fact that possibility of extraction at room temperature is the reason why maceration and percolation stand out among other conventional methods, but long processing time and inefficiency make researchers to approach other methods (Zhang *et al.* 2018). Decoction is the simple and conveniently used extraction technique, as water – 'universal solvent' is mostly used for this purpose. This method was adopted by our ancestors mainly for extracting beneficial compounds from herbs (roots, barks and seeds) as medicines. Boiling for a long period of time (till the mixture reduces to its half volume), many phytochemicals oozes into the water and was consumed orally in concentrated, dilute, or dried forms by our previous generations (Yifan and Jeremy 2010). However, studies proved that drawbacks, like the presence of water, loss of insoluble volatile and heat sensitive antioxidants, long processing time and chances of side reaction due to heat, makes the decoction method inadequate (Pandey and Tripathi 2014).

Among various techniques, Soxhlet Extraction also known as 'Hot Continuous Extraction' is the technique that can successfully compete latest techniques like microwave assisted and supercritical fluid extractions in terms of more extractable sample mass. In 1879, Franz von Soxhlet developed a new system (Soxhlet extractor) for extraction which was originally developed for determining fat in milk and not only has it been used till date, but also this process is kept as a standard to all other leaching techniques. Also, no filtration is required as evaporation of solvent takes place as one of the step. Even though it is a batch process, due to the recirculation of extractant through sample makes it to operate in a continuous manner. Nonetheless, the soxhlet extraction method has various drawbacks as extraction requires long-time run at high temperature with toxic chemicals as solvents which are harmful and can reduce the antioxidant activity and other health benefits of most bioactive components. The most importantdrawbacks are the sample preparation time for solid sample, decomposition of compounds, and wastage of large quantity of solvents which areexpensive to dispose of and also cause environmental problems (De Castro and Priego-Capote 2010).

The first and foremost disadvantage of using these solvents is that their content remains in the final products, which can be harmful to human health. Along with the high processing cost, this is a time consuming process that requires extra steps for the purification of the polyphenols. Additionally, by using pure organic solvents, very polar phenolic acids (benzoic, cinnamic acids) cannot be extracted fully. In such cases, mixtures of alcohol–water or acetone–water are suggested. Waxes, oils, sterols, chlorophyll are highly nonpolar compounds and can be extracted from the material by less polar solvents like dichloromethane, chloroform, hexane and benzene (Stalikas 2007). The yield of the phenolic compound decreases because the process requires high temperature which should be avoided. The basic temperatures at which the processes are being carried out ranges from 20 °C to 50 °C. The temperatures exceeding above 70 °C caused degradation of anthocyanins. Secondly, it is a time consuming process as well. Due to the high demand of the solvents in soxhlet method of extraction, it is not recommended because of the environmental hazards.

Non-conventional or Modern Methods of Extraction

Today, transformation of ideology on every aspect are changing rapidly. Concept of food consumption changed from leisure to health, utilization convenient technologies to modern systems, and many more. Along with these changes, thoughts on 'sustainability' and 'green approach' are dominating. This revolution is reflecting in the field of extraction of compounds also. Traditional methods and other conventional methods are still in use, as they are simpler and has its own advantages. However, accuracy and precision is important in this developing scientific world, where most of the conventional methods fail in their efficiency. Numerous modern technologies are available now in the market for solely extraction purpose. Studies are conducted for improving conventional methods or in development for characterisation and profiling of compounds. Difficulty in efficient extraction, isolation and detection of many antioxidants are still a challenge to the modern world of science. Bottlenecks are consistent in the field of isolating and profiling antioxidants. That is, requirement of derivatization, sensitivity, destruction of samples in many cases, difficulty in handling sophisticated instruments, lack of knowledge about appropriate extraction-detection system, and so on. However, to an extent, these challenges have been overcoming since past few decades (Azmir *et al.* 2013).

Some of the other hyphenated techniques which has been successfully exploited in the laboratories and industries for extraction, characterisation and purification of the antioxidant compounds of plant origin are supercritical fluid extraction, matrix solid-phase dispersion (MSPD), solid-phase micro extraction (SPME), accelerated solvent extraction or pressurized solvent extraction, microwave-assisted and ultra-sonication extraction techniques, chromatographic techniques like High-Performance Liquid Chromatography (HPLC), Supercritical Fluid

Chromatography (SFC), high-speed counter-current chromatography, thin layer chromatography, and Tandem Techniques like GC-MS, LC-MS, LC-DAD, LC-NMR, IR Spectroscopy, MALDI-TOF-MS, UHPLC/Q-TOF-MS, NMR, 1H NMR, HR/MAS and 13C NMR. These techniques have gained higher interest due to their less time taking procedures, simplicity to use and environmental friendly nature. A flow chart showing some of the conventional and non-conventional extraction techniques for characterization and profiling of different antioxidants is given in Fig. (**2**).

Solvent Extraction

Extraction of components are always an important part in the scientific life of human, whether it is natural or artificial process. In order to obtain maximum effect of certain compounds, extraction methods can help us to a certain extend. Methods like decoction, maceration, *etc.*, are some of those cheap and simple practices which had been practiced from our ancestral periods. However, in contemporary world, efficiency is a vital quality we are looking forward to. On top of that, it will be more adequate if we can adopt eco-friendly techniques (use of minimal or no toxic substances as solvents, reducing wastage of solvents in large quantity, *etc.*). Hence,

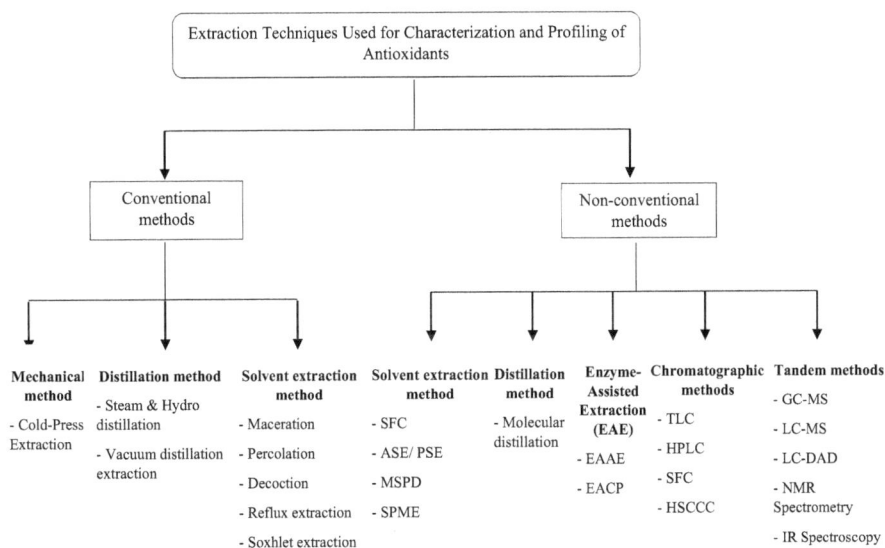

Fig. (2). Illustrates brief extraction methods used for characterization and profiling of antioxidants.

non-conventional methods of extraction possess demand among the scientists and industrialists. Numerous techniques have been developed in this field, where some of them were modified according to present conditions. Some of the techniques are microwave-assisted extraction (MAE), accelerated solvent extraction (ASE), supercritical fluid extraction, pressurized low-polarity water extraction, and so on.

Supercritical Fluid Extraction (SCFE)

SCFE technique is the most suitable of extraction technique for those compounds which are sensitive to the conditions like temperature and pressure because of their mild processing environment. In this technique no oxidation or degradation of compounds occur (King and Bott 1993, Zhou *et al.* 2005). In the field of food and drug industry, government has made stringent rules on the usage of the organic solvents. There are ample number of techniques available that has replaced the conventional methods of isolation of oils and fats, these techniques are environment friendly and produce low toxic wastes. The products obtained from these techniques are of great value in the context of health and nutrition and their bye products are being used during the process itself and in the other industries as well. Research has proved the applications of the supercritical fluid extraction method for various materials and for their determination and quantification of compounds. Since, the high solubility of the compound of interest in the supercritical solvent is essential for the economy of extraction process, practical analyses shall verify if extraction using supercritical fluids is a suitable technique for the isolation of the target compounds (Lack and Simandy 2009). There are several parameters that influence the solubility, mass transfer and the resulting yield of the target compounds in this technique (Kikic *et al.* 1997). Pressure and temperature are the main factors on which the composition of final products depends. Pressure is also an important factor that needs to be considered during the extraction, for the best ratio between solvent amount and extraction time. It is most commercial applications that have been reported in the food sector, which now has extended to the cosmetic and pharma industries for obtaining natural substances at high pressures. This technique has fairy being used in food processing industries because it has been accepted as a clean and environment friendly technique. This could be used as alternative to the organic solvent based extraction of the phenolic compounds. It is used to obtain contamination free and sterilized phenolic compounds. Nutraceutical products can be made chemical free and enantiomeric resolution is obtained. There are multiple applications of this technique including removal of alcohol from wine and beer, removal of fat from food, vitamin (E and C) enrichment from natural sources and extraction and characterization of the functional compounds (Brunner 2005, Xynos *et al.* 2012).

Accelerated Solvent Extraction (ASE)/Pressurized Solvent Extraction (PSE)

Pressurised liquid extraction (PLE), pressurised fluid extraction (PFE), pressurised solvent extraction (PSE) or ASE are same techniques of fluid extraction with different nomenclature (Mustafa and Turner 2011). When the solvent used is water, it is common for all the terms such as subcritical water extraction (SWE), High temperature water extraction (HTWE) and hot water extraction (HWE). In this technique high temperature (9313-473K) is used without reaching the critical point to enhance the speed of the process at high pressure (3.5-20 MPa), to maintain the solvents in their liquid state only. When compared to the traditional soxhlet method, PLE helps to decrease the time consumption and usage of solvent. In comparison to SFE, this technology is a potential alternative due to its various advantages, especially in terms of 'green extraction' as PLE consumes small amount of solvent for whole analysis. Phenolic groups from grape pomace and grape skin; flavonoids from spinach; resveratrol from grape skin, tricin from black bamboo leaf, sulfated polysaccharides (fucoidan) from brown seaweed *Saccharina japonica, etc.* are some of the antioxidant extracted with the help of PLE. However, functioning of this system requires well-trained personnel and cleaning is found to be a hurdle. These are some drawbacks that have to be overcome for the maximum utilization of PLE in future. Some of the major advantages of the process of PSE includes its comparatively non-toxic nature to humans and environment friendly nature as well. PLE based extraction systems are comparatively a low cost compared with the conventional methods of extraction. Management of both the temperature and pressure is relatively easy. Overall, the processing time required id very less and it increases the acceptability of the process to the industrial scale as well.

Matrix Solid-Phase Dispersion (MSPD)

Matrix solid-phase dispersion (MSPD) is a patent-protected process that was first introduced by Barker in the year 1989 based on dispersion of tissues with an SPE column packing material octadecylsiloxane-bonded silica (C18) for the simultaneous disruption and extraction of semi-solid and solid samples (Barker *et al.* 1989). Generally, MSPD follows given steps: blending, transferring to a column, compressing, and elution with solvent. The majority of extraction methods that are available currently includes one or the other extreme conditions. That is, some are working at high pressure, where some others at high temperature or another set requires supplementary energy supplied from assistance (PLE, UAE, or MAE). This is why MSPD stands out from usual solvent extraction techniques as it can be operated at ambient conditions and that also without the assistance of a laboratory equipment. Moreover, this technique provides simplification of sample process (therefore providing ease in sample handling) and in some cases, it assists in purification. Considering its numerous merits, MSPD can be adopted to replace most of the conventional methods as this method is simpler, rapid, environmentally friendly and cost-effective (de Fatima Alpendurada 2000). Advantages and most commercial applications of MSPD are enlisted as follows.

• Isolation of drugs, analysis of herbicides and pesticides
• Comparatively less solvent is used in this technique
• Elimination of the need of precipitation of cellular components
• Centrifugation of undesirable sample components can be avoided
• Process can be completed in minimal time

From past 5 years, MSPD has been is use in the characterization and analysis of antioxidants. Studies have been conducted on determination of flavonoids (anthocyanins, flavanols, isoflavones, flavones, flavanones, and flavonols) from different fruits (mainly citrus) and other samples using MSPD. However, general protocol for the determination of flavonoids and other naturals active compounds are not designed (de Fatima Alpendurada 2000). In most cases, Methanol (MeOH) is used; application of MeOH:water provides better result for target compounds. According to recent studies, ionic liquids, non-ionic detergents, and limonene are considered as 'green solvent' for extracting bioactive components from fruits using MSPD technique (Pérez *et al.* 2020, Visnevschi-Necrasov *et al.* 2015).

Solid-Phase Micro Extraction (SPME)

Solid-Phase Micro extraction technique (SPME) was first introduced in 1990 by Arthur and Pawliszyn, from then it gained its position among the researchers as an effective extraction method. Initially, this system was used in environmental studies like detection of pesticides and herbicides present in water, air and soil. Subsequently other fields like food and natural compounds, theories, *etc.*, came forward to explore this technique. SPME is a highly efficient technique that is used for sample collection, isolation and extraction. It is used to extract the analytes from the liquid, solid and gaseous samples. There are two different partition equilibriums of analytes between the sample matrix and the extraction phase; achievement of equilibrium between these partitions is the basic of SPME technique. It consists of two steps: (i) Partitioning and (ii) Subsequent desorption of extracts. This process can be classified as static in vessel and dynamic inflow micro-extraction. It involves fibres and capillary tubes, but fibre SPME is the most widely used technique for the extraction. In tube, SPME is also an efficient in-flow micro extraction process in which a capillary column is used as extraction device, with the sample analytes in the inner capillary coating. There are other methods for extractions as well *i.e.*, syringe SPME; a syringe tip is used. They may be performed automatically or manually in both the modes.

Unlike other techniques that use different types of solvent, SPME is a solvent-free extraction method and complex equipments and it does not require the assistance of pre-concentration step. These two reason are salient features of SPME as it proves to be a 'green' approach with less input energy as procedure is completed within two steps. One of the best potential of SPME is its automated analysis. Controlling the thickness and polarity of the coating on fibre provides highly consistent, quantifiable results for low concentration analytes (de Fatima Alpendurada 2000). Applications of SPME includes: (Kataoka *et al.* 2000)

1. The analyte is directly extracted into the fibre coating, so, it saves time, solvent and disposal costs.
2. It has been effectively used for separation and detection purpose (*i.e.* for pesticide, food, natural products, pharmaceuticals, toxicology and forensics, *etc.*).
3. Recently applied for on-site sampling and *in vitro* and *in vivo* metabolite analysis process.
4. It can improve the detection limits.
5. It can be used/coupled with other techniques as well, such gas chromatography and mass chromatography.

In the area of profiling different antioxidants, SPME is usually hyphenated with spectrometry, along with head-space (HS) condition to achieve best result. For example, SPME-GC-MS with HS condition was used for the analysis of volatile components in wild mushroom for the identification of biochemical modification (Costa *et al.* 2015) and determination of α- tocopherol from olive oil (Aresta and Zambonin 2017).

Distillation Techniques

Distillation is a traditional unit operation for separating components from a mixture by the principle of partial evaporation. That is, higher the vapour pressure, easily it transfer to its vapour phase. For volatile substances, this property is found to be higher than others as they can transfer their physical form from one to gaseous/ vapour phase. Scientists used this ability for trapping and separation of specific components and till now, they were used as conventional methods (vacuum distillation, steam distillation, *etc*). In present scenario, like other technologies, distillation system also improved for better separation and purification processes. In most of the cases, elevated temperature causes denaturation of biomolecules; mainly antioxidants that are sensitive to heat.

Molecular distillation (MD) is a better alternative for this rather than hydro distillation (HD) - a conventional distillation technique. MD operates at low temperature and the presence of vacuum surrounding helps to attain desired product without any denaturation of molecules. That is, in a molecular distillation, without any collision, vapour molecules will be able to reach the condenser chamber. In initial stages, molecular distillation was developed for separating tocotrienols and other micro-components present in Palm Fatty Acid Distillates (PFAD). Short-path molecular distillation process was used to study antioxidant activity of fractions obtained from oregano essential oils. Nevertheless, for this separation process to be successful, it is necessary to reveal the behaviour of target components in the evaporation process. Some of the advantages of this technique are as follows (Selvamuthukumaran and Shi 2017).

1. Use of low pressure and low temperature helps to maintain the molecular structure of compounds
2. Effective for heat sensitive and complex compounds
3. Used for separation, purification, and concentration of natural products
4. System can be operated at higher vacuum within short time period

Enzyme Assisted Extraction (EAE) Techniques

In some cases, phytochemicals are hidden inside the cell wall that are difficult to obtain through many extraction processes. This reflects in inefficiency of profiling of compounds having antioxidant, antibacterial, *etc*. activities. Therefore, use of suitable enzymes for isolating these active components can improve the accuracy and purpose of characterisation and profiling techniques. Studies states that many bioactive components are dispersed in cytoplasm of cell, whereas, some others have formed complex structures (like polysaccharide-lignin network) with the help of hydrogen bonding or hydrophobic interactions, which hinders the solvent to penetrate. Enzymes (cellulase, α-amylase, and pectinase) helps to disrupt these cell walls or complex molecular structures to enhance the efficiency of different techniques. Hence, enzyme assisted technique can be considered as a novel and excellent pre-treatment. There are two types of EAE are available: Enzyme-assisted aqueous extraction (EAAE) and enzyme-assisted cold pressing (EACP). For better extraction technique, EAAE is used than EACP, because in latter method, enzyme is used to hydrolyse the seed cell wall due to lack of polysaccharide-protein colloid. This advantage is utilised by EAAE method for better extraction of components like seed oil (Concha *et al.* 2004). Then again, some studies have reported that EACP is an alternative method for the seed oil extraction, because it has an upper hand having non-flammable and non-toxic properties. EAAE has been used for in studies related to extraction of polyphenolic compounds from peels, pomace and residues of citrus, *Ribes nigrum* and grapes. Moreover, on quantification of oil extracted, EAE method gives better result in free fatty acids and phosphorous than the solvent-used extraction methods. Some other studies included optimization of lycopene, anthocyanins, non-anthocyanin flavonoids, *etc.* from various fruits like watermelon, raspberry, *etc.*, which has considerably higher positive effect (Selvamuthukumaran and Shi 2017).

Chromatographic Techniques

From the last decade, we come across different types of methods that helps to classify, characterize or purify compounds. Involvement of solvents, time consumption, lack of efficiency and some other factors is why their application is questioned in many cases. There is an increasing demand for highly sensitive and more efficient methods of extraction of compounds like lipids, minerals, polyphenols, *etc.* The majority of extraction techniques are followed by different purification methods that are mostly unreliable. In such cases, chromatographic techniques are advisable. For instance, High Performance Liquid Chromatography (HPLC) is designed for analytical purpose, but simple modification in the system helps to purify the isolated components within short duration. Chromatography is based on the principle where 'molecules in mixture applied onto the surface or into the solid, and fluid stationary phase (stable phase) is separating from each other while moving with the aid of a mobile phase'. Factors like adsorption (liquid-solid), partition (liquid-solid), and affinity or differences among their molecular weights play vital role in determining the efficiency of any chromatographic technique (Cai 2014). Based on adsorption (effective for macromolecules as nucleic acids, and proteins and partition (effective for small molecules such as amino acids, carbohydrates, and fatty acids) principle, different chromatographic methods are designed, developed and modified. In latest applications, for improved efficiency, chromatography and spectroscopy are inter-connected.

Chromatographic techniques have proved their efficacy in science for serving separation, identification and purification applications of both quantitative and qualitative analysis at given time period. However, drawbacks like highly expensive instruments and set-up, occurring of errors due overloaded sample, system operated by highly trained person and also uttermost care is given to the equipment as the instrument is highly sensitive and expensive are not negligible. Ample numbers of techniques are there available today, where some of them can be performed in small scale or laboratory level (paper chromatography, column chromatography, Thin layer chromatography (TLC), *etc.*), while other sophisticated instruments like High-performance liquid chromatography (HPLC),

High-speed counter-current chromatography (HSCCC), Supercritical fluid chromatography (SFC), and thin layer chromatography.

Thin Layer Chromatography (TLC)

Thin Layer Chromatography (TLC), is a similar model of column chromatography, is working on the principle of 'solid-liquid adsorption' and capillary rise of the mobile phase through the stationary phase (a solid adsorbent substance like alumina, silica gel, cellulose, *etc.* are coated on the surface of glass plate) takes place in upward direction of the set-up. TLC is used to separate the non-volatile mixture of polyphenols. There are different ways to perform TLC such as plastic sheet, glass slide or aluminium foil. Any of these modes are used and they are coated with the thin layer of adsorbent material, such as silica gel, cellulose and aluminium oxide. This thin layer of the adsorbent is called as the stationary phase and the sample is being applied to the plate of adsorbent and kept into the solvent medium, which act as a mobile phase. Now after putting the slide into the solvent system it act as a capillary action and the different layers of analytes can be seen on the slide, so separation is achieved (Lewis and Moody 1989). Thin layer chromatography can be used to monitor the results of the reaction, for example,

1. Applicable for the qualitative analytical purpose of alcohols, alkaloids, antibiotics, acids, proteins, amines, fatty acids and ceramides, *etc.*
2. To isolate components from complex mixture.
3. Detection of pesticide and herbicides in the food and water.
4. Identification of medicinal plants and their constituents.
5. Assaying the purity of the chemicals for pharmaceuticals.

A special application of TLC is in the 'characterization of radiolabeled compounds', where it is used to determine radiochemical purity. Even though TLC is a simple technique that can be performed in laboratory on a common basis, existence of limitations are: (Cai 2014)

1. It is a qualitative analytical method; not quantitative.
2. It is not an automated process and poor resolution.
3. Application is limited to non-volatile compounds.
4. Retention factor (R_f) value of all compounds should be known already for identification analysis.
5. Humidity and temperature has great influence on the working efficiency of TLC plate as it is an open system.
6. Limitation of plate length limits the whole separation process.

High-Performance Liquid Chromatography (HPLC)

High-Performance Liquid Chromatography (HPLC) or known as High-Pressure Liquid Chromatography was developed and modified from column chromatography, for separating, characterizing and profiling of active compounds. An HPLC basically consists of (i) two solvents: one is acidified water- solvent A, and second is polar organic solvent- solvent B, (ii) a column containing packed material (stationary phase), (iii) a pump to move the mobile phase, (iv) a detector that helps to show retention time of the molecules. Based on the phase system used, HPLC are of different types (Malviya *et al.* 2010).

- Normal phase HPLC (NP-HPLC) is based on polarity, *i.e.* a polar stationary phase and a non-polar mobile phase is used;
- Reversed phase HPLC (RP-HPLC or RPC) is based on hydrophobic interactions with a non-polar stationary phase and an aqueous or moderately polar mobile phase;
- Size exclusion chromatography (SEC) or gel permeation chromatography or gel filtration chromatography works on the basis of size to separate particles. Applied for determining tertiary structure and quaternary structure of proteins and amino acids and molecular weight of polysaccharides;
- Ion-exchange chromatography is based on the attraction between solute ions and charged sites bound to the stationary phase. Widely used in purification of water and for the analysis of proteins, carbohydrates and oligosaccharides, *etc.*; and
- Bio-affinity chromatography, an effective separation technique based on specific reversible interaction of proteins with ligands. Highly purified components are available in a single step.

For fruits, HPLC is preferred over other techniques for the extraction of antioxidant compounds. For the determination and separation of polyphenols, reverse phase (RP) HPLC is preferred tools with different detection systems, such as diode array detector (HPLC-DAD) & mass spectroscopy (HPLC-MS) (Sakakibara *et al.* 2003). Scientists have determined the polyphenols in foodstuffs simultaneously with HPLC-DAD and made a file that consists of 100 standard chemicals calibration curves. Ample number of phases are present for the analysis of polyphenols like flavonoids, anthocyanins, procyanidins, flavones and phenolic acids. RP-HPLC has changed the process of separation of polyphenols. Limitations of HPLC includes: detection of limited number of phenolic compounds; it is highly sensitive as well; before the analysis with HPLC, an initial pre-concentration and purification from complex matrix is vital in order to simplify the chromatograms, which are prepared for the identification and quantification analysis; and polyphenols are also extracted by the adsorption-desorption processes with the help of efficient sorbents.

Taking these facts into consideration, in most of the works for determining antioxidants, solid phase extraction (SPE) can be used for purification, and the analytes were usually eluted with methanol, ethanol or their aqueous form (Lalaguna 1993). HPLC has been in use from decades for the determination of α-carotene, β-carotene, retinol, vitamin C, vitamin D_2, and other bioactive compounds, among which, most are powerful antioxidant Alternatively, HPLC method coupled with mass spectroscopy (HPLC-MS) is more approachable method for identifying unknown polyphenols and proanthocyanidins present in a biological sample (Shui and Leong 2005), and with the help of coupling reverse phase high pressure liquid chromatography (HPLC) with diode array detection (DAD), of both water- and fat- soluble vitamins can be found proficiently in a single run (Klejdus *et al.* 2004). By using HPLC on normal phase or reverse phase columns low molecular mass antioxidants can be analysed, although it is a time-consuming process along with low resolution and high structural diversity. Liquid Chromatography–Mass Spectrometry (LC–MS) techniques are the best analytical approach to study these days, as the polyphenols from different biological resources, and are the most effective tool in the study of the structure of phenolic compounds (Bureau *et al.* 2009).

Supercritical Fluid Chromatography (SFC)

Supercritical fluids are the fluids that have high densities and dissolving capacities, just like some other liquids, but they have low viscosities and better diffusion properties. So, supercritical fluids are used as mobile phase in the chromatography will act as both the substance carrier and it also dissolve the substances like solvents in HPLC. SFC came into existence at the same time when HPLC came into market. Even if SFC was used in various forms in past decades, present market has demand on packed columns instead of open columns. Packed column SFC has overcome many limitations, where some are remarkable; more environmental friendly and it eliminates solvents that can cause ozone depletion. Also, coupling of FC with mass spectrometry or UV detectors experimentally reliable. When compared to Normal phase HPLC, FC is also working on normal phase system and its orthogonality to reverse phase HPLC makes it an excellent technique for purification analysis. Advantages of SFC over HPLC and some other chromatographic techniques are: (Taylor 2009).

1. Eco-friendly, inert, and more volatile CO_2-based solvent is applicable for large scale separation; hence energy consumption can be reduced.
2. Selectivity, which is similar to reverse HPLC, but more adjustable.
3. Applicable for identification and quantification.
4. Preparative separations.
5. Natural product applications.
6. Analytical scale chiral and achiral separations.

On contrary to its advantages, SFC is mostly used in pharmaceutical field than in any other area so far, whereas as recently, this technique is adopted in food analysis also. For instance, free fatty acid (FFA) analyzed with SFC without ester derivatization. That is, in food analysis, this chromatographic method is applied in two ways: (i) food quality is analyzed by analyzing its active ingredients and (ii) ensure food safety by detecting residual pesticides. Studies (Liu *et al.* 2010, Qu *et al.* 2015, Taguchi *et al.* 2014, Unger *et al.* 2008) prove that antioxidants like lipids (essential oils and phytosterols) are analysed more rapidly (3 min for FFA analysis) by SFC than GC (Gas Chromatography) and HPLC. This is because in GC, isomerization and degradation takes place for non-volatile lipids; lipids that have higher molecular weight and easily volatile are not suitable for GC and in case of HPLC, it requires longer processing time than SFC. Supercritical fluid extraction-SFC (SFE-SFC) is best for bioactive compound analysis such as carotene, coenzyme Q_{10} and ketamine metabolites. This coupling method has proved its supreme efficiency in bioactivity and sensitive quantification of carotenoids and coupling of SFE with SFC-MS reduces overall analysis time. Recent advances in SFC helped in quantification of fat-soluble vitamins (FSVs) like vitamin E (α-tocopherol). Accuracy and precision of quantification analysis makes SFC stand out from HPLC technique. By the combination of SFC and LC (Liquid Chromatography), FSVs (chloroform/methanol (50:50, v/v) can be used a dissolving solvent) and water soluble vitamins (WSVs), like vitamin C (methanol/water (50:50, v/v) as dissolving solvent) which is highly photooxidative can be analyzed easily. Thus, SFC is an efficient chromatographic technique, especially when coupled with other methods. Utilization of this system other than pharmaceutical field is necessary so that newly developed methods with more efficiency and less energy consumption will be possible.

High-speed Counter-current Chromatography (HSCCC)

In classical liquid chromatography, it is difficult to separate all the antioxidants from a plant cell. But, in counter current chromatography (CCC) biphasic liquid system is used to extract the compounds from the mixture. In this, a centrifugal field is made to allow the liquid stationary phase in an open tube. The phase density difference and the centrifugal fields are the only parameters allowing the equilibrium between the two liquid phases. The advantage of the technique in preparative separation is the dual-mode capability of CCC. During the run, the role of the phase can be changed, that is, mobile phase can be made stationary and vice versa.

HSCCC is an advanced technique, which is broadly used for separation of target compounds in large-scale. Application of liquid as stationary phase provides this technique an upper hand over other traditional methods of chromatography as it is face irretrievable adsorption. The capability to couple with analytical instruments inorder to develop hyphenated systems attracts various applications; analytical and/or preparative analysis for separation and purification. HSCCC is used in areas like pharmaceuticals, rare elements, metals, peptides, enantiomer, alkaloids, flavonoids, and phenols. Likewise, factors like pH-zone-refining CCC and pH-gradient elution has major effect on pH alternation, which is not only beneficial for the optimal separation to take place, but also increases sample-loadin--capacity, around ten times. This is useful in cases where electric-charge of analytes depends on pH such as organic acids, alkaloids, amino acids, peptides, *etc*. (Khan and Liu 2018). HSCCC make use of a J shaped coil planet centrifuge to separate the food related polyphenols. The main compounds, which can be effectively separated with the help of HSCCC from the non-fermented green tea includes catechin, esters and caffeine. Furthermore, several food-related polyphenols, such as condensed procyanidins, phenolic acids and flavonol glycosides were clearly separated under the same HSCCC conditions. These separation profiles of HSCCC provide useful information about the hydrophobic diversity of these bioactive polyphenols present in various types of tea and food products. This technique has its own advantages over traditional methods helping the researchers and industrialists in one way or the other to explore the possible utilisation of these products in broad range of food as well as non-food applications. However, more studies are yet to be conducted to explore HSCCC to full of their utilisation and their industrial adoption. Some of its merits are as follows (Wang *et al.* 2018).

1. In this techniques, irreversible adsorption can be eliminated.
2. Risk of denaturation of sample is less.
3. High sample recovery.
4. Preparative capacity is large (or can be increased with pH).
5. Recently, this technique is being successfully used for preparative isolation and purification of many natural products.

On contradict to the advantages of HSCCC, drawbacks like lack of understanding of its working principle, difficulty in gradient elution, selection of solvent system is found to be complex in nature and insufficient number of theoretical plates when compared to HPLC, making it difficult to separate compounds (in 1D HSCCC) having similar k_D values arises question in its practical usage.

Tandem Techniques

Importance of extraction methods for separation, characterization and profiling of antioxidants and other metabolites gave rise to numerous tradition techniques such as supercritical fluid extraction (SFE), HPLC (High-Performance Liquid Chromatography), Gas Chromatography (GC), hydro-distillation, mass spectrometry, and many more. Even though these techniques have established their advantages over other systems, features like specificity, sensitivity, time consumption, *etc.*, are still questioned. Modifications have brought better processing methods, but later studies stated that coupling of analytical techniques are capable to overcome the increasing challenges. Thus, introduction of 'Modern Analytical Techniques' started to replace other traditional methods. Today, wide variety of modern analytical techniques or 'Hyphenated Techniques' are available with an objective of joining separation and detection techniques together with maximum advantage. In addition to this perspective, hyphenated systems are tried to develop on the idea of 'green extraction method'. However, studies are yet to be done in these system so that maximum utilization will be possible in future studies. Some of the multiple tandem techniques for the extraction of polyphenols like NMR, 1H NMR, 13 C NMR, HR/MAS, GC-MS, LC-MS, LC-DAD, IR Spectroscopy, MALDI-TOF-MS.

GC-MS (Gas Chromatography-Mass Spectrometry)

So far, we have seen wide range of technologies for extraction, isolation and identification of different types of antioxidants (phenolics, vitamins, lipids, sugars, *etc*). In terms of efficiency, most of the techniques (like HPLC, capillary electrophoresis (CE), UV/ visible spectrometry, *etc.*) has its own limitations like difficulty in detecting range, lack of satisfactory separation performances, and so on. In such cases, bridging of Capillary Gas Chromatography with Mass Spectrometry (GC-MS) will be supportive. GC-MS, a competent hyphenated system for analytical purpose, which is based on the combined working principle of a Gas-Liquid Chromatography (separation of substances that are volatile and thermally stable) and Mass spectroscopy (detection method). However, in this method, similar separation but based on mass will take place. For more advancement, sometimes, GC-MS is again coupled with MS (GC-MS/MS) (Halket *et al.* 2005). Some of the advantages of this technique, especially over the application of GC alone are as follows (Chauhan *et al.* 2014).

1. GC-MS is functioning on electron impact (EI) and chemical ionization (CI) rather than vapor pressure.
2. In this technique, substances that are having comparatively low volatility and wider range of thermal stability can be successfully analysed.
3. Rapid and highly sensitive instrumentation.
4. Fatty acids, terpenes, alcohols, essential oils, aldehydes, *etc.* present in food and other biological samples are detected.
5. Frequently used in areas for detection of pesticides and biological (narcotics, residual solvents, drugs, adulterations, *etc.*).
6. Efficient for detecting profiling of fatty acid in microbes, presence of free steroids, and metabolites present in serum.
7. Applications in forensic, toxicology, explosive detection system, criminal cases and geo, petro and astro-chemical analysis and medical and pharmaceutical analysis.

This is the technique is mainly used to separate and identify the various types of polyphenols. It is basically developed for the analysis of phenolic compounds in the initial stages. Gas chromatography is highly sensitive and selective when it is combined with the mass spectrometry. Although it is bit difficult to prepare the sample for the Gas Chromatography, including the separation of the lipids from the extracts and the derivation of low volatile polyphenols. Thus, GC-MS technique has some superior hand over common chromatographic methods to an extend for the analysis of piperine, essential oils, lavender oil, spearmint oil, olive oil, lemon oil, peppermint oil, *etc.* On the other hand, GC-MS technique has some inevitable drawbacks such as: (i) derivatization is necessary in order to enhance volatility and range of thermal stability; (ii) direct analysing of nonvolatile, polar or thermally labile compounds are not possible and (iii) involvement of derivatization step makes the system consume more time (Lynch 2017).

Liquid Chromatography-Mass Spectrometry (LC-MS)

Application of MS due to its proficient detection of wide range of compounds are remarkable and thus tandem techniques are developed in present scenario. Also among different chromatographic methods, Liquid Chromatography (LC) has made its own imprint in separation technique. Yet, improvements was made to develop advanced technologies like introduction of LC-MS. Coupling of LC and MS made characterization and profiling of components more convenient, rapid and robust. Existence of LC-MS is as old as GC-MS; lack of progress due to relative incompatibility of MS ion source and continuous liquid stream delayed its advance in both market and laboratories. This situation changed drastically by 1980s with development of 'electron ion spray' and 'matrix assisted laser desorption ionisation'. Adoption of LC-MS over LC is predominantly due to its capability to handle complex molecules and high specificity. Also, its fast scanning speed helps to increase the rate of multiplexing and thus analysis process of more compounds/ samples are possible in a single run (Pitt 2009). Then again, to achieve the above described supremacy, factors like nature of analyte (for determination of optimal ionisation method and polarity used) and Liquid Chromatographic separation. Also, it is advised that optimization of each analyte is essential as they can be independently vary from one instrument to another; similarly to sample matrices. Furthermore, sensitivity of this technique is also depending on capability of instrument and conditions of assay. Therefore, it is necessary to cross-check the sensitivity of LC-MS from time-to-time to achieve desired limit of detection. All these factors are not just a condition for better utilization of the process, but at the same time, a downside that inhibits approach in common laboratory.

These days this technique is used for the study of polyphenols from various kinds of sources. It is also the best tool for the study of structure of phenolic compounds. For the study of the vegetable samples, it is the best technique and the most efficient in the case of anthocyanins. LC-MS allows the characterization of the complex structures such as, tannins, proanthocyanidins and procyanidins. LC-MS is used for estimating the level of resveratrol (an important polyphenol found in the wine with good results) present in wine. Characterization of various vitamins (vitamins A, B_{12}, D, E and K) and related metabolites are also possible through this technique (Priego *et al.* 2007).

Liquid Chromatography-Diode Array Detector (LC-DAD)

Diode Array Detection method was started to use initially for assisting HPLC technique; during the period of UV/ visible spectrometry was extensively using for analytical purpose. Photodiode array detectors are simpler machine with hundreds to thousands of phototubes (light sensing diodes) placed in linear array that are arranged at varying wavelength. When light falls on the sample, it passes through a monochromator, which then falls onto photodiode array detector. This helps to broader the wavelength range of UV/ visible spectrophotometer. Application of DAD with HPLC helps to improvise the characterization and profiling methods in a single run, because scanning speed rate is higher than the conventional HPLC method. This technique is useful mainly for the identification of unknown sample. Even though MS coupled with HPLC provides better sensitive and reliable data, use of DAD coupled to HPLC is common in laboratory practices and among researchers. This is because, latter is cheaper and convenient than the first one (Cuyckens and Claeys 2002). To overcome these issues, HPLC/ESI-MS/UV-DAD is an excellent choice as it gives higher sensitivity; only if it could be affordable for usual researches and studies. For analyzing whole electrolytes or thermally-sensitive samples, liquid chromatography can be used as a stand-alone instrument and is equipped with a diode array detector (DAD), which is capable of acquiring full UV-Vis spectra for better identification of compound spectral signatures. The LC column is also equipped with a fluorescence detector (FLD) allowing for more selective and sensitive compound analysis. The LC-DAD system is mobile and can be moved to be directly coupled to the experiments being performed inside or outside of a glove box.

Coupling DAD with HPLC have wide number of applications especially in determining clinical bioactive components and in biochemistry. Later, this technique was adopted in characterization and profiling of antioxidants. HPLC with DAD provides better separation and peaks can be easily detected. Reports on detection of total and free phenolic acids, flavonoids, coumarins, nicotinic acid, caffeine, trigonelline, linoleic acid and its metabolites, *etc.* are available (Andrade *et al.* 1998, Casal *et al.* 1998, Mattila and Kumpulainen 2002, Melis *et al.* 2001). Along with this, HPLC-DAD-MAS has been used in cases of detecting antioxidants from the peels of sweet orange, berries, and mango (Anagnostopoulou *et al.* 2005, Määttä *et al.* 2003, Schieber *et al.* 2000).

Nuclear Magnetic Resonance (NMR) Spectrometry (^{1}H- and ^{13}C-NMR)

Nuclear Magnetic Resonance (NMR) spectroscopy is the study of molecule, which is placed in a strong magnetic field by recording the interaction between nuclei of molecule and radiofrequency (Rf) electromagnetic radiations. This non-destructive, fast and automated spectroscopic method helps in profiling of molecule through identifying its structure within a very short period of time and less quantity of sample. Other advantages of this technique are low maintenance cost, high reproducibility, ability to use live cell for studying (mainly for continuous lipid analysis) and study of oxidation is also possible. Nevertheless, lack of knowledge and high expense is a barrier for scientists and researchers are great disadvantage. NMR spectroscopy is one, which is being used for food samples, to analyze them for various kinds of components. The first and the foremost advantage of using NMR is, easiness with which its sample is prepared and for the measurement procedures. Standard ^{1}H, ^{13}C and a new high resolution magic angle spinning NMR spectra are the techniques which give information on liquid and semi-solid food stuffs. NMR spectrum act as a fingerprint for vegetables as it can be used to compare, classify and differentiate with other samples. The preparation of food samples is so easy and simple depending on the texture of the sample, whether it is in liquid state or in semi-solid or solid state. There are two common types of NMR: ^{1}H NMR and ^{13}C-NMR. The main difference between ^{1}H-NMR and ^{13}C-NMR is that ^{1}H NMR is used to determine the types and number of hydrogen atoms present in a molecule whereas ^{13}C-NMR is used to determine the type and number of carbon atoms in a molecule. 5-10% of the D20 is being added for the high resolution NMR like, ^{1}H, ^{13}C, HR/MAS for liquids/ aqueous solutions (wines, juices, soups, beer, other drinks *etc*.). In case of solid samples, they are firstly freeze dried and then they are dissolved in the desired solvent. The examples of the freeze dried samples are vegetables, fruits *etc*. With the advantages of NMR, there are few limitations as well, such as the cost of the equipment is very high. It may cost about eight times the cost of HPLC. Second limitation of using NMR is its sensitivity, if we compare it with other techniques like HPLC or GC it is highly sensitive. Along with the upper limitations there are few advantages of using NMR, such as the screening of the food extracts and the power of the structural elucidation of the technique. All the main metabolites can be detected in a single spectrum, such as carbohydrates, fats, amino acids and proteins (Le Gall and Colquhoun 2003).

For the identification antioxidants in the kernel of the walnut, both ^{1}H- and ^{13}C-NMR spectra was used with the solvents like dimethyl sulphoxides and the methanol. ^{1}H- and ^{13}C-NMR has become the preferred choice for the identification of reaction products and for the identification of anthocyanins. Also, studies on metabolic profiling of active components of fruits, quantitative analysis of retinol and retinol palmitate, detection of Omega-3-fatty acids, terpenes and carotenes (Choi *et al.* 2004, Igarashi *et al.* 2000, Jautelat *et al.* 1970) were conducted. Some of the studies on alkaloids were studied by coupling one of the NMR technique with MS.

Infrared (IR) Spectroscopy

IR spectroscopy or infrared spectroscopy deals with the infrared region of electromagnetic spectrum. It has a lower frequency and the longer wavelength than then the visible light. It can be measured in three ways, by measuring the reflection, emission and absorption. An IR spectrum is essentially a graph plotted with the frequency or wavelength on the X-axis against infrared light absorbed on the Y-axis. IR Spectroscopy detects frequencies of infrared light that are absorbed by a molecule. Molecules tend to absorb these specific frequencies of light since they correspond to the frequency of the vibration of bonds in the molecule. IR Spectroscopic technique can be majorly classified as Near-Infrared (NIR) and Mid-infrared (MIR) Spectroscopy. Similar to other tandem techniques, this method is also simple, robust, powerful and fast; but unlike other techniques (except NMR Spectroscopy), it has the advantage of using non-destructive sample. Then again, IR Spectroscopy can dominate NMR Spectrometry, as the latter is highly expensive whereas, the other is convenient method. Because of this reason, most of the traditional chemical analytical methods are being replaced by IR Spectroscopic technique. Salient features of this technique make scientific fields like clinical laboratory (especially which are dealing with live cells), agriculture sectors, food analysis area, *etc*. to rely for supreme efficiency for various analytical purposes. For instance, antioxidants (phenolics, flavonoids and their metabolites, carotenoids, polyphenols, fatty acids and glucosinolates) present in different food sources (wine, cereals, fruits, vegetables, dairy products, spices and herbs) were successfully quantified using IR Spectroscopy (Cozzolino 2015).

CONCLUSION

The advances and potential developments made in the analytical chemistry in the last decade has enabled the scientists to trace the rare compounds of particular interest. These compounds are mostly present in the nature in one or other form and we have been consuming them directly or indirectly since ages based on our traditional food habits. However, particular interest in identification and qualitative analysis of such compounds have gained significant grounds in the recent past. Now the functional importance of specific plant secondary metabolites is well established and continuous studies are underway to reveal their specific health benefits and effect on the target tissues. Their presence in the food sources is long known however, the developments in the instrumentation have enabled us to confirm their physical, chemical and biological nature, the form in which they are present within the plants, their minimum effective concentrations to have specific health benefits and their ultimate extraction and purification. With the tremendous developments in the analytical chemistry, many new novel antioxidant compounds have been identified and isolated successfully for various application. Still the issues like cost of production for small scale industries, technical and handling requirements, compounds specific protocols for better extraction and purification and clear understanding of the working principles of these technologies provides ample scope for the researchers for future developments.

CONFLICT OF INTEREST

The author declares no conflict of interest, financial or otherwise.

ACKNOWLEDGEMENTS

Declared none.

CONSENT FOR PUBLICATION

Not applicable.

REFERENCES

Abascal, K, Ganora, L & Yarnell, E (2005) The effect of freeze-drying and its implications for botanical

medicine: a review. *Phytother Res,* 19, 655-60.
[http://dx.doi.org/10.1002/ptr.1651] [PMID: 16177965]

Ahmad, P, Jaleel, CA, Salem, MA, Nabi, G & Sharma, S (2010) Roles of enzymatic and nonenzymatic antioxidants in plants during abiotic stress. *Crit Rev Biotechnol,* 30, 161-75.
[http://dx.doi.org/10.3109/07388550903524243] [PMID: 20214435]

Al-Majedy, Y, Al-Amiery, A & Kadhum, AA (2017) Antioxidant activity of coumarins. *Systematic Reviews in Pharmacy,* 8, 24.
[http://dx.doi.org/10.5530/srp.2017.1.6]

Anagnostopoulou, MA, Kefalas, P, Kokkalou, E, Assimopoulou, AN & Papageorgiou, VP (2005) Analysis of antioxidant compounds in sweet orange peel by HPLC-diode array detection-electrospray ionization mass spectrometry. *Biomed Chromatogr,* 19, 138-48.
[http://dx.doi.org/10.1002/bmc.430] [PMID: 15515108]

Andrade, PB, Seabra, RM, Valentao, P & Areias, F (1998) Simultaneous determination of flavonoids, phenolic acids, and coumarins in seven medicinal species by HPLC/diode-array detector. *J Liq Chromatogr Relat Technol,* 21, 2813-20.
[http://dx.doi.org/10.1080/10826079808003444]

Aresta, A & Zambonin, C (2017) Determination of α-Tocopherol in Olive Oil by Solid-Phase Microextraction and Gas Chromatography–Mass Spectrometry. *Anal Lett,* 50, 1580-92.
[http://dx.doi.org/10.1080/00032719.2016.1238922]

Ashrafizadeh, M, Ahmadi, Z, Mohammadinejad, R, Kaviyani, N & Tavakol, S (2019) Monoterpenes modulating autophagy: A review study. *Basic Clin Pharmacol Toxicol,* 126, 9-20.
[http://dx.doi.org/10.1111/bcpt.13282] [PMID: 31237736]

Azmir, J, Zaidul, ISM, Rahman, MM, Sharif, KM, Mohamed, A, Sahena, F, Jahurul, MHA, Ghafoor, K, Norulaini, NAN & Omar, AKM (2013) Techniques for extraction of bioactive compounds from plant materials: A review. *J Food Eng,* 117, 426-36.
[http://dx.doi.org/10.1016/j.jfoodeng.2013.01.014]

Bahonar, A, Saadatnia, M, Khorvash, F, Maracy, M & Khosravi, A (2017) Carotenoids as potential antioxidant agents in stroke prevention: a systematic review. *Int J Prev Med,* 8, 70.
[http://dx.doi.org/10.4103/ijpvm.IJPVM_112_17] [PMID: 28983399]

Barker, SA, Long, AR & Short, CR (1989) Isolation of drug residues from tissues by solid phase dispersion. *J Chromatogr A,* 475, 353-61.
[http://dx.doi.org/10.1016/S0021-9673(01)89689-8] [PMID: 2777960]

Bentz, AB (2017) A Review of Quercetin: Chemistry, Antioxident Properties, and Bioavailability. *J Young Investig*

Biesalski, HK, Dragsted, LO, Elmadfa, I, Grossklaus, R, Müller, M, Schrenk, D, Walter, P & Weber, P (2009) Bioactive compounds: definition and assessment of activity. *Nutrition,* 25, 1202-5.
[http://dx.doi.org/10.1016/j.nut.2009.04.023] [PMID: 19695833]

Brewer, MS (2011) Natural antioxidants: sources, compounds, mechanisms of action, and potential applications. *Compr Rev Food Sci Food Saf,* 10, 221-47.
[http://dx.doi.org/10.1111/j.1541-4337.2011.00156.x]

Brunner, G (1994) *Gas Extraction: An Introduction to Fundamentals of Supercritical Fluids and the Application to Separation Processes, Steinkopff: Darmstadt, Germany.*Springer, New York, NY, USA.

Brunner, G (2005) Supercritical fluids: Technology and application to food processing. *J Food Eng,* 67, 21-33.
[http://dx.doi.org/10.1016/j.jfoodeng.2004.05.060]

Bureau, S, Renard, CM, Reich, M, Ginies, C & Audergon, JM (2009) Change in anthocyanin concentrations in red apricot fruits during ripening. *Food Sci Technol (Campinas),* 42, 372-7.

Cai, L (2014) Thin layer chromatography. *Curr Protoc Essent Lab Tech,* 8, 6-3.
[http://dx.doi.org/10.1002/9780470089941.et0603s08]

Çakaloğlu, B, Özyurt, VH & Ötleş, S (2018) Cold press in oil extraction. A review. *Ukr Food J,* 7, 640-54.
[http://dx.doi.org/10.24263/2304-974X-2018-7-4-9]

Casal, S, Oliveira, MB & Ferreira, MA (1998) Development of an HPLC/diode-array detector method for simultaneous determination of trigonelline, nicotinic acid, and caffeine in coffee. *J Liq Chromatogr Relat Technol,* 21, 3187-95.
[http://dx.doi.org/10.1080/10826079808001267]

Chan, JY, Yuen, ACY, Chan, RYK & Chan, SW (2013) A review of the cardiovascular benefits and antioxidant properties of allicin. *Phytother Res,* 27, 637-46.
[http://dx.doi.org/10.1002/ptr.4796] [PMID: 22888009]

Chauhan, A, Goyal, MK & Chauhan, P (2014) GC-MS technique and its analytical applications in science and technology. *J Anal Bioanal Tech,* 5, 222.
[http://dx.doi.org/10.4172/2155-9872.1000222]

Choi, YH, Kim, HK, Wilson, EG, Erkelens, C, Trijzelaar, B & Verpoorte, R (2004) Quantitative analysis of retinol and retinol palmitate in vitamin tablets using 1H-nuclear magnetic resonance spectroscopy. *Anal Chim Acta,* 512, 141-7.
[http://dx.doi.org/10.1016/j.aca.2004.02.024]

Concha, J, Soto, C, Chamy, R & Zuniga, ME (2004) Enzymatic pretreatment on rose-hip oil extraction: hydrolysis and pressing conditions. *J Am Oil Chem Soc,* 81, 549-52.
[http://dx.doi.org/10.1007/s11746-006-0939-y]

Costa, R, De Grazia, S, Grasso, E & Trozzi, A (2015) Headspace-solid-phase microextraction-gas chromatography as analytical methodology for the determination of volatiles in wild mushrooms and evaluation of modifications occurring during storage. *J Anal Methods Chem,* 2015951748
[http://dx.doi.org/10.1155/2015/951748] [PMID: 25945282]

Cozzolino, D (2015) Infrared spectroscopy as a versatile analytical tool for the quantitative determination of antioxidants in agricultural products, foods and plants. *Antioxidants,* 4, 482-97.
[http://dx.doi.org/10.3390/antiox4030482] [PMID: 26783838]

Cruz, KJ, de Oliveira, AR & Marreiro, DdoN (2015) Antioxidant role of zinc in diabetes mellitus. *World J Diabetes,* 6, 333-7.
[http://dx.doi.org/10.4239/wjd.v6.i2.333] [PMID: 25789115]

Cuyckens, F & Claeys, M (2002) Optimization of a liquid chromatography method based on simultaneous electrospray ionization mass spectrometric and ultraviolet photodiode array detection for analysis of flavonoid glycosides. *Rapid Commun Mass Spectrom,* 16, 2341-8.
[http://dx.doi.org/10.1002/rcm.861] [PMID: 12478580]

Dasgupta, A & Acharya, K (2019) Mushrooms: an emerging resource for therapeutic terpenoids. *3 Biotech,* 1, 369.

Luque de Castro, MD & Priego-Capote, F (2010) Soxhlet extraction: Past and present panacea. *J Chromatogr A,* 1217, 2383-9.
[http://dx.doi.org/10.1016/j.chroma.2009.11.027] [PMID: 19945707]

Alpendurada, MF (2000) Solid-phase microextraction: a promising technique for sample preparation in environmental analysis. *J Chromatogr A,* 889, 3-14.
[http://dx.doi.org/10.1016/S0021-9673(00)00453-2] [PMID: 10985530]

Duthie, GG & Brown, KM (1994) *Reducing the risk of cardiovascular disease*
[http://dx.doi.org/10.1007/978-1-4615-2073-3_2]

Franco-Robles, E & López, MG (2015) Implication of fructans in health: immunomodulatory and antioxidant mechanisms. *ScientificWorldJournal,* 2015289267

[http://dx.doi.org/10.1155/2015/289267] [PMID: 25961072]

Guo, JJ, Hsieh, HY & Hu, CH (2009) Chain-breaking activity of carotenes in lipid peroxidation: a theoretical study. *J Phys Chem B,* 113, 15699-708.
[http://dx.doi.org/10.1021/jp907822h] [PMID: 19886649]

Halket, JM, Waterman, D, Przyborowska, AM, Patel, RKP, Fraser, PD & Bramley, PM (2005) Chemical derivatization and mass spectral libraries in metabolic profiling by GC/MS and LC/MS/MS. *J Exp Bot,* 56, 219-43.
[http://dx.doi.org/10.1093/jxb/eri069] [PMID: 15618298]

Hu, S, Yin, J, Nie, S, Wang, J, Phillips, GO, Xie, M & Cui, SW (2016) *In vitro* evaluation of the antioxidant activities of carbohydrates. *Bioactive carbohydrates and dietary fibre,* 7, 19-27.

Igarashi, T, Aursand, M, Hirata, Y, Gribbestad, IS, Wada, S & Nonaka, M (2000) Nondestructive quantitative determination of docosahexaenoic acid and n− 3 fatty acids in fish oils by high-resolution 1 H nuclear magnetic resonance spectroscopy. *J Am Oil Chem Soc,* 77, 737-48.
[http://dx.doi.org/10.1007/s11746-000-0119-0]

Imenshahidi, M & Hosseinzadeh, H (2016) Berberis vulgaris and berberine: an update review. *Phytother Res,* 30, 1745-64.
[http://dx.doi.org/10.1002/ptr.5693] [PMID: 27528198]

Jautelat, M, Grutzner, JB & Roberts, JD (1970) Natural-abundance 13C nuclear magnetic resonance spectra of terpenes and carotenes. *Proc Natl Acad Sci USA,* 65, 288-92.
[http://dx.doi.org/10.1073/pnas.65.2.288] [PMID: 5263764]

Kataoka, H, Lord, HL & Pawliszyn, J (2000) Applications of solid-phase microextraction in food analysis. *J Chromatogr A,* 880, 35-62.
[http://dx.doi.org/10.1016/S0021-9673(00)00309-5] [PMID: 10890509]

Khan, BM & Liu, Y (2018) High speed counter current chromatography: Overview of solvent-system and elution-mode. *J Liq Chromatogr Relat Technol,* 41, 629-36.
[http://dx.doi.org/10.1080/10826076.2018.1499528]

Kikic, I, Lora, M & Bertucco, AA (1997) Thermodynamic Analysis of Three-Phase Equilibria in Binary and Ternary Systems for Applications in Rapid Expansion of a Supercritical Solution (RESS), Particles from Gas-Saturated Solutions (PGSS), and Supercritical Antisolvent (SAS). *Ind Eng Chem Res,* 36, 5507-15.
[http://dx.doi.org/10.1021/ie970376u]

King, MB & Bott, TR (1993) *Extraction of Natural Products Using Near-Critical Solvents* Chapman & Hall, Glasgow, UK 84-100.
[http://dx.doi.org/10.1007/978-94-011-2138-5]

Klejdus, B, Petrlová, J, Potěšil, D, Adam, V, Mikelová, R, Vacek, J, Kizek, R & Kubáň, V (2004) Simultaneous determination of water-and fat-soluble vitamins in pharmaceutical preparations by high-performance liquid chromatography coupled with diode array detection. *Anal Chim Acta,* 520, 57-67.
[http://dx.doi.org/10.1016/j.aca.2004.02.027]

Knez, Z (2016) Food processing using supercritical fluids.*Emerging and Traditional Technologies for Safe Food Engineering Series*Healthy and Quality Food 1571-0297.
[http://dx.doi.org/10.1007/978-3-319-24040-4_20]

Lack, E & Simandy, B (2009) High Pressure technology: Fundamentals and application.*Industrial Chemistry Library* Elsevier, Amsterdam, The Netherlands 537-75.

Lalaguna, F (1993) Purification of fresh cassava root polyphenols by solid-phase extraction with Amberlite XAD-8 resin. *J Chromatogr A,* 657, 445-9.
[http://dx.doi.org/10.1016/0021-9673(93)80301-N]

Le Gall, G & Colquhoun, IJ (2003) NMR spectroscopy in food authentication in food authenticity and traceability.*Food science and technology* 131-56.

Lewis, HW & Moody, CJ (1989)

Li, SH, Zhao, P, Tian, HB, Chen, LH & Cui, LQ (2015) Effect of grape polyphenols on blood pressure: A meta-analysis of randomized controlled trials. *PLoS One,* 10e0137665
[http://dx.doi.org/10.1371/journal.pone.0137665] [PMID: 26375022]

Liu, LX, Zhang, Y, Zhou, Y, Li, GH, Yang, GJ & Feng, XS (2020) The application of supercritical fluid chromatography in food quality and food safety: an overview. *Crit Rev Anal Chem,* 50, 136-60.
[http://dx.doi.org/10.1080/10408347.2019.1586520] [PMID: 30900462]

Lynch, KL (2017) Toxicology: liquid chromatography mass spectrometry.*Mass spectrometry for the clinical laboratory* Academic Press 109-30.
[http://dx.doi.org/10.1016/B978-0-12-800871-3.00006-7]

Määttä, KR, Kamal-Eldin, A & Törrönen, AR (2003) High-performance liquid chromatography (HPLC) analysis of phenolic compounds in berries with diode array and electrospray ionization mass spectrometric (MS) detection: ribes species. *J Agric Food Chem,* 51, 6736-44.
[http://dx.doi.org/10.1021/jf0347517] [PMID: 14582969]

Malviya, R, Bansal, V, Pal, OP & Sharma, PK (2010) High performance liquid chromatography: a short review. *J Glob Pharma Technol,* 2, 22-6.

Matés, JM, Pérez-Gómez, C & Núñez de Castro, I (1999) Antioxidant enzymes and human diseases. *Clin Biochem,* 32, 595-603.
[http://dx.doi.org/10.1016/S0009-9120(99)00075-2] [PMID: 10638941]

Matsui, T, Ebuchi, S, Kobayashi, M, Fukui, K, Sugita, K, Terahara, N & Matsumoto, K (2002) Anti-hyperglycemic effect of diacylated anthocyanin derived from Ipomoea batatas cultivar Ayamurasaki can be achieved through the alpha-glucosidase inhibitory action. *J Agric Food Chem,* 50, 7244-8.
[http://dx.doi.org/10.1021/jf025913m] [PMID: 12452639]

Mattila, P & Kumpulainen, J (2002) Determination of free and total phenolic acids in plant-derived foods by HPLC with diode-array detection. *J Agric Food Chem,* 50, 3660-7.
[http://dx.doi.org/10.1021/jf020028p] [PMID: 12059140]

McDowell, LR, Wilkinson, N, Madison, R & Felix, T (2007) Vitamins and minerals functioning as antioxidants with supplementation considerations *Florida Ruminant Nutrition Symposium,* 30-1.

McHugh, MA & Krukonis, VJ (1986) *Supercritical Fluid Extraction: Principles and Practice.*Butterworths, Stoneham.

Melis, MP, Angioni, E, Carta, G, Murru, E, Scanu, P, Spada, S & Banni, S (2001) Characterization of conjugated linoleic acid and its metabolites by RP-HPLC with diode array detector. *Eur J Lipid Sci Technol,* 103, 617-21.
[http://dx.doi.org/10.1002/1438-9312(200109)103:9<617::AID-EJLT6170>3.0.CO;2-C]

Milner, JA (1994) *Reducing the risk of cancer*
[http://dx.doi.org/10.1007/978-1-4615-2073-3_3]

Mustafa, A & Turner, C (2011) Pressurized liquid extraction as a green approach in food and herbal plants extraction: A review. *Anal Chim Acta,* 703, 8-18.
[http://dx.doi.org/10.1016/j.aca.2011.07.018] [PMID: 21843670]

Ng, RC, Kassim, NK, Yeap, YS & Ee, GC (2018) Isolation of carbazole alkaloids and coumarins from Aegle marmelos and Murraya koenigii and their antioxidant properties. *Sains Malays,* 47, 1749-56.
[http://dx.doi.org/10.17576/jsm-2018-4708-14]

Pandey, A & Tripathi, S (2014) Concept of standardization, extraction and pre phytochemical screening strategies for herbal drug. *J Pharmacogn Phytochem,* •••, 2.

Pérez, RA, Albero, B & Tadeo, JL (2020) Matrix solid phase dispersion.*Solid-Phase Extraction* Elsevier 531-49.

[http://dx.doi.org/10.1016/B978-0-12-816906-3.00019-4]

Pietta, PG (2000) Flavonoids as antioxidants. *J Nat Prod,* 63, 1035-42.
[http://dx.doi.org/10.1021/np9904509] [PMID: 10924197]

Pitt, JJ (2009) Principles and applications of liquid chromatography-mass spectrometry in clinical biochemistry. *Clin Biochem Rev,* 30, 19-34.
[PMID: 19224008]

Priego Capote, F, Jiménez, JR, Granados, JMM & de Castro, MDL (2007) Identification and determination of fat-soluble vitamins and metabolites in human serum by liquid chromatography/triple quadrupole mass spectrometry with multiple reaction monitoring. *Rapid Commun Mass Spectrom,* 21, 1745-54.
[http://dx.doi.org/10.1002/rcm.3014] [PMID: 17486676]

Qiu, Y, Liu, Q & Beta, T (2010) Antioxidant properties of commercial wild rice and analysis of soluble and insoluble phenolic acids. *Food Chem,* 121, 140-7.
[http://dx.doi.org/10.1016/j.foodchem.2009.12.021]

Qu, S, Du, Z & Zhang, Y (2015) Direct detection of free fatty acids in edible oils using supercritical fluid chromatography coupled with mass spectrometry. *Food Chem,* 170, 463-9.
[http://dx.doi.org/10.1016/j.foodchem.2014.08.043] [PMID: 25306372]

Rice-Evans, CA, Miller, NJ & Paganga, G (1996) Structure-antioxidant activity relationships of flavonoids and phenolic acids. *Free Radic Biol Med,* 20, 933-56.
[http://dx.doi.org/10.1016/0891-5849(95)02227-9] [PMID: 8743980]

Roessner, U & Beckles, DM (2009) Metabolite measurements.*Plant Metabolic Networks* 39-69.
[http://dx.doi.org/10.1007/978-0-387-78745-9_3]

Sakakibara, H, Honda, Y, Nakagawa, S, Ashida, H & Kanazawa, K (2003) Simultaneous determination of all polyphenols in vegetables, fruits, and teas. *J Agric Food Chem,* 51, 571-81.
[http://dx.doi.org/10.1021/jf020926l] [PMID: 12537425]

Schieber, A, Ullrich, W & Carle, R (2000) Characterization of polyphenols in mango puree concentrate by HPLC with diode array and mass spectrometric detection. *Innov Food Sci Emerg Technol,* 1, 161-6.
[http://dx.doi.org/10.1016/S1466-8564(00)00015-1]

Selvamuthukumaran, M & Shi, J (2017) Recent advances in extraction of antioxidants from plant by-products processing industries. *Food Quality and Safety,* 1, 61-81.
[http://dx.doi.org/10.1093/fqs/fyx004]

Shui, G & Leong, LP (2005) Screening and identification of antioxidants in biological samples using high-performance liquid chromatography-mass spectrometry and its application on Salacca edulis Reinw. *J Agric Food Chem,* 53, 880-6.
[http://dx.doi.org/10.1021/jf049112q] [PMID: 15712992]

Singh, B, Singh, JP, Kaur, A & Singh, N (2017) Phenolic composition and antioxidant potential of grain legume seeds: A review. *Food Res Int,* 101, 1-16.
[http://dx.doi.org/10.1016/j.foodres.2017.09.026] [PMID: 28941672]

Singh, B, Singh, JP, Singh, N & Kaur, A (2017) Saponins in pulses and their health promoting activities: A review. *Food Chem,* 233, 540-9.
[http://dx.doi.org/10.1016/j.foodchem.2017.04.161] [PMID: 28530610]

Singh, D & Chaudhuri, PK (2018) Structural characteristics, bioavailability and cardioprotective potential of saponins. *Integr Med Res,* 7, 33-43.
[http://dx.doi.org/10.1016/j.imr.2018.01.003] [PMID: 29629289]

Stalikas, CD (2007) Extraction, separation, and detection methods for phenolic acids and flavonoids. *J Sep Sci,* 30, 3268-95.
[http://dx.doi.org/10.1002/jssc.200700261] [PMID: 18069740]

Taguchi, K, Fukusaki, E & Bamba, T (2014) Simultaneous analysis for water- and fat-soluble vitamins by a

novel single chromatography technique unifying supercritical fluid chromatography and liquid chromatography. *J Chromatogr A,* 1362, 270-7.
[http://dx.doi.org/10.1016/j.chroma.2014.08.003] [PMID: 25200530]

Taylor, LT (2009) Supercritical fluid chromatography for the 21st century. *J Supercrit Fluids,* 47, 566-73.
[http://dx.doi.org/10.1016/j.supflu.2008.09.012]

Tinggi, U (2008) Selenium: its role as antioxidant in human health. *Environ Health Prev Med,* 13, 102-8.
[http://dx.doi.org/10.1007/s12199-007-0019-4] [PMID: 19568888]

Unger, KK, Skudas, R & Schulte, MM (2008) Particle packed columns and monolithic columns in high-performance liquid chromatography-comparison and critical appraisal. *J Chromatogr A,* 1184, 393-415.
[http://dx.doi.org/10.1016/j.chroma.2007.11.118] [PMID: 18177658]

Visnevschi-Necrasov, T, Barreira, JC, Cunha, SC, Pereira, G, Nunes, E & Oliveira, MBP (2015) Advances in isoflavone profile characterisation using matrix solid-phase dispersion coupled to HPLC/DAD in Medicago species. *Phytochem Anal,* 26, 40-6.
[http://dx.doi.org/10.1002/pca.2534] [PMID: 25098548]

Wang, D, Song, X, Yan, H, Guo, M, Fu, R, Jiang, H, Zhu, H & Wang, X (2018) Development of online-storage inner-recycling counter-current chromatography for the preparative separation of complex components of alkylphenols from sarcotesta of Ginkgo biloba L. *RSC Advances,* 8, 34321-30.
[http://dx.doi.org/10.1039/C8RA05618H]

Xynos, N, Papaefstathiou, G, Psychis, M, Argyropoulou, A, Aligiannis, N & Leandros, AS (2012) Development of a green extraction procedure with super/subcritical fluids to produce extracts enriched in oleuropein from olive leaves. *J Supercrit Fluids,* 67, 89-93.
[http://dx.doi.org/10.1016/j.supflu.2012.03.014]

Yifan, Y & Jeremy, R (2010) *Theories and concepts in the composition of Chinese herbal formulas*

Yousuf, B, Gul, K, Wani, AA & Singh, P (2016) Health benefits of anthocyanins and their encapsulation for potential use in food systems: a review. *Crit Rev Food Sci Nutr,* 56, 2223-30.
[http://dx.doi.org/10.1080/10408398.2013.805316] [PMID: 25745811]

Zhang, QW, Lin, LG & Ye, WC (2018) Techniques for extraction and isolation of natural products: a comprehensive review. *Chin Med,* 13, 20.
[http://dx.doi.org/10.1186/s13020-018-0177-x] [PMID: 29692864]

Zhou, B, Wu, LM, Yang, L & Liu, ZL (2005) Evidence for alpha-tocopherol regeneration reaction of green tea polyphenols in SDS micelles. *Free Radic Biol Med,* 38, 78-84.
[http://dx.doi.org/10.1016/j.freeradbiomed.2004.09.023] [PMID: 15589374]

CHAPTER 8

Efficacy of Dietary Antioxidants in Diseases Prevention

Khadiga S. Ibrahim[1,*]

[1] *Environmental and Occupational Medicine Department, National Research Centre, Dokki, Cairo, Egypt*

Abstract: Free radicals produced within the body as the inevitable side-effects of standard metabolic procedures of cells, or by exposure to poisons in nature. Excessive levels of free radicals trigger a disorder called oxidative stress, which can destroy cells and contribute to chronic diseases like atherosclerosis, diabetes, rheumatoid arthritis, ocular disease, Alzheimer's disease, deterioration in the immune system, and different kinds of cancer. Antioxidants are materials that counterbalanced free radicals and delay, hinder or remove harm brought about by free radicals. Nutritional antioxidants are commonly distributed in different food forms. Plant foods are major sources of antioxidants. They protect against oxidative stress and reduce the danger of numerous ailments by acting as oxygen and peroxyl radical scavengers. A diet that includes berries, fruits, vegetables, grains, tea, coffee, nuts, and healthy oils has an excellent antioxidant supplement. This combination of multiple detoxifying antioxidants can play a synergistic role in reducing the risk of ailments. Antioxidants including vitamins (A, E, and C), as well as carotenoids and other minerals (zinc, manganese, copper, and selenium) are important for antioxidant enzyme activities. Nutritional polyphenols and flavonoids are also powerful antioxidant compounds. In this chapter, we address the medicinal advantages of various antioxidants in reducing the risk of inflammatory ailments of skin, eye, neurodegenerative, cardiovascular, diabetes and liver diseases.

Keywords: Antioxidants, Cancer, Cardiovascular diseases, Diabetes mellitus, Dietary polyphenols, Eye diseases, Free radicals, Inflammatory diseases, Lipoic acid, Liver diseases, Minerals, Neurodegenerative diseases, Osteoporosis, Vitamins.

INTRODUCTION

Free radicals are produced from both endogenous and exogenous sources. Immune cell activation, irritation, infection, malignant growth, excessive exercise, mental stress, and aging are accountable for endogenous free radical creation for

---

* **Corresponding author Khadiga S. Ibrahim:** Professor of Biochemistry - Department of Environmental & Occupational Medicine - National Research Centre - El-Bohouth St. (Tahrir St. Prev.) Dokki, Cairo-12622, Egypt. E-mail: khadigasalah@yahoo.com

the most part during electron transport in mitochondria. While exogenous free radicals are often produced from exposure to ecological stress or toxins (radiations, heavy metals, and cigarette smoke), and xenobiotics (Young and Woodside 2001, Valko *et al.* 2007).

Under normal conditions, a state of equilibrium between the reactive species and endogenous antioxidants was found. When this equilibrium is disrupted, it results in a situation called oxidative stress where the production of these free radicals exceeds the antioxidant potential of the body (Poljsak *et al.* 2013, Pizzino *et al.*, 2017). The excess production of reactive oxygen species (ROS) damages unsaturated fatty acids membranes, which cause a loss of membrane fluidity and cell degradation (Nimse and Pal 2015). ROS also leads to the formation of several denatured proteins with deleterious assault on nucleic acids, which ultimately results in mutations that can produce malignancy (Davies *et al.* 1987). ROS attacks on carbohydrates cause severe changes in cell receptors, which significantly alter neurotransmitter and hormonal reactions (Dalle-Donne *et al.* 2003). These radicals damage certain cell organelles, particularly the mitochondria, which can cause energy disturbances and create numerous cytotoxic compounds that harm cells. Most chronic diseases are emerging as a result of these deleterious consequences of oxidative stress. Several investigations have shown that many diseases such as atherosclerosis, cataracts, obesity, diabetes, various types of cancers, Alzheimer's disease (AD), cardiovascular disease (CVD), and arthritis are closely linked to oxidative stress (Labat-Robert and Robert 2014, Liu *et al.* 2018). To overcome these harmful impacts of free radicals for restoring the natural body balance between oxidants and antioxidants, the intake of various kinds of antioxidants are necessary. Dietary natural antioxidants (Fig. **1**) are preferred instead of synthetic antioxidants since the latter has numerous unfavorable impacts. Vegetables and fruits are studied extensively and have been appeared to bring down the occurrence of numerous maladies (Slavin and Lloyd 2012). Numerous edible herbs are rich sources of these antioxidants and have an important role in protection against many diseases (Abdel-Azeem *et al.* 2017). The use of a mixture of antioxidants may potentially be more effective than a single antioxidant, as they can act synergistically (Liu 2003, Sonam and Guleria 2017). Vitamins (vitamin A, E, and C), polyphenols (phenolic acids, anthocyanins, flavonoids, lignans, isoflavones, and stilbenes) and, carotenoids (xanthophylls, carotenes, and lycopene) are common plant-based antioxidants (Manach *et al.* 2004, Baiano and del Nobile 2015). Generally, these natural antioxidants, particularly polyphenols and carotenoids, display beneficial biological actions with anti-inflammatory, antibacterial, antiviral, anti-aging, and anticancer activities (Li *et al.* 2014, Zhang *et al.* 2015, Zhou *et al.* 2016, Xu *et al.* 2017).

DIETARY ANTIOXIDANTS

Vitamins

Natural foods are the main sources of many vitamins, of these, vitamin A is a fat-soluble vitamin. Several carotenoids like lutein, canthaxanthin, astaxanthin, lycopene, and neoxanthin have high antioxidant activity. Vitamin A and carotenoids rich foods include cantaloupe melon, mango, liver, carrot, broccoli, sweet potato, butter, spinach, pumpkin, cheddar, apricot, pear, and egg. Thermal treatment facilitates cell-wall disruption and loosened chemical bonding, which increase the bioaccessibility and absorption of carotenoids (Fernandez-Garcia *et al.* 2012). However, combinations with medications, such as aspirin and sulphonamides, decrease the bioavailability of the β-carotene (Castenmiller and West 1997). The recommended dietary allowance (RDA) for vitamin A is 900 µg/day for men and 700 µg/day for women (Olson 1987). Antioxidant effects of vitamin A and carotenoids are due to the hydrophobic chain of polyene units, which quench or neutralize free radicals (Galano 2007). Nevertheless, a significantly high dose of β-carotene has an adverse effect on the incidence of lung cancer in smokers (Druesne-Pecollo *et al.* 2010).

Vitamin E is a collective term for a group of eight fat soluble compounds, four of which are tocopherols and four are tocotrienols (Wang and Quinn 1999). Alpha-tocopherol is the most abundant type of tocopherol in plasma and possesses the best bioavailability. It shields the cell membrane from oxidative damage by neutralizing lipid radicals created in the lipid peroxidation chain response (Lobo *et al.* 2010). Along these lines, it keeps up the integrity of fatty acids within the cell membranes and improves their bioactivity (Rizvi *et al.* 2014). Tocopherol inhibits chronic oxidative stress-related illnesses (Niki 2015). Nuts, asparagus, wheat germ, avocado, egg, spinach, milk, seeds, and entire grain food are the rich sources of tocopherol. The RDA of vitamin E for both genders is 15 mg/day.

Vitamin C is also referred to as ascorbic acid and ascorbate. It is a crucial nutrient necessary for all our body systems to function properly. Vitamin C plays a powerful role in protecting the various tissues against oxidative stress. It works as a cofactor in numerous enzymatic reactions for collagen synthesis because it is a necessary component of collagen hydroxyproline and hydroxylysine synthesis (Darr *et al.* 1993, Akbari *et al.* 2016). Also, it is a vital component for many enzymatic reactions and the proper functioning of the immune system (Carr and Maggini 2017). There is widespread use of vitamin C in medications against a huge number of disorders. Human diseases, which address the essential effect of vitamin C are common cold, cataracts, malignant growth, atherosclerosis, diabetes, and degenerative neurological disorders (Chambial *et al.* 2013).

Ascorbate is a neuromodulator of cholinergic, dopaminergic, GABAergic and glutamatergic transmission and associated behaviors (Harrison and May 2009).

Vitamin C rich sources include strawberries, mustard, broccoli, red or green peppers, cauliflower, turnip greens, potatoes, winter squash, spinach, oranges, lemons, tomatoes, cabbage, guavas, raspberries, grapefruit, and other leafy greens (García-Closas 2004).

Numerous analysts have reported that nonsmoking people require 90–100 mg of vitamin C/day for optimal protection against chronic diseases (Carr and Frei 1999). Pehlivan (2017) has documented that vitamin C can act as a prooxidant, particularly in the presence of transition metals, like iron and copper, causing various harmful free radical reactions.

Dietary Minerals

Minerals are inorganic chemicals that all living organisms required. The majority of the minerals in the human diet are obtained from food and drinking water. Minerals like selenium, copper, zinc, and manganese are components of enzymatic antioxidants. Selenium (Se) is the main component for well-being with a recommended dietary allowance (RDA) of 55 µg/day for men aged 31–50 years and up to 70 µg/day for women on lactation (European Food Safety Authority, 2014). Selenium is a vital component for the antioxidant enzymes like glutathione peroxides (GPx) and thioredoxin reductase (Rayman 2012). Foods rich in Se are mushrooms, seafood (particularly shellfish and tuna), beans, sunflower seeds, meat, poultry, liver, eggs, and brown rice. The deficiency of Se accounts for an increased risk of various diseases like Keshan disease and Kashin-Beck ailment (Fairweather-Tait *et al.* 2011). Se functions as an antioxidant due to its presence in the GPx, an important antioxidant-enzyme (Lobo *et al.* 2010). Through its antioxidant activity, Se protects the cell membranes from the development of free radicals and reduces the danger of cardiovascular and some forms of cancers like colon, prostate, and breast (Brown and Arthur 2001). Wang *et al.* (2017) evaluated the antioxidant role of dietary administration of Se for controlling chronic metabolic disorders, such as hyperlipidemia, hyperglycemia, and hyperphenylalaninemia.

Antioxidant activity by transition metals like zinc (Zn), manganese (Mn), and copper (Cu) has been reported. This effect is attributed to the redox capacity of these metal ions and their capability to modify the physical and chemical properties of the membranes. They could also, displace iron from its binding sites in membranes (Halliwell and Gtteridge 2006). Manganese may hinder lipid peroxidation *in Vivo* and *in vitro*. It is one of the important components of SOD that is responsible for scavenging free radicals. It possesses an important role in the metabolic response of disease prevention and control (Li and Yang 2018).

Zinc is a metal that is fundamental to human physiology. It is a cofactor for SOD antioxidant enzyme. It also significantly activates antioxidant enzymes and inhibits the oxidant-promoting enzymes like inducible nitric acid synthase (Prasad 2014). Clinical manifestations of Zn deficiency include growth-retardation, increased oxidative stress, production of inflammatory cytokines, fertility disorders, and immune dysfunctions (Prasad 2013). The therapeutic level of Zn supplementation effectively decreases the progression of age-related ailments in the elderly (Vishwanathan *et al.* 2013). Zn has been reported to increase the sensitivity of insulin, ultimately reducing chronic hyperglycemia in type 2 diabetes mellitus (Vashum *et al.* 2014). Additionally, Costello and Franklin (2016) reported dietary zinc supplementation might decrease the chance of cancer risk.

The importance of Cu in humans is firmly established by its key role in erythropoiesis and fetal development. RDA for Cu is 0.9 mg/day for 19-70 years old women and men (Food and Nutrition Board 2006). Further, Cu has a vital role in the expression of antioxidant enzymes. Copper is an essential catalytic cofactor for Cu-dependent antioxidant enzymes like Cu-Zn SOD and ceruloplasmin. The activity of such enzymes may be compromised under inadequate Cu levels. Further, the activity of non-Cu-containing antioxidant enzymes such as catalase and selenium peroxidase also decreases due to Cu deficiency. Interestingly, the free radicals scavenging power of metallothioneins and glutathione is substantially altered by the decreased plasma Cu levels (Uriu-Adams and Keen 2005). Though such minerals are essentially required as a cofactor in enzyme activity, they must be utilized in the concentration as low as possible since they interact with certain antioxidants and lead to the creation of free radicals.

Polyphenols

Polyphenols or phenolic compounds can be divided into flavonoids and non-flavonoids. The group flavonoids are flavonols and anthocyanins. The nonflavonoids include phenolic acids (benzoic and hydroxycinnamic acids) and stilbenes (Del Rio *et al.* 2013). The phenolic components curtail the progression of many chronic diseases due to their beneficial properties such as antioxidative (Heima *et al.* 2002), anti-inflammatory (Nichols *et al.* 2010), and neuroprotective effects (Aquilano *et al.* 2008), along with the cardioprotective (Zern *et al.* 2005) and chemopreventive actions (Jafari *et al.* 2014). Furthermore, polyphenols help the body's immune system by acting as anti-inflammatory agents to restrain angiogenesis and prevent tumor development (Tabrez *et al.* 2013).

Polyphenols provide therapeutic effects *via* many actions such as quenching of free radicals, the maintenance and reclamation of other dietary antioxidants (*e.g.* tocopherol), and the chelation of pro-oxidant metals. A phenol group of polyphenols takes an electron to create the most stable phenoxy radicals and suppresses oxidation reactions within the cells. Green tea polyphenols have a strong activity on neurodegenerative ailments such as AD (Oz 2017). Grape seeds contain an immense number of polyphenols. Hokayem *et al.* (2013) affirmed that grape polyphenols could hinder oxidative stress and insulin resistance incited *via* fructose in type II diabetic patients. Also, grape seed polyphenols can hinder the apoptosis of vascular cells through the repression of ROS generated by xanthine oxidase. Farah and Lima (2019) concluded that the antioxidant and anti-inflammatory impacts of chlorogenic acids within coffee are answerable for decreasing the frequency of different degenerative and non-degenerative diseases.

Herbs, spices, and nuts are significant sources of polyphenol. Many investigations revealed numerous plant sources in the antioxidative treatments such as oregano, thyme (TV), sage, cinnamon, rosemary (RM), saffron, ginger, and dried mint leaves. Cinnamon has potent antioxidant activity and is used in the prevention and management of perilous diseases like diabetes and AD. Cinnamon has anticholesterol, and antibacterial activity, and restrains angiogenesis in malignant cell growth (Hamidpour *et al.* 2015). The role of TV and RM against gentamicin (GM) - incited nephrotoxicity in rats was investigated by Abdel-Azeem *et al.* (2017). Both TV and RM showed free radical scavenging capability against GM-induced hepatotoxicity and improved the lipid profile abnormalities in rats (Hegazy *et al.* 2018). Elbahnasawy *et al.* (2019) also showed that TV and RM could present a promising prospect in the prevention of bone resorption and osteoporosis. Besides, ginger, *via* its antioxidant power showed antiaging activity in various age-related maladies through their anti-inflammatory action (Tanaka *et al.* 2015). It can lower the amount of malonaldehyde (MDA) and also reduce the tumor necrotic factor-α.

Alpha-lipoic Acid (ALA)

Alpha-lipoic acid is an organosulfur compound (both water- and fat-soluble) that serves as a strong antioxidant within the body. It may have a role in weight loss, decreased blood glucose levels, diminished inflammation, slowed skin aging, and improved nerve work (Salehi *et al.* 2019). Red meat and organ meats (liver and kidney) are excellent sources of alpha-lipoic acids and also present in many vegetables like broccoli, potatoes, tomatoes, rice bran, green peas, and spinach. Holmquist *et al.* (2007) reported that by the antioxidant activity and through increased production of acetylcholine *via* activation of choline acetyltransferase,

ALA exhibits antidementia or anti-AD properties. Furthermore, ALA could have beneficial impacts on autoimmune diseases (Liu *et al*. 2019).

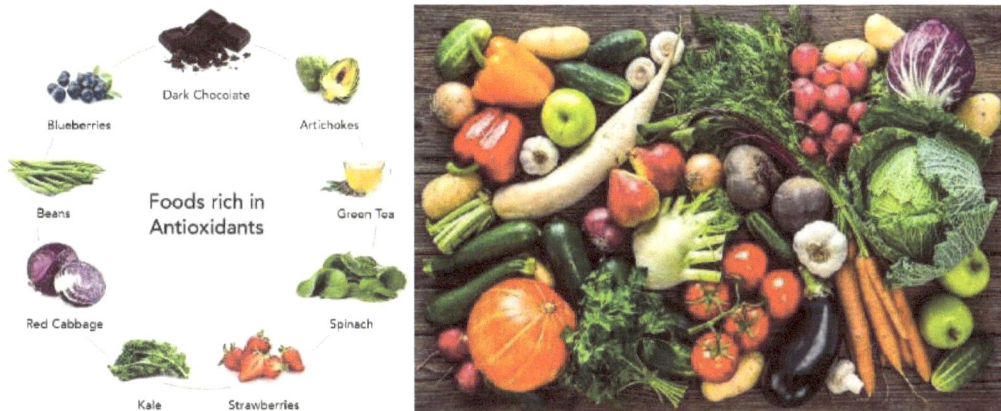

Fig. (1). Foods rich in antioxidants.

ANTIOXIDANTS AND DISEASES MANAGEMENT

Nutritional antioxidants are dispersed in variety of foods and edible herbs. These antioxidants, particularly carotenoids and polyphenols, have a wide scope of biological effects, including anti-aging, anti-atherosclerosis, anti-inflammatory, and anticancer properties.

Ample antioxidants from the foods and herbs are explored as functional foods or potentially as food additives (Hajhashemi *et al*. 2010, Xu *et al*. 2017). Various clinical investigations suggest that the antioxidants in fruits, vegetables, tea, and red wine contribute to reducing the incidence of chronic diseases like cardiovascular disease, inflammatory disease, neurodegenerative diseases, diabetes, and some cancers (Labriola and Livingston 1999, Pandey and Rizvi 2009). So, a balanced diet and dietary antioxidant supplementation have a powerful potential in the management, treatment, and prevention of many diseases.

Antioxidants in Inflammatory Diseases

Vitamin E, A, and C have anti-inflammatory activity and scavenge free radicals that attack lipids and proteins, thus protecting the lipids within cell membranes from peroxidation (McAlindon and Felson 1997).

Pycnogenol plays an important role in the prevention of numerous inflammatoryailments. It increases the intracellular response to scavenge free radicalsby reducing the creation of peroxides by macrophages and shield the cells andtissues from oxidative stress (Rohdewald 2002).

The tea polyphenols inhibit various mechanisms of inflammation. Green tea, *Camellia sinensis*, contains polyphenolic compounds that reduce the arthritis-related inflammation through catechins, which hinder the proteoglycan and collagen breakdown (Adcocks *et al.* 2002, Oz 2017).

Rubin *et al.* (2017) recorded that carotenoids (16 mg/day for 26 days) are inversely correlated with inflammatory markers such as interleukin (IL)- 1 β, tumor necrosis factor-α, IL-6, vascular cell adhesion molecule-1 (VCAM-1), and monocyte chemoattractant protein 1 (MCP-1) in both human and animal models.

Rheumatoid arthritis is a chronic inflammatory disorder that affects the joints and surrounding tissues *via* activated macrophages and infiltration of T-cells (Walston *et al.* 2006, Ostrowska *et al.* 2018). In rheumatoid arthritis, harmful compounds are discharged from the synovium that causes inflammation of the joint tissues leading to the degradation of cartilage. Free radicals at the inflammatory site play an important role in both initiation and development of this condition, as shown by the elevated levels of isoprostane and prostaglandin in the affected patients' synovial fluid (Mahajan and Tandon 2004). Epigallocatechin-3-gallate improves the immune system and joint inflammation through T helper-17 and regulatory T cells, thereby help in the inhibition of osteoclastogenesis (Lee *et al.* 2016). Further, dietary flavonoids may have a possible function in treating patients with inflammatory neutrophil-mediated sicknesses (Nikfarjam *et al.* 2017a, 2017b). Curcumin also has anti-arthritic effects in humans with beneficial effects against inflammatory diseases like osteoarthritis and rheumatoid arthritis (Hewlings and Kalman 2017).

Antioxidants and Diabetes Mellitus (DM) Management

Diabetes mellitus is a chronic disease resulting from the inadequacy or inability of the pancreas to produce insulin. Close to 1.6 million individuals worldwide died in 2016 from diabetes. Type 2 diabetes is the disease's most prevalent form, accounting for almost 90 percent of all cases of diabetes mellitus worldwide (WHO 2019a). Diabetes mellitus is a progressive disease accompanied by complications that include macro- and micro-vascular harm, neuropathy, retinopathy, and nephropathy (Fowler 2011, Chawla *et al.* 2016). Oxidative stress is recognized as a primary risk factor for diabetes development (Ullah *et al.* 2016). Many factors, like aging, obesity, and excessive food consumption, are linked to an increase in oxidative stress and ultimately alter the insulin production by impairing glucose tolerance or fostering insulin resistance (Wang *et al.* 2013). Hyperglycemia is generally associated with diabetes and results in an increase of overall oxidizing conditions (Yan 2014). Different studies have shown that antioxidants in diabetic patients can lower the markers of oxidative stress and lipid peroxidation. Basic carotenoid, astaxanthin, is a potent antioxidant used in diabetes prevention and treatment. Astaxanthin (1.0 mg/mouse/day for 13 weeks) decreases blood glucose levels, increases serum insulin levels, and lowers glucose tolerance in type 2 diabetes rat models (Uchiyama *et al.* 2002). A prospective 10-year examination involving 37,846 people has announced that the high dietary intake of β-carotene (10 ± 4 mg/day) can decrease the danger of type 2 diabetes mellitus (Sluijs *et al.* 2015). The isoflavones genistein and daidzein present in soybean and the byproducts of these compounds help to control diabetes. Also, because of their positive activities on glucose and lipid digestion, dietary phytoestrogens, including isoflavones and lignans, have a useful role in managing both obesity and diabetes. Flaxseed has the best lignan concentration and is also found in seeds, entire grains, and vegetables. Such lignans have been found to possess a crucial role as antioxidants in diabetes control (Bhathena *et al.* 2002). Valdés-Ramos *et al.* (2015) showed that vitamin E, C, and β-carotene insufficiency are also observed in diabetic patients. El-Shobaki *et al.* (2017) demonstrated that the treatment of diabetic rats with formulation containing fenugreek, cinnamon, coffee, ginseng, Jerusalem artichoke, and ste*via* could adjust the hyperglycemia and correct the complications of diabetes.

Antioxidants and Cardiovascular Disease (CVD) Management

In developing countries, CVDs are recognized as the leading cause of high mortality rates. In several CVDs, oxidative stress can be treated as either an essential or an auxiliary reason (Cervantes *et al.* 2017). Kaplan *et al.* (2015) reported that oxidative stress which ultimately increments oxidized low-density lipoprotein (LDL) is the primary cause of blood vessel hypertension, CVDs, atherosclerosis, coronary cardiovascular disease, and cardiopathy.

Other risk factors incorporate lifestyle because of the diet with high fat, energy and cholesterol, tobacco smoking, and physical immobility (Van Gaal *et al.* 2006). Additionally, an individual's genes, gender, and age may play a significant role in CVD. Casas *et al.* (2018) observed potential targets like food patterns, single food, or individual nutrients has beneficial impacts on forestalling CVD.

Vitamin C plays a crucial role in the prevention as well as treatment of CVD *via* increasing the high-density lipoprotein (HDL) (Moser and Chun, 2016) and to some extent by helping to reduce LDL (McRae 2008).

Flavanols from tea, cocoa, and apples substantially minimize the total cholesterol, LDL and increase HDL level (González-Sarrías *et al.* 2017). Low β-carotene levels have been found with an elevated danger of myocardial infarction in smokers (Cook *et al.* 2007).

In addition, several natural compounds in vegetables, fruits, and herbs have been shown to display cardioprotective actions through their antioxidant properties. A good antioxidant source is lycopene, a carotenoid bounteously present within tomatoes. Cheng *et al.* (2019) showed an inverse relationship between lycopene consumption and the risk of CVD. Also, grape proanthocyanidin had remarkable heart protection ability (Martín-Fernández *et al.* 2014). Turmeric extracts also mask doxorubicin toxicity on the heart (EL-Sayed *et al.* 2011).

These natural antioxidants can shield the heart by activating the Nrf2 transcription factor through the upregulation of gene expression for phase II detoxification enzymes and proteins like GST, glutamylcysteine synthase, and ferritin (Chen and Kunsch 2004). Ninić *et al.* (2019) concurred with this theory and demonstrated that gene expression for Cu/Zn (Cu/Zn SOD) and Mn (Mn-SOD) enzymes may downregulate with the oxidative stress in patients suffering from coronary artery disease.

Antioxidants and Liver Diseases Management

Within the body, the liver is an essential organ that helps in reductive biotransformation of both xenobiotic and endogenous compounds. It is therefore a key focus for many disorders, such as oxidative stress, which can contribute to liver diseases (Eapen 2019). Many organelles can produce ROS in liver parenchymal cells, like the mitochondrion. ROS can increase collagen production and its synthesis by hepatic stellate cells, which cause liver fibrosis and cirrhosis (Cichoż-Lach and Michalak 2014). Antioxidant supplementation is therefore crucial to the defense of the liver against different chronic ailments and various degenerative diseases through the regulation of cell apoptosis, gene expression, protein building, and action of stellate cells (Singal *et al.* 2011).

Nonalcoholic fatty liver disease (NAFLD) is characterized by the accumulation of excess liver fatty acids. Vitamin E has been clinically exhibited to be a promising medication for NAFLD. Further, tea leaves can treat NAFLD caused by incessant ethanol drinking through their flavonoids and polyphenolic compounds (Xu *et al.* 2019). Rosemary and thyme extracts that are rich in many polyphenols could also protect the liver from gentamicin toxicity in rats (Hegazy *et al.* 2018). While ginger gives hepatic defense against acetaminophen toxicity (Abdel-Azeem *et al.* 2013). Melatonin, a hormone that is primarily secreted *via* the pineal gland and also found in several foods, is more effective than tocopherol in preventing cholestasis (Bonomini *et al.* 2018). Melatonin has a strong capacity for removing ROS and nitrogen species and downregulates the gene expression of pro-inflammatory cytokines. Curcumin has hepatoprotective ability against liver cirrhosis and prevents malignant growths (Wang *et al.* 2012). It increases the mRNA levels and expression of antioxidant enzymes (Farzaei *et al.* 2018). Quercetin, a flavonoid found within the onion and apple, has been demonstrated to show hepatoprotective action by downregulating the level of profibrogenic genes and increasing the gene expression of antioxidant enzymes, like, SOD and catalase (El Faras and Elsawaf 2017).

Coffee and green tea intake is inversely associated with liver disorders, through their antioxidant potential, and decreased profibrogenic cytokine production (Salomone *et al.* 2017, Budryn *et al.* 2018).

Antioxidants in Cancer Management

Carcinogenesis begins by converting a normal cell into a cancerous cell. This transition includes initiation, development, and progression (Halliwell 2000). Dietary phytochemicals can interact with each of the above-mentioned stages to prevent the development of cancer. Polyphenols found mainly in fruits, vegetables, tea, coffee, chocolates, legumes, cereals, have anticarcinogenic and antimutagenic actions and may interfere with a specific stage of cancer, thereby reducing the hazard of certain malignant growths especially of the stomach and respiratory tracts (Surh 2003). It has appeared that grape seed proanthocyanidin extract possesses a beneficial effect against various stages of neoplastic processes and carcinogenesis (Bagchi *et al.* 2014).

Lycopene scavenges free radicals to prevent lipid and DNA damage and has anticarcinogenic properties (Kelkel *et al.* 2011). Many examinations have discovered that the intake of fruits and vegetables rich in carotenoids can forestall cancers like prostate and cervical (Satomi 2017, Hoang *et al.* 2018). A diet of high plant-based foods is generally known to be good for the prevention of malignant growth. Furthermore, Pan *et al.* (2011) recommended that dietary supplementation of β-carotene, tocopherol, vitamin C, and Zn reduce the risk of breast cancer. In addition, several dietary antioxidants have a vital role in the prevention of skin cancer (Katta and Brown 2015). Curcumin also has anticancer effects on a variety of malignant growths like prostate, breast, and colorectal cancers (Tomeh *et al.* 2019).

Resveratrol has a chemopreventive action against prostate cancer cells *via* apoptotic induction (Jasiński *et al.* 2013). Additionally, isothiocyanates from cruciferous vegetables have chemopreventive actions against many cancers (Robin *et al.* 2015, Mitsiogianni *et al.* 2019). Also, α-lipoic acid induces apoptosis in lung cancer (Moungjaroen *et al.* 2006), breast cancer (Dozio *et al.* 2010), and colon cancer (Trivedi and Jena 2013).

Dietary Antioxidants and Osteoporosis

Osteoporosis is the most severe metabolic bone condition, which is characterized by low bone mass and increased bone fragility (International Foundation for Osteoporosis 2017). By reducing oxidative stress, carotenoids could forestall bone injuries. Osteoclastogenesis and osteoblasts apoptosis is triggered by the oxidative stress and ultimately contribute to bone resorption (Almeida *et al.* 2007). Furthermore, epidemiological investigations have discovered that dietary intake of carotenoids can lower the risk of osteoporosis (Dai *et al.* 2014) and improve bone mineral density and thickness (Zhang *et al.* 2016).

Tominari *et al.* (2017) demonstrated that lutein suppresses the resorption of osteoclastic bone and promotes bone formation. High levels of serum lutein and zeaxanthin increase bone thickness in healthy young adults, recommending their key role in ideal bone health (Bovier and Hammond 2017).

Antioxidants and Eye Disorders

Radiations, smoke, and other contaminants are oxidative factors that the eye, particularly the retina, is often exposed to. Different eye diseases, like age-related macular degeneration (AMD), cataract, glaucoma, and diabetic retinopathy (DR), have been associated with oxidative stress (Nita and Grzybowski 2016). Acetyl--carnitine dietary enrichment is an important therapy against homocysteine-induced lens damage (Yang *et al.* 2015). Besides, Braakhuis *et al.* (2017) have shown that fruits and vegetables-rich diets prevent cataracts, glaucoma, and AMD. Pretreatment with a low concentration of flavonoids (kaempferol) protect the retina cells against AMD oxidative damage (Du *et al.* 2018). Furthermore, carotenoids have been shown to be protective agents for the eye (Bungau *et al.* 2019). In cataracts, zeaxanthin and lutein treatment have yielded significant benefits (Liu *et al.* 2014). The consumption of carotenoids reduce oxidative stress and have beneficial role in eye safety and performance (Hammond *et al.* 2014). Additionally, after nine months of treatment, N-acetylcarnosine eye drops enhanced the vision quality in cataract patients. Ample doses of vitamins C, E, and β-carotene, however, had been demonstrated to have insignificant effects against cataracts (Toh *et al.* 2007). In this sense, Garica-Medina *et al.* (2011) showed that antioxidant supplements delay the chronic or acute injury to the retina.

Antioxidants and Neurological Disorders Management

Some investigations suggest that many neurodegenerative disorders like Parkinson's disease, Alzheimer's disease (AD), amyotrophic lateral sclerosis (ALS), multiple sclerosis, depression, and memory loss are correlated with ROS and oxidative stress (Patten *et al*. 2010, Niedzielska *et al*. 2016). Alzheimer's disease is the most prevalent type of dementia, accounting for about 60-70 percent of cases (WHO 2019b). Many experimental and clinical forms of research in AD, demonstrated that oxidative damage plays a crucial role in neuron loss and dementia development (Förstermann 2008). β-amyloid, a toxic peptide commonly found in the brain of AD patients is formed by free radical activity and responsible for neurodegeneration seen during the initiation and progression of AD (Oz 2017).

The brain has some characteristics for its particular susceptibility to oxidative damage. For instance, it has a high metabolic rate and higher levels of polyunsaturated lipids (Cobley *et al*. 2018) which are the key trigger for lipid peroxidation. Antioxidants can be involved in regulating the symptoms of neurological disorders and related problems (Kim *et al*. 2015). Dietary supplements with vitamin E can minimize dyskinesia. In addition, vitamin E and C supplementation inhibits the development of AD and Parkinsons's disease (Bhatti *et al*. 2016). A few herbs, like *Calamintha Officinalis*, have demonstrated neuromodulatory effects in epilepsy with their enzymatic and non-enzymatic antioxidant constituents (Moattar *et al*. 2016). Green tea catechin diminished the frequency of infarction and modulated apoptosis of neurons (Han *et al*. 2014). Potential neuroprotective impacts of the phytochemicals present in fruits and vegetables against PD are documented (Mazo *et al*. 2017). Epicatechin (EC), a brain-permeable compound, has been exhibited to be advantageous for vascular and cognitive function in people (Chang *et al*. 2014). EC lessens cell death caused by intracerebral hemorrhage prompted with the perihematomal edema, decreases the expression of HO-1 protein and iron deposition, and decreases oxidative brain damage. It has been shown that the major polyphenolic compound of rhizomes of turmeric, curcumin, protect the brain from ischemia (Yang *et al*. 2009). Curcumin encompasses a potential neuroprotective effect against Parkinsonss disease (Mythri and Bharath 2012). An isothiocyanate, sulforaphane, in cruciferous vegetables significantly diminished the localized necrosis within the ischemic animal model (Ping *et al*. 2010). Resveratrol (in grape seed), and lycopene (a carotenoid in tomatoes and carrots) showed comparative neuroprotective properties similar to EC within the ischemic brain (Sun *et al*. 2017). As well, Lakey-Beitia *et al*. (2019) demonstrated that carotenoids are effective anti-amyloidogenic agents and can play an essential role in forestalling AD. In addition, the hot pepper capsaicin demonstrated improved effects within the AD by decreasing amyloid-beta protein deposition (Shalaby *et al*. 2019). In addition, garlic allylsulfides decrease levels of amyloid-beta (Aβ) and secure neurons from Aβ-mediated neurotoxicity (Farooqui 2017). Table **1** summarizes the dietary antioxidants and their main clinical effects in diseases.

Table 1. Some of the nutritional antioxidants and their main clinical effects in diseases.

Antioxidant	Dietary Sources	Main Clinical Effects	References
Curcumin	Turmeric	Anti-inflammatory Antimicrobial and wound healing Neuroprotective Anti-carcinogenic Anti-arthritic effects	Aggarwal and Harikumar (2009), Hewlings and Kalman (2017) Krausz *et al.* (2015) Mythri and Bharath (2012) Tomeh *et al.* (2019) Chandran and Goel (2012)
Resveratrol	Purple wine, grapes, and peanuts	Managing diabetes Cardiovasculardiseases Neurological diseases.	Nanjan and Betz (2014) Bonnefont-Rousselot (2016) Andrade *et al.* (2018)
Catchines	Green tea	Antimicrobial Anti-inflammatory, Neuroprotection Antidiabetic, Anti-carcinogenic	Reygaert *et al.* (2018) Ohishi *et al.* (2016) Khalatbary and Khademi (2018) Fu *et al.* (2017) Yang *et al.* (2016)
Quercetin	Leafy vegetables, red onions, garlic, grapes, berries, citrus fruits, black and green tea, pepper, coriander, fennel, radish, broccoli, tomatoes, apples, nuts, and red wine	prevention/management of diseases (diabetes, hypertension and neurodegenerative diseases) Anti-inflammatory	Oboh *et al.* (2016), Shi *et al.* (2016), Costa *et al.* (2019) Li *et al.*(2016)
Lycopene	Tomatoes, watermelon, papaya, apricot, and pink grapefruit	Reduce CVD risk Improvement of clinical asthma	Song *et al.* (2017), Cheng *et al.* (2019) Wood *et al.* (2012)
Carotenoids	All color fruits and vegetables, sweet potatoes, cantaloupe, corn, carrots, orange, mango, peppers, nuts, fish, salmon, eggs	Anti-carcinogenic, Preventing cardiovascular disease Preventing eye diseases Neurodegenerative	Gerster (1993), Linnewiel-Hermoni *et al.* (2015) Di Pietro *et al.* (2016) Bungau *et al.* (2019) Lakey-Beitia *et al.* (2019)
Lipoic acid	Red and organ meats, vegetables (broccoli, potatoes, tomatoes, rice bran, green peas, and spinach)	Protected neurons against ROS Anti-AD properties Used in diabetes and other diseases	Molz and Schroder (2017) Holmquist *et al.* (2007) Gomes and Negrato (2014)
Anthocyanin	Strawberries, black rice	Preserved neuromuscular junctions and muscle function	Winter *et al.* (2018)
Vitamin A	Eggs, dairy products, orange, colored fruits, green leafy and yellow-colored vegetables	Treatment of infectious illnesses. Treatment of skin illnesses Treat dry eyes	Huang *et al.* (2018) Beckenbach *et al.* (2015) Moy *et al.* (2015)

(Table 1) cont.....

Antioxidant	Dietary Sources	Main Clinical Effects	References
Vitamin C	Kakadu peach, acerola cherry, sweet and hot pepper, guavas, parsley, cabbage, lemon, Grapefruit, broccoli, and orange	Prevention and treatment of CVD, cancer, atherosclerosis, diabetes Neurodegenerative disease	Moser and Chun (2016) Chambial *et al.* (2013) Han *et al.* (2018)
Vitamin E	All nuts and seeds, asparagus, wheat germ, avocado, kiwifruit, Butternut Squash, egg, spinach, milk, olive oil, whole grain food, meat, animal fat, shrimp, trout	Ameliorated nonalcoholic steatohepatitis Protection against membrane lipid peroxidation	Sumida *et al.* (2013) Schneider (2005)
Selenium	Tuna, oyster, salmon, eggs, green peas, pepper, onion, pork, beef	Management of hyperlipidemia, hyperglycemia	Wang *et al.* (2017)
Zinc	Meat, Shellfish like oysters, crab, mussels, shrimp, Legumes, and Nuts	Reduces the hyperglycemia in type 2 diabetes Diminish the risk of malignant	Vashum *et al.* (2014) Costello and Franklin (2016)

HARMFULNESS OF ANTIOXIDANTS

Antioxidant harmfulness, particularly tocopherol, β-carotene, and lipoic acid, has been extensively studied and assessed when delivered in patients as intravenous injections or by mouth. High concentrations of vitamin A, vitamin C, and tocopherol can have an undesirable pro-oxidant effect leading to the increased possibility of lethal myocardial infarctions. β-carotene and tocopherol in greater doses, more than RDA, has also be linked with increased mortality (Bjelakovic *et al.* 2013). Tocopherol is often metabolized to quinone derivatives that are harmful to cells and create radicals of oxygen. β-carotene is the precursor of vitamin A whose excessive administration increases the incidence of cancer in smokers. Vitamin A administration can quicken bone loss and danger of hip fracture potentially because of vitamin A-induced osteoclasts incitement and inhibits new bone development increasing osteoporosis vulnerability (Binkley and Krueger 2000). Lipoic acid has antioxidant activity, however, in its reduced form (dihydrolipoic acid) it shows a pro-oxidant effect (Middha *et al.* 2019). Also, high doses of exogenous antioxidants can cause chronic diseases through pro-oxidant induced-oxidative damage over a long period (Hosseini *et al.* 2014).

CONCLUSION

The dietary antioxidants support the endogenous defense system if it fails to provide protection against oxidative stress and free radicals induced diseases. Polyphenols, vitamins A, C, and E, essential minerals, and lipoic acid are the various sources of dietary antioxidants. Antioxidants play a fundamental role in the scavenging of free radicals, the upregulation of antioxidant genes, and the improvement of our body immune system. The principal sources of antioxidants are vegetables, fruits, and herbs. It is preferable to use a mixture of antioxidants for disease management or prevention over a single one. The mixture of polyphenols, minerals, and vitamins play a significant role in the avoidance of infectious diseases, cancers, osteoporosis, CVDs, DM, eye and neurodegenerative disorders. It is worth noting that during the treatment of diseases, the utilization of dietary antioxidants should be increased not only to maintain health but also as an adjuvant to conventional treatments. However, too high doses of antioxidants have major adverse effects. Therefore, standardized non-toxic doses should be administered under medical supervision to get the necessary benefits.

CONFLICT OF INTEREST

The authors have no conflicts of interest

ACKNOWLEDGEMENTS

The authors sincerely thank the National Research Center Board of Directors for enabling them to complete this chapter.

CONSENT FOR PUBLICATION

None

REFERENCES

Abdel-Azeem, AS, Hegazy, AM, Ibrahim, KS, Farrag, AR & El-Sayed, EM (2013) Hepatoprotective, antioxidant, and ameliorative effects of ginger (Zingiber officinale Roscoe) and vitamin E in acetaminophen treated rats. *J Diet Suppl,* 10, 195-209.
[http://dx.doi.org/10.3109/19390211.2013.822450] [PMID: 23927622]

Abdel-Azeem, AS, Hegazy, AM, Zeidan, HM, Ibrahim, KS & El-Sayed, EM (2017) Potential renoprotective effects of rosemary and thyme against gentamicin toxicity in rats. *J Diet Suppl,* 14, 380-94.
[http://dx.doi.org/10.1080/19390211.2016.1253632] [PMID: 27973970]

Adcocks, C, Collin, P & Buttle, DJ (2002) Catechins from green tea (Camellia sinensis) inhibit bovine and human cartilage proteoglycan and type II collagen degradation *in vitro. J Nutr,* 132, 341-6.
[http://dx.doi.org/10.1093/jn/132.3.341] [PMID: 11880552]

Aggarwal, BB & Harikumar, KB (2009) Potential therapeutic effects of curcumin, the anti-inflammatory agent, against neurodegenerative, cardiovascular, pulmonary, metabolic, autoimmune and neoplastic diseases. *Int J Biochem Cell Biol,* 41, 40-59.
[http://dx.doi.org/10.1016/j.biocel.2008.06.010] [PMID: 18662800]

Akbari, A, Jelodar, G, Nazifi, S & Sajedianfard, J (2016) An Overview of the Characteristics and Function of Vitamin C in Various Tissues: Relying on its Antioxidant Function. *Zahedan J Res Med Sci,* 18e4037
[http://dx.doi.org/10.17795/zjrms-4037]

Almeida, M, Han, L, Martin-Millan, M, O'Brien, CA & Manolagas, SC (2007) Oxidative stress antagonizes Wnt signaling in osteoblast precursors by diverting beta-catenin from T cell factor- to forkhead box O-

mediated transcription. *J Biol Chem,* 282, 27298-305.
[http://dx.doi.org/10.1074/jbc.M702811200] [PMID: 17623658]

Andrade, S, Ramalho, MJ, Pereira, MDC & Loureiro, JA (2018) Resveratrol Brain Delivery for Neurological Disorders Prevention and Treatment. *Front Pharmacol,* 9, 1261.
[http://dx.doi.org/10.3389/fphar.2018.01261] [PMID: 30524273]

Aquilano, K, Baldelli, S, Rotilio, G & Ciriolo, MR (2008) Role of nitric oxide synthases in Parkinson's disease: a review on the antioxidant and anti-inflammatory activity of polyphenols. *Neurochem Res,* 33, 2416-26.
[http://dx.doi.org/10.1007/s11064-008-9697-6] [PMID: 18415676]

Bagchi, D, Swaroop, A, Preuss, HG & Bagchi, M (2014) Free radical scavenging, antioxidant and cancer chemoprevention by grape seed proanthocyanidin: an overview. *Mutat Res,* 768, 69-73.
[http://dx.doi.org/10.1016/j.mrfmmm.2014.04.004] [PMID: 24751946]

Baiano, A & Del Nobile, MA (2016) Antioxidant compounds from vegetable matrices: Biosynthesis, occurrence, and extraction systems. *Crit Rev Food Sci Nutr,* 56, 2053-68.
[http://dx.doi.org/10.1080/10408398.2013.812059] [PMID: 25751787]

Beckenbach, L, Baron, JM, Merk, HF, Löffler, H & Amann, PM (2015) Retinoid treatment of skin diseases. *Eur J Dermatol,* 25, 384-91.
[http://dx.doi.org/10.1684/ejd.2015.2544] [PMID: 26069148]

Bhathena, SJ & Velasquez, MT (2002) Beneficial role of dietary phytoestrogens in obesity and diabetes. *Am J Clin Nutr,* 76, 1191-201.
[http://dx.doi.org/10.1093/ajcn/76.6.1191] [PMID: 12450882]

Bhatti, AB, Usman, M, Ali, F & Satti, SA (2016) Vitamin supplementation as an adjuvant treatment for Alzheimer's disease. *J Clin Diagn Res,* 10, OE07-11.
[http://dx.doi.org/10.7860/JCDR/2016/20273.8261] [PMID: 27656493]

Binkley, N & Krueger, D (2000) Hypervitaminosis A and bone. *Nutr Rev,* 58, 138-44.
[http://dx.doi.org/10.1111/j.1753-4887.2000.tb01848.x] [PMID: 10860393]

Bjelakovic, G, Nikolova, D & Gluud, C (2013) Meta-regression analyses, meta-analyses, and trial sequential analyses of the effects of supplementation with beta-carotene, vitamin A, and vitamin E singly or in different combinations on all-cause mortality: do we have evidence for lack of harm? *PLoS One,* 8e74558
[http://dx.doi.org/10.1371/journal.pone.0074558] [PMID: 24040282]

Bonnefont-Rousselot, D (2016) Resveratrol and Cardiovascular Diseases. *Nutrients,* 8, 250.
[http://dx.doi.org/10.3390/nu8050250] [PMID: 27144581]

Bonomini, F, Borsani, E, Favero, G, Rodella, LF & Rezzani, R (2018) Dietary Melatonin Supplementation Could Be a Promising Preventing/Therapeutic Approach for a Variety of Liver Diseases. *Nutrients,* 10, 1135.
[http://dx.doi.org/10.3390/nu10091135] [PMID: 30134592]

Bovier, ER & Hammond, BR (2017) The macular carotenoids lutein and zeaxanthin are related to increased bone density in young healthy adults. *Foods,* 6, 78.
[http://dx.doi.org/10.3390/foods6090078] [PMID: 28880221]

Braakhuis, A, Raman, R & Vaghefi, E (2017) The association between dietary intake of antioxidants and ocular disease. *Diseases,* 5, 3.
[http://dx.doi.org/10.3390/diseases5010003] [PMID: 28933356]

Brown, KM & Arthur, JR (2001) Selenium, selenoproteins and human health: a review. *Public Health Nutr,* 4, 593-9.
[http://dx.doi.org/10.1079/PHN2001143] [PMID: 11683552]

Budryn, G, Żyżelewicz, D, Buko, V, Lukivskaya, O, Naruta, E, Belonovskaya, E, Moroz, V, Kirko, S, Grzelczyk, J, Bojczuk, M & Falih, M (2018) Evaluation of antifibrotic effects of coffee and cocoa extracts in rats with thioacetamide-induced fibrosis. *Eur Food Res Technol,* 244, 2107-15.

[http://dx.doi.org/10.1007/s00217-018-3119-z]

Bungau, S, Abdel-Daim, MM, Tit, DM, Ghanem, E, Sato, S, Maruyama-Inoue, M, Yamane, S & Kadonosono, K (2019) Health Benefits of Polyphenols and Carotenoids in Age-Related Eye Diseases. *Oxid Med Cell Longev,* 20199783429
[http://dx.doi.org/10.1155/2019/9783429] [PMID: 30891116]

Carr, AC & Frei, B (1999) Toward a new recommended dietary allowance for vitamin C based on antioxidant and health effects in humans. *Am J Clin Nutr,* 69, 1086-107.
[http://dx.doi.org/10.1093/ajcn/69.6.1086] [PMID: 10357726]

Carr, AC & Maggini, S (2017) Vitamin C and Immune Function. *Nutrients,* 9, 1211.
[http://dx.doi.org/10.3390/nu9111211] [PMID: 29099763]

Casas, R, Castro-Barquero, S, Estruch, R & Sacanella, E (2018) Nutrition and Cardiovascular Health. *Int J Mol Sci,* 19, 3988.
[http://dx.doi.org/10.3390/ijms19123988] [PMID: 30544955]

Castenmiller, JJM & West, CE (1997) Bioavailability of carotenoids. *Pure Appl Chem,* 69, 2145-50.
[http://dx.doi.org/10.1351/pac199769102145]

Cervantes Gracia, K, Llanas-Cornejo, D & Husi, H (2017) CVD and Oxidative Stress. *J Clin Med,* 6, 22.
[http://dx.doi.org/10.3390/jcm6020022] [PMID: 28230726]

Chambial, S, Dwivedi, S, Shukla, KK, John, PJ & Sharma, P (2013) Vitamin C in disease prevention and cure: an overview. *Indian J Clin Biochem,* 28, 314-28.
[http://dx.doi.org/10.1007/s12291-013-0375-3] [PMID: 24426232]

Chandran, B & Goel, A (2012) A randomized, pilot study to assess the efficacy and safety of curcumin in patients with active rheumatoid arthritis. *Phytother Res,* 26, 1719-25.
[http://dx.doi.org/10.1002/ptr.4639] [PMID: 22407780]

Chang, CF, Cho, S & Wang, J (2014) (-)-Epicatechin protects hemorrhagic brain *via* synergistic Nrf2 pathways. *Ann Clin Transl Neurol,* 1, 258-71.
[http://dx.doi.org/10.1002/acn3.54] [PMID: 24741667]

Chawla, A, Chawla, R & Jaggi, S (2016) Microvasular and macrovascular complications in diabetes mellitus: Distinct or continuum? *Indian J Endocrinol Metab,* 20, 546-51.
[http://dx.doi.org/10.4103/2230-8210.183480] [PMID: 27366724]

Chen, XL & Kunsch, C (2004) Induction of cytoprotective genes through Nrf2/antioxidant response element pathway: a new therapeutic approach for the treatment of inflammatory diseases. *Curr Pharm Des,* 10, 879-91.
[http://dx.doi.org/10.2174/1381612043452901] [PMID: 15032691]

Cheng, HM, Koutsidis, G, Lodge, JK, Ashor, AW, Siervo, M & Lara, J (2019) Lycopene and tomato and risk of cardiovascular diseases: A systematic review and meta-analysis of epidemiological evidence. *Crit Rev Food Sci Nutr,* 59, 141-58.
[http://dx.doi.org/10.1080/10408398.2017.1362630] [PMID: 28799780]

Christen, Y (2000) Oxidative stress and Alzheimer disease. *Am J Clin Nutr,* 71, 621S-9S.
[http://dx.doi.org/10.1093/ajcn/71.2.621s] [PMID: 10681270]

Cichoż-Lach, H & Michalak, A (2014) Oxidative stress as a crucial factor in liver diseases. *World J Gastroenterol,* 20, 8082-91.
[http://dx.doi.org/10.3748/wjg.v20.i25.8082] [PMID: 25009380]

Cobley, JN, Fiorello, ML & Bailey, DM (2018) 13 reasons why the brain is susceptible to oxidative stress. *Redox Biol,* 15, 490-503.
[http://dx.doi.org/10.1016/j.redox.2018.01.008] [PMID: 29413961]

Cook, NR, Albert, CM, Gaziano, JM, Zaharris, E, MacFadyen, J, Danielson, E, Buring, JE & Manson, JE (2007) A randomized factorial trial of vitamins C and E and beta carotene in the secondary prevention of

cardiovascular events in women: results from the Women's Antioxidant Cardiovascular Study. *Arch Intern Med,* 167, 1610-8.
[http://dx.doi.org/10.1001/archinte.167.15.1610] [PMID: 17698683]

Costa, LG, Garrick, JM, Roquè, PJ & Pellacani, C (2016) Mechanisms of Neuroprotection by Quercetin: Counteracting Oxidative Stress and More. *Oxid Med Cell Longev,* 20162986796
[http://dx.doi.org/10.1155/2016/2986796] [PMID: 26904161]

Costello, LC & Franklin, RB (2016) A comprehensive review of the role of zinc in normal prostate function and metabolism; and its implications in prostate cancer. *Arch Biochem Biophys,* 611, 100-12.
[http://dx.doi.org/10.1016/j.abb.2016.04.014] [PMID: 27132038]

Dai, Z, Wang, R, Ang, LW, Low, YL, Yuan, JM & Koh, WP (2014) Protective effects of dietary carotenoids on risk of hip fracture in men: the Singapore Chinese Health Study. *J Bone Miner Res,* 29, 408-17.
[http://dx.doi.org/10.1002/jbmr.2041] [PMID: 23857780]

Dalle-Donne, I, Rossi, R, Giustarini, D, Milzani, A & Colombo, R (2003) Protein carbonyl groups as biomarkers of oxidative stress. *Clin Chim Acta,* 329, 23-38.
[http://dx.doi.org/10.1016/S0009-8981(03)00003-2] [PMID: 12589963]

Darr, D, Combs, S & Pinnell, S (1993) Ascorbic acid and collagen synthesis: rethinking a role for lipid peroxidation. *Arch Biochem Biophys,* 307, 331-5.
[http://dx.doi.org/10.1006/abbi.1993.1596] [PMID: 8274018]

Davies, KJA, Lin, SW & Pacifici, RE (1987) Protein damage and degradation by oxygen radicals. IV. Degradation of denatured protein. *J Biol Chem,* 262, 9914-20.
[http://dx.doi.org/10.1016/S0021-9258(18)48021-0] [PMID: 3036878]

Del Rio, D, Rodriguez-Mateos, A, Spencer, JPE, Tognolini, M, Borges, G & Crozier, A (2013) Dietary (poly)phenolics in human health: structures, bioavailability, and evidence of protective effects against chronic diseases. *Antioxid Redox Signal,* 18, 1818-92.
[http://dx.doi.org/10.1089/ars.2012.4581] [PMID: 22794138]

Di Pietro, N, Di Tomo, P & Pandolfi, A (2016) Carotenoids in Cardiovascular Disease Prevention. *JSM Atherosclerosis,* 1, 1002.

Dozio, E, Ruscica, M, Passafaro, L, Dogliotti, G, Steffani, L, Marthyn, P, Pagani, A, Demartini, G, Esposti, D, Fraschini, F & Magni, P (2010) The natural antioxidant alpha-lipoic acid induces p27(Kip1)-dependent cell cycle arrest and apoptosis in MCF-7 human breast cancer cells. *Eur J Pharmacol,* 641, 29-34.
[http://dx.doi.org/10.1016/j.ejphar.2010.05.009] [PMID: 20580704]

Druesne-Pecollo, N, Latino-Martel, P, Norat, T, Barrandon, E, Bertrais, S, Galan, P & Hercberg, S (2010) Beta-carotene supplementation and cancer risk: a systematic review and metaanalysis of randomized controlled trials. *Int J Cancer,* 127, 172-84.
[http://dx.doi.org/10.1002/ijc.25008] [PMID: 19876916]

Du, W, An, Y, He, X, Zhang, D & He, W (2018) Protection of Kaempferol on Oxidative Stress-Induced Retinal Pigment Epithelial Cell Damage. *Oxid Med Cell Longev,* 20181610751
[http://dx.doi.org/10.1155/2018/1610751] [PMID: 30584457]

Eapen, CE (2019) The liver: Oxidative stress and dietary antioxidants. *Indian J Med Res,* 149, 81.
[http://dx.doi.org/10.4103/ijmr.IJMR_2098_18] [PMID: 31571633]

El Faras, AA & Elsawaf, AL (2017) Hepatoprotective activity of quercetin against paracetamol induced liver toxicity in rats. *Tanta Med J,* 45, 92-8.
[http://dx.doi.org/10.4103/tmj.tmj_43_16]

Elbahnasawy, AS, Valeeva, ER, El-Sayed, EM & Rakhimov, II (2019) *The Impact of Thyme and Rosemary on Prevention of Osteoporosis in Rats*
[http://dx.doi.org/10.1155/2019/1431384]

(2011) Cardioprotective effects of curcuma longa L. Extracts against doxorubicininduced cardiotoxicity in rats. *J Med Plants Res,* 5, 4049-58.

El-Shobaki, FA, Abdel-Azeem, AS, Hegazy, AM, Hassouna, HZ & Badawy, IH (2017) Amelioration of hyperglycemia and associated health hazards using two dietary formulas composed of multiple ingredients. *Am J Food Technol,* 12, 227-35.
[http://dx.doi.org/10.3923/ajft.2017.227.235]

(2014) Scientific opinion on dietary reference values for selenium. *EFSA J,* 12, 3846.
[http://dx.doi.org/10.2903/j.efsa.2014.3846]

Fairweather-Tait, SJ, Bao, Y, Broadley, MR, Collings, R, Ford, D, Hesketh, JE & Hurst, R (2011) Selenium in human health and disease. *Antioxid Redox Signal,* 14, 1337-83.
[http://dx.doi.org/10.1089/ars.2010.3275] [PMID: 20812787]

Farah, A & Lima, JD (2019) Consumption of Chlorogenic Acids through Coffee and Health Implications. *Beverages,* 5, 11.
[http://dx.doi.org/10.3390/beverages5010011]

Farooqui, AA & Farooqui, T (2017) *Garlic and its Effects in Neurological Disorders" in Farooqui, T, Farooqui AA" Neuroprotective Effects of Phytochemicals in Neurological Disorders.*John Wiley & Sons, Inc..
[http://dx.doi.org/10.1002/9781119155195]

Farzaei, MH, Zobeiri, M, Parvizi, F, El-Senduny, FF, Marmouzi, I, Coy-Barrera, E, Naseri, R, Nabavi, SM, Rahimi, R & Abdollahi, M (2018) Curcumin in Liver Diseases: A Systematic Review of the Cellular Mechanisms of Oxidative Stress and Clinical Perspective. *Nutrients,* 10, 855.
[http://dx.doi.org/10.3390/nu10070855] [PMID: 29966389]

Fernandez-Garcia, E, Carvajal-Lerida, I, Jaren-Galan, M, Garrido-Fernández, J, Pérez-Gálvez, A & Hornero-Méndez, D (2012) Carotenoids bioavailability from foods: From plant pigments to efficient biological activities. *Food Res Int,* 46, 438-50.
[http://dx.doi.org/10.1016/j.foodres.2011.06.007]

(2006)

Förstermann, U (2008) Oxidative stress in vascular disease: causes, defense mechanisms and potential therapies. *Nat Clin Pract Cardiovasc Med,* 5, 338-49.
[http://dx.doi.org/10.1038/ncpcardio1211] [PMID: 18461048]

Fowler, MJ (2011) Microvascular and macrovascular complications of diabetes. *Clin Diabetes,* 29, 116-22.
[http://dx.doi.org/10.2337/diaclin.29.3.116]

Fu, QY, Li, QS, Lin, XM, Qiao, RY, Yang, R, Li, XM, Dong, ZB, Xiang, LP, Zheng, XQ, Lu, JL, Yuan, CB, Ye, JH & Liang, YR (2017) Antidiabetic Effects of Tea. *Molecules,* 22, 849.
[http://dx.doi.org/10.3390/molecules22050849] [PMID: 28531120]

Galano, A (2007) Relative antioxidant efficiency of a large series of carotenoids in terms of one electron transfer reactions. *J Phys Chem B,* 111, 12898-908.
[http://dx.doi.org/10.1021/jp074358u] [PMID: 17941663]

García-Closas, R, Berenguer, A, José Tormo, M, José Sánchez, M, Quirós, JR, Navarro, C, Arnaud, R, Dorronsoro, M, Dolores Chirlaque, M, Barricarte, A, Ardanaz, E, Amiano, P, Martinez, C, Agudo, A & González, CA (2004) Dietary sources of vitamin C, vitamin E and specific carotenoids in Spain. *Br J Nutr,* 91, 1005-11.
[http://dx.doi.org/10.1079/BJN20041130] [PMID: 15182404]

Garcia-Medina, JJ, Pinazo-Duran, MD, Garcia-Medina, M, Zanon-Moreno, V & Pons-Vazquez, S (2011) A 5-year follow-up of antioxidant supplementation in type 2 diabetic retinopathy. *Eur J Ophthalmol,* 21, 637-43.
[http://dx.doi.org/10.5301/EJO.2010.6212] [PMID: 21218388]

Gerster, H (1993) Anticarcinogenic effect of common carotenoids. *Int J Vitam Nutr Res,* 63, 93-121.
[PMID: 8407171]

Gomes, MB & Negrato, CA (2014) Alpha-lipoic acid as a pleiotropic compound with potential therapeutic use in diabetes and other chronic diseases. *Diabetol Metab Syndr,* 6, 80.
[http://dx.doi.org/10.1186/1758-5996-6-80] [PMID: 25104975]

González-Sarrías, A, Combet, E, Pinto, P, Mena, P, Dall'Asta, M, Garcia-Aloy, M, Rodríguez-Mateos, A, Gibney, ER, Dumont, J, Massaro, M, Sánchez-Meca, J, Morand, C & García-Conesa, M-T (2017) A Systematic Review and Meta-Analysis of the Effects of Flavanol-Containing Tea, Cocoa and Apple Products on Body Composition and Blood Lipids: Exploring the Factors Responsible for Variability in Their Efficacy. *Nutrients,* 9, 746.
[http://dx.doi.org/10.3390/nu9070746]

Hajhashemi, V, Vaseghi, G, Pourfarzam, M & Abdollahi, A (2010) Are antioxidants helpful for disease prevention? *Res Pharm Sci,* 5, 1-8.
[PMID: 21589762]

Halliwell, B (2000) The antioxidant paradox. *Lancet,* 355, 1179-80.
[http://dx.doi.org/10.1016/S0140-6736(00)02075-4] [PMID: 10791396]

Halliwill, B & Gtteridge, JMC (2006) *Free Radicals in Biology and Medicine* Clarendon Press, Oxford.

Hamidpour, R, Hamidpour, M, Hamidpour, S & Shahlari, M (2015) Cinnamon from the selection of traditional applications to its novel effects on the inhibition of angiogenesis in cancer cells and prevention of Alzheimer's disease, and a series of functions such as antioxidant, anticholesterol, antidiabetes, antibacterial, antifungal, nematicidal, acaracidal, and repellent activities. *J Tradit Complement Med,* 5, 66-70.
[http://dx.doi.org/10.1016/j.jtcme.2014.11.008] [PMID: 26151013]

Hammond, BR, Fletcher, LM, Roos, F, Wittwer, J & Schalch, W (2014) A double-blind, placebo-controlled study on the effects of lutein and zeaxanthin on photostress recovery, glare disability, and chromatic contrast. *Invest Ophthalmol Vis Sci,* 55, 8583-9.
[http://dx.doi.org/10.1167/iovs.14-15573] [PMID: 25468896]

Han, J, Wang, M, Jing, X, Shi, H, Ren, M & Lou, H (2014) (-)-Epigallocatechin gallate protects against cerebral ischemia-induced oxidative stress *via* Nrf2/ARE signaling. *Neurochem Res,* 39, 1292-9.
[http://dx.doi.org/10.1007/s11064-014-1311-5] [PMID: 24792731]

Han, QQ, Shen, TT, Wang, F, Wu, PF & Chen, JG (2018) Preventive and Therapeutic Potential of Vitamin C in Mental Disorders. *Curr Med Sci,* 38, 1-10.
[http://dx.doi.org/10.1007/s11596-018-1840-2] [PMID: 30074145]

Harrison, FE & May, JM (2009) Vitamin C function in the brain: vital role of the ascorbate transporter SVCT2. *Free Radic Biol Med,* 46, 719-30.
[http://dx.doi.org/10.1016/j.freeradbiomed.2008.12.018] [PMID: 19162177]

Hegazy, AM, Abdel-Azeem, AS, Zeidan, HM, Ibrahim, KS & Sayed, EE (2018) Hypolipidemic and hepatoprotective activities of rosemary and thyme in gentamicin-treated rats. *Hum Exp Toxicol,* 37, 420-30.
[http://dx.doi.org/10.1177/0960327117710534] [PMID: 28534439]

Heim, KE, Tagliaferro, AR & Bobilya, DJ (2002) Flavonoid antioxidants: chemistry, metabolism and structure-activity relationships. *J Nutr Biochem,* 13, 572-84.
[http://dx.doi.org/10.1016/S0955-2863(02)00208-5] [PMID: 12550068]

Hewlings, SJ & Kalman, DS (2017) Curcumin: A Review of Its Effects on Human Health. *Foods,* 6, 92.
[http://dx.doi.org/10.3390/foods6100092] [PMID: 29065496]

Van Hoang, D, Pham, NM, Lee, AH, Tran, DN & Binns, CW (2018) Dietary carotenoid intakes and prostate cancer risk: A case-control study from Vietnam. *Nutrients,* 10, 70.
[http://dx.doi.org/10.3390/nu10010070] [PMID: 29324670]

Hokayem, M, Blond, E, Vidal, H, Lambert, K, Meugnier, E, Feillet-Coudray, C, Coudray, C, Pesenti, S, Luyton, C, Lambert-Porcheron, S, Sauvinet, V, Fedou, C, Brun, JF, Rieusset, J, Bisbal, C, Sultan, A, Mercier, J, Goudable, J, Dupuy, AM, Cristol, JP, Laville, M & Avignon, A (2013) Grape polyphenols prevent fructose-induced oxidative stress and insulin resistance in first-degree relatives of type 2 diabetic patients.

Diabetes Care, 36, 1454-61.
[http://dx.doi.org/10.2337/dc12-1652] [PMID: 23275372]

Holmquist, L, Stuchbury, G, Berbaum, K, Muscat, S, Young, S, Hager, K, Engel, J & Münch, G (2007) Lipoic acid as a novel treatment for Alzheimer's disease and related dementias. *Pharmacol Ther,* 113, 154-64.
[http://dx.doi.org/10.1016/j.pharmthera.2006.07.001] [PMID: 16989905]

Hosseini, A, Shafiee-Nick, R & Mousavi, SH (2014) Combination of Nigella sativa with Glycyrrhiza glabra and Zingiber officinale augments their protective effects on doxorubicin-induced toxicity in h9c2 cells. *Iran J Basic Med Sci,* 17, 993-1000.
[PMID: 25859303]

Huang, Z, Liu, Y, Qi, G, Brand, D & Zheng, SG (2018) Role of Vitamin A in the Immune System. *J Clin Med,* 7, 258.
[http://dx.doi.org/10.3390/jcm7090258] [PMID: 30200565]

(2017) *Facts and Statistics.*https://www.iofbonehealth.org/facts-statistics

Jafari, S, Saeidnia, S & Abdollahi, M (2014) Role of natural phenolic compounds in cancer chemoprevention *via* regulation of the cell cycle. *Curr Pharm Biotechnol,* 15, 409-21.
[http://dx.doi.org/10.2174/1389201015666140813124832] [PMID: 25312621]

Jasiński, M, Jasińska, L & Ogrodowczyk, M (2013) Resveratrol in prostate diseases - a short review. *Cent European J Urol,* 66, 144-9.
[PMID: 24579014]

Kaplan, TB, Berkowitz, AL & Samuels, MA (2015) Cardiovascular dysfunction in multiple sclerosis. *Neurologist,* 20, 108-14.
[http://dx.doi.org/10.1097/NRL.0000000000000064] [PMID: 26671744]

Katta, R & Brown, DN (2015) Diet and skin cancer: the potential role of dietary antioxidants in nonmelanoma skin cancer prevention. *J Skin Cancer,* 2015893149
[http://dx.doi.org/10.1155/2015/893149] [PMID: 26583073]

Kelkel, M, Schumacher, M, Dicato, M & Diederich, M (2011) Antioxidant and anti-proliferative properties of lycopene. *Free Radic Res,* 45, 925-40.
[http://dx.doi.org/10.3109/10715762.2011.564168] [PMID: 21615277]

Khalatbary, AR & Khademi, E (2018) The green tea polyphenolic catechin epigallocatechin gallate and neuroprotection. *Nutr Neurosci,* 25, 1-14.
[PMID: 30043683]

Kim, GH, Kim, JE, Rhie, SJ & Yoon, S (2015) The role of oxidative stress in neurodegenerative diseases. *Exp Neurobiol,* 24, 325-40.
[http://dx.doi.org/10.5607/en.2015.24.4.325] [PMID: 26713080]

Krausz, AE, Adler, BL, Cabral, V, Navati, M, Doerner, J, Charafeddine, RA, Chandra, D, Liang, H, Gunther, L, Clendaniel, A, Harper, S, Friedman, JM, Nosanchuk, JD & Friedman, AJ (2015) Curcumin-encapsulated nanoparticles as innovative antimicrobial and wound healing agent. *Nanomedicine,* 11, 195-206.
[http://dx.doi.org/10.1016/j.nano.2014.09.004] [PMID: 25240595]

Labat-Robert, J & Robert, L (2014) Longevity and aging. Role of free radicals and xanthine oxidase. A review. *Pathol Biol (Paris),* 62, 61-6.
[http://dx.doi.org/10.1016/j.patbio.2014.02.009] [PMID: 24650523]

Labriola, D & Livingston, R (1999) Possible interactions between dietary antioxidants and chemotherapy. *Oncology (Williston Park),* 13, 1003-8.
[PMID: 10442346]

Lakey-Beitia, J, Kumar D, J, Hegde, ML & Rao, KS (2019) Carotenoids as Novel Therapeutic Molecules Against Neurodegenerative Disorders: Chemistry and Molecular Docking Analysis. *Int J Mol Sci,* 20E5553 [http://dx.doi.org/10.3390/ijms20225553] [PMID: 31703296]

Lee, SY, Jung, YO, Ryu, JG, Oh, HJ, Son, HJ, Lee, SH, Kwon, JE, Kim, EK, Park, MK, Park, SH, Kim, HY & Cho, ML (2016) Epigallocatechin-3-gallate ameliorates autoimmune arthritis by reciprocal regulation of T helper-17 regulatory T cells and inhibition of osteoclastogenesis by inhibiting STAT3 signaling. *J Leukoc Biol,* 100, 559-68.
[http://dx.doi.org/10.1189/jlb.3A0514-261RR] [PMID: 26957211]

Li, AN, Li, S, Zhang, YJ, Xu, XR, Chen, YM & Li, HB (2014) Resources and biological activities of natural polyphenols. *Nutrients,* 6, 6020-47.
[http://dx.doi.org/10.3390/nu6126020] [PMID: 25533011]

Li, L & Yang, X (2018) The Essential Element Manganese, Oxidative Stress, and Metabolic Diseases: Links and Interactions. *Oxid Med Cell Longev,* 20187580707
[http://dx.doi.org/10.1155/2018/7580707] [PMID: 29849912]

Li, Y, Yao, J, Han, C, Yang, J, Chaudhry, MT, Wang, S, Liu, H & Yin, Y (2016) Quercetin, Inflammation and Immunity. *Nutrients,* 8, 167.
[http://dx.doi.org/10.3390/nu8030167] [PMID: 26999194]

Linnewiel-Hermoni, K, Khanin, M, Danilenko, M, Zango, G, Amosi, Y, Levy, J & Sharoni, Y (2015) The anti-cancer effects of carotenoids and other phytonutrients resides in their combined activity. *Arch Biochem Biophys,* 572, 28-35.
[http://dx.doi.org/10.1016/j.abb.2015.02.018] [PMID: 25711533]

Liu, RH (2003) Health benefits of fruit and vegetables are from additive and synergistic combinations of phytochemicals. *Am J Clin Nutr,* 78 (Suppl.), 517S-20S.
[http://dx.doi.org/10.1093/ajcn/78.3.517S] [PMID: 12936943]

Liu, W, Shi, L & Li, S (2019) *The Immunomodulatory Effect of Alpha-Lipoic Acid in Autoimmune Diseases*
[http://dx.doi.org/10.1155/2019/8086257]

Liu, Z, Ren, Z, Zhang, J, Chuang, C-C, Kandaswamy, E, Zhou, T & Zuo, L (2018) Role of ROS and Nutritional Antioxidants in Human Diseases. *Front Physiol,* 9, 477.
[http://dx.doi.org/10.3389/fphys.2018.00477] [PMID: 29867535]

Liu, XH, Yu, RB, Liu, R, Hao, Z-X, Han, C-C, Zhu, Z-H & Ma, L (2014) Association between lutein and zeaxanthin status and the risk of cataract: a meta-analysis. *Nutrients,* 6, 452-65.
[http://dx.doi.org/10.3390/nu6010452] [PMID: 24451312]

Lobo, V, Patil, A, Phatak, A & Chandra, N (2010) Free radicals, antioxidants and functional foods: Impact on human health. *Pharmacogn Rev,* 4, 118-26.
[http://dx.doi.org/10.4103/0973-7847.70902] [PMID: 22228951]

Mahajan, A & Tandon, VR (2004) Antioxidants and rheumatoid arthritis. *Journal of Indian Rheumatology Association,* 12, 139-42.

Manach, C, Scalbert, A, Morand, C, Rémésy, C & Jiménez, L (2004) Polyphenols: food sources and bioavailability. *Am J Clin Nutr,* 79, 727-47.
[http://dx.doi.org/10.1093/ajcn/79.5.727] [PMID: 15113710]

Martín-Fernández, B, de las Heras, N, Valero-Muñoz, M, Ballesteros, S, Yao, YZ, Stanton, PG, Fuller, PJ & Lahera, V (2014) Beneficial effects of proanthocyanidins in the cardiac alterations induced by aldosterone in rat heart through mineralocorticoid receptor blockade. *PLoS One,* 9e111104
[http://dx.doi.org/10.1371/journal.pone.0111104] [PMID: 25353961]

Mazo, NA, Echeverria, V, Cabezas, R, Avila-Rodriguez, M, Tarasov, VV, Yarla, NS, Aliev, G & Barreto, GE (2017) Medicinal plants as protective strategies against Parkinson's Disease. *Curr Pharm Des,* 23, 4180-8.
[http://dx.doi.org/10.2174/1381612823666170316142803] [PMID: 28302024]

McAlindon, T & Felson, DT (1997) Nutrition: risk factors for osteoarthritis. *Ann Rheum Dis,* 56, 397-400.

[http://dx.doi.org/10.1136/ard.56.7.397] [PMID: 9485998]

McRae, MP (2008) Vitamin C supplementation lowers serum low-density lipoprotein cholesterol and triglycerides: a meta-analysis of 13 randomized controlled trials. *J Chiropr Med,* 7, 48-58.
[http://dx.doi.org/10.1016/j.jcme.2008.01.002] [PMID: 19674720]

Middha, P, Weinstein, SJ, Männistö, S, Albanes, D & Mondul, AM (2019) β-Carotene Supplementation and Lung Cancer Incidence in the Alpha-Tocopherol, Beta-Carotene Cancer Prevention Study: The Role of Tar and Nicotine. *Nicotine Tob Res,* 21, 1045-50.
[http://dx.doi.org/10.1093/ntr/nty115] [PMID: 29889248]

Mitsiogianni, M, Koutsidis, G, Mavroudis, N, Trafalis, DT, Botaitis, S, Franco, R, Zoumpourlis, V, Amery, T, Galanis, A, Pappa, A & Panayiotidis, MI (2019) The Role of Isothiocyanates as Cancer Chemo-Preventive, Chemo-Therapeutic and Anti-Melanoma Agents. *Antioxidants,* 8, 106.
[http://dx.doi.org/10.3390/antiox8040106] [PMID: 31003534]

Moattar, FS, Sariri, R, Yaghmaee, P & Giahi, M (2016) Enzymatic and non-enzymatic antioxidants of calaminthaofficinalismoench extracts. *Journal of Applied Biotechnology Reports,* 3, 489-94.

Molz, P & Schröder, N (2017) Potential therapeutic effects of lipoic acid on memory deficits related to aging and neurodegeneration. *Front Pharmacol,* 8, 849.
[http://dx.doi.org/10.3389/fphar.2017.00849] [PMID: 29311912]

Moser, MA & Chun, OK (2016) Vitamin C and heart health: a review based on findings from epidemiologic studies. *Int J Mol Sci,* 17, 1328.
[http://dx.doi.org/10.3390/ijms17081328] [PMID: 27529239]

Moungjaroen, J, Nimmannit, U, Callery, PS, Wang, L, Azad, N, Lipipun, V, Chanvorachote, P & Rojanasakul, Y (2006) Reactive oxygen species mediate caspase activation and apoptosis induced by lipoic acid in human lung epithelial cancer cells through Bcl-2 down-regulation. *J Pharmacol Exp Ther,* 319, 1062-9.
[http://dx.doi.org/10.1124/jpet.106.110965] [PMID: 16990509]

Moy, A, McNamara, NA & Lin, MC (2015) Effects of isotretinoin on meibomian glands. *Optom Vis Sci,* 92, 925-30.
[http://dx.doi.org/10.1097/OPX.0000000000000656] [PMID: 26154692]

Mythri, RB & Bharath, MM (2012) Curcumin: a potential neuroprotective agent in Parkinson's disease. *Curr Pharm Des,* 18, 91-9.
[http://dx.doi.org/10.2174/138161212798918995] [PMID: 22211691]

Nanjan, MJ & Betz, J (2014) Resveratrol for the Management of Diabetes and its Downstream Pathologies. *Eur Endocrinol,* 10, 31-5.
[http://dx.doi.org/10.17925/EE.2014.10.01.31] [PMID: 29872461]

Nichols, JA & Katiyar, SK (2010) Skin photoprotection by natural polyphenols: anti-inflammatory, antioxidant and DNA repair mechanisms. *Arch Dermatol Res,* 302, 71-83.
[http://dx.doi.org/10.1007/s00403-009-1001-3] [PMID: 19898857]

Niedzielska, E, Smaga, I, Gawlik, M, Moniczewski, A, Stankowicz, P, Pera, J & Filip, M (2016) Oxidative Stress in Neurodegenerative Diseases. *Mol Neurobiol,* 53, 4094-125.
[http://dx.doi.org/10.1007/s12035-015-9337-5] [PMID: 26198567]

Nikfarjam, BA, Adineh, M, Hajiali, F & Nassiri-Asl, M (2017) Treatment with rutin-A therapeutic strategyfor neutrophil-mediated inflammatory and autoimmune diseases: - Anti-inflammatory effects of rutin on neutrophils. *J Pharmacopuncture,* 20, 52-6. a
[http://dx.doi.org/10.3831/KPI.2017.20.003] [PMID: 28392963]

Nikfarjam, BA, Hajiali, F, Adineh, M & Nassiri-Asl, M (2017) Anti-inflammatory Effects of Quercetin and Vitexin on Activated Human Peripheral Blood Neutrophils: - The effects of quercetin and vitexin on human neutrophils. *J Pharmacopuncture,* 20, 127-31. b
[PMID: 30087790]

Niki, E (2015) Evidence for beneficial effects of vitamin E. *Korean J Intern Med (Korean Assoc Intern Med)*, 30, 571-9.
[http://dx.doi.org/10.3904/kjim.2015.30.5.571] [PMID: 26354050]

Nimse, SB & Pal, D (2015) Free radicals, natural antioxidants, and their reaction mechanisms. *RSC Advances*, 5, 27986-8006.
[http://dx.doi.org/10.1039/C4RA13315C]

Ninić, A, Bogavac-Stanojević, N, Sopić, M, Munjas, J, Kotur-Stevuljević, J, Miljković, M, Gojković, T, Kalimanovska-Oštrić, D & Spasojević-Kalimanovska, V (2019) Superoxide Dismutase Isoenzymes Gene Expression in Peripheral Blood Mononuclear Cells in Patients with Coronary Artery Disease. *J Med Biochem*, 38, 284-91.
[http://dx.doi.org/10.2478/jomb-2018-0041] [PMID: 31156338]

Nita, M & Grzybowski, A (2016) The role of the reactive oxygen species and oxidative stress in the pathomechanism of the age-related ocular diseases and other pathologies of the anterior and posterior eye segments in adults. *Oxid Med Cell Longev*, 20163164734
[http://dx.doi.org/10.1155/2016/3164734] [PMID: 26881021]

Oboh, G, Ademosun, AO & Ogunsuyi, OB (2016) Quercetin and Its Role in Chronic Diseases. *Adv Exp Med Biol*, 929, 377-87.
[http://dx.doi.org/10.1007/978-3-319-41342-6_17] [PMID: 27771934]

Ohishi, T, Goto, S, Monira, P, Isemura, M & Nakamura, Y (2016) Anti-inflammatory Action of Green Tea. *Antiinflamm Antiallergy Agents Med Chem*, 15, 74-90.
[http://dx.doi.org/10.2174/1871523015666160915154443] [PMID: 27634207]

Olson, JA (1987) Recommended dietary intakes (RDI) of vitamin A in humans. *Am J Clin Nutr*, 45, 704-16.
[http://dx.doi.org/10.1093/ajcn/45.4.704] [PMID: 3565297]

Ostrowska, M, Maśliński, W, Prochorec-Sobieszek, M, Nieciecki, M & Sudoł-Szopińska, I (2018) Cartilage and bone damage in rheumatoid arthritis. *Reumatologia*, 56, 111-20.
[http://dx.doi.org/10.5114/reum.2018.75523] [PMID: 29853727]

Oz, HS (2017) Chronic inflammatory diseases and green tea polyphenols. *Nutrients*, 9, 561.
[http://dx.doi.org/10.3390/nu9060561] [PMID: 28587181]

Pan, SY, Zhou, J, Gibbons, L, Morrison, H & Wen, SW (2011) Antioxidants and breast cancer risk- a population-based case-control study in Canada. *BMC Cancer*, 11, 372.
[http://dx.doi.org/10.1186/1471-2407-11-372] [PMID: 21864361]

Pandey, KB & Rizvi, SI (2009) Plant polyphenols as dietary antioxidants in human health and disease. *Oxid Med Cell Longev*, 2, 270-8.
[http://dx.doi.org/10.4161/oxim.2.5.9498] [PMID: 20716914]

Patten, DA, Germain, M, Kelly, MA & Slack, RS (2010) Reactive oxygen species: stuck in the middle of neurodegeneration. *J Alzheimers Dis*, 20 (Suppl. 2), S357-67.
[http://dx.doi.org/10.3233/JAD-2010-100498] [PMID: 20421690]

Pehlivan, FE (2017) Vitamin C: An antioxidant agent.*Vitamin C*.IntechOpen.
[http://dx.doi.org/10.5772/intechopen.69660]

Ping, Z, Liu, W, Kang, Z, Cai, J, Wang, Q, Cheng, N, Wang, S, Wang, S, Zhang, JH & Sun, X (2010) Sulforaphane protects brains against hypoxic-ischemic injury through induction of Nrf2-dependent phase 2 enzyme. *Brain Res*, 1343, 178-85.
[http://dx.doi.org/10.1016/j.brainres.2010.04.036] [PMID: 20417626]

Pizzino, G, Irrera, N, Cucinotta, M, Pallio, G, Mannino, F, Arcoraci, V, Squadrito, F, Altavilla, D & Bitto, A (2017) Oxidative Stress: Harms and Benefits for Human Health. *Oxid Med Cell Longev*, 20178416763
[http://dx.doi.org/10.1155/2017/8416763] [PMID: 28819546]

Poljsak, B, Šuput, D & Milisav, I (2013) Achieving the balance between ROS and antioxidants: when to use

the synthetic antioxidants. *Oxid Med Cell Longev,* 2013956792
[http://dx.doi.org/10.1155/2013/956792] [PMID: 23738047]

Prasad, AS (2013) Discovery of human zinc deficiency: its impact on human health and disease. *Adv Nutr,* 4, 176-90.
[http://dx.doi.org/10.3945/an.112.003210] [PMID: 23493534]

Prasad, AS (2014) Zinc is an Antioxidant and Anti-Inflammatory Agent: Its Role in Human Health. *Front Nutr,* 1, 14.
[http://dx.doi.org/10.3389/fnut.2014.00014] [PMID: 25988117]

Rayman, MP (2012) Selenium and human health. *Lancet,* 379, 1256-68.
[http://dx.doi.org/10.1016/S0140-6736(11)61452-9] [PMID: 22381456]

Reygaert, WC (2018) Green Tea Catechins: Their Use in Treating and Preventing Infectious Diseases. *BioMed Res Int,* 20189105261
[http://dx.doi.org/10.1155/2018/9105261] [PMID: 30105263]

Rizvi, S, Raza, ST, Ahmed, F, Ahmad, A, Abbas, S & Mahdi, F (2014) The role of vitamin e in human health and some diseases. *Sultan Qaboos Univ Med J,* 14, e157-65.
[PMID: 24790736]

Robin, Arora (2015) Inhibition of DNA oxidative damage and antimutagenic activity by dichloromethane extract of *Brassica rapa* var. *rapa* L. seeds. *Ind Crops Prod,* 74, 585-91.
[http://dx.doi.org/10.1016/j.indcrop.2015.05.038]

Rohdewald, P (2002) A review of the French maritime pine bark extract (Pycnogenol), a herbal medication with a diverse clinical pharmacology. *Int J Clin Pharmacol Ther,* 40, 158-68.
[http://dx.doi.org/10.5414/CPP40158] [PMID: 11996210]

Rubin, LP, Ross, AC, Stephensen, CB, Bohn, T & Tanumihardjo, SA (2017) Metabolic effects of inflammation on vitamin A and carotenoids in humans and animal models. *Adv Nutr,* 8, 197-212.
[http://dx.doi.org/10.3945/an.116.014167] [PMID: 28298266]

Salehi, B, Berkay Yılmaz, Y, Antika, G, Boyunegmez Tumer, T, Fawzi Mahomoodally, M, Lobine, D, Akram, M, Riaz, M, Capanoglu, E, Sharopov, F, Martins, N, Cho, WC & Sharifi-Rad, J (2019) Insights on the Use of α-Lipoic Acid for Therapeutic Purposes. *Biomolecules,* 9, 356.
[http://dx.doi.org/10.3390/biom9080356] [PMID: 31405030]

Salomone, F, Galvano, F & Li Volti, G (2017) Molecular Bases Underlying the Hepatoprotective Effects of Coffee. *Nutrients,* 9, 85.
[http://dx.doi.org/10.3390/nu9010085] [PMID: 28124992]

Schneider, C (2005) Chemistry and biology of vitamin E. *Mol Nutr Food Res,* 49, 7-30.
[http://dx.doi.org/10.1002/mnfr.200400049] [PMID: 15580660]

Shalaby, MA, Nounou, HA & Deif, MM (2019) The potential value of capsaicin in modulating cognitive functions in a rat model of streptozotocin-induced Alzheimer's disease. *Egypt J Neurol Psychiat Neurosurg,* 55, 48.
[http://dx.doi.org/10.1186/s41983-019-0094-7]

Shi, GJ, Li, Y, Cao, QH, Wu, HX, Tang, XY, Gao, XH, Yu, JQ, Chen, Z & Yang, Y (2019) *In vitro* and *in Vivo* evidence that quercetin protects against diabetes and its complications: A systematic review of the literature. *Biomed Pharmacother,* 109, 1085-99.
[http://dx.doi.org/10.1016/j.biopha.2018.10.130] [PMID: 30551359]

Singal, AK, Jampana, SC & Weinman, SA (2011) Antioxidants as therapeutic agents for liver disease. *Liver Int,* 31, 1432-48.
[http://dx.doi.org/10.1111/j.1478-3231.2011.02604.x] [PMID: 22093324]

Slavin, JL & Lloyd, B (2012) Health benefits of fruits and vegetables. *Adv Nutr,* 3, 506-16.
[http://dx.doi.org/10.3945/an.112.002154] [PMID: 22797986]

Sluijs, I, Cadier, E, Beulens, JW, van der A, DL, Spijkerman, AM & van der Schouw, YT (2015) Dietary intake of carotenoids and risk of type 2 diabetes. *Nutr Metab Cardiovasc Dis,* 25, 376-81.
[http://dx.doi.org/10.1016/j.numecd.2014.12.008] [PMID: 25716098]

Sonam, KS & Guleria, S (2017) Synergistic Antioxidant Activity of Natural Products. *Ann Pharmacol Pharm,* 2, 1086.

Song, B, Liu, K, Gao, Y, Zhao, L, Fang, H, Li, Y, Pei, L & Xu, Y (2017) Lycopene and risk of cardiovascular diseases: A meta-analysis of observational studies. *Mol Nutr Food Res,* 61
[http://dx.doi.org/10.1002/mnfr.201601009] [PMID: 28318092]

Sumida, Y, Naito, Y, Tanaka, S, Sakai, K, Inada, Y, Taketani, H, Kanemasa, K, Yasui, K, Itoh, Y, Okanoue, T & Yoshikawa, T (2013) Long-term (>=2 yr) efficacy of vitamin E for non-alcoholic steatohepatitis. *Hepatogastroenterology,* 60, 1445-50.
[PMID: 23933938]

Sun, Y, Yang, T, Leak, RK, Chen, J & Zhang, F (2017) Preventive and protective roles of dietary Nrf2 activators against central nervous system diseases. *CNS Neurol Disord Drug Targets,* 16, 326-38.
[http://dx.doi.org/10.2174/1871527316666170102120211] [PMID: 28042770]

Surh, YJ (2003) Cancer chemoprevention with dietary phytochemicals. *Nat Rev Cancer,* 3, 768-80.
[http://dx.doi.org/10.1038/nrc1189] [PMID: 14570043]

Tabrez, S, Priyadarshini, M, Urooj, M, Shakil, S, Ashraf, GM, Khan, MS, Kamal, MA, Alam, Q, Jabir, NR, Abuzenadah, AM, Chaudhary, AG & Damanhouri, GA (2013) Cancer chemoprevention by polyphenols and their potential application as nanomedicine. *J Environ Sci Health Part C Environ Carcinog Ecotoxicol Rev,* 31, 67-98.
[http://dx.doi.org/10.1080/10590501.2013.763577] [PMID: 23534395]

Tanaka, K, Arita, M, Sakurai, H, Ono, N & Tezuka, Y (2015) *Analysis of chemical properties of edible and medicinal ginger by metabolomics approach*
[http://dx.doi.org/10.1155/2015/671058]

Toh, T, Morton, J, Coxon, J & Elder, MJ (2007) Medical treatment of cataract. *Clin Exp Ophthalmol,* 35, 664-71.
[http://dx.doi.org/10.1111/j.1442-9071.2007.01559.x] [PMID: 17894689]

Tomeh, MA, Hadianamrei, R & Zhao, X (2019) A Review of Curcumin and Its Derivatives as Anticancer Agents. *Int J Mol Sci,* 20, 1033.
[http://dx.doi.org/10.3390/ijms20051033] [PMID: 30818786]

Tominari, T, Matsumoto, C, Watanabe, K, Hirata, M, Grundler, FMW, Inada, M & Miyaura, C (2017) Lutein, a carotenoid, suppresses osteoclastic bone resorption and stimulates bone formation in cultures. *Biosci Biotechnol Biochem,* 81, 302-6.
[http://dx.doi.org/10.1080/09168451.2016.1243983] [PMID: 27776451]

Trivedi, PP & Jena, GB (2013) Role of α-lipoic acid in dextran sulfate sodium-induced ulcerative colitis in mice: studies on inflammation, oxidative stress, DNA damage and fibrosis. *Food Chem Toxicol,* 59, 339-55.
[http://dx.doi.org/10.1016/j.fct.2013.06.019] [PMID: 23793040]

Uchiyama, K, Naito, Y, Hasegawa, G, Nakamura, N, Takahashi, J & Yoshikawa, T (2002) Astaxanthin protects beta-cells against glucose toxicity in diabetic db/db mice. *Redox Rep,* 7, 290-3.
[http://dx.doi.org/10.1179/135100002125000811] [PMID: 12688512]

Asmat, U, Abad, K & Ismail, K (2016) Diabetes mellitus and oxidative stress-A concise review. *Saudi Pharm J,* 24, 547-53.
[http://dx.doi.org/10.1016/j.jsps.2015.03.013] [PMID: 27752226]

Uriu-Adams, JY & Keen, CL (2005) Copper, oxidative stress, and human health. *Mol Aspects Med,* 26, 268-98.
[http://dx.doi.org/10.1016/j.mam.2005.07.015] [PMID: 16112185]

Valdés-Ramos, R, Guadarrama-López, AL, Martínez-Carrillo, BE & Benítez-Arciniega, AD (2015) Vitamins and type 2 diabetes mellitus. *Endocr Metab Immune Disord Drug Targets,* 15, 54-63.
[http://dx.doi.org/10.2174/1871530314666141111103217] [PMID: 25388747]

Valko, M, Leibfritz, D, Moncol, J, Cronin, MT, Mazur, M & Telser, J (2007) Free radicals and antioxidants in normal physiological functions and human disease. *Int J Biochem Cell Biol,* 39, 44-84.
[http://dx.doi.org/10.1016/j.biocel.2006.07.001] [PMID: 16978905]

Van Gaal, LF, Mertens, IL & De Block, CE (2006) Mechanisms linking obesity with cardiovascular disease. *Nature,* 444, 875-80.
[http://dx.doi.org/10.1038/nature05487] [PMID: 17167476]

Vashum, KP, McEvoy, M, Milton, AH, Islam, MR, Hancock, S & Attia, J (2014) Is serum zinc associated with pancreatic beta cell function and insulin sensitivity in pre-diabetic and normal individuals? Findings from the Hunter Community Study. *PLoS One,* 9e83944
[http://dx.doi.org/10.1371/journal.pone.0083944] [PMID: 24416185]

Vishwanathan, R, Chung, M & Johnson, EJ (2013) A systematic review on zinc for the prevention and treatment of age-related macular degeneration. *Invest Ophthalmol Vis Sci,* 54, 3985-98.
[http://dx.doi.org/10.1167/iovs.12-11552] [PMID: 23652490]

Walston, J, Xue, Q, Semba, RD, Ferrucci, L, Cappola, AR, Ricks, M, Guralnik, J & Fried, LP (2006) Serum antioxidants, inflammation, and total mortality in older women. *Am J Epidemiol,* 163, 18-26.
[http://dx.doi.org/10.1093/aje/kwj007] [PMID: 16306311]

Wang, ME, Chen, YC, Chen, IS, Hsieh, SC, Chen, SS & Chiu, CH (2012) Curcumin protects against thioacetamide-induced hepatic fibrosis by attenuating the inflammatory response and inducing apoptosis of damaged hepatocytes. *J Nutr Biochem,* 23, 1352-66.
[http://dx.doi.org/10.1016/j.jnutbio.2011.08.004] [PMID: 22221674]

Wang, N, Tan, HY, Li, S, Xu, Y, Guo, W & Feng, Y (2017) Supplementation of Micronutrient Selenium in Metabolic Diseases: Its Role as an Antioxidant. *Oxid Med Cell Longev,* 20177478523
[http://dx.doi.org/10.1155/2017/7478523] [PMID: 29441149]

Wang, X & Quinn, PJ (1999) Vitamin E and its function in membranes. *Prog Lipid Res,* 38, 309-36.
[http://dx.doi.org/10.1016/S0163-7827(99)00008-9] [PMID: 10793887]

Wang, J, Light, K, Henderson, M, O'Loughlin, J, Mathieu, ME, Paradis, G & Gray-Donald, K (2014) Consumption of added sugars from liquid but not solid sources predicts impaired glucose homeostasis and insulin resistance among youth at risk of obesity. *J Nutr,* 144, 81-6.
[http://dx.doi.org/10.3945/jn.113.182519] [PMID: 24198307]

(2019) https://www.who.int/news-room/fact-sheets/detail/diabetes a

(2019) https://www.who.int/news-room/fact-sheets/detail/dementia b

Winter, AN, Ross, EK, Wilkins, HM, Stankiewicz, TR, Wallace, T, Miller, K & Linseman, DA (2018) An anthocyanin-enriched extract from strawberries delays disease onset and extends survival in the hSOD1[G93A] mouse model of amyotrophic lateral sclerosis. *Nutr Neurosci,* 21, 414-26.
[http://dx.doi.org/10.1080/1028415X.2017.1297023] [PMID: 28276271]

Wood, LG, Garg, ML, Smart, JM, Scott, HA, Barker, D & Gibson, PG (2012) Manipulating antioxidant intake in asthma: a randomized controlled trial. *Am J Clin Nutr,* 96, 534-43.
[http://dx.doi.org/10.3945/ajcn.111.032623] [PMID: 22854412]

Xu, DP, Li, Y, Meng, X, Zhou, T, Zhou, Y, Zheng, J, Zhang, JJ & Li, HB (2017) Natural antioxidants in foods and medicinal plants: extraction, assessment and resources. *Int J Mol Sci,* 18, 96.
[http://dx.doi.org/10.3390/ijms18010096] [PMID: 28067795]

Xu, XY, Zheng, J, Meng, JM, Gan, RY, Mao, QQ, Shang, A, Li, BY, Wei, XL & Li, HB (2019) Effects of Food Processing on *In Vivo* Antioxidant and Hepatoprotective Properties of Green Tea Extracts. *Antioxidants,* 8, 572.

[http://dx.doi.org/10.3390/antiox8120572] [PMID: 31766414]

Yan, LJ (2014) Pathogenesis of chronic hyperglycemia: from reductive stress to oxidative stress. *J Diabetes Res,* 2014137919
[http://dx.doi.org/10.1155/2014/137919] [PMID: 25019091]

Yang, C, Zhang, X, Fan, H & Liu, Y (2009) Curcumin upregulates transcription factor Nrf2, HO-1 expression and protects rat brains against focal ischemia. *Brain Res,* 1282, 133-41.
[http://dx.doi.org/10.1016/j.brainres.2009.05.009] [PMID: 19445907]

Yang, CS & Wang, H (2016) Cancer Preventive Activities of Tea Catechins. *Molecules,* 21, 1679.
[http://dx.doi.org/10.3390/molecules21121679] [PMID: 27941682]

Yang, SP, Yang, XZ & Cao, GP (2015) Acetyl-l-carnitine prevents homocysteine-induced suppression of Nrf2/Keap1 mediated antioxidation in human lens epithelial cells. *Mol Med Rep,* 12, 1145-50.
[http://dx.doi.org/10.3892/mmr.2015.3490] [PMID: 25776802]

Young, IS & Woodside, JV (2001) Antioxidants in health and disease. *J Clin Pathol,* 54, 176-86.
[http://dx.doi.org/10.1136/jcp.54.3.176] [PMID: 11253127]

Zern, TL & Fernandez, ML (2005) Cardioprotective effects of dietary polyphenols. *J Nutr,* 135, 2291-4.
[http://dx.doi.org/10.1093/jn/135.10.2291] [PMID: 16177184]

Zhang, YJ, Gan, RY, Li, S, Zhou, Y, Li, AN, Xu, DP & Li, HB (2015) Antioxidant phytochemicals for the prevention and treatment of chronic diseases. *Molecules,* 20, 21138-56.
[http://dx.doi.org/10.3390/molecules201219753] [PMID: 26633317]

Zhang, ZQ, Cao, WT, Liu, J, Cao, Y, Su, YX & Chen, YM (2016) Greater serum carotenoid concentration associated with higher bone mineral density in Chinese adults. *Osteoporos Int,* 27, 1593-601.
[http://dx.doi.org/10.1007/s00198-015-3425-2] [PMID: 26753540]

Zhou, Y, Zheng, J, Li, Y, Xu, DP, Li, S, Chen, YM & Li, HB (2016) Natural polyphenols for prevention and treatment of cancer. *Nutrients,* 8, 515.
[http://dx.doi.org/10.3390/nu8080515] [PMID: 27556486]

CHAPTER 9

Dietary Antioxidants and their Molecular Targets in Oxidative Stress Mediated Cancer Progression

Sandeep Kumar[1] and **Yogendra Padwad**[1,*]

[1] *Pharmacology and Toxicology Lab, Block-J, CSIR- Institute of Himalayan Bioresource Technology Palampur-176061, India*

Abstract: Cancer is a complex disease and is currently the leading cause of mortality and morbidity across the globe. Dysregulated bioenergetics is one of the hallmarks of cancer cells and is characterized by increased activity of several enzymes of metabolic pathways. Consequently, cancer cells produce higher levels of reactive oxygen species (ROS) which contribute to their enhanced proliferation and survival over normal cells. Elevated levels of ROS cause oxidative stress, redox imbalance, DNA damage, activation of oncogenes, chronic inflammation and eventually cancer. Additionally, ROS mediated oxidative stress activates several oncogenic signaling cascades including PI3K/Akt pathway, NF-κB pathway, cyclooxygenase pathway, JAK/STAT pathway, angiogenesis and metastasis. To maintain redox balance and neutralize the detrimental effects of ROS, normal cells exhibit an antioxidant defence system, comprising of both enzymatic and non-enzymatic division. Activation of Nrf2 signaling pathway is the key regulatory pathway that helps in restoring the cellular redox homeostasis. Extensive research in the past decades has witnessed the potential health benefits of dietary antioxidants alone or in combination in the prevention of several chronic diseases, including cancer. A number of antioxidants from dietary backgrounds such as epigallocatechin gallate, resveratrol, curcumin, phloretin, berberine and lycopene have shown appreciable potential as a chemopreventive agent without causing significant toxicity. This chapter presents an extensive analysis of existing knowledge on the protective effects of various dietary antioxidants against cancer with a focus on oxidative stress, redox homeostasis and dysregulated cellular signaling leading to cancer cell proliferation, survival and metastasis.

Keywords: Antioxidants, Cancer, Oxidative stress, Reactive oxygen species, Redox homeostasis.

---

* **Corresponding author Yogendra Padwad:** Pharmacology and Toxicology Lab, Block-J, CSIR-IHBT Palampur-176061, India. E-mail: yogendra@ihbt.res.in

Pardeep Kaur, Rajendra G. Mehta, Robin, Tarunpreet Singh Thind and Saroj Arora (Eds.)

INTRODUCTION

Cancer represents one of the major public health problems of the 21st century and is currently the second leading cause of mortality across the globe (Bray *et al.* 2018). In 2018, nearly 9.6 million deaths and 18.1 million new cases of cancer were expected across the globe. There are approximately 6.06 lakh deaths and 1.8 million new cancer cases are expected in 2020 in the United States alone (Siegel *et al.* 2020). Genetic and environmental factors, several of which are associated with socio-economic development have been recognised as risk factors for cancer development (Dean *et al.* 2018, Herceg *et al.* 2018). The striking finding about displacement of cancers caused by infection or poverty with cancers which are largely diagnosed in developed countries (Europe, America, high income countries in Asia), is an indicator of adoption of westernised lifestyle in these countries (Bray *et al.* 2018). This emphasises, albeit indirect, that a large proportion of cancer types can be prevented simply by modifying lifestyle related factors such as diet, physical exercise, smoking and alcohol consumption. These factors play a crucial role in promoting or suppressing carcinogenesis *via* modulation of levels of reactive oxygen species (ROS) and associated redox signaling pathways. Perturbed redox status and subsequently altered redox signaling is a common hallmark of all cancers (Bakalova *et al.* 2013). Free radical generation is a general physiological process, resulting from different biological functions, including metabolism and inflammation. The increased engagement of cancer cells towards metabolic activities generates high levels of cellular ROS and eventually oxidative stress. The enhanced oxidative stress causes genomic instability, genetic mutations in genes whose products keep a check on cell divisions. Additionally, oxidative stress causes aberrant activation of several key signaling cascades such as NF-κB signaling pathway, PI3K/Akt pathway, cyclooxygenase pathway, JAK/STAT pathway aiding cancer cell proliferation and survival, angiogenesis and metastasis. Mitochondria represent the main centre for production of ROS under physiological conditions which subsequently plays a major role in metabolic regulation, cell proliferation and survival mechanisms. To balance ROS, certain defence molecules are present in the cell called "antioxidants". These cellular antioxidants are divided into two major categories: enzymatic and non-enzymatic antioxidants. The enzymatic antioxidant system includes superoxide dismutase (SOD), catalase, glutathione peroxidase (Gpx) and glutathione-S-transferase. The non-enzymatic antioxidant defence system is comprised of vitamin C and E, flavonoids, carotenoids, lipoic acid and others (Watson 2013). In addition to the cellular antioxidant system, regular consumption of foods containing high content of antioxidants also protects against oxidative stress mediated genetic insults and subsequently cancer development.

A series of chemotherapeutic agents have been devised to treat cancers of different origins. However, none of these agents is effective in eradicating cancers of advanced stages. Furthermore, several major adverse effects of chemotherapeutic drugs such as cardiac myopathy, haematological, gastrointestinal, neural, renal and liver damages have been recorded (Pearce *et al.* 2017, Nurgali *et al.* 2018). In this scenario, chemoprevention seems to be a promising window to curb the ever-increasing cancer burden. Moreover, a shift in the perspective of the general public about the origin of medicine has been observed. The acceptance rate of medicines of herbal origin is now gaining more priority over the synthetic ones. The traditional knowledge has indicated the crucial role of diet in promoting or delaying several human diseases including cancer. The idea of preventing most human diseases through certain modifications in diet was suggested by Hippocrates and dates back 2500 years ago . His famous phrase "Let food be thy medicine and medicine be thy food" clearly indicates the critical role of diet in human health and endorses the consumption of food items containing medicinal properties (Langner and Rzeski 2012). Moreover, epidemiological reports have suggested that daily consumption of fruits, vegetables, nuts, flax seeds and fatty fish has an inverse relationship with cancer incidence (Boeing *et al.* 2012, Grosso *et al.* 2013). It has been shown that cancer incidence is half in individuals consuming fruits and vegetables five serves in a day (Surh 2003). Phytochemical analysis of these fruits, vegetables, sea foods revealed the presence of certain kind of bioactive compounds of antioxidant nature including polyphenols, flavonoids, carotenoids and alkaloids. Examples of dietary phytochemicals with chemopreventive activity include epigallocatechin gallate, resveratrol, curcumin, phloretin, berberine and lycopene. The chemopreventive potential of above-mentioned dietary phytochemicals has been supported by numerous pre-clinical and clinical studies (Chikara *et al.* 2018, Choi 2019, Grabowska *et al.* 2019). Additionally, dietary phytochemicals are cost effective, easily administered and are generally recognized as pharmacologically safe. Most of the dietary phytochemicals are suggested to exert their chemopreventive action *via* targeting ROS and associated redox signaling pathways. Daily consumption of dietary compounds enhances cellular antioxidant status, neutralization of free radical species, suppresses expression of proteins regulating cell cycle, inflammation, neovascularization and promotes detoxification of carcinogen and apoptosis of cancer cells. Therefore, targeting ROS signaling pathway and redox homeostasis in cancer cells is a novel approach for the prevention of cancer development. In this chapter, we discuss the basic mechanism of ROS generation, redox signaling mechanism and redox sensitive transcription factors and how dietary phytochemicals target this complex pathway to prevent cancer development. Also, this chapter provides key finding on clinical efficacy of selected dietary phytochemicals in high-risk populations (Table **1**).

BASIC CONCEPT OF ROS GENERATION AND BIOLOGICAL FUNCTION

Oxygen plays a vital role in the metabolism of sugar, lipids, proteins and other food components. However, participation of oxygen in metabolism produces certain highly reactive species termed as ROS. Mitochondria is a central hub of ROS production such as superoxide ($O^{2 \cdot \cdot}$), hydroxyl radicals ($OH^{\cdot}$), hydrogen peroxide (H_2O_2), and singlet oxygen ($1O_2$) (Agnihotri *et al.* 2015). During oxidative phosphorylation, the leaked electrons from the electron transport chain react with molecular oxygen and produce $O_2^{(\cdot)}$ termed as superoxide free radical. The $O_2^{(\cdot)}$ acts as the main precursor for most of the ROS and rapidly converts into H_2O_2. In addition to mitochondria, NADPH oxidase is also a major producer of superoxide $O_2^{(\cdot)}$. Moreover, a small amount of ROS is produced by xanthine oxidase, lipoxygenases, cyclooxygenases, cytochrome p450 and peroxisomes in the cytoplasm (Qian *et al.* 2019). The intracellular ROS thus generated are tackled by ROS-detoxification system, comprised of both enzymatic and non-enzymatic antioxidants (Valko *et al.* 2007). The enzymatic antioxidant system includes superoxide dismutase (SOD), catalase (CAT), peroxiredoxin (PRX), glutathione peroxidase (GPX) and thioredoxin while non-enzymatic antioxidant system is comprised of cellular glutathione, flavonoids and vitamins (C, E, A) (Kurutas 2016). Different isoforms of superoxide dismutases such as cytoplasmic (SOD1), mitochondrial (SOD2) and extracellular matrix (SOD3) efficiently convert ROS to H_2O_2 (McCord and Fridovich 1969, Abreu and Cabelli 2010) which is further converted to water *via* CAT, PRX and GPX system. In the presence of iron/copper, H_2O_2 can be further converted to $OH^{\cdot}$ *via* Fenton reaction (Winterbourn 1995, Salgado *et al.* 2013). Moreover, transcription factor nuclear factor erythrocyte 2 related factor (Nrf2) plays a central role in maintaining cellular redox homeostasis (Chen *et al.* 2008, Basak *et al.* 2017). Normally, Nrf2 is expressed at a low level in the cytoplasm and is targeted for proteosomal degradation on binding to Kelch like ECH association Protein 1 (KEAP-1). Enhanced ROS levels cause dissociation of Nrf-2/KEAP-1 complex in cytoplasm, allowing Nrf-2 to bind to antioxidant response elements (AREs) in the nucleus and upregulate the expression of GSH, PRX and TRX encoding genes and thereby lowers ROS levels and protect the cells from ROS mediated cell death (Kobayashi and Yamamoto 2005).

ROS control different biological processes in a concentration dependent manner. At low concentration, ROS acts as a secondary messenger and stimulates cell proliferation, differentiation and stress-responsive survival mechanisms by regulating a series of membrane receptors including G-coupled receptors, cytokines receptors and serine/threonine kinase receptors (Bartosz 2009, Ray *et al.* 2012, Kumari *et al.* 2018). In contrast, high levels of ROS could be cytotoxic to cells due to their strong oxidizing capacity (Bartosz 2009). ROS react with cysteine residues (Cys-SH) of membrane proteins and produce sulfenic acid (Cys-SOH) and thus altering the structural and functional properties of proteins (Hurd *et al.* 2007). The reversible nature of this process allows Cys-SOH to get reduced back to Cys-SH form by TRX and GRX for restoring the protein function (Berndt *et al.* 2008). The continuous increase in ROS levels results in higher production of sulfenic acid, which damages cellular macromolecules such as phospholipids, membrane proteins and nucleic acids (Schumacker 2006, Pan *et al.* 2009). This accounts the double face nature of ROS, which mostly depends upon concentration and duration of exposure in determining the fate of cell to proliferate or die (Fig. **1**). Therefore, modulation of pathways linked to generation and detoxification of intracellular ROS levels with natural products seems an attractive approach to prevent cancer.

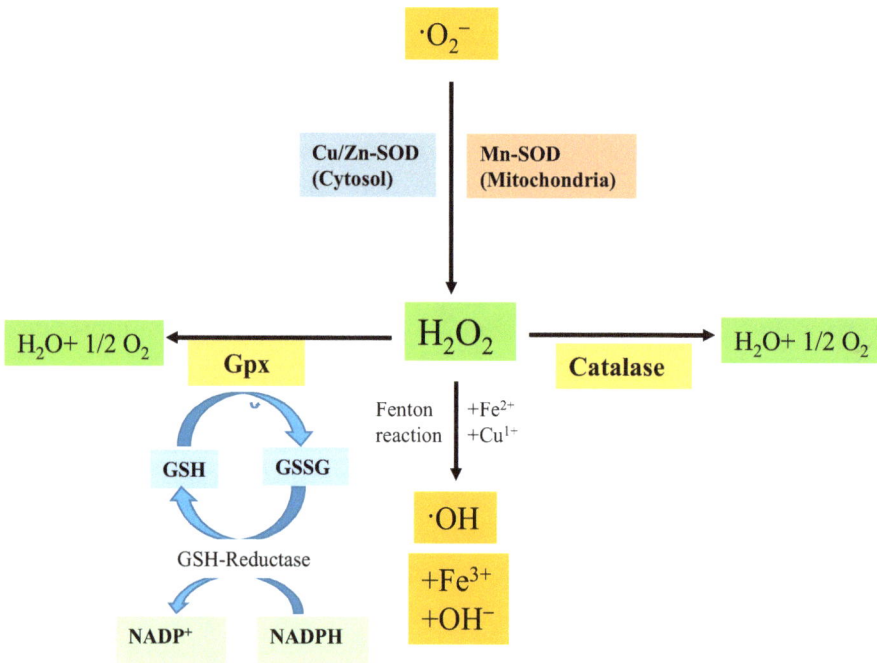

Fig. (1). Basic mechanism of ROS generation and its detoxification in cell.

ROLE OF ROS AND OXIDATIVE STRESS IN CANCER

Increased ROS production and oxidative stress represent the major contributing factor for neoplastic transformation and tumor growth. During initiation phase, oxidative stress causes mutation(s) in genes called proto-oncogenes and tumor suppressors. The products of these genes regulate cell division and thus maintain tissue homeostasis. ROS mediated mutations in proto-oncogene KRAS and tumor suppressor TP53 gene are most widely observed in the cancer patients (Lee and Muller 2010). Oxidative stress mediated formation of DNA adduct *i.e.* 8-hydrox--2'-deoxyguanosine (8-OHdG) is used as indicator of oxidative stress and promotes neoplastic transformation of normal cells (Valavanidis *et al.* 2009). The elevated levels of 8-OHdG are commonly observed in formalin fixed tumor tissues compared to adjacent normal tissue. In addition to genetic mutations, ROS react with lipid components of membrane causing lipid peroxidation (Ayala *et al.* 2014). In this connection, 4 hydroxylnonenal (4HNE), an end product of lipid peroxidation is also reported to cause mutations in TP53 gene (Hu 2002). Moreover, increased 4-HNE level has been linked to development of multiple cancer types (Shoeb *et al.* 2013, Zhong and Yin 2015).

Further progress in redox biology demonstrated that oxidative stress also trigger dysregulation of multiple signaling pathways controlling cell survival, apoptosis, invasion and epithelial to mesenchymal transition pathway (Tong *et al.* 2015). The key signaling pathways regulated by oxidative stress include Nrf2/Keap 1 pathway (Jaramillo and Zhang 2013), Ras/Raf/MEK (McCubrey *et al.* 2007), PI3K/Akt pathway (Koundouros and Poulogiannis, 2018), NF-κB pathway (Hoesel and Schmid 2013), JAK/STAT pathway (Bharadwaj *et al.* 2020), VEGF receptor pathway (Ushio *et al.* 2008) and epithelial to mesenchymal pathway (Wang *et al.* 2010).

Anticancer Effects of Natural Products *via* Targeting ROS and Oxidative Stress

As described above, oxidative stress may promote or suppress the tumor progression depending upon the concentration. Most of the tumor cells are adapted to proliferate and survive under higher basal ROS levels compared to normal cells. Furthermore, elevated ROS levels in cancer cells increase the cellular antioxidants to maintain redox balance as well as to avert the excessive oxidative stress mediated cell death (Perillo *et al.* 2020). Therefore, disrupting the redox adaptation of cancer cells by reducing or increasing the ROS levels can be an effective approach in cancer prevention or cancer therapy. Natural products have long history in preventing various human diseases including cancer and are currently gaining substantial attention from scientific community. A series of natural products have recently been isolated and shown to exhibit strong anticancer potential both in cell lines and pre-clinical studies (Pratheeshkumar *et al.* 2012, Majolo *et al.* 2019). However, the precise pharmacological mechanism of action of most of these natural compounds is limited as majority of the research is carried out on crude extract of plant material. According to the literature, majority of natural compounds exert chemopreventive action *via* ROS regulation.

In this section, we summarize the current information on chemopreventive effect of selected dietary compounds, their mechanism of action with an emphasis on ROS and associated signaling pathways in cancer progression (Fig. **2**).

Epigallocatechin-3-gallate

Tea is the most widely consumed beverage across the globe. Tea is derived from plant *Camellia sinensis* and is generally produced as black, oolong or green tea depending upon the extent of fermentation (Green tea is non-fermented, oolong is partly fermented while black tea is completely fermented). The protective effect of green tea against oxidative stress was first described in a randomized control study where daily consumption of four cups of decaffeinated green tea in heavy smokers for a period of 4 months reduced 8-OHdG levels by 31% (Hakim *et al.* 2003). Additionally, consumption of 2-3 cups of tea per day showed protective effects against several cancers including esophageal (Gao *et al.* 1994), breast (Imai *et al.* 1997, Shrubsole *et al.* 2009, Huang *et al.* 2017, Filippi *et al.* 2018), lung (Izdebska *et al.* 2015, Rawangkan *et al.* 2018, Guo *et al.* 2019), colon (Wang *et al.* 2013, Chen *et al.* 2017, Hao *et al.* 2017) and prostate cancer (Guo *et al.* 2017).

Green tea contains several bioactive compounds collectively termed as catechins which have been shown to possess anticancer activity (Rahmani *et al.* 2015, Shimizu *et al.* 2015, Cao *et al.* 2016, Ullah *et al.* 2016). The most abundant catechins in green tea are epicatechin, epigallocatechin-3-gallate (EGCG) and epigallocatechin. Of these, EGCG is the major and potent anticancer catechin present in green tea (Fujiki *et al.* 2018, Gan *et al.* 2018, Negri *et al.* 2018, Saeki *et al.* 2018). The anticancer properties of EGCG are attributed to its strong antioxidant potential. EGCG has been shown to suppress H_2O_2 mediated cytotoxicity in HepG2 liver carcinoma by increasing GSH levels (Murakami *et al.* 2002). In an orthotopic mouse model, EGCG has been reported to inhibit the colon carcinogenesis as well as its metastasis probably *via* activating Nrf2-UGTA1 signaling pathway (Yuan *et al.* 2007). Similarly, EGCG has shown protective effect against oxalate induced migration of kidney tubular cells *via* activation of Nrf 2/Keap-1 pathway (Kanlaya *et al.* 2016). Recently, EGCG has also been shown to exhibit chemosensitizing properties (Datta and Sinha 2019). EGCG pre-treatment to lung cancer cells not only enhanced sensitivity of lung cancer cells for etoposide but also maintained the redox homeostasis by regulating Nrf2/Keap-1 signaling pathway. The study also showed that EGCG may re-orient Nrf2/Keap-1 pathway both in positive and negative direction to exert its protective effect. The chemopreventive effect of EGCG has also been demonstrated in several pre-clinical studies. Mice administered with EGCG 50-100 mg/kg/day for four weeks exhibited suppressed breast cancer growth *via* inhibition of NF-κB, HIF-1α and VEGF expression (Gu *et al.* 2013). Recently, EGCG induced apoptosis in colon cancer cells *via* activation of endoplasmic reticulum or inhibiting notch signaling pathway (Jin *et al.* 2013, Nesran *et al.* 2019).

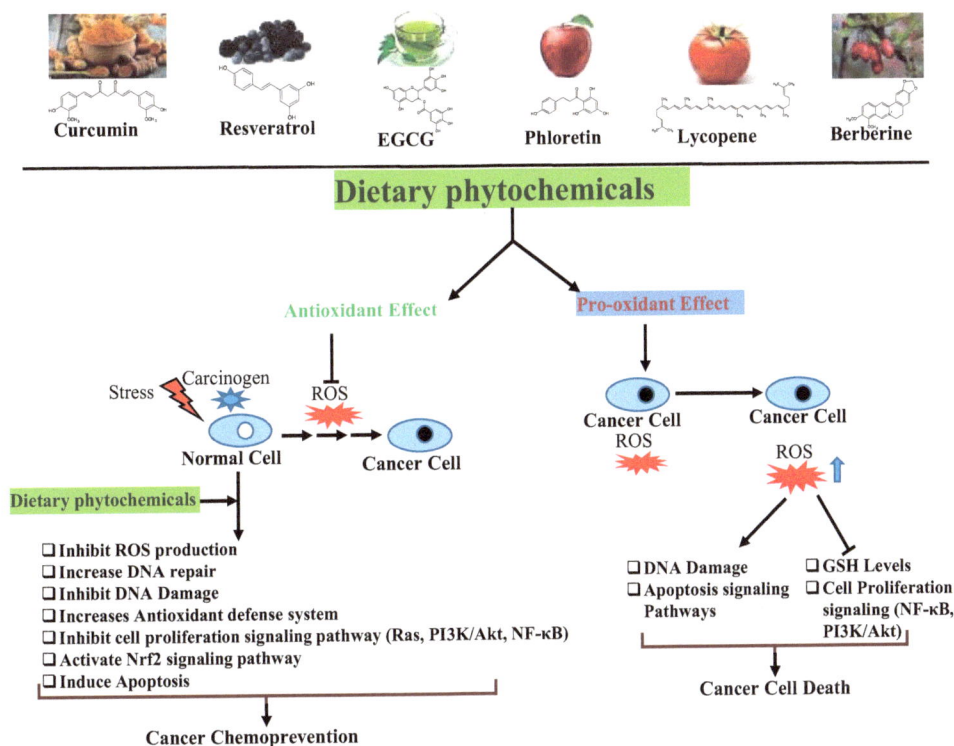

Fig. (2). The antioxidant and pro-oxidant activity of dietary bioactive compounds. The chemopreventive potential of dietary agents is observed in normal cells where these bioactive compounds inhibit ROS mediated DNA damage, neoplastic transformation and clonal expansion of cancer cells *via* activating cellular antioxidant defense system. On the other hand, dietary bioactive compounds in combination with standard chemotherapeutic drugs heighten oxidative stress beyond threshold levels which eventually leads to cancer cell death.

The clinical application of EGCG as chemopreventive as well as chemotherapeutic agent has a remarkable success. Oral administration of EGCG generated a response to treatment in patients suffering from B-cell lymphoma (Shanafelt *et al.* 2006). A phase II clinical trial showed chemopreventive efficacy of tea catechins consumption (1.3 g/day) for six weeks against prostate cancer (McLarty *et al.* 2009). There was a marked reduction in several tumor promoting factors such as serum levels of VEGF, HGF and activated AKT and c-Met in patients who consumed green tea catechins. Another phase II clinical trial conducted in Italy demonstrated that EGCG administration on daily basis delayed prostate cancer development in males suffering from advanced intraepithelial neoplasia in prostate gland (Bettuzzi *et al.* 2006). Neo-angiogenesis is considered as one of the key step in tumor metastasis. In this regard, a phase II randomized placebo-controlled trial was conducted to evaluate the clinical efficacy of green tea catechins in patients at increased risk of premalignant oral lesions (Tsao *et al.* 2009). The patients receiving 0.5 - 1 g/m^2 of catechins for a period of 12 weeks showed reduced levels of VEGF which play a vital role in metastatic spread of tumors. Recently, topical application of EGCG has been reported to ameliorate the radiation induced acute skin damage in breast cancer patients undergoing adjuvant radiotherapy (Zhu *et al.* 2016). Taken together, these findings clearly demonstrate the effectiveness of EGCG as a chemopreventive agent or an adjuvant in chemotherapy.

Resveratrol

Resveratrol ($C_{14}H_{12}O_3$) is a natural phytoalexin present abundantly in blue berries, cranberries, grapes and nuts. Two enantiomeric forms of resveratrol have been identified to exist *i.e.* cis and trans isoforms. Biological assay studies suggested that trans resveratrol is more active than its cis counterpart (Trela and Waterhouse 1996, Gambini *et al.* 2015). Red wine serves as a good source of trans resveratrol (1.9±1.7 mg/L) depending upon the quality of grape cultivar, geographical conditions and process of preparation (Weiskirchen and Weiskirchen 2016). Jang *et al.* in 1997 were first to report that resveratrol is effective in preventing all the three stages of carcinogenesis. Moreover, epidemiological studies have shown a reduction of 50% or more in breast cancer cases in women consuming two or more serves per day of grapes (Levi *et al.* 2005). Building on this research, researchers across the globe have demonstrated the cancer chemopreventive/anti-cancer effect of resveratrol in several pre-clinical studies including breast, colon, lung, prostate and hepatocellular carcinoma (Signorelli and Ghidoni 2005, Athar *et al.* 2007, Aluyen *et al.* 2012, Colica *et al.* 2018). The chemopreventive activity of resveratrol is attributed to its antioxidant properties. In breast epithelial cell lines, resveratrol suppressed migration and transformation *via* inhibiting 4-hydroxyestradiol induced ROS and downstream activation of Akt, ERK and NF-κB signaling pathway (Fernandez *et al.* 2006). Similarly, resveratrol suppressed hypergylcemia induced metastatic potential of pancreatic cancer cells *via* inhibition of ROS (Chen *et al.* 2016). On the other hand, resveratrol protected prostate cancer cells from H_2O_2 induced ROS, oxidative stress and cytotoxicity (Chen *et al.* 2005). This was followed by transcriptional upregulation of hemeoxygenase-1 (HO-1), a vital antioxidant enzyme, *via* activating Nrf-2 signaling pathway. Resveratrol effectively suppressed estrogen induced breast cancer through upregulation of antioxidant genes such as SOD3, NQO1 and DNA damage repair enzyme, in a Nrf-2 dependent manner (Singh *et al.* 2014). These antioxidant enzymes confer protection against oxidative stress mediated DNA damage. Moreover, the efficacy of resveratrol was greatly appreciated even at low dose (200 mg/kg body weight) in preventing 1,2-dimethylhydrazine induced colon carcinogenesis in rodents (Tessitore *et al.* 2000, Sengottuvelan and Nalini 2006). The studies suggested that intake of resveratrol even at low doses present in grapes or red wine can be of significant therapeutic value. In a diethylnitrosamine (DENA)-induced liver tumorigenesis, resveratrol was reported to reduce expression of 3-nitrotyrosine containing proteins and inducible nitric oxide synthase, marker of oxidative damage and inflammation respectively (Bishayee *et al.* 2010). Resveratrol has also been shown a protective effect against cigarette smoking induced ROS/oxidative stress mediated cell death in lung epithelial cells (Kode *et al.* 2008). Further studies revealed that resveratrol enables the transcriptional upregulation of GSH in Nrf-2 dependent way. Overall, resveratrol exerts its chemopreventive action *via* activation of Nrf-2 signaling pathway.

In one clinical trial involving 40 healthy volunteers, daily consumption of resveratrol for 29 days was shown safe even at a dose of 5 g/day (Brown *et al.* 2010). Constitutive activation of Wnt signaling pathway has been testified in more than 85% of colorectal patients (Bienz and Clevers 2000). A phase 1 clinical trial suggested that consumption of grapes (150 g to 450 g/day) for 14 days significantly reduced the constitutive Wnt activation and subsequent mucosal proliferation (Holcombe *et al.* 2015). Similarly, another phase 1 clinical trial suggested protective effect of grape powder with resveratrol as major constituent (80 g/day) against colon cancer by inhibiting Wnt signaling (Nguyen *et al.* 2009). A formulation of resveratrol (SRT501) was also investigated as chemotherapeutic agent in a double blind randomized trial in colon cancer patients (n=9) with hepatic metastatic condition (Howells *et al.* 2011). The trial demonstrated that a daily intake of SRT501 (5 g/per day) for two weeks showed a significant increase in apoptosis of cancer cell in hepatic tissue, as depicted by caspase-3 activity. In another phase I/III clinical trial, resveratrol consumption was correlated with at least 5% reduction in tumor size in colon cancer patients (Patel *et al.* 2010). Recently, Singh *et al.* (2019) reviewed the detailed clinical data on potential health benefits of resveratrol in human diseases. Collectively, these studies warrant resveratrol a potential chemopreventive agent for cancers of multiple origin.

Curcumin

Curcumin represents the most abundant bioactive phytochemicals called curcuminoids found in Indian dietary spice turmeric (*Curcuma longa*). The yellow color of turmeric is due to the presence of curcumin, accounting about 2-5% of it (Tayyem *et al.* 2006). The most noticeable point of curcumin related to its anticancer activity is its selective killing of ROS mediated cancer cell proliferation as compared to their healthy counterparts (Aggarwal *et al.* 2007, Epstein *et al.* 2010). Interestingly, no toxicity in healthy tissue caused on curcumin administration even at a high doses (8 g/day) further warrants the efficacy of curcumin as valuable chemopreventive agent (Chen *et al.* 2001). Curcumin has been reported to suppress ROS mediated activation of certain transcription factors including NF-κB and ERK1/2 as a mechanism to inhibit metastatic potential of cancer cells (Cao *et al.* 2016). In lung cancer cells, curcumin has been shown to trigger anoikis mediated apoptosis in ROS dependent manner, as the pro-apoptotic effect of curcumin was nullified on treatment with Mn(III)tetrakis(4-benzoic acid)porphyrin chloride, a superoxide anion scavenger (Pongrakhananon *et al.* 2010). The promising chemopreventive potential of curcumin has been demonstrated in several preclinical studies including cancer of colon (Reuhl *et al.* 1994, Park 2010), stomach (Azuine and Bhide 1994), liver (Chuang 2000, Darvesh *et al.* 2011), skin cancer (Tsai *et al.* 2012) as well as head and neck cancer (Wilken *et al.* 2011). Molecular studies have shown that curcumin exerts its chemopreventive action through activation of Nrf2 signaling pathway, a principal transcription factor responsible for detoxification of ROS generated during carcinogenesis (Zhao *et al.* 2013, Greenwald *et al.* 2017). In mouse model of lymphoma, long term consumption of curcumin resulted in reduced tumor invasion and liver metastasis by inhibiting MMPs, VEGF and PKCα levels (Das and Vinayak 2014). Further investigations revealed that curcumin administration upregulated the expression of cellular antioxidant enzymes such as HO-1 and SOD and a concomitant decrease in ROS producing enzyme (NOX) in liver, as a mechanism of action of curcumin. The notion that curcumin primarily exploits the cellular redox status to exert its protective/chemopreventive effect was strengthened by a study where curcumin was shown to ameliorate radiation induced ROS and tissue damage in murine derived primary pulmonary cells *via* upregulating HO-1 expression (Lee *et al.* 2010). Curcumin also showed protective effect against ROS induced DNA damage in mouse fibroblast cells (Shih and Lin 1993) and human mononuclear cells (Chan and Wu 2006). On the other hand, several recent reports have indicated the pro-oxidant nature of curcumin and probable mechanism of action to cause cytotoxicity selectively in cancer cells (Kim *et al.* 2016, Wang *et al.* 2017, 2019, Huang *et al.* 2017). Curcumin has also been shown to synergistically improve cytotoxic effect of other anticancer agents (Batra *et al.* 2019).

Regarding the clinical trials, several phase trials were conducted to evaluate beneficial effects of curcumin alone or in combination for cancer management (Salehi *et al.* 2019). Curcumin administration emphatically provided symptomatic relief and more importantly restore the levels of various tumor biomarkers to their physiological range (Gupta *et al.* 2013, Salehi *et al.* 2019). A phase I clinical trial on oral administration of curcumin (3.6 g/day) upto 4 months in patients with advance stage colorectal cancer significantly decreased inducible PGE2 generation in blood, an important biomarker in colon cancer progression (Sharma *et al.* 2004). A phase II trial on pancreatic cancer patients (n=25) demonstrated that long term oral consumption of curcumin (8 g/day) significantly downregulated NF-κB, COX-2, STAT3 levels (Dhillon *et al.* 2008). Kuriakose and colleagues conducted a randomised double-blind placebo controlled phase II trial (n=223) to investigate the effectiveness of curcumin as a treatment strategy for leukoplakia, a malignancy of oral cavity (Kuriakose *et al.* 2016). The trial showed that curcumin was well tolerated and its daily consumption (3.6 g/day) for six months significantly reduced the NF-κB/COX-2 levels, potent molecule for oral carcinogenesis. Recently, in a randomized phase IIa trial, curcumin in combination with FOLFOX chemotherapy is reported to be safe, tolerable in colorectal cancer patients (Howells *et al.* 2019).

Despite the giant success of curcumin as promising anticancer drug in numerous pre-clinical studies, several concerns have been raised regarding the bioavailability, therapeutic potential as well as pharmacological safety. Pharmacokinetic studies of curcumin at oral dose of 10-12 g in healthy volunteers (n=12) revealed that only one subject showed a 50 ng/ml limit of detection which questioned about bioavailability of this compound (Vareed *et al.* 2008). It was found that curcumin when taken orally is readily metabolized in intestine and liver, limiting its desired concentration in blood and tissue (Ireson *et al.* 2001, 2002). In this regard, several attempts have been devised to improve bioavailability of curcumin (Sanidad *et al.* 2019). The use of piperine, an alkaloid from black pepper represents one of the earliest strategies to increase bioavailability of curcumin and approved for clinical trial (Shoba *et al.* 1998). Curcumin has also been reported to act as an efficient iron chelator, which warrants its use as chemopreventive or chemotherapeutic agent in patients with suboptimal iron status (Jiao *et al.* 2009).

Phloretin

Phloretin ($C_{15}H_{14}O_5$) represents the major bioactive polyphenol present in apple fruit (*Malus domestica*). Due to the presence of unsaturation and phenolic moieties, phloretin has been categorised as chalcone. The presence of hydroxyl group (OH) at 2' position of phloretin is responsible for scavenging free radicals and thus indicating its antioxidant nature. A low value of bond dissociation enthalpy (BDE) for OH group is considered as an indicator of antioxidant capacity. Based on computational modelling studies Mendes *et al.* (2018) have suggested that phloretin has a lower BDE value compared to some of well-known antioxidants and thus exhibit higher antioxidant capacity. Further, phloretin was shown to inhibit lipid peroxidation *via* scavenging peroxynitrite radicals and confirmed its antioxidant capacity (Rezk *et al.* 2002). In human colon cancer cell lines, apple juice extract majorly containing phloretin has been demonstrated to inhibit ROS mediated DNA damage by restoring cellular glutathione levels (Schaefer *et al.* 2006). Similarly, phloretin treatment ameliorated ROS mediated oxidative stress in rat hepatocytes *via* activation of Nrf2/HO-1 signaling pathway, a redox sensitive signaling pathway (Yang *et al.* 2011). The study also revealed that phloretin treatment instrumented ERK mediated activation of Nrf2 and subsequent GSH synthesis. Recently, pro-oxidant nature of phloretin has also been demonstrated as a mechanism of killing cancer cells. Kim *et al.* (2020) have shown that phloretin treatment reduced the viability index of human prostate cancer cells through the generation of ROS and a concomitant reduction in cellular catalase, SOD2, GPX1 and GPX3 levels.

Tanaka and colleagues, first of all, reported the anticarcinogenic potential of phloretin. The authors showed that phloretin inhibited the phorbol acetate mediated neoplastic transformation of mouse fibroblast cells (Tanaka *et al.* 1986). Thereafter, phloretin has been extensively explored for its anticancer activity in a wide range of *in vitro* and *in vivo* studies (Choi 2019). Oral administration of phloretin inhibited DMBA induced buccal cavity cancer in Syrina golden hamsters (Anand and Suresh 2014). Phloretin has been demonstrated to suppress colorectal cancer development and ensuing colonic inflammation *via* inhibition of *Escherichia coli* biofilm formation (Lee *et al.* 2011). Moreover, phloretin treatment effectively reduced size of tumor xenografts of multiple origins in SCID mice including liver (Wu *et al.* 2009), colon (Lin *et al.* 2016), lung (Min *et al.* 2015) and breast cancer (Wu *et al.* 2018). Phloretin has been reported to possess anti-inflammatory properties. For example, phloretin treatment reduced the expression of principle mediators of inflammation such as NF-κB, COX-2, STAT-3 and IL-8 (Jung *et al.* 2009). LPS exposure stimulates murine macrophages to secrete various pro-inflammatory cytokines and upregulate the expression of *i*NOS and COX-2. Pre-treatment with phloretin attenuated LPS induced production of inflammatory cytokines including NO, IL-6, PGE2 and TNF-α vis a vis inhibited NF-κB and MAP kinase signaling pathways (Chang *et al.* 2012). Phloretin has recently been investigated for its chemo-sensitizing potential in chemotherapeutic regimens. Phloretin treatment effectively reverted chemoresistance of breast cancer cells and mouse lymphoma cells by mitigated P-gp activity, a principle drug efflux pump on cancer cell membrane and is responsible for acquired drug resistance (Molnár *et al.* 2010). Interestingly, phloretin facilitated cisplatin induced apoptosis in non small cell lung cancer cells (Ma *et al.* 2016) while inhibited cisplatin induced toxicity in normal auditory cells

(Choi *et al.* 2011). Recently, Zhou *et al.* (2018) investigated the efficacy of atorvastatin, a lipid lowering drug, with phloretin against human colon cancer cells. The authors demonstrated that combination of phloretin and atorvastatin showed synergistic effect in inhibiting cancer cell proliferation than treatment with individual compound.

Lycopene

Lycopene ($C_{40}H_{56}$) is a natural pigment and is responsible for red pigmentation in fruits and vegetables. Lycopene is soluble in organic solvents such as hexane, acetone; it is slightly soluble in ethanol and methanol while insoluble in water (Gutiérrez *et al.* 2007). The major sources of lycopene include red guava, watermelon, tomato, carrot, rose-hip, pumpkin and apricot (Bramley 2000, Shi and Maguer 2000). An expected variation in lycopene content has been observed which depends upon the variety, maturation, harvesting and storage methods. Tomatoes represents the most cost-effective source of lycopene and comprise about 80-90% of all carotenoids (Kelkel *et al.* 2011). Lycopene exhibit highest antioxidant potential among carotenoids (lycopene > tocopherol > carotene > cryptoxanthin > zeaxanthin =β-carotene > lutein) and protects cells by its extraordinary capacity to quench free radicals (Heber and Lu 2002). The anticancer activity of lycopene against oxidative stress mediated cellular damage and neoplastic transformation has been verified in numerous pre-clinical and clinical investigations (Grabowska *et al.* 2019, Saini *et al.* 2020). Lycopene supplementation in diet has shown beneficial effect against fluoride induced apoptosis in ameloblasts *via* increasing SOD, GPx activity and Bcl-2 expression (Li *et al.* 2017). Wan and colleagues investigated the impact of lycopene feeding on about 200 genes related to the early prostate cancer in transgenic mouse model (Wan *et al.* 2014). The authors showed that lycopene supplementation in diet significantly downregulated genes related to androgen metabolism and signaling in prostate cancer. Differential expression studies specifically androgen metabolism related showed that Srd5a1 gene was downregulated by 2.5 times. The product of this gene *i.e.*, steroid 5α-reductase is responsible for conversion of testosterone into 5-α-dihydrotestosterone, a potent activator of androgen receptor (Gao *et al.* 2005). Evidence from *in vitro* experiments suggested that lycopene treatment caused cell cycle arrest and growth inhibition of prostate cancer cells (Rafi *et al.* 2013, Soares *et al.* 2013). Variation in β-carotene 9′,10′-oxygenase (Bco2) activity is a crucial factor which may alter the overall beneficial effects of tomato or lycopene consumption against prostate cancer. Bco2 acts as tumor suppressor by inhibiting NF-κB phosphorylation and its nuclear translocation. Deletion of Bco2 genes in prostate cancer cells resulted in complete failure in lycopene anticancer effect. This observation further underpinned Bco2 as principle target of lycopene to exert anti-neoplastic activity (Tan *et al.* 2017).

Lycopene supplementation (2.2 and 6.6 mg/kg) in diet suppressed 4-(N-methy--N-nitrosamine)-1-(3-pyridyl)-1-butanone (NNK), the potent tobacco carcinogen, in liver and lung of ferrets (Aizawa *et al.* 2016). One of the xenograft study demonstrated that lycopene consumption significantly suppressed tumor growth and expression of inflammatory makers such COX-2, PGE2 and phosphorylated ERK1/2 within this xenograft model (Tang *et al.* 2011). Together, these results suggested that lycopene can effectively inhibit the process of carcinogenesis.

Several clinical trials regarding the health benefits of lycopene have been conducted across the globe. Lycopene (15-120 mg/day) was evaluated in a phase I/II trial for toxicity profile in patients (n=36) with biochemical relapse of prostate cancer (Clark *et al.* 2006). Out of 36 patients enrolled in this trial, only one patient developed diarrhoea while others did not show any significant toxicity. In another phase II clinical trial conducted on Chinese population indicated that lycopene consumption can reduce prostate specific antigen (Zhang *et al.* 2014). Gann *et al.* evaluated the protective effect of lycopene rich tomato extract in a phase II randomized trial in prostate cancer patients (Gann *et al.* 2015). Recently, a phase II randomized placebo-controlled trial entitled 'ProDiet' has been conducted to analyse chemopreventive potential of lycopene in combination with green tea catechins in individuals at high risk of prostate cancer (Lane *et al.* 2018). In this trial, daily consumption of 600 mg EGCG and 15 mg lycopene for six months was shown protective against prostate cancer.

Berberine

Berberine ($C_{20}H_{18}NO_4$) is natural alkaloid found in plants belonging to berberidaceae, rutaceae and papaveraceae family. Berberine or source of berberine such as stem, bark and roots of Berberis plants are used traditionally in various Ayurvedic and Chinese medicines for its anti-oxidative, anti-inflammation, antimicrobial, anti-diarrhoea, anti-diabetic properties. Research in the recent decades has demonstrated anti-tumor activity of berberine in multiple types of cancer (Mantena *et al.* 2006b, 2006a, Hsu *et al.* 2007, Kim *et al.* 2010, Sharma *et al.* 2014, Jin *et al.* 2016, Zhang *et al.* 2020). The *in vitro* biological assessment such as cellular thiobarbituric acid reactive species (TBARS) formation, free radical scavenging capacity, diphenyl-α-picrylhydrazyl (DPPH) oxidation, Gpx and SOD activity suggested that berberine is a potent antioxidant (Wahab *et al.* 2013). Further, berberine (50 mg/kg body weight p.o.) mitigated cyclophosphamide-induced liver toxicity by modulating antioxidant status (Germoush and Mahmoud 2014). It was evident from biochemical results that berberine significantly inhibited ROS mediated lipid peroxidation, COX-2 and serum TNF-α levels vis a vis increased the cellular SOD, Gpx activity and GSH content. Sun *et al.* (2017) showed that berberine is capable of ameliorating fatty acid induced oxidative stress in hepatocellular carcinoma. In several studies, however, pro-oxidant activity of berberine has also been reported as a mechanism of anticancer effect. Berberine treatment augmented ROS production, mitochondrial dysfunction and also accompanied ER stress collectively to inhibit the growth of human breast and brain cancer cells (Eom *et al.* 2010, Xie *et al.* 2015). Moreover, Hou and colleagues showed that berberine is capable to downregulate homologous recombinant DNA repair and thus DNA damage *via* increasing ROS production in ovarian cancer cells (Hou *et al.* 2017). Berberine has been reported to radiosensitize hepatoma cell *via* downregulating Nrf2 expression, a vital signaling pathway to combat oxidative stress (You *et al.* 2019). Similarly, berberine has been shown to chemosensitize HER(+) breast cancer cells to lapatinib by increasing ROS production (Zhang *et al.* 2016).

Table 1. Summary of plant based antioxidants and their molecular mechanism in cancer chemoprevention.

Plant Based Antioxidant	Preventable Cancer/Study	Molecular Mechanism	Outcome	References
EGCG	Liver carcinoma	• Enhanced the GSH level	• Suppressed the liver carcinoma cell growth	Murakami *et al.* (2002)
	Orthotopic mouse model of colon cancer	• Activating Nrf2-UGTA1 pathway	• Reduced the colon cancer cell proliferation and metastatic potential	Yuan *et al.* (2007)
	Kidney tubular cells	• Activating Nrf2/Keap-1 pathway	• Inhibited the migration of kidney tubular cell	Kanlaya *et al.* (2016)
	Lung cancer	• Restored the redox homeostasis • Activation of Nrf2/Keap-1 pathway	• Enhanced the chemotherapeutic efficacy of etoposide	Datta and Sinha (2019)
	Breast cancer	• Suppressed NF-κB, HIF-1α and VEGF expression	• Suppressed the breast cancer cell proliferation and metastasis	Gu *et al.* (2013)
	Colon cancer	• Targeting ER stress mediated apoptosis	• Induced apoptosis in colon cancer cells	Jin *et al.* (2013)
	Colon cancer	• Notch signaling	• Induced apoptosis in colon cancer cells	Nesran *et al.* (2019)
	Prostate cancer (Phase II)	• Reduced levels of VEGF, HGF, phosphorylated AKT and c-Met	• EGCG could be a option for prevention of prostate cancer	McLarty *et al.* (2009)
	Prostate cancer (Phase II)	• Reduced the PSA levels	• Delayed Prostate cancer development	Bettuzzi *et al.* (2006)
	Premalignant oral lesions	• Reduced levels of VEGF	• Suppressed the metastatic spread of tumors	Tsao *et al.* (2009)
	Advanced breast cancer	• Reduced the pain, burning feeling, itching and tenderness	• Suppressed skin damage in breast cancer patients undergoing adjuvant radiotherapy	Zhu *et al.* (2016)

(Table 1) cont.....

Plant Based Antioxidant	Preventable Cancer/Study	Molecular Mechanism	Outcome	References
Resveratrol	Breast epithelial cell lines	• Inhibiting ROS, Akt, EKR and NF-κB signaling pathway	• Suppressed neoplastic transformation and migration	Fernandez *et al.* (2006)
	Pancreatic cancer	• Inhibition of ROS	• Suppressed hyperglycemia induced metastasis	Chen *et al.* (2016)
	Prostate Cancer	• Inhibition of ROS • Upregulation of HO-1 • Activation of Nrf2 pathway	• Protected cancer cells from ROS mediated cell death	Chen *et al.* (2005)
	Breast cancer	• Activation of SOD3, NQO1 and DNA damage repair • Activation of Nrf2 pathway	• Delayed the breast cancer progression	Singh *et al.* (2014)
	Colon cancer	• Induction of apoptosis • Inhibition of ACF in colon	• Depressed the colon cancer progression	Tessitore *et al.* (2000), Sengottuvelan and Nalini (2006)
	Liver cancer	• Inhibition of 3-Nitrotyrosine containing proteins • Inhibition of *i*NOS	• Delayed liver cancer cell proliferation	Bishayee *et al.* (2010)
	Lung epithelial cells	• Inihibtion of ROS • Upregulation of GSH • Activation of Nrf2 pathway • Inhibited cell death	• Protected lung epithelial cells from cigarette smoking induced cell death	Kode *et al.* (2008)
	Colon cancer (Phase I)	• Inhibition of Wnt activation • ACF formation	• Suppressed mucosal cell proliferation	Holcombe *et al.* (2015) Nguyen *et al.* (2009)
	Hepatic metastatic cancer SRT501 (a formulation of Resveratrol, 5 g/day)	• Induction of apoptosis in cancer cells • Increased Caspase-3 activity	• Suppressed the metastatic potential of hepatic cancer cells	Howells *et al.* (2011)
	Colon cancer (Phase I/III)	• Inhibition of tumor growth	• Reduction in tumor size	Patel *et al.* (2010)

(Table 1) cont.....

Plant Based Antioxidant	Preventable Cancer/Study	Molecular Mechanism	Outcome	References
Curcumin	Pancreatic cancer	• Inhibition of NF-κB and ERK activity	• Reduced the invasion and migration of pancreatic cancer	Cao *et al.* (2016)
	Non small cell lung cancer	• Induction of apoptosis • Downregulation of Bcl-2 expression	• Chemosensitized the tumor cells to Bcl-2 therapy	Pongrakhananon *et al.* (2010)
	Lymphoma	• Inhibition of MMPs, VEGF ad PKCα • Activation of HO-1 and SOD levels	• Reduced the tumor invasion and liver metastasis	Das and Vinayak (2014)
	Mouse derived primary pulmonary cells	• Uprgulation of HO-1 expression	• Protection against ROS mediated tissue damage	Lee *et al.* (2010)
	Mouse fibroblasts	• Inhibition of 8-hydroxydeoxyguanosine formation	• Protection against ROS mediated DNA damage	Shih and Lin *et al.* (1993)
	Human mononuclear cells	• Inhibition of methylglyoxal induced apoptosis	• Protection against ROS mediated DNA damage	Chan and Wu (2006)
	Cervical cancer	• Selective induction of ER stress in cancer cells • Selective induction of apoptosis in cancer cells	• Suppressed cervical cancer cell proliferation	Kim *et al.* (2016)
	Gastric cancer	• Restoration of ROS mediated depletion of DNA polymerase γ	• Inhibited the gastric tumor growth, proliferation and colony formation	Wang *et al.* (2017)
	Non small cell lung cancer	• Induction of ER stress mediated apoptosis • Cell cycle arrest at G2/M phase	• Suppressed the lung cancer growth and proliferation	Wang *et al.* (2019)
	Colorectal cancer	• Generation of ER stress • Induction of apoptosis	• Enhanced the effect of irinotecan	Huang *et al.* (2017)
	Colorectal cancer (Phase I trial)	• Reduction in serum PGE$_2$ Levels • Suppression of DNA adduct formation	• Inference for chemopreventive potential of curcumin	Sharma *et al.* (2004)
	Pancreatic cancer (Phase II trial)	• Inhibition of NF-κB, COX-2 and STAT3 levels	• Oral curcumin is well tolerated • Curcumin showed biological activity in some of patients	Dhillon *et al.* (2008)
	Leukoplakia (Double blind Placebo Phase IIb)	• Reduced the levels of NF-κB and COX-2 levels	• Significant and durable clinical response for 6 months	Kuriakose *et al.* (2016)
	Colorectal cancer (Randomized Phase IIa trial)	• CXCL1 levels were unchanged	• Safe and tolerable in CRC for FOLFOX chemotherapy	Howells *et al.* (2019)

(Table 1) cont.....

Plant Based Antioxidant	Preventable Cancer/Study	Molecular Mechanism	Outcome	References
Phloretin	Colon cancer	• Inhibition of ROS generation • Restoration of cellular glutathione levels	• Suppressed oxidative DNA damage	Schaefer *et al.* (2006)
	Murine hepatocyte	• Reduction of ROS generation • Activation of Nrf2/HO-1 pathway • Stimulated GSH synthesis	• Protected rat hepatocytes against oxidative DNA damage	Yang *et al.* (2011)
	Prostate cancer	• Selective generation of ROS in cancer cells • Selective depletion of cellular catalase, SOD, GPX in cancer cells	• Suppressed the prostate cancer cell proliferation	Kim *et al.* (2019)
	Mouse fibroblast	• Inhibition of protein kinase C	• Inhibited the neoplastic transformation of murine fibroblasts	Tanaka *et al.* (1986)
	Buccal cavity cancer	• Reduction in lipid peroxidation levels • Restored the cellular antioxidants and Phase I and Phase II enzyme activity	• Prevented buccal cavity cancer progression *via* restoring antioxidant and detoxification enzyme status	Anand and Suresh (2014)
	Colorectal cancer	• Inhibition of *E. coli* biofilm formation	• Suppressed *E. coli* mediated CRC development	Lee *et al.* (2011)
	Liver cancer	• Reduction in tumor size	• Suppressed xenograft tumor growth in SCID mice	Wu *et al.* (2009)
	Colon cancer	• Reduction in tumor size	• Suppressed xenograft tumor growth in SCID mice	Lin *et al.* (2016)
	Lung cancer	• Reduction in tumor size	• Suppressed xenograft tumor growth in SCID mice	Min *et al.* (2015)
	Breast cancer	• Reduction in tumor size	• Suppressed xenograft tumor growth in SCID mice	Wu *et al.* (2018)
	Breast cancer	• Mitigated p-gp activity	• Reversed the chemoresistance in cancer cells	Molnár *et al.* (2010)
	Mouse lymphoma	• Mitigated p-gp activity	• Reversed the chemoresistance in cancer cells	Molnár *et al.* (2010)
	Non small cell lung cancer	• Increased the caspase-3 expression • Reduction in Bcl-2 and MMPs expression	• Improved the therapeutic efficacy of cisplatin	Ma *et al.* (2016)
	Normal auditory cells	• Activation of Nrf2-HO-1 pathway	• Reduced cisplatin induced tissue toxicity	Choi *et al.* (2011)
	Colon cancer	• Augmented apoptosis • G2/M Cell cycle arrest	• Improved the efficacy of atorvastatin	Zhou *et al.* (2018)

(Table 1) cont.....

Plant Based Antioxidant	Preventable Cancer/Study	Molecular Mechanism	Outcome	References
Lycopene	Prostate cancer	• Downregulated Srd5a1 gene expression	• Reduced early onset of prostate cancer	Wan *et al.* (2014)
	Prostate cancer	• Induction of apoptosis • Augmented PPARγ effect	• Improved the efficacy of PPARγ agonists	Rafi *et al.* (2013)
	Prostate cancer	• Induction of apoptosis • Increased Bax/Bcl-2 ratio • Arrested cell cycle at G0/G1 phase	• Suppressed prostate cancer cell proliferation	Soares *et al.* (2013)
	Prostate cancer	• Acted as Bco2 agonist	• Suppressed the prostate cancer development	Tan *et al.* (2017)
	Lung cancer	• Reduction in tobacco carcinogen accumulation	• Delayed lung cancer development	Aizawa *et al.* (2016)
	Colon cancer	• Downregulated COX-2, PGE_2 and ERK1/2 expression	• Effectively inhibited xenografted tumor growth in SCID mice	Tang *et al.* (2011)
	Prostate cancer (Phase II trial)	• Reduction in prostate cancer antigen levels	• Consumption of lycopene could be effective in preventing prostate cancer	Zhang *et al.* (2014)
	Prostate cancer (Phase II randomized trial)	• No significant change in MCM-2 and p27 expression	• Further studies are warranted to reach on conclusion	Gann *et al.* (2015)
	Prostate Cancer (ProDiet, a phase II randomized placebo control trial)	• No significant alteration in PSA levels	• Combination clinical trials can be performed	Lane *et al.* (2018)

(Table 1) cont.....

Plant Based Antioxidant	Preventable Cancer/Study	Molecular Mechanism	Outcome	References
Berberine	Prostate cancer	• Induction of apoptosis • Cell cycle arrest at G1 phase	• Delayed prostate cancer cell proliferation	Mantena *et al.* (2006a)
	Epidermoid carcinoma	• Induction of apoptosis • Cell cycle arrest at G1 phase	• Inhibited epidermal cancer cell proliferation	Mantena *et al.* (2006b)
	Colon cancer	• Induction of apoptosis • ROS generation • Activation of JNK/p38/MAPK pathway	• Suppressed the colon cancer cell proliferation	Hsu *et al.* (2007)
	Breast cancer	• Cell cycle arrest at G0/G1 phase	• Inhibited breast cancer cell growth and proliferation	Kim *et al.* (2010)
	Epidermal carcinoma cells	• Induction of apoptosis • Cell cycle arrest at G1 phase	• Suppressed the epidermal carcinoma development	Sharma *et al.* (2014)
	Hepatocellular carcinoma	• Reduction of oxidative stress	• Inhibited the liver cancer cell proliferation	Sun *et al.* (2017)
	Brain cancer	• Increased production of ROS and Ca^{2+} release • Induction of apoptosis through ER stress and mitochondrial dysfunction	• Suppressed the growth and proliferation of glioblastoma cells	Eom *et al.* (2010)
	Breast cancer	• Induction of mitochondrial related apoptosis • Increased production of ROS	• Inhibited breast cancer cell colony formation	Xie *et al.* (2015)
	Ovarian cancer	• Increased oxidative DNA damage • Augmented apoptotic potential of niraparib	• Increased the therapeutic efficacy of niraparib in ovarian cancer	Hou *et al.* (2017)
	Liver cancer	• Downregulation of Nrf2 signaling pathway	• Increased the radiosensitivity of hepatoma cells	You *et al.* (2019)
	Breast cancer	• Increased production of ROS • Induction of apoptosis	• Improved the chemotherapeutic efficacy of lapatinib	Zhang *et al.* (2016)
	Lung cancer	• Inhibition of NF-κB signaling pathway	• Suppressed lung cancer cell proliferation and migration	Pandey *et al.* (2008)
	Leukemia	• Inhibition of NF-κB signaling pathway	• Suppressed proliferation of leukemia cells	Pandey *et al.* (2008)
	Multiple myeloma	• Inhibition of NF-κB signaling pathway	• Suppressed growth and proliferation of myeloma cells	Pandey *et al.* (2008)
	Primary effusion lymphoma	• Suppression of NF-κB signaling pathway	• Inhibited growth and invasion of primary effusion lymphoma	Goto *et al.* (2012)
	Hepatocellular carcinoma	• Downregulation of NF-κB activity	• Suppressed the growth and proliferation of hepatocellular carcinoma	Li *et al.* (2017)
	Cholangio-carcinoma	• Cell cycle arrest at G1 phase • Downregulation of NF-κB and STAT3	• Inhibited the growth and proliferation of cholangiocarcinoma cells	Puthdee *et al.* (2017)
	Cervical cancer	• Inhibition of NFκB, HIF1A and NFE2L2/AP-1 pathways	• Suppressed the growth and proliferation of HeLa cell lines	Belanova *et al.* (2018)
	Colon cancer	• Inhibition of NF-κB signaling	• Increased the therapeutic efficacy of irinotecan	Yu *et al.* (2014)
	Gastric cancer	• Inhibition of survivin and STAT3	• Increased the chemotherapeutic efficacy of 5-FU	Pandey *et al.* (2015)
	Lung cancer (randomized double-blind trial)	• Reduction in ICAM-1 and TGF-β levels	• Protected against radiation induced lung injury	Liu *et al.* (2008)
	Colorectal cancer (a multicentre, double-blinded, randomised controlled study)	• Inhibited the recurrence of CRC	• Could be used as an option for chemoprevention of CRC after polypectomy	Chen *et al.* (2020)

In addition to ROS, researchers also identified several other cellular targets of berberine to kill cancer cells. Berberine also inhibited aberrant activation of NF-κB in different cancer cell types, indicating its anti-inflammatory properties (Pandey *et al.* 2008, Goto *et al.* 2012, Li *et al.* 2017, Puthdee *et al.* 2017, Belanova *et al.* 2018). Phytochemical analysis of plant extracts showing NF-κB inhibition has revealed the presence of berberine as major constituent of extract (Muralimanoharan *et al.* 2009, Diab *et al.* 2015, Sharma *et al.* 2019). Moreover, berberine enhanced the chemosensitivity of tumor cells to standard drugs such as 5-FU and irinotecan (Yu *et al.* 2014, Pandey *et al.* 2015). Protective effects of berberine were evaluated in a randomized double blind placebo controlled trial on radiation induced tissue damage in lung cancer patients (Liu *et al.* 2008). Out of 90 patients, trial group (n=42) showed a significant reduction in soluble ICAM-1 and TGFβ-1 compared to control patients (n=43), suggesting the health benefits of berberine consumption during radiation therapy. In a double blind randomized placebo controlled trial, chemopreventive potential and safety of berberine was examined in 891 patients with colorectal adenoma recurrence (Chen *et al.* 2020). This trial suggested that consumption of berberine (300 mg) twice a day was safe and effective in preventing recurrence of colorectal adenoma.

CONCLUSION

In conclusion, perturbation of redox homeostasis; increased oxidative stress is a critical event in setting up the stage for carcinogenesis. Therefore, inhibition of oxidative stress with the use of dietary phytochemicals appears an effective approach in preventing neoplastic transformation of normal cells. Activation of Nrf2 pathway plays a central role in dietary antioxidant mediated inhibition of carcinogenesis. On the other hand, tumor cells exhibit elevated oxidative stress compared to normal cells. In this condition, a further increase in oxidative stress beyond a threshold level using ROS generating natural compounds make cancer cells vulnerable to excessive oxidative stress mediated cell death. Therefore, increasing endogenous antioxidants is a promising strategy for preventing tumorigenesis while increasing the oxidative stress causing cell death is an attractive strategy for treatment of cancer.

In this chapter, several dietary compounds have been discussed for their anticancer potential. Detailed literature survey revealed that these natural compounds possess both pro-oxidant and antioxidant properties to show anticancer activity. What actually determine the antioxidant and pro-oxidant effect is largely unknown. However, several factors such as cancer cell milieu (cellular pH), concentration of phytochemical and p53 activation have been recognized which determine the antioxidant or pro-oxidant effect of these natural compounds in prevention or chemotherapeutic regimens. Taken together, dietary compounds exhibit strong anticancer potential which can be integrated to well-designed pre-clinical and clinical studies for cancer treatment.

CONFLICT OF INTEREST

Authors declare no conflict of interest.

ACKNOWLEDGEMENT

Sandeep Kumar sincerely thanks to Indian Council of Medical Research, New Delhi, India for providing ICMR RA Fellowship (File No. 45/31/2019-BIO/BMS). The authors also acknowledge Council of Scientific and Industrial Research Institute of Himalayan Bioresource Technology Palampur-176061, Himachal Pradesh, India for providing necessary facilities for this work.

CONSENT FOR PUBLICATION

None

REFERENCES

Abreu, IA & Cabelli, DE (2010) Superoxide dismutases-a review of the metal-associated mechanistic variations. *Biochim Biophys Acta,* 1804, 263-74.
[http://dx.doi.org/10.1016/j.bbapap.2009.11.005] [PMID: 19914406]

Aggarwal, BB, Surh, YJ & Shishodia, S (2007) *The Molecular Targets and Therapeutic Uses of Curcumin in Health and Disease*
[http://dx.doi.org/10.1007/978-0-387-46401-5]

Agnihotri, N, Rani, I & Kumar, S (2015) Targeting Mitochondria: A Powerhouse Approach to Cancer Treatment.*Multi-Targeted Approach to Treatment of Cancer* Springer International Publishing Switzerland 263-76.
[http://dx.doi.org/10.1007/978-3-319-12253-3_16]

Aizawa, K, Liu, C, Tang, S, Veeramachaneni, S, Hu, KQ, Smith, DE & Wang, XD (2016) Tobacco carcinogen induces both lung cancer and non-alcoholic steatohepatitis and hepatocellular carcinomas in ferrets which can be attenuated by lycopene supplementation. *Int J Cancer,* 139, 1171-81.
[http://dx.doi.org/10.1002/ijc.30161] [PMID: 27116542]

Aluyen, JK, Ton, QN, Tran, T, Yang, AE, Gottlieb, HB & Bellanger, RA (2012) Resveratrol: potential as anticancer agent. *J Diet Suppl,* 9, 45-56.
[http://dx.doi.org/10.3109/19390211.2011.650842] [PMID: 22432802]

Anand, MA & Suresh, K (2014) Biochemical profiling and chemopreventive activity of phloretin on 7,12-Dimethylbenz (a) anthracene induced oral carcinogenesis in male golden Syrian hamsters. *Toxicol Int,* 21, 179-85.
[http://dx.doi.org/10.4103/0971-6580.139805] [PMID: 25253928]

Athar, M, Back, JH, Tang, X, Kim, KH, Kopelovich, L, Bickers, DR & Kim, AL (2007) Resveratrol: a review of preclinical studies for human cancer prevention. *Toxicol Appl Pharmacol,* 224, 274-83.
[http://dx.doi.org/10.1016/j.taap.2006.12.025] [PMID: 17306316]

Ayala, A, Muñoz, MF & Argüelles, S (2014) Lipid peroxidation: production, metabolism, and signaling mechanisms of malondialdehyde and 4-hydroxy-2-nonenal. *Oxid Med Cell Longev,* 2014360438

[http://dx.doi.org/10.1155/2014/360438] [PMID: 24999379]

Azuine, MA & Bhide, SV (1994) Adjuvant chemoprevention of experimental cancer: catechin and dietary turmeric in forestomach and oral cancer models. *J Ethnopharmacol,* 44, 211-7.
[http://dx.doi.org/10.1016/0378-8741(94)01188-5] [PMID: 7898128]

Bakalova, R, Zhelev, Z, Aoki, I & Saga, T (2013) Tissue redox activity as a hallmark of carcinogenesis: from early to terminal stages of cancer. *Clin Cancer Res,* 19, 2503-17.
[http://dx.doi.org/10.1158/1078-0432.CCR-12-3726] [PMID: 23532887]

Bartosz, G (2009) Reactive oxygen species: destroyers or messengers? *Biochem Pharmacol,* 77, 1303-15.
[http://dx.doi.org/10.1016/j.bcp.2008.11.009] [PMID: 19071092]

Basak, P, Sadhukhan, P, Sarkar, P & Sil, PC (2017) Perspectives of the Nrf-2 signaling pathway in cancer progression and therapy. *Toxicol Rep,* 4, 306-18.
[http://dx.doi.org/10.1016/j.toxrep.2017.06.002] [PMID: 28959654]

Batra, H, Pawar, S & Bahl, D (2019) Curcumin in combination with anti-cancer drugs: A nanomedicine review. *Pharmacol Res,* 139, 91-105.
[http://dx.doi.org/10.1016/j.phrs.2018.11.005] [PMID: 30408575]

Belanova, A, Beseda, D, Chmykhalo, V, Stepanova, A, Belousova, M, Khrenkova, V, Gavalas, N & Zolotukhin, P (2019) Berberine Effects on NFκB, HIF1A and NFE2L2/AP-1 Pathways in HeLa Cells. *Anticancer Agents Med Chem,* 19, 487-501.
[http://dx.doi.org/10.2174/1871520619666181211121405] [PMID: 30526471]

Berndt, C, Lillig, CH & Holmgren, A (2008) Thioredoxins and glutaredoxins as facilitators of protein folding. *Biochim Biophys Acta,* 1783, 641-50.
[http://dx.doi.org/10.1016/j.bbamcr.2008.02.003] [PMID: 18331844]

Bettuzzi, S, Brausi, M, Rizzi, F, Castagnetti, G, Peracchia, G & Corti, A (2006) Chemoprevention of human prostate cancer by oral administration of green tea catechins in volunteers with high-grade prostate intraepithelial neoplasia: a preliminary report from a one-year proof-of-principle study. *Cancer Res,* 66, 1234-40.
[http://dx.doi.org/10.1158/0008-5472.CAN-05-1145] [PMID: 16424063]

Bharadwaj, U, Kasembeli, MM, Robinson, P & Tweardy, DJ (2020) Targeting janus kinases and signal transducer and activator of transcription 3 to treat inflammation, fibrosis, and cancer: Rationale, progress, and caution. *Pharmacol Rev,* 72, 486-526.
[http://dx.doi.org/10.1124/pr.119.018440] [PMID: 32198236]

Bienz, M & Clevers, H (2000) Linking colorectal cancer to Wnt signaling. *Cell,* 103, 311-20.
[http://dx.doi.org/10.1016/S0092-8674(00)00122-7] [PMID: 11057903]

Bishayee, A, Barnes, KF, Bhatia, D, Darvesh, AS & Carroll, RT (2010) Resveratrol suppresses oxidative stress and inflammatory response in diethylnitrosamine-initiated rat hepatocarcinogenesis. *Cancer Prev Res (Phila),* 3, 753-63.
[http://dx.doi.org/10.1158/1940-6207.CAPR-09-0171] [PMID: 20501860]

Boeing, H, Bechthold, A, Bub, A, Ellinger, S, Haller, D, Kroke, A, Leschik-Bonnet, E, Müller, MJ, Oberritter, H, Schulze, M, Stehle, P & Watzl, B (2012) Critical review: vegetables and fruit in the prevention of chronic diseases. *Eur J Nutr,* 51, 637-63.
[http://dx.doi.org/10.1007/s00394-012-0380-y] [PMID: 22684631]

Bramley, PM (2000) Is lycopene beneficial to human health? *Phytochemistry,* 54, 233-6.
[http://dx.doi.org/10.1016/S0031-9422(00)00103-5] [PMID: 10870177]

Bray, F, Ferlay, J, Soerjomataram, I, Siegel, RL, Torre, LA & Jemal, A (2018) Global cancer statistics 2018: GLOBOCAN estimates of incidence and mortality worldwide for 36 cancers in 185 countries. *CA Cancer J Clin,* 68, 394-424.
[http://dx.doi.org/10.3322/caac.21492] [PMID: 30207593]

Brown, VA, Patel, KR, Viskaduraki, M, Crowell, JA, Perloff, M, Booth, TD, Vasilinin, G, Sen, A, Schinas,

AM, Piccirilli, G, Brown, K, Steward, WP, Gescher, AJ & Brenner, DE (2010) Repeat dose study of the cancer chemopreventive agent resveratrol in healthy volunteers: safety, pharmacokinetics, and effect on the insulin-like growth factor axis. *Cancer Res,* 70, 9003-11.
[http://dx.doi.org/10.1158/0008-5472.CAN-10-2364] [PMID: 20935227]

Cao, J, Han, J, Xiao, H, Qiao, J & Han, M (2016) Effect of tea polyphenol compounds on anticancer drugs in terms of anti-tumor activity, toxicology, and pharmacokinetics. *Nutrients,* 8, 1-12.
[http://dx.doi.org/10.3390/nu8120762] [PMID: 27983622]

Cao, L, Chen, X, Xiao, X; Ma, Q & Li, W (2016) Resveratrol inhibits hyperglycemia-driven ROS-induced invasion and migration of pancreatic cancer cells *via* suppression of the ERK and p38 MAPK signaling pathways. *Int J Oncol,* 49, 735-43.
[http://dx.doi.org/10.3892/ijo.2016.3559] [PMID: 27278736]

Cao, L, Liu, J, Zhang, L, Xiao, X & Li, W (2016) Curcumin inhibits H2O2-induced invasion and migration of human pancreatic cancer *via* suppression of the ERK/NF-κB pathway. *Oncol Rep,* 36, 2245-51.
[http://dx.doi.org/10.3892/or.2016.5044] [PMID: 27572503]

Chan, WH & Wu, HJ (2006) Protective effects of curcumin on methylglyoxal-induced oxidative DNA damage and cell injury in human mononuclear cells. *Acta Pharmacol Sin,* 27, 1192-8.
[http://dx.doi.org/10.1111/j.1745-7254.2006.00374.x] [PMID: 16923340]

Cheng, AL, Hsu, CH, Lin, JK, Hsu, MM, Ho, YF, Shen, TS, Ko, JY, Lin, JT, Lin, BR, Ming-Shiang, W, Yu, HS, Jee, SH, Chen, GS, Chen, TM, Chen, CA, Lai, MK, Pu, YS, Pan, MH, Wang, YJ, Tsai, CC & Hsieh, CY (2001) Phase I clinical trial of curcumin, a chemopreventive agent, in patients with high-risk or pre-malignant lesions. *Anticancer Res,* 21, 2895-900.
[PMID: 11712783]

Chen, CY, Jang, JH, Li, MH & Surh, YJ (2005) Resveratrol upregulates heme oxygenase-1 expression *via* activation of NF-E2-related factor 2 in PC12 cells. *Biochem Biophys Res Commun,* 331, 993-1000.
[http://dx.doi.org/10.1016/j.bbrc.2005.03.237] [PMID: 15882976]

Chen, J, Kinter, M, Shank, S, Cotton, C, Kelley, TJ & Ziady, AG (2008) Dysfunction of Nrf-2 in CF epithelia leads to excess intracellular H2O2 and inflammatory cytokine production. *PLoS One,* 3e3367
[http://dx.doi.org/10.1371/journal.pone.0003367] [PMID: 18846238]

Chen, Y, Wu, Y, Du, M, Chu, H, Zhu, L, Tong, N, Zhang, Z, Wang, M, Gu, D & Chen, J (2017) An inverse association between tea consumption and colorectal cancer risk. *Oncotarget,* 8, 37367-76.
[http://dx.doi.org/10.18632/oncotarget.16959] [PMID: 28454102]

Chen, YX, Gao, QY, Zou, TH, Wang, BM, Liu, SD, Sheng, JQ, Ren, JL, Zou, XP, Liu, ZJ, Song, YY, Xiao, B, Sun, XM, Dou, XT, Cao, HL, Yang, XN, Li, N, Kang, Q, Zhu, W, Xu, HZ, Chen, HM, Cao, XC & Fang, JY (2020) Berberine *versus* placebo for the prevention of recurrence of colorectal adenoma: a multicentre, double-blinded, randomised controlled study. *Lancet Gastroenterol Hepatol,* 5, 267-75.
[http://dx.doi.org/10.1016/S2468-1253(19)30409-1] [PMID: 31926918]

Chikara, S, Nagaprashantha, LD, Singhal, J, Horne, D, Awasthi, S & Singhal, SS (2018) Oxidative stress and dietary phytochemicals: Role in cancer chemoprevention and treatment. *Cancer Lett,* 413, 122-34.
[http://dx.doi.org/10.1016/j.canlet.2017.11.002] [PMID: 29113871]

Choi, BM, Chen, XY, Gao, SS, Zhu, R & Kim, BR (2011) Anti-apoptotic effect of phloretin on cisplatin-induced apoptosis in HEI-OC1 auditory cells. *Pharmacol Rep,* 63, 708-16.
[http://dx.doi.org/10.1016/S1734-1140(11)70582-5] [PMID: 21857081]

Choi, BY (2019) Biochemical basis of anti-cancer-effects of phloretin—a natural dihydrochalcone. *Molecules,* 24, 1-14.
[http://dx.doi.org/10.3390/molecules24020278] [PMID: 30642127]

Chuang, SE, Kuo, ML, Hsu, CH, Chen, CR, Lin, JK, Lai, GM, Hsieh, CY & Cheng, AL (2000) Curcumin-containing diet inhibits diethylnitrosamine-induced murine hepatocarcinogenesis. *Carcinogenesis,* 21, 331-5.
[http://dx.doi.org/10.1093/carcin/21.2.331] [PMID: 10657978]

Clark, PE, Hall, MC, Borden, LS, Jr, Miller, AA, Hu, JJ, Lee, WR, Stindt, D, D'Agostino, R, Jr, Lovato, J, Harmon, M & Torti, FM (2006) Phase I-II prospective dose-escalating trial of lycopene in patients with biochemical relapse of prostate cancer after definitive local therapy. *Urology,* 67, 1257-61.
[http://dx.doi.org/10.1016/j.urology.2005.12.035] [PMID: 16765186]

Colica, C, Milanović, M, Milić, N, Aiello, V, De Lorenzo, A & Abenavoli, L (2018) A systematic review on natural antioxidant properties of resveratrol. *Nat Prod Commun,* 13, 1195-203.
[http://dx.doi.org/10.1177/1934578X1801300923]

Darvesh, AS, Aggarwal, BB & Bishayee, A (2012) Curcumin and liver cancer: a review. *Curr Pharm Biotechnol,* 13, 218-28.
[http://dx.doi.org/10.2174/138920112798868791] [PMID: 21466422]

Das, L & Vinayak, M (2014) Long term effect of curcumin in regulation of glycolytic pathway and angiogenesis *via* modulation of stress activated genes in prevention of cancer. *PLoS One,* 9e99583
[http://dx.doi.org/10.1371/journal.pone.0099583] [PMID: 24932681]

Datta, S & Sinha, D (2019) EGCG maintained Nrf2-mediated redox homeostasis and minimized etoposide resistance in lung cancer cells. *J Funct Foods,* 62, 1-13.
[http://dx.doi.org/10.1016/j.jff.2019.103553]

Dean, LT, Gehlert, S, Neuhouser, ML, Oh, A, Zanetti, K, Goodman, M, Thompson, B, Visvanathan, K & Schmitz, KH (2018) Social factors matter in cancer risk and survivorship. *Cancer Causes Control,* 29, 611-8.
[http://dx.doi.org/10.1007/s10552-018-1043-y] [PMID: 29846844]

Dhillon, N, Aggarwal, BB, Newman, RA, Wolff, RA, Kunnumakkara, AB, Abbruzzese, JL, Ng, CS, Badmaev, V & Kurzrock, R (2008) Phase II trial of curcumin in patients with advanced pancreatic cancer. *Clin Cancer Res,* 14, 4491-9.
[http://dx.doi.org/10.1158/1078-0432.CCR-08-0024] [PMID: 18628464]

Diab, S, Fidanzi, C, Léger, DY, Ghezali, L, Millot, M, Martin, F, Azar, R, Esseily, F, Saab, A, Sol, V, Diab-Assaf, M & Liagre, B (2015) Berberis libanotica extract targets NF-κB/COX-2, PI3K/Akt and mitochondrial/caspase signalling to induce human erythroleukemia cell apoptosis. *Int J Oncol,* 47, 220-30.
[http://dx.doi.org/10.3892/ijo.2015.3012] [PMID: 25997834]

Eom, KS, Kim, HJ, So, HS, Park, R & Kim, TY (2010) Berberine-induced apoptosis in human glioblastoma T98G cells is mediated by endoplasmic reticulum stress accompanying reactive oxygen species and mitochondrial dysfunction. *Biol Pharm Bull,* 33, 1644-9.
[http://dx.doi.org/10.1248/bpb.33.1644] [PMID: 20930370]

Epstein, J, Sanderson, IR & Macdonald, TT (2010) Curcumin as a therapeutic agent: the evidence from in vitro, animal and human studies. *Br J Nutr,* 103, 1545-57.
[http://dx.doi.org/10.1017/S0007114509993667] [PMID: 20100380]

Fernandez, SV, Russo, IH & Russo, J (2006) Estradiol and its metabolites 4-hydroxyestradiol and 2-hydroxyestradiol induce mutations in human breast epithelial cells. *Int J Cancer,* 118, 1862-8.
[http://dx.doi.org/10.1002/ijc.21590] [PMID: 16287077]

Filippi, A, Picot, T, Aanei, CM, Nagy, P, Szöllősi, J, Campos, L, Ganea, C & Mocanu, MM (2018) Epigallocatechin-3-O-gallate alleviates the malignant phenotype in A-431 epidermoid and SK-BR-3 breast cancer cell lines. *Int J Food Sci Nutr,* 69, 584-97.
[http://dx.doi.org/10.1080/09637486.2017.1401980] [PMID: 29157036]

Fujiki, H, Watanabe, T, Sueoka, E, Rawangkan, A & Suganuma, M (2018) Cancer prevention with green tea and its principal constituent, EGCG: From early investigations to current focus on human cancer stem cells. *Mol Cells,* 41, 73-82.
[http://dx.doi.org/10.14348/molcells.2018.2227] [PMID: 29429153]

Gambini, J, Inglés, M, Olaso, G, Lopez-Grueso, R, Bonet-Costa, V, Gimeno-Mallench, L, Mas-Bargues, C, Abdelaziz, KM, Gomez-Cabrera, MC, Vina, J & Borras, C (2015) Properties of Resveratrol: *In Vitro* and *In vivo* Studies about Metabolism, Bioavailability, and Biological Effects in Animal Models and Humans. *Oxid*

Med Cell Longev, 2015837042
[http://dx.doi.org/10.1155/2015/837042] [PMID: 26221416]

Gan, RY, Li, HB, Sui, ZQ & Corke, H (2018) Absorption, metabolism, anti-cancer effect and molecular targets of epigallocatechin gallate (EGCG): An updated review. *Crit Rev Food Sci Nutr,* 58, 924-41.
[http://dx.doi.org/10.1080/10408398.2016.1231168] [PMID: 27645804]

Gann, PH, Deaton, RJ, Rueter, EE, van Breemen, RB, Nonn, L, Macias, V, Han, M & Ananthanarayanan, V (2015) A Phase II Randomized Trial of Lycopene-Rich Tomato Extract Among Men with High-Grade Prostatic Intraepithelial Neoplasia. *Nutr Cancer,* 67, 1104-12.
[http://dx.doi.org/10.1080/01635581.2015.1075560] [PMID: 26422197]

Gao, W, Bohl, CE & Dalton, JT (2005) Chemistry and structural biology of androgen receptor. *Chem Rev,* 105, 3352-70.
[http://dx.doi.org/10.1021/cr020456u] [PMID: 16159155]

Gao, YT, McLaughlin, JK, Blot, WJ, Ji, BT, Dai, Q & Fraumeni, JF, Jr (1994) Reduced risk of esophageal cancer associated with green tea consumption. *J Natl Cancer Inst,* 86, 855-8.
[http://dx.doi.org/10.1093/jnci/86.11.855] [PMID: 8182766]

Germoush, MO & Mahmoud, AM (2014) Berberine mitigates cyclophosphamide-induced hepatotoxicity by modulating antioxidant status and inflammatory cytokines. *J Cancer Res Clin Oncol,* 140, 1103-9.
[http://dx.doi.org/10.1007/s00432-014-1665-8] [PMID: 24744190]

Goto, H, Kariya, R, Shimamoto, M, Kudo, E, Taura, M, Katano, H & Okada, S (2012) Antitumor effect of berberine against primary effusion lymphoma *via* inhibition of NF-κB pathway. *Cancer Sci,* 103, 775-81.
[http://dx.doi.org/10.1111/j.1349-7006.2012.02212.x] [PMID: 22320346]

Grabowska, M, Wawrzyniak, D, Rolle, K, Chomczyński, P, Oziewicz, S, Jurga, S & Barciszewski, J (2019) Let food be your medicine: nutraceutical properties of lycopene. *Food Funct,* 10, 3090-102.
[http://dx.doi.org/10.1039/C9FO00580C] [PMID: 31120074]

Ben Yehuda Greenwald, M, Frušić-Zlotkin, M, Soroka, Y, Ben Sasson, S, Bitton, R, Bianco-Peled, H & Kohen, R (2017) Curcumin Protects Skin against UVB-Induced Cytotoxicity *via* the Keap1-Nrf2 Pathway: The Use of a Microemulsion Delivery System. *Oxid Med Cell Longev,* 20175205471
[http://dx.doi.org/10.1155/2017/5205471] [PMID: 28757910]

Grosso, G, Buscemi, S, Galvano, F, Mistretta, A, Marventano, S, La Vela, V, Drago, F, Gangi, S, Basile, F & Biondi, A (2013) Mediterranean diet and cancer: epidemiological evidence and mechanism of selected aspects. *BMC Surg,* 13 (Suppl. 2), S14.
[http://dx.doi.org/10.1186/1471-2482-13-S2-S14] [PMID: 24267672]

Gu, JW, Makey, KL, Tucker, KB, Chinchar, E, Mao, X, Pei, I, Thomas, EY & Miele, L (2013) EGCG, a major green tea catechin suppresses breast tumor angiogenesis and growth *via* inhibiting the activation of HIF-1α and NFκB, and VEGF expression. *Vasc Cell,* 5, 1-9.
[http://dx.doi.org/10.1186/2045-824X-5-9] [PMID: 23316704]

Guo, Y, Zhi, F, Chen, P, Zhao, K, Xiang, H, Mao, Q, Wang, X & Zhang, X (2017) Green tea and the risk of prostate cancer: A systematic review and meta-analysis. *Medicine (Baltimore),* 96e6426
[http://dx.doi.org/10.1097/MD.0000000000006426] [PMID: 28353571]

Guo, Z, Jiang, M, Luo, W, Zheng, P, Huang, H & Sun, B (2019) Association of lung cancer and tea-drinking habits of different subgroup populations: Meta-analysis of case-control studies and cohort studies. *Iran J Public Health,* 48, 1566-76.
[PMID: 31700812]

Gupta, SC, Patchva, S & Aggarwal, BB (2013) Therapeutic roles of curcumin: lessons learned from clinical trials. *AAPS J,* 15, 195-218.
[http://dx.doi.org/10.1208/s12248-012-9432-8] [PMID: 23143785]

Gutiérrez, JMR & Castro, MDL (2007) Lycopene: The need for better methods for characterization and determination. *Trends Analyt Chem,* 26, 163-70.

[http://dx.doi.org/10.1016/j.trac.2006.11.013]

Hakim, IA, Harris, RB, Brown, S, Chow, HHS, Wiseman, S, Agarwal, S & Talbot, W (2003) Effect of increased tea consumption on oxidative DNA damage among smokers: a randomized controlled study. *J Nutr*, 133, 3303S-9S.
[http://dx.doi.org/10.1093/jn/133.10.3303S] [PMID: 14519830]

Hao, X, Xiao, H, Ju, J, Lee, MJ, Lambert, JD & Yang, CS (2017) Green Tea Polyphenols Inhibit Colorectal Tumorigenesis in Azoxymethane-Treated F344 Rats. *Nutr Cancer*, 69, 623-31.
[http://dx.doi.org/10.1080/01635581.2017.1295088] [PMID: 28323438]

Heber, D & Lu, QY (2002) Overview of mechanisms of action of lycopene. *Exp Biol Med (Maywood)*, 227, 920-3.
[http://dx.doi.org/10.1177/153537020222701013] [PMID: 12424335]

Herceg, Z, Ghantous, A, Wild, CP, Sklias, A, Casati, L, Duthie, SJ, Fry, R, Issa, JP, Kellermayer, R, Koturbash, I, Kondo, Y, Lepeule, J, Lima, SCS, Marsit, CJ, Rakyan, V, Saffery, R, Taylor, JA, Teschendorff, AE, Ushijima, T, Vineis, P, Walker, CL, Waterland, RA, Wiemels, J, Ambatipudi, S, Degli Esposti, D & Hernandez-Vargas, H (2018) Roadmap for investigating epigenome deregulation and environmental origins of cancer. *Int J Cancer*, 142, 874-82.
[http://dx.doi.org/10.1002/ijc.31014] [PMID: 28836271]

Hoesel, B & Schmid, JA (2013) The complexity of NF-κB signaling in inflammation and cancer. *Mol Cancer*, 12, 86.
[http://dx.doi.org/10.1186/1476-4598-12-86] [PMID: 23915189]

Holcombe, RF, Martinez, M, Planutis, K & Planutiene, M (2015) Effects of a grape-supplemented diet on proliferation and Wnt signaling in the colonic mucosa are greatest for those over age 50 and with high arginine consumption. *Nutr J*, 14, 62.
[http://dx.doi.org/10.1186/s12937-015-0050-z] [PMID: 26085034]

Hou, D, Xu, G, Zhang, C, Li, B, Qin, J, Hao, X, Liu, Q, Zhang, X, Liu, J, Wei, J, Gong, Y, Liu, Z & Shao, C (2017) *Berberine induces oxidative DNA damage and impairs homologous recombination repair in ovarian cancer cells to confer increased sensitivity to PARP inhibition*
[http://dx.doi.org/10.1038/cddis.2017.471]

Howells, LM, Berry, DP, Elliott, PJ, Jacobson, EW, Hoffmann, E, Hegarty, B, Brown, K, Steward, WP & Gescher, AJ (2011) Phase I randomized, double-blind pilot study of micronized resveratrol (SRT501) in patients with hepatic metastases--safety, pharmacokinetics, and pharmacodynamics. *Cancer Prev Res (Phila)*, 4, 1419-25.
[http://dx.doi.org/10.1158/1940-6207.CAPR-11-0148] [PMID: 21680702]

Howells, LM, Iwuji, COO, Irving, GRB, Barber, S, Walter, H, Sidat, Z, Griffin-Teall, N, Singh, R, Foreman, N, Patel, SR, Morgan, B, Steward, WP, Gescher, A, Thomas, AL & Brown, K (2019) Curcumin combined with FOLFOX chemotherapy is safe and tolerable in patients with metastatic colorectal cancer in a randomized phase IIa trial. *J Nutr*, 149, 1133-9.
[http://dx.doi.org/10.1093/jn/nxz029] [PMID: 31132111]

Hsu, WH, Hsieh, YS, Kuo, HC, Teng, CY, Huang, HI, Wang, CJ, Yang, SF, Liou, YS & Kuo, WH (2007) Berberine induces apoptosis in SW620 human colonic carcinoma cells through generation of reactive oxygen species and activation of JNK/p38 MAPK and FasL. *Arch Toxicol*, 81, 719-28.
[http://dx.doi.org/10.1007/s00204-006-0169-y] [PMID: 17673978]

Hu, W, Feng, Z, Eveleigh, J, Iyer, G, Pan, J, Amin, S, Chung, FL & Tang, MS (2002) The major lipid peroxidation product, trans-4-hydroxy-2-nonenal, preferentially forms DNA adducts at codon 249 of human p53 gene, a unique mutational hotspot in hepatocellular carcinoma. *Carcinogenesis*, 23, 1781-9.
[http://dx.doi.org/10.1093/carcin/23.11.1781] [PMID: 12419825]

Huang, CY, Han, Z, Li, X, Xie, HH & Zhu, SS (2017) Mechanism of EGCG promoting apoptosis of MCF-7 cell line in human breast cancer. *Oncol Lett*, 14, 3623-7.
[http://dx.doi.org/10.3892/ol.2017.6641] [PMID: 28927122]

Huang, YF, Zhu, DJ, Chen, XW, Chen, QK, Luo, ZT, Liu, CC, Wang, GX, Zhang, WJ & Liao, NZ (2017) Curcumin enhances the effects of irinotecan on colorectal cancer cells through the generation of reactive oxygen species and activation of the endoplasmic reticulum stress pathway. *Oncotarget,* 8, 40264-75.
[http://dx.doi.org/10.18632/oncotarget.16828] [PMID: 28402965]

Hurd, TR, Prime, TA, Harbour, ME, Lilley, KS & Murphy, MP (2007) Detection of reactive oxygen species-sensitive thiol proteins by redox difference gel electrophoresis: implications for mitochondrial redox signaling. *J Biol Chem,* 282, 22040-51.
[http://dx.doi.org/10.1074/jbc.M703591200] [PMID: 17525152]

Imai, K, Suga, K & Nakachi, K (1997) Cancer-preventive effects of drinking green tea among a Japanese population. *Prev Med,* 26, 769-75.
[http://dx.doi.org/10.1006/pmed.1997.0242] [PMID: 9388788]

Ireson, C, Orr, S, Jones, DJL, Verschoyle, R, Lim, CK, Luo, JL, Howells, L, Plummer, S, Jukes, R, Williams, M, Steward, WP & Gescher, A (2001) Characterization of metabolites of the chemopreventive agent curcumin in human and rat hepatocytes and in the rat *in vivo*, and evaluation of their ability to inhibit phorbol ester-induced prostaglandin E2 production. *Cancer Res,* 61, 1058-64.
[PMID: 11221833]

Ireson, CR, Jones, DJL, Orr, S, Coughtrie, MW, Boocock, DJ, Williams, ML, Farmer, PB, Steward, WP & Gescher, AJ (2002) Metabolism of the cancer chemopreventive agent curcumin in human and rat intestine. *Cancer Epidemiol Biomarkers Prev,* 11, 105-11.
[PMID: 11815407]

Izdebska, M, Klimaszewska-Wiśniewska, A, Hałas, M, Gagat, M & Grzanka, A (2015) Green tea extract induces protective autophagy in A549 non-small lung cancer cell line. *Postepy Hig Med Dosw,* 69, 1478-84.
[http://dx.doi.org/10.5604/01.3001.0009.6617] [PMID: 27259219]

Jang, M, Cai, L, Udeani, GO, Slowing, KV, Thomas, CF, Beecher, CWW, Fong, HHS, Farnsworth, NR, Kinghorn, AD, Mehta, RG, Moon, RC & Pezzuto, JM (1997) Cancer chemopreventive activity of resveratrol, a natural product derived from grapes. *Science,* 275, 218-20.
[http://dx.doi.org/10.1126/science.275.5297.218] [PMID: 8985016]

Jaramillo, MC & Zhang, DD (2013) The emerging role of the Nrf2-Keap1 signaling pathway in cancer. *Genes Dev,* 27, 2179-91.
[http://dx.doi.org/10.1101/gad.225680.113] [PMID: 24142871]

Jiao, Y, Wilkinson, J, IV, Di, X, Wang, W, Hatcher, H, Kock, ND, D'Agostino, R, Jr, Knovich, MA, Torti, FM & Torti, SV (2009) Curcumin, a cancer chemopreventive and chemotherapeutic agent, is a biologically active iron chelator. *Blood,* 113, 462-9.
[http://dx.doi.org/10.1182/blood-2008-05-155952] [PMID: 18815282]

Jin, H, Gong, W, Zhang, C & Wang, S (2013) Epigallocatechin gallate inhibits the proliferation of colorectal cancer cells by regulating Notch signaling. *OncoTargets Ther,* 6, 145-53.
[http://dx.doi.org/10.2147/OTT.S40914] [PMID: 23525843]

Jin, Y, Khadka, DB & Cho, WJ (2016) Pharmacological effects of berberine and its derivatives: a patent update. *Expert Opin Ther Pat,* 26, 229-43.
[http://dx.doi.org/10.1517/13543776.2016.1118060] [PMID: 26610159]

Jung, M, Triebel, S, Anke, T, Richling, E & Erkel, G (2009) Influence of apple polyphenols on inflammatory gene expression. *Mol Nutr Food Res,* 53, 1263-80.
[http://dx.doi.org/10.1002/mnfr.200800575] [PMID: 19764067]

Kanlaya, R, Khamchun, S, Kapincharanon, C & Thongboonkerd, V (2016) Protective effect of epigallocatechin-3-gallate (EGCG) *via* Nrf2 pathway against oxalate-induced epithelial mesenchymal transition (EMT) of renal tubular cells. *Sci Rep,* 6, 30233.
[http://dx.doi.org/10.1038/srep30233] [PMID: 27452398]

Kelkel, M, Schumacher, M, Dicato, M & Diederich, M (2011) Antioxidant and anti-proliferative properties of

lycopene. *Free Radic Res,* 45, 925-40.
[http://dx.doi.org/10.3109/10715762.2011.564168] [PMID: 21615277]

Kim, B, Kim, HS, Jung, EJ, Lee, JY, K Tsang, B, Lim, JM & Song, YS (2016) Curcumin induces ER stress-mediated apoptosis through selective generation of reactive oxygen species in cervical cancer cells. *Mol Carcinog,* 55, 918-28.
[http://dx.doi.org/10.1002/mc.22332] [PMID: 25980682]

Kim, JB, Yu, JH, Ko, E, Lee, KW, Song, AK, Park, SY, Shin, I, Han, W & Noh, DY (2010) The alkaloid Berberine inhibits the growth of Anoikis-resistant MCF-7 and MDA-MB-231 breast cancer cell lines by inducing cell cycle arrest. *Phytomedicine,* 17, 436-40.
[http://dx.doi.org/10.1016/j.phymed.2009.08.012] [PMID: 19800775]

Kim, U, Kim, CY, Lee, JM, Oh, H, Ryu, B, Kim, J & Park, JH (2020) Phloretin Inhibits the Human Prostate Cancer Cells Through the Generation of Reactive Oxygen Species. *Pathol Oncol Res,* 26, 977-84.
[http://dx.doi.org/10.1007/s12253-019-00643-y] [PMID: 30937835]

Kobayashi, M & Yamamoto, M (2005) Molecular mechanisms activating the Nrf2-Keap1 pathway of antioxidant gene regulation. *Antioxid Redox Signal,* 7, 385-94.
[http://dx.doi.org/10.1089/ars.2005.7.385] [PMID: 15706085]

Kode, A, Rajendrasozhan, S, Caito, S, Yang, SR, Megson, IL & Rahman, I (2008) Resveratrol induces glutathione synthesis by activation of Nrf2 and protects against cigarette smoke-mediated oxidative stress in human lung epithelial cells. *Am J Physiol Lung Cell Mol Physiol,* 294, L478-88.
[http://dx.doi.org/10.1152/ajplung.00361.2007] [PMID: 18162601]

Koundouros, N & Poulogiannis, G (2018) Phosphoinositide 3-Kinase/Akt signaling and redox metabolism in cancer. *Front Oncol,* 8, 160.
[http://dx.doi.org/10.3389/fonc.2018.00160] [PMID: 29868481]

Kumari, S, Badana, AK, G, MM, G, S & Malla, R (2018) Reactive Oxygen Species: A Key Constituent in Cancer Survival. *Biomark Insights,* 131177271918755391
[http://dx.doi.org/10.1177/1177271918755391] [PMID: 29449774]

Kuriakose, MA, Ramdas, K, Dey, B, Iyer, S, Rajan, G, Elango, KK, Suresh, A, Ravindran, D, Kumar, RR, R, P, Ramachandran, S, Kumar, NA, Thomas, G, Somanathan, T, Ravindran, HK, Ranganathan, K, Katakam, SB, Parashuram, S, Jayaprakash, V & Pillai, MR (2016) A randomized double-blind placebo-controlled phase iib trial of curcumin in oral leukoplakia. *Cancer Prev Res (Phila),* 9, 683-91.
[http://dx.doi.org/10.1158/1940-6207.CAPR-15-0390] [PMID: 27267893]

Kurutas, EB (2016) The importance of antioxidants which play the role in cellular response against oxidative/nitrosative stress: current state. *Nutr J,* 15, 71.
[http://dx.doi.org/10.1186/s12937-016-0186-5] [PMID: 27456681]

Lane, JA, Er, V, Avery, KNL, Horwood, J, Cantwell, M, Caro, GP, Crozier, A, Smith, GD, Donovan, JL, Down, L, Hamdy, FC, Gillatt, D, Holly, J, Macefield, R, Moody, H, Neal, DE, Walsh, E, Martin, RM & Metcalfe, C (2018) ProDiet: A Phase II Randomized Placebo-controlled Trial of Green Tea Catechins and Lycopene in Men at Increased Risk of Prostate Cancer. *Cancer Prev Res (Phila),* 11, 687-96.
[http://dx.doi.org/10.1158/1940-6207.CAPR-18-0147] [PMID: 30309839]

Langner, E & Rzeski, W (2012) Dietary derived compounds in cancer chemoprevention. *Contemp Oncol (Pozn),* 16, 394-400.
[http://dx.doi.org/10.5114/wo.2012.31767] [PMID: 23788916]

Lee, EYHP & Muller, WJ (2010) Oncogenes and tumor suppressor genes. *Cold Spring Harb Perspect Biol,* 2a003236
[http://dx.doi.org/10.1101/cshperspect.a003236] [PMID: 20719876]

Lee, JC, Kinniry, PA, Arguiri, E, Serota, M, Kanterakis, S, Chatterjee, S, Solomides, CC, Javvadi, P, Koumenis, C, Cengel, KA & Christofidou-Solomidou, M (2010) Dietary curcumin increases antioxidant defenses in lung, ameliorates radiation-induced pulmonary fibrosis, and improves survival in mice. *Radiat Res,* 173, 590-601.

[http://dx.doi.org/10.1667/RR1522.1] [PMID: 20426658]

Lee, JH, Regmi, SC, Kim, JA, Cho, MH, Yun, H, Lee, CS & Lee, J (2011) Apple flavonoid phloretin inhibits Escherichia coli O157:H7 biofilm formation and ameliorates colon inflammation in rats. *Infect Immun*, 79, 4819-27.
[http://dx.doi.org/10.1128/IAI.05580-11] [PMID: 21930760]

Levi, F, Pasche, C, Lucchini, F, Ghidoni, R, Ferraroni, M & La Vecchia, C (2005) Resveratrol and breast cancer risk. *Eur J Cancer Prev*, 14, 139-42.
[http://dx.doi.org/10.1097/00008469-200504000-00009] [PMID: 15785317]

Lin, ST, Tu, SH, Yang, PS, Hsu, SP, Lee, WH, Ho, CT, Wu, CH, Lai, YH, Chen, MY & Chen, LC (2016) Apple Polyphenol Phloretin Inhibits Colorectal Cancer Cell Growth *via* Inhibition of the Type 2 Glucose Transporter and Activation of p53-Mediated Signaling. *J Agric Food Chem*, 64, 6826-37.
[http://dx.doi.org/10.1021/acs.jafc.6b02861] [PMID: 27538679]

Liu, Y, Yu, H, Zhang, C, Cheng, Y, Hu, L, Meng, X & Zhao, Y (2008) Protective effects of berberine on radiation-induced lung injury *via* intercellular adhesion molecular-1 and transforming growth factor-beta-1 in patients with lung cancer. *Eur J Cancer*, 44, 2425-32.
[http://dx.doi.org/10.1016/j.ejca.2008.07.040] [PMID: 18789680]

Ma, L, Wang, R, Nan, Y, Li, W, Wang, Q & Jin, F (2016) Phloretin exhibits an anticancer effect and enhances the anticancer ability of cisplatin on non-small cell lung cancer cell lines by regulating expression of apoptotic pathways and matrix metalloproteinases. *Int J Oncol*, 48, 843-53.
[http://dx.doi.org/10.3892/ijo.2015.3304] [PMID: 26692364]

Majolo, F, de Oliveira Becker Delwing, LK, Marmitt, DJ, Bustamante-Filho, IC & Goettert, MI (2019) Medicinal plants and bioactive natural compounds for cancer treatment: Important advances for drug discovery. *Phytochem Lett*, 31, 196-207.
[http://dx.doi.org/10.1016/j.phytol.2019.04.003]

Mantena, SK, Sharma, SD & Katiyar, SK (2006) Berberine, a natural product, induces G1-phase cell cycle arrest and caspase-3-dependent apoptosis in human prostate carcinoma cells. *Mol Cancer Ther*, 5, 296-308. a
[http://dx.doi.org/10.1158/1535-7163.MCT-05-0448] [PMID: 16505103]

Mantena, SK, Sharma, SD & Katiyar, SK (2006) Berberine inhibits growth, induces G1 arrest and apoptosis in human epidermoid carcinoma A431 cells by regulating Cdki-Cdk-cyclin cascade, disruption of mitochondrial membrane potential and cleavage of caspase 3 and PARP. *Carcinogenesis*, 27, 2018-27. b
[http://dx.doi.org/10.1093/carcin/bgl043] [PMID: 16621886]

McCord, JM & Fridovich, I (1969) Superoxide dismutase. An enzymic function for erythrocuprein (hemocuprein). *J Biol Chem*, 244, 6049-55.
[http://dx.doi.org/10.1016/S0021-9258(18)63504-5] [PMID: 5389100]

McCubrey, JA, Steelman, LS, Chappell, WH, Abrams, SL, Wong, EWT, Chang, F, Lehmann, B, Terrian, DM, Milella, M, Tafuri, A, Stivala, F, Libra, M, Basecke, J, Evangelisti, C, Martelli, AM & Franklin, RA (2007) Roles of the Raf/MEK/ERK pathway in cell growth, malignant transformation and drug resistance. *Biochim Biophys Acta*, 1773, 1263-84.
[http://dx.doi.org/10.1016/j.bbamcr.2006.10.001] [PMID: 17126425]

McLarty, J, Bigelow, RLH, Smith, M, Elmajian, D, Ankem, M & Cardelli, JA (2009) Tea polyphenols decrease serum levels of prostate-specific antigen, hepatocyte growth factor, and vascular endothelial growth factor in prostate cancer patients and inhibit production of hepatocyte growth factor and vascular endothelial growth factor in vitro. *Cancer Prev Res (Phila)*, 2, 673-82.
[http://dx.doi.org/10.1158/1940-6207.CAPR-08-0167] [PMID: 19542190]

Nesran, ZNM, Shafie, NH, Ishak, AH, Esa, MN, Ismail, A & Tohid, MSF (2019) Induction of Endoplasmic Reticulum Stress Pathway by Green Tea Epigallocatechin-3-Gallate (EGCG) in Colorectal Cancer Cells: Activation of PERK/p-eIF2 α /ATF4 and IRE1 α. *BioMed Res Int*, 2019, 1-9.
[http://dx.doi.org/10.1155/2019/3480569]

Nguyen, AV, Martinez, M, Stamos, MJ, Moyer, MP, Planutis, K, Hope, C & Holcombe, RF (2009) Results

of a phase I pilot clinical trial examining the effect of plant-derived resveratrol and grape powder on Wnt pathway target gene expression in colonic mucosa and colon cancer. *Cancer Manag Res,* 1, 25-37.
[http://dx.doi.org/10.2147/CMAR.S4544] [PMID: 21188121]

Mendes, RA, E Silva, BLS, Takeara, R, Freitas, RG, Brown, A & de Souza, GLC (2018) Probing the antioxidant potential of phloretin and phlorizin through a computational investigation. *J Mol Model,* 24, 101.
[http://dx.doi.org/10.1007/s00894-018-3632-9] [PMID: 29569097]

Min, J, Huang, K, Tang, H, Ding, X, Qi, C, Qin, X, Xu, Z & Xu, Z (2015) Phloretin induces apoptosis of non-small cell lung carcinoma A549 cells *via* JNK1/2 and p38 MAPK pathways. *Oncol Rep,* 34, 2871-9.
[http://dx.doi.org/10.3892/or.2015.4325] [PMID: 26503828]

Molnár, J, Engi, H, Hohmann, J, Molnár, P, Deli, J, Wesolowska, O, Michalak, K & Wang, Q (2010) Reversal of multidrug resitance by natural substances from plants. *Curr Top Med Chem,* 10, 1757-68.http://www.ncbi.nlm.nih.gov/pubmed/20645919
[http://dx.doi.org/10.2174/156802610792928103] [PMID: 20645919]

Murakami, C, Hirakawa, Y, Inui, H, Nakano, Y & Yoshida, H (2002) Effect of tea catechins on cellular lipid peroxidation and cytotoxicity in HepG2 cells. *Biosci Biotechnol Biochem,* 66, 1559-62.
[http://dx.doi.org/10.1271/bbb.66.1559] [PMID: 12224642]

Muralimanoharan, SB, Kunnumakkara, AB, Shylesh, B, Kulkarni, KH, Haiyan, X, Ming, H, Aggarwal, BB, Rita, G & Kumar, AP (2009) Butanol fraction containing berberine or related compound from nexrutine inhibits NFkappaB signaling and induces apoptosis in prostate cancer cells. *Prostate,* 69, 494-504.
[http://dx.doi.org/10.1002/pros.20899] [PMID: 19107816]

Negri, A, Naponelli, V, Rizzi, F & Bettuzzi, S (2018) Molecular targets of epigallocatechin—gallate (EGCG): A special focus on signal transduction and cancer. *Nutrients,* 10, 1-24.
[http://dx.doi.org/10.3390/nu10121936] [PMID: 30563268]

Nurgali, K, Jagoe, RT & Abalo, R (2018) Editorial: Adverse effects of cancer chemotherapy: Anything new to improve tolerance and reduce sequelae? *Front Pharmacol,* 9, 245.
[http://dx.doi.org/10.3389/fphar.2018.00245] [PMID: 29623040]

Pan, JS, Hong, MZ & Ren, JL (2009) Reactive oxygen species: a double-edged sword in oncogenesis. *World J Gastroenterol,* 15, 1702-7.
[http://dx.doi.org/10.3748/wjg.15.1702] [PMID: 19360913]

Pandey, A, Vishnoi, K, Mahata, S, Tripathi, SC, Misra, SP, Misra, V, Mehrotra, R, Dwivedi, M & Bharti, AC (2015) Berberine and Curcumin Target Survivin and STAT3 in Gastric Cancer Cells and Synergize Actions of Standard Chemotherapeutic 5-Fluorouracil. *Nutr Cancer,* 67, 1293-304.
[http://dx.doi.org/10.1080/01635581.2015.1085581] [PMID: 26492225]

Pandey, MK, Sung, B, Kunnumakkara, AB, Sethi, G, Chaturvedi, MM & Aggarwal, BB (2008) Berberine modifies cysteine 179 of IkappaBalpha kinase, suppresses nuclear factor-kappaB-regulated antiapoptotic gene products, and potentiates apoptosis. *Cancer Res,* 68, 5370-9.
[http://dx.doi.org/10.1158/0008-5472.CAN-08-0511] [PMID: 18593939]

Park, J & Conteas, CN (2010) Anti-carcinogenic properties of curcumin on colorectal cancer. *World J Gastrointest Oncol,* 2, 169-76.
[http://dx.doi.org/10.4251/wjgo.v2.i4.169] [PMID: 21160593]

Patel, KR, Brown, VA, Jones, DJL, Britton, RG, Hemingway, D, Miller, AS, West, KP, Booth, TD, Perloff, M, Crowell, JA, Brenner, DE, Steward, WP, Gescher, AJ & Brown, K (2010) Clinical pharmacology of resveratrol and its metabolites in colorectal cancer patients. *Cancer Res,* 70, 7392-9.
[http://dx.doi.org/10.1158/0008-5472.CAN-10-2027] [PMID: 20841478]

Pearce, A, Haas, M, Viney, R, Pearson, SA, Haywood, P, Brown, C & Ward, R (2017) Incidence and severity of self-reported chemotherapy side effects in routine care: A prospective cohort study. *PLoS One,* 12e0184360
[http://dx.doi.org/10.1371/journal.pone.0184360] [PMID: 29016607]

Perillo, B, Di Donato, M, Pezone, A, Di Zazzo, E, Giovannelli, P, Galasso, G, Castoria, G & Migliaccio, A (2020) ROS in cancer therapy: the bright side of the moon. *Exp Mol Med,* 52, 192-203.
[http://dx.doi.org/10.1038/s12276-020-0384-2] [PMID: 32060354]

Pongrakhananon, V, Nimmannit, U, Luanpitpong, S, Rojanasakul, Y & Chanvorachote, P (2010) Curcumin sensitizes non-small cell lung cancer cell anoikis through reactive oxygen species-mediated Bcl-2 downregulation. *Apoptosis,* 15, 574-85.
[http://dx.doi.org/10.1007/s10495-010-0461-4] [PMID: 20127174]

Pratheeshkumar, P, Sreekala, C, Zhang, Z, Budhraja, A, Ding, S, Son, YO, Wang, X, Hitron, A, Hyun-Jung, K, Wang, L, Lee, JC & Shi, X (2012) Cancer prevention with promising natural products: mechanisms of action and molecular targets. *Anticancer Agents Med Chem,* 12, 1159-84.
[http://dx.doi.org/10.2174/187152012803833035] [PMID: 22583402]

Puthdee, N, Seubwai, W, Vaeteewoottacharn, K, Boonmars, T, Cha'on, U, Phoomak, C & Wongkham, S (2017) Berberine induces cell cycle arrest in cholangiocarcinoma cell lines *via* inhibition of NF-κB and STAT3 pathways. *Biol Pharm Bull,* 40, 751-7.
[http://dx.doi.org/10.1248/bpb.b16-00428] [PMID: 28566619]

Qian, Q, Chen, W, Cao, Y, Cao, Q, Cui, Y, Li, Y & Wu, J (2019) Targeting Reactive Oxygen Species in Cancer *via* Chinese Herbal Medicine. *Oxid Med Cell Longev,* 20199240426
[http://dx.doi.org/10.1155/2019/9240426] [PMID: 31583051]

Rafi, MM, Kanakasabai, S, Reyes, MD & Bright, JJ (2013) Lycopene modulates growth and survival associated genes in prostate cancer. *J Nutr Biochem,* 24, 1724-34.
[http://dx.doi.org/10.1016/j.jnutbio.2013.03.001] [PMID: 23746934]

Rahmani, AH, Al Shabrmi, FM, Allemailem, KS, Aly, SM & Khan, MA (2015) Implications of green tea and its constituents in the prevention of cancer *via* the modulation of cell signalling pathway. *BioMed Res Int,* 2015925640
[http://dx.doi.org/10.1155/2015/925640] [PMID: 25977926]

Rawangkan, A, Wongsirisin, P, Namiki, K, Iida, K, Kobayashi, Y, Shimizu, Y, Fujiki, H & Suganuma, M (2018) Green tea catechin is an alternative immune checkpoint inhibitor that inhibits PD-l1 expression and lung tumor growth. *Molecules,* 23, 1-12.
[http://dx.doi.org/10.3390/molecules23082071] [PMID: 30126206]

Ray, PD, Huang, BW & Tsuji, Y (2012) Reactive oxygen species (ROS) homeostasis and redox regulation in cellular signaling. *Cell Signal,* 24, 981-90.
[http://dx.doi.org/10.1016/j.cellsig.2012.01.008] [PMID: 22286106]

Huang, MT, Lou, YR, Ma, W, Newmark, HL, Reuhl, KR & Conney, AH (1994) Inhibitory effects of dietary curcumin on forestomach, duodenal, and colon carcinogenesis in mice. *Cancer Res,* 54, 5841-7.
[PMID: 7954412]

Rezk, BM, Haenen, GRMM, van der Vijgh, WJF & Bast, A (2002) The antioxidant activity of phloretin: the disclosure of a new antioxidant pharmacophore in flavonoids. *Biochem Biophys Res Commun,* 295, 9-13.
[http://dx.doi.org/10.1016/S0006-291X(02)00618-6] [PMID: 12083758]

Saeki, K, Hayakawa, S, Nakano, S, Ito, S, Oishi, Y, Suzuki, Y & Isemura, M (2018) *In Vitro* and in silico studies of the molecular interactions of epigallocatechin-3-o-gallate (egcg) with proteins that explain the health benefits of green tea. *Molecules,* 23, 1-24.
[http://dx.doi.org/10.3390/molecules23061295] [PMID: 29843451]

Saini, RK, Rengasamy, KRR, Mahomoodally, FM & Keum, YS (2020) Protective effects of lycopene in cancer, cardiovascular, and neurodegenerative diseases: An update on epidemiological and mechanistic perspectives. *Pharmacol Res,* 155104730
[http://dx.doi.org/10.1016/j.phrs.2020.104730] [PMID: 32126272]

Salehi, B, Stojanović-Radić, Z, Matejić, J, Sharifi-Rad, M, Anil Kumar, NV, Martins, N & Sharifi-Rad, J (2019) The therapeutic potential of curcumin: A review of clinical trials. *Eur J Med Chem,* 163, 527-45.

[http://dx.doi.org/10.1016/j.ejmech.2018.12.016] [PMID: 30553144]

Salgado, P, Melin, V, Contreras, D, Moreno, Y & Mansilla, HD (2013) Fenton reaction driven by iron ligands. *J Chil Chem Soc,* 58, 2096-101.
[http://dx.doi.org/10.4067/S0717-97072013000400043]

Sanidad, KZ, Sukamtoh, E, Xiao, H, McClements, DJ & Zhang, G (2019) Curcumin: Recent Advances in the Development of Strategies to Improve Oral Bioavailability. *Annu Rev Food Sci Technol,* 10, 597-617.
[http://dx.doi.org/10.1146/annurev-food-032818-121738] [PMID: 30633561]

Schaefer, S, Baum, M, Eisenbrand, G, Dietrich, H, Will, F & Janzowski, C (2006) Polyphenolic apple juice extracts and their major constituents reduce oxidative damage in human colon cell lines. *Mol Nutr Food Res,* 50, 24-33.
[http://dx.doi.org/10.1002/mnfr.200500136] [PMID: 16317784]

Schumacker, PT (2006) Reactive oxygen species in cancer cells: live by the sword, die by the sword. *Cancer Cell,* 10, 175-6.
[http://dx.doi.org/10.1016/j.ccr.2006.08.015] [PMID: 16959608]

Sengottuvelan, M & Nalini, N (2006) Dietary supplementation of resveratrol suppresses colonic tumour incidence in 1,2-dimethylhydrazine-treated rats by modulating biotransforming enzymes and aberrant crypt foci development. *Br J Nutr,* 96, 145-53.
[http://dx.doi.org/10.1079/BJN20061789] [PMID: 16870003]

Shanafelt, TD, Lee, YK, Call, TG, Nowakowski, GS, Dingli, D, Zent, CS & Kay, NE (2006) Clinical effects of oral green tea extracts in four patients with low grade B-cell malignancies. *Leuk Res,* 30, 707-12.
[http://dx.doi.org/10.1016/j.leukres.2005.10.020] [PMID: 16325256]

Sharma, A, Tirpude, NV, Kulurkar, PM, Sharma, R & Padwad, Y (2020) Berberis lycium fruit extract attenuates oxi-inflammatory stress and promotes mucosal healing by mitigating NF-κB/c-Jun/MAPKs signalling and augmenting splenic Treg proliferation in a murine model of dextran sulphate sodium-induced ulcerative colitis. *Eur J Nutr,* 59, 2663-81.
[http://dx.doi.org/10.1007/s00394-019-02114-1] [PMID: 31620885]

Sharma, RA, Euden, SA, Platton, SL, Cooke, DN, Shafayat, A, Hewitt, HR, Marczylo, TH, Morgan, B, Hemingway, D, Plummer, SM, Pirmohamed, M, Gescher, AJ & Steward, WP (2004) Phase I clinical trial of oral curcumin: biomarkers of systemic activity and compliance. *Clin Cancer Res,* 10, 6847-54.
[http://dx.doi.org/10.1158/1078-0432.CCR-04-0744] [PMID: 15501961]

Sharma, SD, Mantena, SK & Katiyar, SK (2014) *Berberine, a natural product, inhibits growth and induces G1 arrest and caspase-3-dependent apoptosis accompanied with loss of mitochondrial membrane potential in human epidermoid carcinoma A431 cells*

Shi, J & Le Maguer, M (2000) Lycopene in tomatoes: chemical and physical properties affected by food processing. *Crit Rev Biotechnol,* 20, 293-334.
[http://dx.doi.org/10.1080/07388550091144212] [PMID: 11192026]

Shih, CA & Lin, JK (1993) Inhibition of 8-hydroxydeoxyguanosine formation by curcumin in mouse fibroblast cells. *Carcinogenesis,* 14, 709-12.
[http://dx.doi.org/10.1093/carcin/14.4.709] [PMID: 8472336]

Shimizu, M, Shirakami, Y, Sakai, H, Kubota, M, Kochi, T, Ideta, T, Miyazaki, T & Moriwaki, H (2015) Chemopreventive potential of green tea catechins in hepatocellular carcinoma. *Int J Mol Sci,* 16, 6124-39.
[http://dx.doi.org/10.3390/ijms16036124] [PMID: 25789501]

Shoba, G, Joy, D, Joseph, T, Majeed, M, Rajendran, R & Srinivas, PS (1998) Influence of piperine on the pharmacokinetics of curcumin in animals and human volunteers. *Planta Med,* 64, 353-6.
[http://dx.doi.org/10.1055/s-2006-957450] [PMID: 9619120]

Shoeb, M, Ansari, NH, Srivastava, SK & Ramana, KV (2014) 4-Hydroxynonenal in the pathogenesis and progression of human diseases. *Curr Med Chem,* 21, 230-7.
[http://dx.doi.org/10.2174/09298673113209990181] [PMID: 23848536]

Shrubsole, MJ, Lu, W, Chen, Z, Shu, XO, Zheng, Y, Dai, Q, Cai, Q, Gu, K, Ruan, ZX, Gao, YT & Zheng, W (2009) Drinking green tea modestly reduces breast cancer risk. *J Nutr,* 139, 310-6.
[http://dx.doi.org/10.3945/jn.108.098699] [PMID: 19074205]

Siegel, RL, Miller, KD & Jemal, A (2020) Cancer statistics, 2020. *CA Cancer J Clin,* 70, 7-30.
[http://dx.doi.org/10.3322/caac.21590] [PMID: 31912902]

Signorelli, P & Ghidoni, R (2005) Resveratrol as an anticancer nutrient: molecular basis, open questions and promises. *J Nutr Biochem,* 16, 449-66.
[http://dx.doi.org/10.1016/j.jnutbio.2005.01.017] [PMID: 16043028]

Singh, AP, Singh, R, Verma, SS, Rai, V, Kaschula, CH, Maiti, P & Gupta, SC (2019) Health benefits of resveratrol: Evidence from clinical studies. *Med Res Rev,* 39, 1851-91.
[http://dx.doi.org/10.1002/med.21565] [PMID: 30741437]

Singh, B, Shoulson, R, Chatterjee, A, Ronghe, A, Bhat, NK, Dim, DC & Bhat, HK (2014) Resveratrol inhibits estrogen-induced breast carcinogenesis through induction of NRF2-mediated protective pathways. *Carcinogenesis,* 35, 1872-80.
[http://dx.doi.org/10.1093/carcin/bgu120] [PMID: 24894866]

Soares, NdaC, Teodoro, AJ, Oliveira, FL, Santos, CADN, Takiya, CM, Junior, OS, Bianco, M, Junior, AP, Nasciutti, LE, Ferreira, LB, Gimba, ERP & Borojevic, R (2013) Influence of lycopene on cell viability, cell cycle, and apoptosis of human prostate cancer and benign hyperplastic cells. *Nutr Cancer,* 65, 1076-85.
[http://dx.doi.org/10.1080/01635581.2013.812225] [PMID: 24053141]

Sun, Y, Yuan, X, Zhang, F, Han, Y, Chang, X, Xu, X, Li, Y & Gao, X (2017) Berberine ameliorates fatty acid-induced oxidative stress in human hepatoma cells. *Sci Rep,* 7, 11340.
[http://dx.doi.org/10.1038/s41598-017-11860-3] [PMID: 28900305]

Surh, YJ (2003) Cancer chemoprevention with dietary phytochemicals. *Nat Rev Cancer,* 3, 768-80.
[http://dx.doi.org/10.1038/nrc1189] [PMID: 14570043]

Tan, HL, Thomas-Ahner, JM, Moran, NE, Cooperstone, JL, Erdman, JW, Jr, Young, GS & Clinton, SK (2017) β-Carotene 90,100 oxygenase modulates the anticancer activity of dietary tomato or lycopene on prostate carcinogenesis in the TRAMP model. *Cancer Prev Res (Phila),* 10, 161-9.
[http://dx.doi.org/10.1158/1940-6207.CAPR-15-0402] [PMID: 27807077]

Tanaka, K, Ono, T & Umeda, M (1986) Inhibition of biological actions of 12-O-tetradecanoylphorbol-13-acetate by inhibitors of protein kinase C. *Jpn J Cancer Res,* 77, 1107-13.
[PMID: 3025144]

Tang, FY, Pai, MH & Wang, XD (2011) Consumption of lycopene inhibits the growth and progression of colon cancer in a mouse xenograft model. *J Agric Food Chem,* 59, 9011-21.
[http://dx.doi.org/10.1021/jf2017644] [PMID: 21744871]

Tayyem, RF, Heath, DD, Al-Delaimy, WK & Rock, CL (2006) Curcumin content of turmeric and curry powders. *Nutr Cancer,* 55, 126-31.
[http://dx.doi.org/10.1207/s15327914nc5502_2] [PMID: 17044766]

Tessitore, L, Davit, A, Sarotto, I & Caderni, G (2000) Resveratrol depresses the growth of colorectal aberrant crypt foci by affecting bax and p21(CIP) expression. *Carcinogenesis,* 21, 1619-22.
[http://dx.doi.org/10.1093/carcin/21.5.619] [PMID: 10910967]

Tong, L, Chuang, CC, Wu, S & Zuo, L (2015) Reactive oxygen species in redox cancer therapy. *Cancer Lett,* 367, 18-25.
[http://dx.doi.org/10.1016/j.canlet.2015.07.008] [PMID: 26187782]

Trela, BC & Waterhouse, AL (1996) Resveratrol: Isomeric molar absorptivities and stability. *J Agric Food Chem,* 44, 1253-7.
[http://dx.doi.org/10.1021/jf9504576]

Tsai, KD, Lin, JC, Yang, SM, Tseng, MJ, Hsu, JD, Lee, YJ & Cherng, JM (2012) Curcumin protects against

UVB-induced skin cancers in SKH-1 hairless mouse: Analysis of early molecular markers in carcinogenesis. *Evid Based Complement Alternat Med,* 2012593952
[http://dx.doi.org/10.1155/2012/593952] [PMID: 22888366]

Tsao, AS, Liu, D, Martin, J, Tang, XM, Lee, JJ, El-Naggar, AK, Wistuba, I, Culotta, KS, Mao, L, Gillenwater, A, Sagesaka, YM, Hong, WK & Papadimitrakopoulou, V (2009) Phase II randomized, placebo-controlled trial of green tea extract in patients with high-risk oral premalignant lesions. *Cancer Prev Res (Phila),* 2, 931-41.
[http://dx.doi.org/10.1158/1940-6207.CAPR-09-0121] [PMID: 19892663]

Ullah, N, Ahmad, M, Aslam, H, Tahir, MA, Aftab, M, Bibi, N & Ahmad, S (2016) Green tea phytocompounds as anticancer: A review. *Asian Pac J Trop Dis,* 6, 330-6.
[http://dx.doi.org/10.1016/S2222-1808(15)61040-4]

Ushio-Fukai, M & Nakamura, Y (2008) Reactive oxygen species and angiogenesis: NADPH oxidase as target for cancer therapy. *Cancer Lett,* 266, 37-52.
[http://dx.doi.org/10.1016/j.canlet.2008.02.044] [PMID: 18406051]

Valavanidis, A, Vlachogianni, T & Fiotakis, C (2009) 8-hydroxy-2′-deoxyguanosine (8-OHdG): A critical biomarker of oxidative stress and carcinogenesis. *J Environ Sci Health Part C Environ Carcinog Ecotoxicol Rev,* 27, 120-39.
[http://dx.doi.org/10.1080/10590500902885684] [PMID: 19412858]

Valko, M, Leibfritz, D, Moncol, J, Cronin, MTD, Mazur, M & Telser, J (2007) Free radicals and antioxidants in normal physiological functions and human disease. *Int J Biochem Cell Biol,* 39, 44-84.
[http://dx.doi.org/10.1016/j.biocel.2006.07.001] [PMID: 16978905]

Vareed, SK, Kakarala, M, Ruffin, MT, Crowell, JA, Normolle, DP, Djuric, Z & Brenner, DE (2008) Pharmacokinetics of curcumin conjugate metabolites in healthy human subjects. *Cancer Epidemiol Biomarkers Prev,* 17, 1411-7.
[http://dx.doi.org/10.1158/1055-9965.EPI-07-2693] [PMID: 18559556]

Abd El-Wahab, AE, Ghareeb, DA, Sarhan, EEM, Abu-Serie, MM & El Demellawy, MA (2013) *In Vitro* biological assessment of Berberis vulgaris and its active constituent, berberine: antioxidants, anti-acetylcholinesterase, anti-diabetic and anticancer effects. *BMC Complement Altern Med,* 13, 218.
[http://dx.doi.org/10.1186/1472-6882-13-218] [PMID: 24007270]

Wan, L, Tan, HL, Thomas-Ahner, JM, Pearl, DK, Erdman, JW, Jr, Moran, NE & Clinton, SK (2014) Dietary tomato and lycopene impact androgen signaling- and carcinogenesis-related gene expression during early TRAMP prostate carcinogenesis. *Cancer Prev Res (Phila),* 7, 1228-39.
[http://dx.doi.org/10.1158/1940-6207.CAPR-14-0182] [PMID: 25315431]

Wang, C, Song, X, Shang, M, Zou, W, Zhang, M, Wei, H & Shao, H (2019) Curcumin exerts cytotoxicity dependent on reactive oxygen species accumulation in non-small-cell lung cancer cells. *Future Oncol,* 15, 1243-53.
[http://dx.doi.org/10.2217/fon-2018-0708] [PMID: 30843426]

Wang, L, Chen, X, Du, Z, Li, G, Chen, M, Chen, X, Liang, G & Chen, T (2017) Curcumin suppresses gastric tumor cell growth *via* ROS-mediated DNA polymerase γ depletion disrupting cellular bioenergetics. *J Exp Clin Cancer Res,* 36, 47.
[http://dx.doi.org/10.1186/s13046-017-0513-5] [PMID: 28359291]

Wang, ZJ, Ohnaka, K, Morita, M, Toyomura, K, Kono, S, Ueki, T, Tanaka, M, Kakeji, Y, Maehara, Y, Okamura, T, Ikejiri, K, Futami, K, Maekawa, T, Yasunami, Y, Takenaka, K, Ichimiya, H & Terasaka, R (2013) Dietary polyphenols and colorectal cancer risk: the Fukuoka colorectal cancer study. *World J Gastroenterol,* 19, 2683-90.
[http://dx.doi.org/10.3748/wjg.v19.i17.2683] [PMID: 23674876]

Wang, Z, Li, Y & Sarkar, FH (2010) Signaling mechanism(s) of reactive oxygen species in Epithelial-Mesenchymal Transition reminiscent of cancer stem cells in tumor progression. *Curr Stem Cell Res Ther,* 5, 74-80.

[http://dx.doi.org/10.2174/157488810790442813] [PMID: 19951255]

Watson, J (2013) Oxidants, antioxidants and the current incurability of metastatic cancers. *Open Biol,* 3120144
[http://dx.doi.org/10.1098/rsob.120144] [PMID: 23303309]

Weiskirchen, S & Weiskirchen, R (2016) Resveratrol: How much wine do you have to drink to stay healthy? *Adv Nutr,* 7, 706-18.
[http://dx.doi.org/10.3945/an.115.011627] [PMID: 27422505]

Wilken, R, Veena, MS, Wang, MB & Srivatsan, ES (2011) Curcumin: A review of anti-cancer properties and therapeutic activity in head and neck squamous cell carcinoma. *Mol Cancer,* 10, 12.
[http://dx.doi.org/10.1186/1476-4598-10-12] [PMID: 21299897]

Winterbourn, CC (1995) Toxicity of iron and hydrogen peroxide: the Fenton reaction. *Toxicol Lett,* 82-83, 969-74.
[http://dx.doi.org/10.1016/0378-4274(95)03532-X] [PMID: 8597169]

Wu, CH, Ho, YS, Tsai, CY, Wang, YJ, Tseng, H, Wei, PL, Lee, CH, Liu, RS & Lin, SY (2009) *In Vitro* and *in vivo* study of phloretin-induced apoptosis in human liver cancer cells involving inhibition of type II glucose transporter. *Int J Cancer,* 124, 2210-9.
[http://dx.doi.org/10.1002/ijc.24189] [PMID: 19123483]

Wu, KH, Ho, CT, Chen, ZF, Chen, LC, Whang-Peng, J, Lin, TN & Ho, YS (2018) The apple polyphenol phloretin inhibits breast cancer cell migration and proliferation *via* inhibition of signals by type 2 glucose transporter. *J Food Drug Anal,* 26, 221-31.
[http://dx.doi.org/10.1016/j.jfda.2017.03.009] [PMID: 29389559]

Xie, J, Xu, Y, Huang, X, Chen, Y, Fu, J, Xi, M & Wang, L (2015) Berberine-induced apoptosis in human breast cancer cells is mediated by reactive oxygen species generation and mitochondrial-related apoptotic pathway. *Tumour Biol,* 36, 1279-88.
[http://dx.doi.org/10.1007/s13277-014-2754-7] [PMID: 25352028]

Yang, YC, Lii, CK, Lin, AH, Yeh, YW, Yao, HT, Li, CC, Liu, KL & Chen, HW (2011) Induction of glutathione synthesis and heme oxygenase 1 by the flavonoids butein and phloretin is mediated through the ERK/Nrf2 pathway and protects against oxidative stress. *Free Radic Biol Med,* 51, 2073-81.
[http://dx.doi.org/10.1016/j.freeradbiomed.2011.09.007] [PMID: 21964506]

You, X, Cao, X & Lin, Y (2019) *Berberine enhances the radiosensitivity of hepatoma cells by Nrf2 pathway*
[http://dx.doi.org/10.2741/4775]

Yu, M, Tong, X, Qi, B, Qu, H, Dong, S, Yu, B, Zhang, N, Tang, N, Wang, L & Zhang, C (2014) Berberine enhances chemosensitivity to irinotecan in colon cancer *via* inhibition of NF-κB. *Mol Med Rep,* 9, 249-54.
[http://dx.doi.org/10.3892/mmr.2013.1762] [PMID: 24173769]

Yuan, JH, Li, YQ & Yang, XY (2007) Inhibition of epigallocatechin gallate on orthotopic colon cancer by upregulating the Nrf2-UGT1A signal pathway in nude mice. *Pharmacology,* 80, 269-78.
[http://dx.doi.org/10.1159/000106447] [PMID: 17657175]

Zhang, C, Sheng, J, Li, G, Zhao, L, Wang, Y, Yang, W, Yao, X, Sun, L, Zhang, Z & Cui, R (2020) Effects of berberine and its derivatives on cancer: A systems pharmacology review. *Front Pharmacol,* 10, 1461.
[http://dx.doi.org/10.3389/fphar.2019.01461] [PMID: 32009943]

Zhang, R, Qiao, H, Chen, S, Chen, X, Dou, K, Wei, L & Zhang, J (2016) Berberine reverses lapatinib resistance of HER2-positive breast cancer cells by increasing the level of ROS. *Cancer Biol Ther,* 17, 925-34.
[http://dx.doi.org/10.1080/15384047.2016.1210728] [PMID: 27416292]

Zhang, X, Yang, Y & Wang, Q (2014) Lycopene can reduce prostate-specific antigen velocity in a phase II clinical study in Chinese population. *Chin Med J (Engl),* 127, 2143-6.
[http://dx.doi.org/10.3760/cma.j.issn.0366-6999.20132829] [PMID: 24890168]

Zhao, R, Yang, B, Wang, L, Xue, P, Deng, B, Zhang, G, Jiang, S, Zhang, M, Liu, M, Pi, J & Guan, D (2013) Curcumin protects human keratinocytes against inorganic arsenite-induced acute cytotoxicity through an

NRF2-dependent mechanism. *Oxid Med Cell Longev,* 2013412576
[http://dx.doi.org/10.1155/2013/412576] [PMID: 23710286]

Zhong, H & Yin, H (2015) Role of lipid peroxidation derived 4-hydroxynonenal (4-HNE) in cancer: focusing on mitochondria. *Redox Biol,* 4, 193-9.
[http://dx.doi.org/10.1016/j.redox.2014.12.011] [PMID: 25598486]

Zhou, M, Zheng, J, Bi, J, Wu, X, Lyu, J & Gao, K (2018) Synergistic inhibition of colon cancer cell growth by a combination of atorvastatin and phloretin. *Oncol Lett,* 15, 1985-92.
[http://dx.doi.org/10.3892/ol.2017.7480] [PMID: 29399200]

Zhu, W, Jia, L, Chen, G, Zhao, H, Sun, X, Meng, X, Zhao, X, Xing, L, Yu, J & Zheng, M (2016) Epigallocatechin-3-gallate ameliorates radiation-induced acute skin damage in breast cancer patients undergoing adjuvant radiotherapy. *Oncotarget,* 7, 48607-13.
[http://dx.doi.org/10.18632/oncotarget.9495] [PMID: 27224910]

CHAPTER 10

Therapeutic Potential of Probiotics on Oxidative Stress and their Role in Human Health

Ajay Kumar[1], Sandeep Kaur[1,2], Samiksha [5], Sharad Thakur[3,4], Neha Sharma[1], Kritika Pandit[1], Satwinder Kaur Sohal[5] and Satwinderjeet Kaur[1,*]

[1] *Department of Botanical and Environmental Sciences, Guru Nanak Dev University, Amritsar-143005, Punjab, India*

[2] *PG Department of Botany, Khalsa College, Amritsar-143005, Punjab, India*

[3] *Department of Molecular Biology and Biochemistry, Guru Nanak Dev University, Amritsar-143005, Punjab, India*

[4] *PG Department of Agriculture, Khalsa College, Amritsar-143005, Punjab, India*

[5] *Department of Zoology, Guru Nanak Dev University, Amritsar-143005, Punjab, India*

Abstract: In the industrialized world, functional foods have become part of a diet that provide potential health benefits by curbing various diseases. Currently, the most commonly used functional foods are probiotics which reduce damages caused by oxidative stress and reactive oxygen species (ROS). Probiotics are live microbes used as a therapeutic food with fewer side effects in comparison to other therapeutic agents. The incorporation of probiotics in foods shows many medicinal properties by acting as antioxidant, anti-inflammatory, anti-bacterial and anti-cancer agents. As such probiotic foods (fermented dairy products, drinks, fruits, vegetables, *etc.*) can affect the individual by raising the existing gastrointestinal flora with live microbial nutritional supplements and improve the microbial balance of *Lactobacillus*, *Bifidobacterium* and several other microbial species in the gastrointestinal tract, which causes an alteration in carcinogen metabolism as well as regulation of the immune system. Accumulating evidence highlighted that probiotics have therapeutic effects with a reduction of invasion and metastasis in cancer cells by modulating key signaling pathways. Globally probiotics market extent was valued at $ 48.38 billion in 2018 and expanded at 6.9% annually which indicates the rising demand for probiotics worldwide. Hence, the chapter sheds light on the current state of probiotics and their potential applications for human health and in the development of modern therapeutic drugs for the treatment of diseases.

Keywords: Antioxidant, Immunity, Metastasis, Oxidative stress, Probiotics, ROS.

* **Corresponding author Satwinderjeet Kaur:** Genetic Toxicology Laboratory, Department of Botanical and Environmental Sciences, Guru Nanak Dev University, Amritsar-143005, (Punjab) India. E-mails: satwinderjeet.botenv@gndu.ac.in and sjkaur2011@gmail.com

Pardeep Kaur, Rajendra G. Mehta, Robin, Tarunpreet Singh Thind and Saroj Arora (Eds.)

INTRODUCTION

Functional foods are supplements or dietary foods usually consumed to get some beneficial results from them. Probiotics are considered as functional food's ideal group with rising large marketable interest and market shares (Mishra *et al.* 2019). Probiotics bacteria have the capacity to colonize the colonic mucosa. These bacteria have the potential to prevent and treat various diseases *viz.* gastrointestinal infections, lactose intolerance, inflammatory bowel disease, urogenital infections, allergies, cancers, cystic fibrosis, reduction of side effects of antibiotics, in oral health like the curing of dental problems and periodontal diseases (Singh *et al.* 2013). However, the alteration in the structure of this defending microbial flora by certain eating and environmental factors makes the host prone to diseases by minimizing its food utilization efficacy (Fuller 1989). Probiotics are used in the treatment of distressed microflora of the intestine and raise gut porousness which are the major features of several intestinal disorders in warm-blooded organisms. The basic action mechanism of probiotics is its ability to compete for the adherence sites on the intestinal epithelium and mucosa and also produce bactericidal substances to neutralize the harmful effects of pathogens and other related toxins (Vanderpool *et al.* 2008).

Probiotics (yogurt and fruits) intake in acceptable quantities has useful health benefits on the host (Fernandez and Marette 2017). The relationship between human beings and live-microbial diet has been well known in history and antedate to the millennium of years ago (Nazir *et al.* 2018). Parker in 1974 used the terms probiotic for the first time and defined as the association of substances and organisms which have a positive influence on their host by maintaining the equilibrium of gastrointestinal flora (Tannock 1999). Metchnikoff and coworkers reported the first study on probiotic and demonstrated the positive impact of the fermented milk on human health. Till now, scientific studies on the valuable outcomes of probiotics on the human have been investigated for treatment and mitigation of gut-related illnesses like indigestion, bowel diseases, stomach swelling and diarrhea (Kim *et al.* 2019). According to the data of PUBMED search, there were 26,207 papers indexed to the term "probiotic" as of March 03, 2020, in comparison to the 714 papers prior to the year 2000. Due to its importance, there is a great increase in the demand for probiotic-based nutrients. In 2017, for probiotic worth, the global market was 42.55 billion US\$ and in 2025, it is observed to augment by 74.69 billion US\$ (Fortune Business Insights 2019). To date, only scarce information is available about probiotics possessing antioxidative, anti-inflammatory, anticancer and gastroprotective properties. Furthermore, probiotics exhibited the health encouraging efficacy in maintaining hypersensitive, inflammatory and infectious diseases by modifying the functioning of the gut and by enhancing homeostatic immune defenses.

Although probiotics can be found useful in specific clinical applications and human health, the mechanisms behind the modulation of the immune function are understood poorly. Probiotics are usually not necessarily considered as commensal bacteria. They are commonly lactic acid bacteria (LAB), utmost *Bifidobacteria* and *Lactobacilli* species, while *Enterococcus* and *Lactococcus* species of non-pathogenic strains are also identified as probiotics. Though, the available works on the beneficial effects of pro-biotic on these diseases are still controversial and limited. In addition, many studies are not able to sufficiently address the mechanisms through which probiotics treat, reduce and modulate the progression of diseases. Recently, several literature findings showed an upsurge in exploring the beneficial effects of various probiotics in protecting and managing the different human disorders and diseases (Table **1**). Besides the importance of yeasts in the fermentation of beverages and food, it also showed some beneficial effects in promoting human health. Therefore, this chapter will highlight the role of probiotics in averting the incidence of the above-mentioned illnesses besides suggesting its main mechanisms of action.

PROBIOTICS AS ANTIOXIDANT

Oxidative stress (OS) is normally induced due to the formation of ROS. It usually occurs due to disturbance in the equilibrium of antioxidant molecules and pro-oxidant generation (Hussain *et al.* 2012). The main health benefits of probiotics are to improve the antioxidant defense capacity of the human body as these are reported to enhance the total GSH level in the plasma (Mishra *et al.* 2015). Pro-oxidants mostly consist of one or more unpaired electron that is unstable. Mostly, the production of ROS constantly in the cell system can cause damage to the proteins, fats, starches and nucleic acid. Several endogenous sources also generate ROS *i.e.,* xanthine oxidase, mitochondria (Sisein 2014), inflammation, peroxisomes, phagocytosis, exercise (Hussain *et al.* 2012), respiratory burst and free metal ions (Takashima *et al.* 2012). The exogenous sources include industrial solvents, cigarette smoke, UV irradiation and environmental pollutants. The partial reduction of unreactive dioxygen leads to the generation of reactive oxygen species (ROS) (Kumar *et al.* 2014). In OS, cellular mitochondria generate ROS with the reduction in the expression of enzymatic antioxidants and nonenzymatic antioxidants. The elevation in the level of ROS generates oxidative stress and leads to the progression of several chronic diseases, including diabetes, cancer and aging (Valko *et al.* 2007). The antioxidants bind with the free radicals formed in the cells and the chain reaction gets ended before its completion preventing impairment to the vital molecules (Mishra *et al.* 2015). All of these molecules in the body perform diverse physiological roles by suppressing the process of oxidation. All chain reactions are stopped by the antioxidants through the inhibition of free radicals. Therefore, it is crucial to find natural antioxidants that provide protection to the human body from the accumulation of ROS to overcome the development of certain diseases (Fig. **1**). Attributed to the perceptional changes of the consumer to the therapeutic value of foods, there are food-based supplements and ingredients available which contain antioxidants. Probiotics show extensive therapeutic uses and have been developed as a source of effective and natural antioxidants with no side effects. (Mishra *et al.* 2015). The importance of probiotics as an antioxidant is keenly being investigated. Probiotics have the crucial property of inhabiting the stomach, so as to improve metabolic diseases, including diabetes and obesity by controlling the micro-organisms community in the intestine (Homayouni *et al.* 2016). Probiotic strains are also able to restore the natural intestinal microflora and their enzymatic activity.

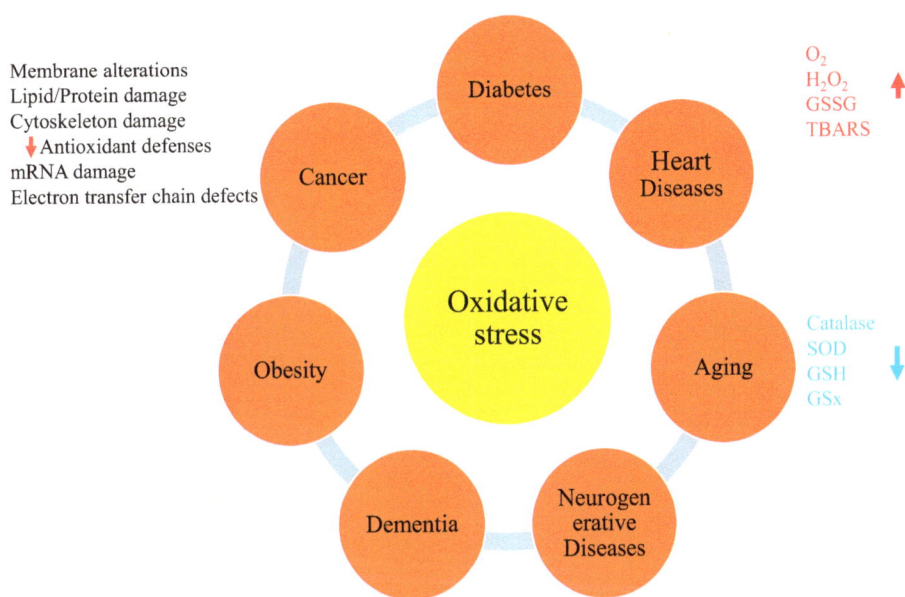

Fig. (1). The outcome of oxidative stress and the gathering of ROS leads to mRNA damage, decreasing antioxidant defenses and ultimately produces more oxidative stress.

Table 1. Examples of probiotics acting as protective agents against various diseases and their molecular targets.

Bacteria	Mechanism/molecular Targets	References
Lactobacillus salivarius	*L. salivarius* showed anti-inflammatory effect with local IL-10 production, which is abolished in NOD2-deficient mice.	Fernandez *et al.* (2011)

(Table 1) cont.....

Bacteria	Mechanism/molecular Targets	References
Bifidobacterium breve Lactobacillus rhamnosus Lactobacillus casei	*B. breve* strain produced a lesser amount of the pro-inflammatory cytokine IFN-γ than *L. rhamnosus* and *L. casei*. Moreover, *B. breve* and lactobacilli generated cytokines in a TLR9-dependent manner, and the lower inflammatory profile of *B. breve* is due to inhibitory effects of TLR2.	Plantinga *et al.* (2011)
Lactobacillus casei	*L. casei* has capacity to bind three heterocyclic aromatic amines (IQ, MelQx and PhIP) *in vitro* and decrease genotoxicity of Heterocyclic aromatic amines (HCA).	Nowak and Libudzisz (2009)
Lactobacillus acidophilus Bifidobacterium animalis	Lactic acid bacteria (LAB) strains detoxify the contaminants and protect humans or animals against the adverse health effects of compounds namely ochratoxin A (OTA) and patulin (PAT).	Fuchs and Sontag (2008)
Pediococcus pentosaceus, Lactobacillus salivarius, Lactobacillus salivarius, and Enterococcus faecium	These bacteria showed antiproliferative effects against colon cancer cells and may serve as a suitable alternative with bioprophylactic and biotherapeutic strategy for the treatment of colon cancer.	Thirabunyanon and Hongwittayakorn (2012)
Lactobacillus casei	*L. casei* showed an inhibitory effect on colorectal cancer and bladder cancer with immunomodulatory effects and can support the immune defense of the host by inducing IL-12 (interleukin-12) generation *via* phagocytes.	Molska and Reguła (2019)
Lactobacillus fermentum	*L. fermentum* showed antiproliferative effect and has the capacity to modulate hyperinsulinemia, insulin resistance, hyper cholesterolemia, and hypertriglyceridemia.	
Saccharomyces cerevisiae	*S. cerevisiae* showed anti-inflammatory and antibacterial effects by stimulating the secretion of immunoglobulin A (IgA) and maintaining the integrity of the epithelial barrier. It helps in the treatment of travelers' diarrhea.	
Lactobacillus acidophilus Bifidobacterium bifidum	*L. acidophilus* and *B. bifidum* showed significant improvement in stool evenness, and also decreased radiotherapy-induced diarrhea.	Chitapanarux *et al.* (2010)
Lactobacillus rhamnosus GG	Reduced apoptosis in epithelial cells *via* downregulation of TNF-α expression.	Gogineni *et al.* (2013)
L. acidophilus	*L. acidophilus* can block the communication between pathogenic bacteria *via* secreting different molecules which block quorum sensing signaling.	

(Table 1) cont.....

Bacteria	Mechanism/molecular Targets	References
L. casei Shirota (LcS)	L-lactic acid and LcS culture supernatant inhibited NF-κB activation, increased TNF-α mRNA expression, and TNF-α protein secretion in cells treated with lipopolysaccharide (LPS) in *in vivo* and *in vitro* system.	Watanabe *et al.* (2009)

PROBIOTICS AS ANTI-INFLAMMATORY

The anti-inflammatory properties of probiotics suppress the production of proinflammatory cytokines and inflammatory mediators. It was investigated that the probiotics-supplemented diet in infants delivers defense against the development of eczema and also ameliorates the development of inflammatory response in allergic diseases (Laiho *et al.* 2002). It was evaluated that no other dietary supplement was as efficient and safe as the use of prebiotics and probiotics in providing a natural remedy for the treatment of atopic dermatitis (Schlichte *et al.* 2016). The combination of three probiotics strains viz. *Bifidobacterium bifidum* MF 20/5, *Lactobacillus gasseri* PA 16/8 and *Bifidobacterium longum* SP 07/3 along with minerals and vitamins showed potent effects in combating the incidence or sternness of recurrent and acute respirational tract infections (Kalyuzhin and coauthors 2016). Lichtenstein and coworkers (2016) reported the efficacy of probiotics and prebiotics in the inhibition of pouchitis by manipulating the composition of pouch flora and restoring the proctocolectomy for colitis ulcer. The study had reported the differences in the composition of gut microbiota between both obese and non-obese patients. It was observed that an increment in the growth of *Bifidobacteria* causes a reduction in weight but enhances the obesity-related parameters like the adipogenic effects of diet and inflammation. Obesity is considered to be caused due to alterations in the metabolism and in the ingestion and storing of dietary lipids, which varies with the conformation of gut microbiota (da Silva *et al.* 2013). Pothoulakis (2009) reported a probiotic, *Saccharomyces boulardii,* which showed diverse pathophysiological effects against gastrointestinal inflammatory diseases like bacteria mediated or enterotoxin-mediated inflammation and diarrhea and other inflammatory bowel diseases. The results obtained demonstrated the secretion of proteins by *S. boulardii* that inhibit pro-inflammatory cytokines production by interfering with the intermediary of inflammation nuclear factor kappa B, and also exhibited modulatory effects on the action of mitogen-activated protein kinases ERK1/2.

PROBIOTICS AS IMMUNOMODIFIER

Certain destabilizing factors like antibiotics disturb the colonic microbial community. There exists a relationship among the mucosal immunity and mucosal microbial colonization of the different biotopes of the body. Carter and coworkers (2016) reported the role of probiotics as dietary supplements in promoting health benefits by curing the human immunodeficiency virus infection. The data obtained suggested management in the level of CD4 count, diarrhea and bacterial vaginosis. *Lactobacillus plantarum* L67, available as dietary supplement and as yogurt starters, was found helpful in inhibiting the allergic inflammatory response and other allergy-related immune disorders in bisphenol treated the rat basophilic leukemia 2H3 cells and mouse splenocytes. The results obtained revealed that L67 protein-induced interleukin and interferon IFN-γ in cultured splenocytes and also significantly ameliorate the T helper 2-linked cytokines IL-1β, IL-6, and IL-10 expression analyzed using ELISA and western blotting (Song *et al.* 2016). Ben Salah *et al.* (2013) evaluated the immunomodulatory effect of six isolated lactic acid bacteria on the mononuclear cells of the peripheral blood in Wistar rats. The data obtained revealed the health-improving effects of *Lactobacillus plantarum* TN8 strain as compared to all the other strains and found that TN8 induced the secretion of anti-inflammatory cytokine IL-10 whereas decreased the production of pro-inflammatory cytokine IL-12, IFN-γ and TNF-α. The crucial role of probiotics in the immunomodulation of intestinal epithelial cells contributes to diminishing the intestinal inflammation and infections by reducing the accessibility of pathogenic organism adherence to the intestinal epithelial cells (Mack and Lebel 2004). Gorbach (2000) evaluated that *Lactobacillus rhamnosus* GG (LGG) showed a wide range of applications when consumed as dairy products. LGG promoted health benefits by colonizing the gastrointestinal tract in 3-7 days. LGG acts as immunoadjuvant in oral vaccines and enhance the numbers of IgA and other immunoglobulin-secreting cells to improve intestinal immunity. LGG was also found effective in antibiotic-associated diarrhea, Traveler's diarrhea and relapsing *Clostridium difficile* colitis. It was investigated that there was no long-term effect of probiotics like *Lactobacillus paracasei* subsp. *paracasei* F19 (LF19) on the IgE sensitization, airway inflammation and other prevalent allergic diseases such as eczema, asthma, allergic rhinitis and food allergy in the 8-9 years aged children (West *et al.* 2013).

PROBIOTICS AS GASTROPROTECTIVE

The probiotics as gastroprotective agents improve the digestive enzyme activity and maintain microbial balance to treat and prevent the diseases related to the gastrointestinal tract. The gastroprotective efficacy of *Escherichia coli* Nissle strain, a probiotic bacteria, against stress-induced gastric erosion in rats was reported (Konturek *et al.* 2009). It was investigated that the non-antigenic fractions of probiotics were found effective in suppressing/reducing the bacterial and viral infections in tumor cells induced inbred strain of mice (Nutini *et al.* 1982). Reid *et al.* (1990) found that protective effect of *Lactobacillus acidophilus* against pathogen-induced intestinal and urogenital infectious diseases is due to due to the interference of bacteria which involves the secretion of inhibitory substances like bacteriocins and competitive exclusion. Katelaris (1996) reported the efficacy of probiotics in the prevention and treatment of diarrheal diseases by preventing the pathogens from colonizing the gut. Hayes and Vargas (2016) evaluated the safety and effectiveness of probiotics in pediatric (0-18 years age) to whom antibiotics are prescribed frequently and are suffering from antibiotic-associated diarrhea due to the alterations in the gastrointestinal tract microbial balance. It was found that that the specified strain and the appropriate dose of probiotics as dietary supplements help to restore the gut microflora. Hidalgo-Cantabrana *et al.* (2017) reported the importance of *Bifidobacteria* in the promotion of human health as it is the first microbial colonizer of the newborn's intestines and also predominant in adults. Kirpich and McClain (2012) identified the positive effects of probiotics on the liver ailments by modifying the intestinal microflora and immune system. Baryshnikova (2012) investigated that the addition of the probiotic to the *Helicobacter pylori* strain showed a sign of improvements as this strain causes higher levels of duodenal ulcer and chronic gastroduodenitis in patients. Administration of the mixture of two probiotics, *Bacillus subtilis* strains *viz.* L10 and G1 in equal amounts for 8 weeks to shrimp showed a reduction in the cumulative mortality and an improvement in the growth, digestive enzyme activity and resistance to diseases by enhancing the response of the immune system as related to the control shrimp (Zokaeifar *et al.* 2012). Moslehi-Jenabian *et al.* (2010) found that the food-borne and probiotics yeast causes the hydrolysis of folate biofortification and phytate and mycotoxins detoxification due to its binding to the surface of the yeast cell wall and thereby found helpful in treating intestinal diseases and modulating the immune system. Teanpaisan and Piwat (2014) evaluated that the daily short-term ingestion of *Lactobacillus paracasei* SD1, which is a human-derived probiotic cause a reduction in the number of salivary mutans streptococci.

PROBIOTICS AS ANTICANCER

The anticancer activity of probiotics inhibits the proliferation of cancer cells by acting as natural anti-metastatic agents. Im *et al.* (2009) reported that the probiotics bacterium, *Bacillus polyfermenticus* ameliorates the expression level of inflammatory molecules in colonic cells. The results obtained demonstrated the reduction of apoptosis and promotion of migration and proliferation in colonic epithelial cells as analyzed using a terminal deoxynucleotidyl transferase dUTP nick end labeling assay and caspase-3 or seperation of poly (ADP-ribose) polymerase. The study had reported the beneficial effects of probiotics in curing the development of colon cancer, acute rotavirus diarrhea, subjects with colonic disorders, food allergy and patients undergoing pelvic radiotherapy (Strus 1997).

Nouri *et al.* (2016) investigated the anticancer potential of a group of *Lactobacilli* probiotics such as *Lactobacillus rhamnosus* supernatant and *Lactobacillus crispatus* supernatant against the human cervical cancer (HeLa) and colon adenocarcinoma (HT-29) cell lines. It was further demonstrated that the administration of these two probiotics was found effective in delaying/postponing the later stage of cancer by acting as anti-proliferative and anti-metastatic agents. Elise *et al.* (2015) reported that probiotic *Bifidobacterium* showed anticancer activity by suppressing the tumor growth in female CD-1 nude mice and found cytotoxic towards HT-29, HeLa, Caco-375, DLD-1, MCF-7, and A549 cell lines.

PROBIOTICS AS ANTI-MICROBIALS

WHO defines probiotics as "live microorganisms which when administered in adequate amounts confer a health benefit on the host" (Hotel and Cordoba 2001). Considerable scientific evidence has accumulated over the few decades for the practice of probiotics on humans because of the suitable properties of probiotic bacteria for well-being. Continuously rising consumer awareness related to gut health and due to the rising levels of fitness the concept of defensive health care is growing in the form of probiotic food, beverages and nutritional enhancements. Probiotics have developed progressively in the food industry. LAB, particularly *Lactobacillus*, bacteria used as probiotics because of the awareness that they are needed for the abdominal microflora and these microorganisms are "Generally Recognized As Safe" (GRAS) grade. The infections such as inflammatory bowel disease and diarrhea could be because of the lack of gut micro-flora and probiotics that have proven beneficial in the treatment. The therapy used for the inflammatory bowel disease (IBD) for quite some time is the fecal transplant. *Clostridium difficile* is the causative agent for the recurrent *C. difficile* infection (CDI), which may be due to the extreme use of the antibiotics. The antibiotics execute the important bacteria in the gut foremost to the CDI infection. Fecal replacement from a healthy donor into the gastrointestinal tract resolved the recurring *C. difficile* colitis (Rohlke and Stollman 2012).

Probiotics' ability to bear the normal acidic environment of the gastric juices of the bile duct along with the generation of lactic acid that prevent the evolution of extra bacteria leads to its enhancement in the intestinal tract (Prabhurajeshwar and Chandrakanth 2019). The health of the female vagina is predominantly dependent upon the *Lactobacillus* bacteria colonizing the vagina of a healthy woman. The beneficial *Lactobacilli* do not allow other opportunistic infection-causing bacteria to establish and cause bacterial vaginosis. Probiotics yield an extensive variety of antimicrobial metabolites. The bacteriocins are active proteins that prevent the development of pathogenic bacteria, particularly in the gastrointestinal tract. Thus, probiotics act as anti-microbials by regulating the growth of microorganisms and by inhibiting the growth of the pathogenic bacteria (Atassi *et al.* 2019). *Lactobacilli* are the predominant microflora of the human intestine and the urogenital flora. Lactic acid bacteria can produce both narrow spectrum (effect on the limited microorganisms) and broad-spectrum bacteriocins (effect on many microorganisms). Lactobacilli also compete for the food and space with the pathogenic bacteria. Hence, *Lactobacilli*, concluded antagonistic connections with pathogenic bacteria, keep the intestinal balance. Probiotics are incorporated into various kinds of foods and are living, health-promoting microorganisms. Yogurt holding viable bacteria recovers lactose absorption and amends the signs of lactose intolerance. The probiotic bacteria that have commercial value in products are primarily members of the genera *Lactobacillus* and *Bifidobacterium* (Karimi *et al.* 2018).

PROBIOTICS AS ANTIDEPRESSANT

The gut microbiota maintains the homeostasis of the microorganism that suppresses the development of various ailments: inflammatory diseases of gastro-intestinal, metabolic disorders, and autoimmune diseases (Lankelma *et al.* 2015). The microbiome, contains approximately 10,000 billion microorganisms, maintain the abdominal lining and supports its maintenance (Mangiola *et al.* 2016). The gut microbiota is affected by numerous factors, including age (Yatsunenko *et al.* 2012), diet (David *et al.* 2014), stress (O'Mahony *et al.* 2009) and genetic factors (Goodrich *et al.* 2014). Several studies suggested that mental stress can rise the absorptivity of the gastrointestinal layer (Meddings and Swain 2000) and microbiota can influence and moderate emotional behavior (Rhee *et al.* 2009).

Over the past few years, adequate studies highlighted that several bacterial strains affect the working of the central nervous system (CNS) and performance of humans and animals (Yunes *et al.* 2019). The microbiota of the gut can impact the CNS *via* the gut-brain axis and improve ailments of the nervous system (Foster *et al.* 2013). Probiotics are used with a combination of several drugs to cure various illnesses (Linares *et al.* 2016). Probiotics that influence the CNS are known as psychobiotics, when consumed in acceptable quantities, confer mental health benefits (Sarkar *et al.* 2016, Bermúdez-Humarán *et al.* 2019). The several compounds generated by gut-bacteria are neuroactive compounds which helps to maintain the working of the nervous system with mediators between bacteria and their hosts (Averina *et al.* 2017).

CONCLUSION

Several evidences demonstrated the role of nutraceuticals and functional foods in the prevention and treatment of various ailments as well as developing eco-friendly and acceptable natural products for controlling various diseases. Probiotics as nutraceutical are crucial in the prevention and treatment of many infectious diseases related to the gastrointestinal tract and colon and thereby provide overall health benefits to individuals. Probiotics possess antioxidant, anti-inflammatory, immune modifying, antimicrobial, anticancer and gastroprotective properties to overcome the incidence of conflicting health issues. Thereby, safety and affordable bioavailability, quality and quantity control, of these nutraceutical products are crucial in getting rid of various unexpected side effects in humans.

CONFLICT OF INTEREST

The authors declare that there are no conflicts of interest.

ACKNOWLEDGMENT

This work was supported by the University Grants Commission (UGC) - Basic Scientific Research (BSR), and DST-PURSE Programme, Department of Science and Technology (DST) and Fund for Improvement of S & T Infrastructure (FIST) programme of DST and DRS-SAP (II) Programme of University Grants Commission, New Delhi (India).

CONSENT FOR PUBLICATION

None

REFERENCES

Atassi, F, Pho Viet Ahn, DL, Lievin-Le Moal, V & Moal, LL (2019) Diverse expression of antimicrobial activities against bacterial vaginosis and urinary tract infection pathogens by cervicovaginal microbiota strains of *Lactobacillus gasseri* and *Lactobacillus crispatus*. *Front Microbiol,* 10, 2900.
[http://dx.doi.org/10.3389/fmicb.2019.02900] [PMID: 31921075]

Averina, OV & Danilenko, VN (2017) Human intestinal microbiota: Role in development and functioning of the nervous system. *Mikrobiologiia,* 86, 5-24.
[PMID: 30207138]

Baryshnikova, NV (2012) Helicobacter pylori-associated gastroenterological diseases: genetic features and probiotic treatment. *Benef Microbes,* 3, 157-61.
[http://dx.doi.org/10.3920/BM2011.0023] [PMID: 22683837]

Bermúdez-Humarán, LG, Salinas, E, Ortiz, GG, Ramirez-Jirano, LJ, Morales, JA & Bitzer-Quintero, OK (2019) From probiotics to psychobiotics: live beneficial bacteria which act on the Brain-Gut axis. *Nutrients,* 11, 1-22.
[http://dx.doi.org/10.3390/nu11040890] [PMID: 31010014]

Carter, GM, Esmaeili, A, Shah, H, Indyk, D, Johnson, M, Andreae, M & Sacks, HS (2016) Probiotics in human immunodeficiency virus infection: a systematic review and evidence synthesis of benefits and risks. *Open Forum Infect Dis,* 3ofw164
[http://dx.doi.org/10.1093/ofid/ofw164] [PMID: 27747250]

da Silva, ST, dos Santos, CA & Bressan, J (2013) Intestinal microbiota; relevance to obesity and modulation by prebiotics and probiotics. *Nutr Hosp,* 28, 1039-48.

[PMID: 23889619]

David, LA, Maurice, CF, Carmody, RN, Gootenberg, DB, Button, JE, Wolfe, BE, Ling, AV, Devlin, AS, Varma, Y, Fischbach, MA, Biddinger, SB, Dutton, RJ & Turnbaugh, PJ (2014) Diet rapidly and reproducibly alters the human gut microbiome. *Nature,* 505, 559-63.
[http://dx.doi.org/10.1038/nature12820] [PMID: 24336217]

Macho Fernandez, E, Valenti, V, Rockel, C, Hermann, C, Pot, B, Boneca, IG & Grangette, C (2011) Anti-inflammatory capacity of selected lactobacilli in experimental colitis is driven by NOD2-mediated recognition of a specific peptidoglycan-derived muropeptide. *Gut,* 60, 1050-9.
[http://dx.doi.org/10.1136/gut.2010.232918] [PMID: 21471573]

Fernandez, MA & Marette, A (2017) Potential health benefits of combining yogurt and fruits based on their probiotic and prebiotic properties. *Adv Nutr,* 8, 155S-64S.
[http://dx.doi.org/10.3945/an.115.011114] [PMID: 28096139]

Fortune Business Insights (2019)   https://www.fortunebusinessinsights.com/industry-reports/probiotic--market-100083

Foster, JA & McVey Neufeld, KA (2013) Gut-brain axis: how the microbiome influences anxiety and depression. *Trends Neurosci,* 36, 305-12.
[http://dx.doi.org/10.1016/j.tins.2013.01.005] [PMID: 23384445]

Fuchs, S, Sontag, G, Stidl, R, Ehrlich, V, Kundi, M & Knasmüller, S (2008) Detoxification of patulin and ochratoxin A, two abundant mycotoxins, by lactic acid bacteria. *Food Chem Toxicol,* 46, 1398-407.
[http://dx.doi.org/10.1016/j.fct.2007.10.008] [PMID: 18061329]

Fuller, R (1989) Probiotics in man and animals. *J Appl Bacteriol,* 66, 365-78.
[http://dx.doi.org/10.1111/j.1365-2672.1989.tb05105.x] [PMID: 2666378]

Gogineni, VK, Morrow, LE & Malesker, MA (2013) Probiotics: Mechanisms of Action and Clinical Applications. *J Prob Health,* 1, 1-11.
[http://dx.doi.org/10.4172/2329-8901.1000101]

Goodrich, JK, Waters, JL, Poole, AC, Sutter, JL, Koren, O, Blekhman, R, Beaumont, M, Van Treuren, W, Knight, R, Bell, JT, Spector, TD, Clark, AG & Ley, RE (2014) Human genetics shape the gut microbiome. *Cell,* 159, 789-99.
[http://dx.doi.org/10.1016/j.cell.2014.09.053] [PMID: 25417156]

Hayes, SR & Vargas, AJ (2016) Probiotics for the prevention of pediatric antibiotic-associated diarrhea. *Explore (NY),* 12, 463-6.
[http://dx.doi.org/10.1016/j.explore.2016.08.015] [PMID: 27688016]

Hidalgo-Cantabrana, C, Delgado, S, Ruiz, L, Ruas-Madiedo, P, Sánchez, B & Margolles, A (2018) Bifidobacteria and their health-promoting effects. *Bugs as Drugs: Therapeutic Microbes for the Prevention and Treatment of Disease,* 73-98.

Homayouni-Rad, A, Soroush, AR, Khalili, L, Norouzi-Panahi, L, Kasaie, Z & Ejtahed, HS (2017) Diabetes management by probiotics: current knowledge and future pespective. *Int J Vitam Nutr Res,* 1, 1-13.
[PMID: 28436760]

Hotel, AC & Cordoba, A (2001) Health and nutritional properties of probiotics in food including powder milk with live lactic acid bacteria. *Prevention,* 5, 1-0.
[http://dx.doi.org/] [PMID:]

Im, E, Choi, YJ, Pothoulakis, C & Rhee, SH (2009) *Bacillus polyfermenticus* ameliorates colonic inflammation by promoting cytoprotective effects in colitic mice. *J Nutr,* 139, 1848-54.
[http://dx.doi.org/10.3945/jn.109.108613] [PMID: 19675103]

Kalyuzhin, OV, Afanasyev, SS & Bykov, AS (2016) [Probiotics as stimulators of immune response against pathogens in the respiratory tract]. *Ter Arkh,* 88, 118-24.
[http://dx.doi.org/10.17116/terarkh2016885118-124] [PMID: 27458629]

Karimi, S, Azizi, F, Nayeb-Aghaee, M & Mahmoodnia, L (2018) The antimicrobial activity of probiotic bacteria *Escherichia coli* isolated from different natural sources against hemorrhagic *E. coli* O157:H7. *Electron Physician,* 10, 6548-53.
[http://dx.doi.org/10.19082/6548] [PMID: 29765581]

Katelaris, PH (1996) Probiotic control of diarrhoeal disease. *Asia Pac J Clin Nutr,* 5, 39-43.
[PMID: 24394465]

Kim, SK, Guevarra, RB, Kim, YT, Kwon, J, Kim, H, Cho, JH, Kim, HB & Lee, JH (2019) Role of probiotics in human gut microbiome-associated diseases. *J Microbiol Biotechnol,* 29, 1335-40.
[http://dx.doi.org/10.4014/jmb.1906.06064] [PMID: 31434172]

Kirpich, IA & McClain, CJ (2012) Probiotics in the treatment of the liver diseases. *J Am Coll Nutr,* 31, 14-23.
[http://dx.doi.org/10.1080/07315724.2012.10720004] [PMID: 22661622]

Konturek, PC, Sliwowski, Z, Koziel, J, Ptak-Belowska, A, Burnat, G, Brzozowski, T & Konturek, SJ (2009) Probiotic bacteria *Escherichia coli* strain Nissle 1917 attenuates acute gastric lesions induced by stress. *J Physiol Pharmacol,* 60 (Suppl. 6), 41-8.
[PMID: 20224150]

Kumar, P, Mishra, S, Malik, A & Satya, S (2014) Biocontrol potential of essential oil monoterpenes against housefly, Musca domestica (Diptera: Muscidae). *Ecotoxicol Environ Saf,* 100, 1-6.
[http://dx.doi.org/10.1016/j.ecoenv.2013.11.013] [PMID: 24433784]

Laiho, K, Ouwehand, A, Salminen, S & Isolauri, E (2002) Inventing probiotic functional foods for patients with allergic disease. *Ann Allergy Asthma Immunol,* 89 (Suppl. 1), 75-82.
[http://dx.doi.org/10.1016/S1081-1206(10)62128-X] [PMID: 12487210]

Lankelma, JM, Nieuwdorp, M, de Vos, WM & Wiersinga, WJ (2015) The gut microbiota in internal medicine: implications for health and disease. *Neth J Med,* 73, 61-8.
[PMID: 25753070]

Lichtenstein, L, Avni-Biron, I & Ben-Bassat, O (2016) The current place of probiotics and prebiotics in the treatment of pouchitis. *Best Pract Res Clin Gastroenterol,* 30, 73-80.
[http://dx.doi.org/10.1016/j.bpg.2016.02.003] [PMID: 27048898]

Linares, DM, Ross, P & Stanton, C (2016) Beneficial Microbes: The pharmacy in the gut. *Bioengineered,* 7, 11-20.
[http://dx.doi.org/10.1080/21655979.2015.1126015] [PMID: 26709457]

Ma, EL, Choi, YJ, Choi, J, Pothoulakis, C, Rhee, SH & Im, E (2010) The anticancer effect of probiotic Bacillus polyfermenticus on human colon cancer cells is mediated through ErbB2 and ErbB3 inhibition. *Int J Cancer,* 127, 780-90.
[PMID: 19876926]

Mack, DR & Lebel, S (2004) Role of probiotics in the modulation of intestinal infections and inflammation. *Curr Opin Gastroenterol,* 20, 22-6.
[http://dx.doi.org/10.1097/00001574-200401000-00006] [PMID: 15703616]

Mangiola, F, Ianiro, G, Franceschi, F, Fagiuoli, S, Gasbarrini, G & Gasbarrini, A (2016) Gut microbiota in autism and mood disorders. *World J Gastroenterol,* 22, 361-8.
[http://dx.doi.org/10.3748/wjg.v22.i1.361] [PMID: 26755882]

Markowiak, P & Śliżewska, K (2017) Effects of probiotics, prebiotics, and synbiotics on human health. *Nutrients,* 9, 1-30.
[http://dx.doi.org/10.3390/nu9091021] [PMID: 28914794]

Meddings, JB & Swain, MG (2000) Environmental stress-induced gastrointestinal permeability is mediated by endogenous glucocorticoids in the rat. *Gastroenterology,* 119, 1019-28.
[http://dx.doi.org/10.1053/gast.2000.18152] [PMID: 11040188]

Mishra, V, Shah, C, Mokashe, N, Chavan, R, Yadav, H & Prajapati, J (2015) Probiotics as potential

antioxidants: a systematic review. *J Agric Food Chem,* 63, 3615-26.
[http://dx.doi.org/10.1021/jf506326t] [PMID: 25808285]

Molska, M & Reguła, J (2019) Potential Mechanisms of Probiotics Action in the Prevention and Treatment of Colorectal Cancer. *Nutrients,* 11, 1-17.
[http://dx.doi.org/10.3390/nu11102453] [PMID: 31615096]

Moslehi-Jenabian, S, Pedersen, LL & Jespersen, L (2010) Beneficial effects of probiotic and food borne yeasts on human health. *Nutrients,* 2, 449-73.
[http://dx.doi.org/10.3390/nu2040449] [PMID: 22254033]

Nazir, Y, Hussain, SA, Abdul Hamid, A & Song, Y (2018) Probiotics and their potential preventive and therapeutic role for cancer, high serum cholesterol, and allergic and HIV diseases. *BioMed Res Int,* 20183428437
[http://dx.doi.org/10.1155/2018/3428437] [PMID: 30246019]

Nouri, Z, Karami, F, Neyazi, N, Modarressi, MH, Karimi, R, Khorramizadeh, MR, Taheri, B & Motevaseli, E (2016) Dual anti-metastatic and anti-proliferative activity assessment of two probiotics on HeLa and HT-29 cell lines. *Cell J,* 18, 127-34.
[PMID: 27551673]

Nutini, LG, Sperti, GS, Fardon, JC, Duarte, AG & Freidel, JF (1982) Probiotics: nonantigenic tissue fractions in cancer control. *J Surg Oncol,* 19, 233-7.
[http://dx.doi.org/10.1002/jso.2930190412] [PMID: 7078176]

O'Mahony, SM, Marchesi, JR, Scully, P, Codling, C, Ceolho, AM, Quigley, EM, Cryan, JF & Dinan, TG (2009) Early life stress alters behavior, immunity, and microbiota in rats: implications for irritable bowel syndrome and psychiatric illnesses. *Biol Psychiatry,* 65, 263-7.
[http://dx.doi.org/10.1016/j.biopsych.2008.06.026] [PMID: 18723164]

Plantinga, TS, van Maren, WW, van Bergenhenegouwen, J, Hameetman, M, Nierkens, S, Jacobs, C, de Jong, DJ, Joosten, LA, van't Land, B, Garssen, J, Adema, GJ & Netea, MG (2011) Differential Toll-like receptor recognition and induction of cytokine profile by Bifidobacterium breve and Lactobacillus strains of probiotics. *Clin Vaccine Immunol,* 18, 621-8.
[http://dx.doi.org/10.1128/CVI.00498-10] [PMID: 21288993]

Pothoulakis, C (2009) Review article: anti-inflammatory mechanisms of action of Saccharomyces boulardii. *Aliment Pharmacol Ther,* 30, 826-33.
[http://dx.doi.org/10.1111/j.1365-2036.2009.04102.x] [PMID: 19706150]

Prabhurajeshwar, C & Chandrakanth, K (2019) Evaluation of antimicrobial properties and their substances against pathogenic bacteria *in-vitro* by probiotic Lactobacilli strains isolated from commercial yoghurt. *Clin Nutr Exp,* 23, 97-115.
[http://dx.doi.org/10.1016/j.yclnex.2018.10.001]

Rahal, A, Kumar, A, Singh, V, Yadav, B, Tiwari, R, Chakraborty, S & Dhama, K (2014) Oxidative stress, prooxidants, and antioxidants: the interplay. *BioMed Res Int,* 2014761264
[http://dx.doi.org/10.1155/2014/761264] [PMID: 24587990]

Reid, G, Bruce, AW, McGroarty, JA, Cheng, KJ & Costerton, JW (1990) Is there a role for lactobacilli in prevention of urogenital and intestinal infections? *Clin Microbiol Rev,* 3, 335-44.
[http://dx.doi.org/10.1128/CMR.3.4.335] [PMID: 2224835]

Rhee, SH, Pothoulakis, C & Mayer, EA (2009) Principles and clinical implications of the brain-gut-enteric microbiota axis. *Nat Rev Gastroenterol Hepatol,* 6, 306-14.
[http://dx.doi.org/10.1038/nrgastro.2009.35] [PMID: 19404271]

Rohlke, F & Stollman, N (2012) Fecal microbiota transplantation in relapsing Clostridium difficile infection. *Therap Adv Gastroenterol,* 5, 403-20.
[http://dx.doi.org/10.1177/1756283X12453637] [PMID: 23152734]

Roshan, H, Ghaedi, E, Rahmani, J, Barati, M, Najafi, M, Karimzedeh, M & Nikpayam, O (2019) Effects of

probiotics and synbiotic supplementation on antioxidant status: A meta-analysis of randomized clinical trials. *Clin Nutr ESPEN,* 30, 81-8.
[http://dx.doi.org/10.1016/j.clnesp.2019.02.003] [PMID: 30904233]

Ben Salah, R, Trabelsi, I, Hamden, K, Chouayekh, H & Bejar, S (2013) Lactobacillus plantarum TN8 exhibits protective effects on lipid, hepatic and renal profiles in obese rat. *Anaerobe,* 23, 55-61.
[http://dx.doi.org/10.1016/j.anaerobe.2013.07.003] [PMID: 23891961]

Sarkar, A, Lehto, SM, Harty, S, Dinan, TG, Cryan, JF & Burnet, PWJ (2016) Psychobiotics and the manipulation of bacteria–gut–brain signals. *Trends Neurosci,* 39, 763-81.
[http://dx.doi.org/10.1016/j.tins.2016.09.002] [PMID: 27793434]

Schlichte, MJ, Vandersall, A & Katta, R (2016) Diet and eczema: a review of dietary supplements for the treatment of atopic dermatitis. *Dermatol Pract Concept,* 6, 23-9.
[http://dx.doi.org/10.5826/dpc.0603a06] [PMID: 27648380]

Singh, VP, Sharma, J, Babu, S, Rizwanulla, SA & Singla, A (2013) Role of probiotics in health and disease: a review. *J Pak Med Assoc,* 63, 253-7.
[PMID: 23894906]

Sisein, EA (2014) Biochemistry of free radicals and antioxidants. *Scholars Acad J Biosci,* 2, 110-8.

Song, S, Lee, SJ, Park, DJ, Oh, S & Lim, KT (2016) The anti-allergic activity of Lactobacillus plantarum L67 and its application to yogurt. *J Dairy Sci,* 99, 9372-82.
[http://dx.doi.org/10.3168/jds.2016-11809] [PMID: 27743673]

Strus, M (1997) [The significance of lactic acid bacteria in treatment and prophylaxis of digestive tract disorders]. *Postepy Hig Med Dosw,* 51, 605-19.
[PMID: 9481894]

Takashima, M, Horie, M, Shichiri, M, Hagihara, Y, Yoshida, Y & Niki, E (2012) Assessment of antioxidant capacity for scavenging free radicals *in vitro* : a rational basis and practical application. *Free Radic Biol Med,* 52, 1242-52.
[http://dx.doi.org/10.1016/j.freeradbiomed.2012.01.010] [PMID: 22306582]

Tan, BL, Norhaizan, ME, Liew, WP & Sulaiman Rahman, H (2018) Antioxidant and oxidative stress: A mutual interplay in age-related diseases. *Front Pharmacol,* 9, 1162.
[http://dx.doi.org/10.3389/fphar.2018.01162] [PMID: 30405405]

Tannock, GW (1999) Probiotics: a critical review. *J Antimicrob Chemother,* 43, 849-52.
[http://dx.doi.org/10.1093/jac/43.6.849]

Tauber, AI (1992) The birth of immunology. III. The fate of the phagocytosis theory. *Cell Immunol,* 139, 505-30.
[http://dx.doi.org/10.1016/0008-8749(92)90089-8] [PMID: 1733516]

Teanpaisan, R & Piwat, S (2014) *Lactobacillus paracasei* SD1, a novel probiotic, reduces mutans streptococci in human volunteers: a randomized placebo-controlled trial. *Clin Oral Investig,* 18, 857-62.
[http://dx.doi.org/10.1007/s00784-013-1057-5] [PMID: 23892501]

Valko, M, Leibfritz, D, Moncol, J, Cronin, MT, Mazur, M & Telser, J (2007) Free radicals and antioxidants in normal physiological functions and human disease. *Int J Biochem Cell Biol,* 39, 44-84.
[http://dx.doi.org/10.1016/j.biocel.2006.07.001] [PMID: 16978905]

Vanderpool, C, Yan, F & Polk, DB (2008) Mechanisms of probiotic action: Implications for therapeutic applications in inflammatory bowel diseases. *Inflamm Bowel Dis,* 14, 1585-96.
[http://dx.doi.org/10.1002/ibd.20525] [PMID: 18623173]

Watanabe, T, Nishio, H, Tanigawa, T, Yamagami, H, Okazaki, H, Watanabe, K, Tominaga, K, Fujiwara, Y, Oshitani, N, Asahara, T, Nomoto, K, Higuchi, K, Takeuchi, K & Arakawa, T (2009) Probiotic Lactobacillus casei strain Shirota prevents indomethacin-induced small intestinal injury: involvement of lactic acid. *Am J Physiol Gastrointest Liver Physiol,* 297, G506-13.

[http://dx.doi.org/10.1152/ajpgi.90553.2008] [PMID: 19589943]

West, CE, Hammarström, ML & Hernell, O (2013) Probiotics in primary prevention of allergic disease--follow-up at 8-9 years of age. *Allergy,* 68, 1015-20.
[http://dx.doi.org/10.1111/all.12191] [PMID: 23895631]

Yatsunenko, T, Rey, FE, Manary, MJ, Trehan, I, Dominguez-Bello, MG, Contreras, M, Magris, M, Hidalgo, G, Baldassano, RN, Anokhin, AP & Heath, AC (2012) Human gut microbiome viewed across age and geography. *nature,* 486, 222-7.

Yunes, RA, Poluektova, EU, Vasileva, EV, Odorskaya, MV, Marsova, MV, Kovalev, GI & Danilenko, VN (2019) A Multi-strain Potential Probiotic Formulation of GABA-Producing Lactobacillus plantarum 90sk and Bifidobacterium adolescentis 150 with Antidepressant Effects. *Probiotics Antimicrob Proteins,* •••, 1-7.
[http://dx.doi.org/10.1007/s12602-019-09601-1] [PMID: 31677091]

Zokaeifar, H, Balcázar, JL, Saad, CR, Kamarudin, MS, Sijam, K, Arshad, A & Nejat, N (2012) Effects of Bacillus subtilis on the growth performance, digestive enzymes, immune gene expression and disease resistance of white shrimp, Litopenaeus vannamei. *Fish Shellfish Immunol,* 33, 683-9.
[http://dx.doi.org/10.1016/j.fsi.2012.05.027] [PMID: 22659618]

CHAPTER 11

Expression of miRNA in Regulating Cancer: Role of Phytoconstituents

Shivani Attri[1], **Prabhjot Kaur**[1], **Davinder Singh**[1], **Farhana Rashid**[1], **Harneetpal kaur**[1], **Avinash Kumar**[1], **Kirandeep Kaur**[2], **Neena Bedi**[2], **Balbir Singh**[2] and **Saroj Arora**[1,*]

[1] *Department of Botanical and Environmental Sciences, Guru Nanak Dev University, Amritsar, Punjab, India*

[2] *Department of Pharmaceutical Sciences, Guru Nanak Dev University, Amritsar, Punjab, India*

Abstract: MicroRNAs (miRNAs) are short, non-coding and functional 18-22 nucleotide sequences, which bind to 3' UTR region of the mRNA and modify mRNA expression by degrading them or modulating their translation process. Besides, miRNAs act as either suppressors or inducers of tumor depending upon binding with the target site. The action of miRNAs is reported for controlling the various important functions like metastasis, angiogenesis, apoptosis and tumor growth. They play an important role in suppressing cancer cell proliferation or invasion by targeting caspases and other factors involved in programmed cell death (apoptosis). So, the application of miRNA is proved to be a novel approach for cancer prevention. According to literature, numerous phytoconstituents isolated from medicinal plants or other botanicals modulate the functioning of different miRNAs which are involved in the pathology and biology of cancer. Therefore, the regulation of miRNA by botanicals or isolated compounds is a new model for researchers to develop/formulate a novel drug to combat this devastating disease. An attempt has been made in this chapter to explore the role of phytoconstituents to control the process of carcinogenesis targeting miRNAs.

Keywords: Apoptosis, Carcinogenesis, Metastasis, miRNA, Oxidative stress, Phytoconstituents, Proliferation, ROS.

INTRODUCTION

The human genome is a set of nucleotides that contains both coding as well as non-coding sequences. The total number of coding and non-coding genes is 19,000-20,000 and 46,831 respectively. Besides this, approximately 1.5% of the genome contains micro-RNA coding sequences. The first microRNA (miRNAs) was discovered by Victor Ambros laboratory in 1993 from *Caenorhabditis*

---

* **Corresponding author Saroj Arora:** Department of Botanical and Environmental Sciences, Guru Nanak Dev University, Amritsar, Punjab, India. E-mail: sarojarora.gndu@gmail.com

Pardeep Kaur, Rajendra G. Mehta, Robin, Tarunpreet Singh Thind and Saroj Arora (Eds.)

elegans (Peng and Croce 2016). miRNA are small group of non-coding sequences consisting of 19-22 nucleotides that regulate the various functions such as differentiation, development, cell proliferation, apoptosis, and stress responses. It may induce or suppress the tumor depending upon its specific binding sites to mRNA by its mature region called seed region (Ryan *et al.* 2010, Reddy 2010).

Mainly 50% miRNA genes are localized in cancer-associated genomic regions or the delicate sites which are prone to mutations (Bandyopadhyay *et al.* 2016). The mutations like amplification, deletion, epigenetic silencing and inhibition of transcription factors in the fragile region of miRNA lead to cancer of prostate, ovary, lungs, pancreas, tongue, colon, liver and diffuse large B-cell lymphoma as well as neurodegenerative disorders, cardiovascular diseases and viral conditions (Pan *et al.* 2010, Kosaka *et al.* 2010). The same kinds of miRNA may act as tumor suppressor genes depending upon their gene expression pattern. It has been reported that miRNA-29 is an oncogene in case of breast cancer whereas the same miRNA-29 acts as tumor suppressor gene in lung cancer. Furthermore, the loss of function of miRNA-23b leads to invasion and migration of bladder cancer cells but if the expression of same miRNA-29 gets knock down then it can reduce the invasion and in turn, promote apoptosis in renal cell carcinoma cell lines (Reddy 2010). The synthesis of miRNA takes place in two compartments *i.e.*, nucleus and cytoplasm. It involves various endonuclease enzymes like poly II, poly III and transcriptional factors (c-Myc, p53, MEF 2, PU.1 and REST) (Davis-Dusenbery *et al.* 2010). Any change or mutation in any type of transcriptional factors like c-Myc and p53 can induce different kinds of cancers. Besides this, miRNAs play a vital role in apoptosis. miRNAs modulate the cancer progression or suppression by targeting either extrinsic or intrinsic pathways of apoptosis. In this natural or programmed cell death, various intracellular and extracellular receptors are involved, which receive signal and transmit it to the effector caspases (cleave substrate at aspartic residue) involved in cell death. Due to their significant role in cancer initiation and proliferation, targeting miRNAs has been considered an effective treatment for cancer. According to literature, phytochemicals have a significant role in the intonation of miRNA expression which in turn directly affects tumor inducer, suppressor and cancer-related protein expression. So in this way, phytoconstituents inhibit tumor growth, suppress metastasis and reverse epithelial-mesenchymal transition *via* regulating miRNAs. Moreover, various phytoconstituents isolated from plants either singly or in a mixture may target different types of cancer by inhibiting oncogenes or inducing tumor suppressor genes to modulate cell proliferation. Modulating ROS production and oxidative stress by miRNAs is very crucial for the normal and better functioning of a cell. Due to the significant role of miRNAs in cancer initiation and proliferation coupled with the vital role of phytoconstituents in its inhibition, it is imperative to recognize the modulation of microRNA expression as the potential target for controlling the abnormal signaling pathways of cancer cells.

MICRO-RNA: BIOSYNTHESIS AND FUNCTION

Biogenesis of the human miRNA occurs in the nucleus and cytoplasm. The synthesis involves various enzymes and transcriptional factors that lead to the formation of a complete, mature and functional miRNA. The graphical presentation of the synthesis of miRNA is shown in Fig. (**1**). The transcription of intergenic miRNA containing both exons and introns is catalysed by poly II or poly III form pri-miRNA. The pri-mRNA having a stem-loop structure, single strands overhang at both ends complementary to the target sequence and forms functional miRNA. Then, RNAase and its cofactors *i.e.*, DROSHA and DGCR8 lead to the formation of pre-miRNA consisting of 70 nucleotides sequence and stem-loop structure (Hogg *et al.* 2014, Suzuki *et al.* 2012, Hata *et al.* 2015). This precursor product (pre-miRNA) moves to the cytoplasm for further processing by Exportin 5 and RNA-GTP. In the cytoplasm, the stem-loop structure of pre-miRNA is cleaved by RNAase DICER and double-stranded RNA binding protein TRBP which result in the formation of 22 nucleotides containing functional double-stranded RNA. Then this double-stranded RNA is cleaved by enzyme helicase into two single-stranded RNA. One strand is degraded and the other strand is mainly bound to RISC (RNA Inducing Silencing Complex) and performs numerous functions like mRNA cleavage, translational activation and translational repression. The selection and rejection of the miRNA strand is mainly dependent upon the thermal stability of the strand (Iorio and Croce 2012). The mature and functional sequence of the miRNA is highly conserved among species and it regulates various functions such as apoptosis, development, differentiation and cell proliferation (Suzuki *et al.* 2013). Mutation in any step of miRNA synthesis *i.e.* mutations in the promoter region, functional enzyme, transcriptional factors (Drosha, Dicer1, TARBP2 and XPO5), growth factor receptors, chromatin remodelling and any change in apoptosis regulators or signal transducers lead to various types of cancer (Jansson *et al.* 2012, MacFarlane *et al.* 2010).

miRNAs as Oncogene and Tumor Suppressor Gene

Cancer is an uncontrolled division of cells in which normal cells transform into malignant cells due to changes in genetic material. The development of cancer involves multiple biological networks which include: hyper proliferation of tissues, self-sustained growth factors, insensitivity of growth signals, anti-apoptotic activity, induced angiogenesis, replicative immortality, invasion and metastasis. Any mutation/change in miRNAs may function as a tumor suppressor (gain-of-function mutation) or oncogene (loss-of-function mutation) depending upon the target (Iorio and Croce 2012).

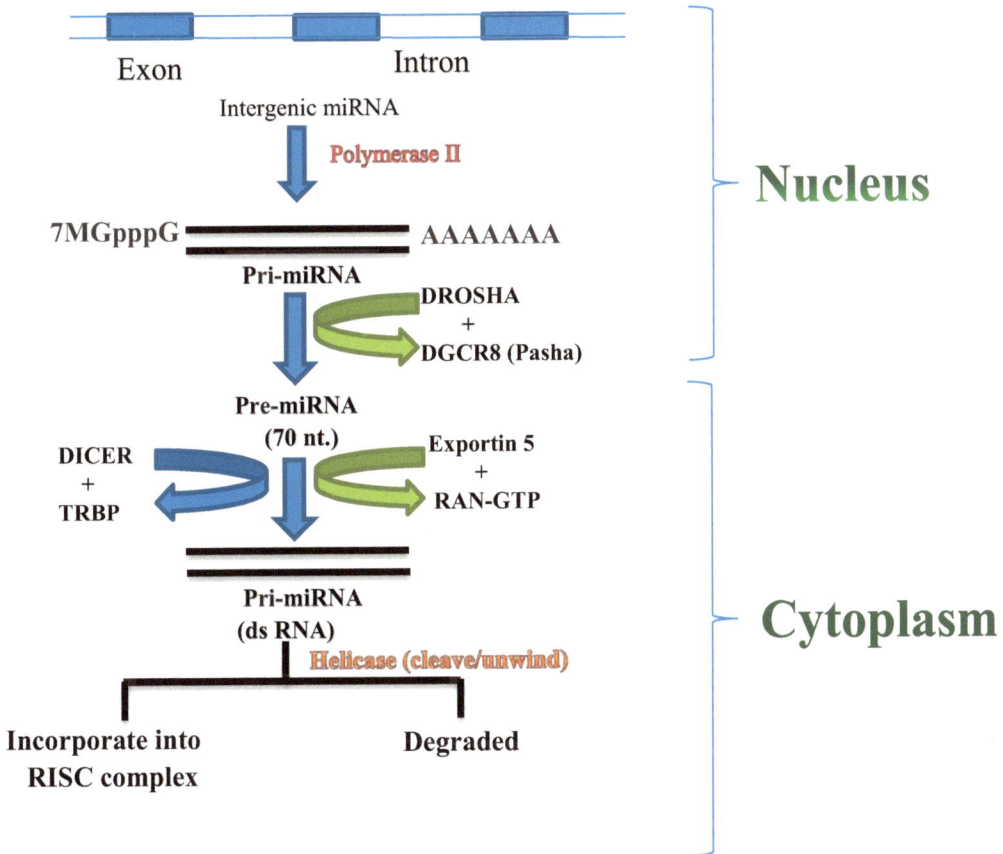

Fig. (1). Biogenesis of miRNA.

Major causes of miRNAs mutations are DNA methylation and histone modification (Suzuki *et al.* 2013). Therefore, dysregulation of miRNAs expression leads to the initiation, regulation and proliferation of tumors as well as angiogenesis, invasiveness, metastasis and even drug resistance in some cases of cancer (Ross *et al.* 2011). miRNA-21 which acts as an oncogene targets tropomyosin 1 programmed cell death 4 and phosphate and tensin homologue in different cancer cells while let-7 targets RAS, CDC25A, CDK6, whereas mir-15a and mir-16-1 downregulate the expression of BCL-2 gene (Babashah *et al.* 2011). Moreover, the miRNA (miR-127-3p, miR-148b, miR-4093p, miR-652, and miR-801) are the biomarkers to identify the onset or progression of breast cancer in women. These miRNAs are reported to be deregulated in the plasma of women having breast cancer (Cuk *et al.* 2013). Adding on, the miRNA-127 regulates the level of Rtl1 gene through RNAi-mediated post-transcriptional degradation. The knockdown of miRNA-127 in mice has been reported to cause defects associated with labyrinthine zone involved in maternal fetal nutrient transfer (Ito *et al.* 2015). Furthermore, down regulation of miRNA-127 after the partial hepatectomy due to methylation of its promoter genes facilitates the release of BCL-6 and Setd8 (Pan *et al.* 2012) miR-127, miR-205 and miR-218 are highly expressive and hence are the promising tumor markers in cervical cancer (You *et al.* 2015). The miR-12-3p has also been reported to be suppressed in giant cell tumor of bone *via* COA1 pathway (Fellenberg *et al.* 2016).

Role of miRNAs in Programmed Cell Death (Apoptosis)

Apoptosis is defined as programmed cell death which involves some morphological changes in cells like cellular shrinkage, plasma membrane blebbing, condensation of chromatin and nuclear fragmentation. This is a gene regulated process in which any mutation/change/disturbance leads to various human cancers, autoimmune disorders and neurogenerative diseases (Lowe *et al.* 2000). Caspases are reported to have an important function to cut peptide sequence of aspartic residue on its carboxyl side. There are 14 types of caspases, in which some act as initiators and others are effectors or executioners (Strasser *et al.* 2000). In the recent past, miRNAs have been found to play a key role in the modulation of cancer through apoptosis. miR-21 acts as an oncogene and promotes cell proliferation, angiogenesis, immortal replication and resists programmed cell death. Its overexpression inhibits the binding of Pdcd4 with eIF4e, resulting in increased invasion in colorectal cancer cells (Buscaglia *et al.* 2011). Despite this, miR-21 targets various other markers like SPRY1 and SPRY2, PTEN, TPM1, RECK, BCL-2, SMARCA4, THRB, and FASLG which lead to tumor progression by acting on extrinsic/intrinsic pathways of cell death. Similarly, Glioblastoma (GBM) is one of the dangerous brain cancers with no curative treatment. The expression of miR-211 in GBM is epigenetically suppressed when the promoter region is methylated. The expression of miR-211 and MMP-9 (pM) is inversely related to each other. Overexpression of miR-211 and treatment of pM lead to activation of intrinsic mitochondrial/Caspase-9/-mediated apoptotic pathway in glioma cells as well as cancer stem cells (Asuthkar *et al.* 2012). Besides these miRNAs, miR-146a also regulates osteoarthritis pathogenesis by targeting the apoptotic pathway. Overexpression of IL-1β responsive miR-146a leads to upregulation of VEGF, downregulation of Smad4 *via* impairment of TGF-β signaling pathway and induces apoptosis of chondrocytes (Li *et al.* 2012). Further, the expression of anti-apoptotic protein Bcl-xL is also negatively regulated by the let-7 miRNAs (let-7c or let-7g) in hepatocellular carcinoma. Moreover, in the presence of an anti-cancer drug that target Mcl-1 (another Bcl-2 protein), the overexpression of let-7c leads to the enhanced apoptosis of cancer cells with downregulation of Mcl-1 expression (Shimizu *et al.* 2010). Also, the overexpressed miR-221 and miR-222 significantly augment the antiproliferative effect by apoptotic induction in gastrointestinal stromal tumors (GISTs) *via* signalling cascade encompassing KIT, Akt and Bcl-2 (Ihle *et al.* 2015). Conclusively, various types of miRNAs are involved in the modulation of signaling pathways *via* targeting numerous pro-apoptotic and anti-apoptotic genes in cancer.

ROLE OF VARIOUS PHYTOCONSTITUENTS IN MODULATING THE CANCER BY TARGETING MIRNAS

Many phyto-based extracts, fractions and even single active constituent have been reported to possess a superlative anticancer activity. In the study conducted by Subramaniam *et al.* (2012), curcumin downregulated the Notch-1 specific microRNAs such as miR-21 and miR-34a with increased expression of let-7a miRNA leading to the apoptosis of esophageal cancer cells. In another study, curcumin also induced apoptosis and inhibited the growth of the pancreatic cancer cells *via* downregulation of miR-22 and overexpression of miRNA199a (Subramaniam *et al.* 2012). Moreover, the potent phytoconstituent and histone deacetylase inhibitor, sulforaphane, obtained from the cruciferous vegetables demonstrated the excellent anti-cancer activity in colorectal cells by downregulating the oncogenic miRNAs *i.e.*, miR-21, hTERT and HDAC (Martin *et al.* 2018). Another potential use of sulforaphane is observed by suppression of gastric carcinoma by alterating miR-9, miR-326, CDX1 and CDX2 expression (Kiani *et al.* 2018). Furthermore, isoflavone genistein known as an anti-angiogenic agent is involved in the knockdown of miR-21 and induced overexpression of p-21 and p-38 MAP kinase genes, which lead to apoptosis of renal cancer cells with reduced migration, invasion and induced cell cycle arrest *via* inhibition of cyclin E2 (Zaman *et al.* 2012).

Table 1. Involvement of various kind of microRNAs in cancer progression in different organs.

MiRNA	Tissue/cell line	Markers/mechanism Involved	Location of Cancer	References
miRNA-127	MHCC97H cells		Liver cancer	(Yang *et al.* 2013b, Tryndyak *et al.* 2009)
	OVCAR-3, Caov-3, SKOV-3, ES-2, PA-4 and HS-832 (non-tumorogenic)		Ovarian cancer	(Bi *et al.* 2016)
	TE-1 ECA109		Esophageal cancer	(Gao *et al.* 2016)
	CaPan-1, PANC-1	BAG-5 (target gene)	Pancreatic cancer	(Yu *et al.* 2016)

(Table 1) cont.....

MiRNA	Tissue/cell line	Markers/mechanism Involved	Location of Cancer	References
miRNA-127	MHCC97H cells		Liver cancer	(Yang *et al.* 2013, Tryndyak *et al.* 2009)
	OVCAR-3, Caov-3, SKOV-3, ES-2, PA-4 and HS-832 (non-tumorogenic)		Ovarian cancer	(Bi *et al.* 2016)
	TE-1 ECA109		Esophageal cancer	(Gao *et al.* 2016)
	CaPan-1, PANC-1	BAG-5 (target gene)	Pancreatic cancer	(Yu *et al.* 2016)
	GCTB	miRNA-127-3P, miRNA-376-3P COA1/PD1A6 Reduce tumor colonisation	Bone Tumor	(Herr *et al.* 2017)
	W1-38, IMR-90	miRNA BCL-6/Cyclin D1 Arrest G0/G1 phase Increase cellular senescence/aging	Cellular senescence/aging	(Chen *et al.* 2013)
	MCF-7, MDA-MB-231	miRNA BCL-6/Cyclin D1 Dephosphorylation of PRb at Sar 780 Reduce breast cancer progression	Breast cancer	(Cuk *et al.* 2013, Wang *et al.* 2014)
	HEP-G2		Hepatic cancer	(Willers *et al.* 2012)
	MHCC97H MHCC97L		Hepatic cancer	(Pan *et al.* 2012)
	LN229, T98G		Glioblastoma	(Jiang *et al.* 2014)
	HGC-27	miRNA-127 Integration with oncogenic cell factors such as KRAS and MAPK4 Progression of cell cycle Migration and invasion of cells	Gastric cancer	(Guo *et al.* 2013)
	HT3C33A,SiHa	miRNA-127 binds with FOXD and upregulates POU3F3 Knockdown of non coding RNA (lncRNA POU3F3) Later one leads to multiplication and metastasis of cervical tumor cells	Cervical cancer	(Chang *et al.* 2019)
	------------	PIK3R1 pathway	Bladder cancer	(Xu *et al.* 2015)
	MG-63, OS-732, SaOS, G292, and 143B and hFOB1.19	Target gene of miRNA-127 is ZEB1. Overexpression of miRNA-127 results impairs cell growth and metastasis, whereas process reversed when ZEB1 is overexpressed.	Osteosarcoma	(Wang and Kong 2018)
	ESCC cell lines and normal esophageal epithelium cell line	Regulation of oncogene FMNL3	Esophageal squamous cell carcinoma	(Gao *et al.* 2016)

(Table 1) cont.....

MiRNA	Tissue/cell line	Markers/mechanism Involved	Location of Cancer	References
miRNA-21	----------		Non-small cell lung cancer	(Yang *et al.* 2013a)
	MDA-MB-468 (Triple negative breast cancer cells)	miR-21 downregulates PTEN proliferation and invasion of cells miR-21 antisense oligonucleotides inhibit the overexpression of miR-21	Breast cancer	(Fang *et al.* 2017, Chen and Bourguignon 2014)
miRNA-17-92	SW480 and HT29	c-myc induced apoptosis	Colon cancer	(Tsuchida *et al.* 2011)
	CCLP1, SG231, HuCCT1, and TFK1, and human cholangiocyte cell line (H69)		Cholangiocarcinoma	(Zhu *et al.* 2014)
	SHEP-TR-miR-17-92 and SHEP-TR cells		Neuroblastoma	(Mestdagh *et al.* 2010)
	KMS28PE, OCI-My5 and XG1 cell lines		Multiple myeloma	(Chen *et al.* 2011)
miRNA-155	HeLa and SiHa cells	miR-155↑ Target LKB1↓ (Tumor suppressor gene) Cervical cancer	Cervical cancer	(Lao *et al.* 2014)
	MDA-MB-231 cells		Breast cancer	(Jiang *et al.* 2012, Jiang *et al.* 2010, Sun *et al.* 2012)
	MCF-7	Ki-67↑ and p53↓ resulted miR-155↑ showed high proliferative activity and decreased apoptotic capability	Breast cancer	(Liu *et al.* 2013, Sochor *et al.* 2014)
	MKN45	IL-6/STAT3 pathway	Gastric carcinoma	(Han *et al.* 2015)
	----------	Downregulation of SOCS1 gene, Caspase-3 and TP53BP1	lung cancer (NSCLC)	(Yang *et al.* 2013a)

(Table 1) cont.....

MiRNA	Tissue/cell line	Markers/mechanism Involved	Location of Cancer	References
miRNA-126	HEK293 cells and MCF-7, MDA-MB-231	miR-126 (overexpression) IRS-1 (translation level) Inhibit cell growth in cancerous cell lines	Breast cancer	(Zhang *et al.* 2008)
	HT-29, HCT-116, SW480 and SW620	miRNA-126 target VEGF and downregulates its expression and results in inhibition of cell proliferation, metastasis and angiogenesis	Colorectal carcinoma	(Zhou *et al.* 2013, Zhang *et al.* 2013)
	NCI-N87, SGC-7901, BGC-823, MKN-45 AGS and MKN-28	miR-126↑ Crk↓ Inhibit gastric cancer	Gastric cancer	(Feng *et al.* 2010)
	ASPC-1, MiaPaca-2, BxPC3, Panc-1, and KLM-1	miR-126 target ADAM9 and results in reduced cellular migration, invasion, and induction of epithelial marker E-cadherin	Pancreatic Cancer	(Hamada *et al.* 2012)
	H226 (squamous), A549 (adenocarcinoma), H1703 (squamous), H358 (bronchoalveolar cell), and DMS 53 (small cell)	miR-126 targets Crk and results in reduction in adhesion, migration, and invasion	Non-small cell lung carcinoma	(Crawford *et al.* 2008)
miRNA-335	-----------	MiR-335 targets the SOX4 and extracellular matrix component tenascin C	Breast cancer	(Yang *et al.* 2011)
	PC-3	MiR-335 and MiR-543 mutate seed region of eNOS	Prostate cancer	(Fu *et al.* 2015)
	-------------	Expression of MiR-335 in Primary gall bladder carcinoma patients is lower as compared to the non-PGC patients	Gall bladder carcinoma	(Peng *et al.* 2013)
	RWPE-1 (non-malignant epithelial prostate cell line) and DU145, LNCaP and PC-3	miR-335 is directly leads to prostate cancer when its activity is low but their overexpression suppress tumor proliferation, penetration and relocation of prostate tumor cells	Prostate cancer	(Xiong *et al.* 2013)
	SW480, HT29, SW620, and LOVO	miR-335 directly target the 3'UTR luciferase reporter ZEB2 gene	Colorectal cancer	(Sun *et al.* 2014)
miRNA-34	BJ, A549, NCI-H460, NCI-H596, Calu-3, NCI-H1650, SW-900, HCC2935, NCI-H226, NCI-H1299, NCI-H522, TE353.sk and Wi-38.	MiR-34 act as a tumor suppressor	Lung cancer	(Wiggins *et al.* 2010)
	Lung epithelial cells	miR-34a target Met and BCL-2 genes	Lung Adenocarcinoma	(Kasinski and Slack 2012)
	SNU-5 and HGC27	Increase in phosphorylated EGFR and MMP7	Gastric cancer	(Liu *et al.* 2014)
	MCF-7, MDA-MB-231)	MiR-34a targets both BCL-2 and CCND1 in docetaxel-resistant cells	Breast cancer	(Kastl *et al.* 2012)

(Table 1) cont.....

MiRNA	Tissue/cell line	Markers/mechanism Involved	Location of Cancer	References
miRNA-205	MCF-7	Induce apoptosis	Breast cancer	(Liu *et al.* 2013)

In another study by Lin *et al.* (2018), the mushroom extract of *Antrodia cinnamomea* inhibited the growth of tamoxifen-resistant breast cancer cells *via* suppressing the mRNA expression of skp2 by augmenting the miR-26-5p, miR-30-5p and miR21-5p expression. Furthermore, the *Urtica dioica* extract inhibited breast cancer cell migration by downregulating the expression of miR-21, MMP1, MMP9, MMP13, vimentin and CXCR-4 and increased E-cadherin expression (Mansoori *et al.* 2017). On similar lines the extract of *Ilex rotunda* containing caffeic acid showed an anti-cancerous potential against colitis associated cancer *via* downregulation of TNF-α and IL-6 as well as restoration of the miR-31-5p level (Chen *et al.* 2019). The kanglaite injection (extracted from *Coixla crymajobi*) administered to patients with advanced lung cancer resisted the growth of lungs cancer cells by downregulating miR-21 expression (Wu *et al.* 2018). On similar lines, the proliferation of lung cancer cells was also inhibited by the *Artemesino liveriana* extract *via* change in miR-192s expression and other associated genes such as Bax, BCL-2, Caspase-3 and Caspase-9 (Fard *et al.* 2018). Conclusively, many plant based products such oleuropin from *Olea europaea* leaves, extract of *Stellera chamaejasme*, grape seed proanthocyanidins extract, extract fraction of *Phaleria marocarpa* fruit, Nimbolide (a limonoid from *Azadirachta indica*) and extract fraction of *Scutellaria barbata* have been reported to inhibit glioblastoma, hepatocellular carcinoma, pancreatic cancer, breast cancer, oral cancer, colorectal cancer and lung cancer respectively *via* modulation of miRNA expression (Tezcan *et al.* 2019, Liu *et al.* 2018, Ma *et al.* 2015, Kavitha *et al.* 2018, Kavitha *et al.* 2018, Zhang *et al.* 2017, Mao *et al.* 2016). Considering the data in Table **1** and **2**, the modulation of miRNA seems to play a major role in the progression/suppression of various types of cancer.

Table 2. Role of phytoconstituents in different cancer by targeting miRNA.

S.No.	Phytoconstituent	miRNA Involved	Target Cancer	References
1	Curcumin	Downregulate: miR-21 and miR-34 Upregulate: let-7a miRNA	Esophageal cancer	(Subramaniam *et al.* 2012)
2	Curcumin	Downregulate: miR22 Overexpress: miRNA 199a	Pancreatic cancer	(Subramaniam *et al.* 2012)
3	Sulforaphane	Downregulate: miR-21, hTERT, HDAC	Colorectal cancer	(Martin *et al.* 2018)
4	Sulforaphane	miR-9, miR-326	Gastric carcinoma	(Kiani *et al.* 2018)

(Table 2) cont.....

S.No.	Phytoconstituent	miRNA Involved	Target Cancer	References
5	Isoflavone genistein	Downregulate: miR-21	Renal Carcinoma	(Zaman *et al.* 2012)
6	*Antrodia cinnamomea* extract	Overexpression: miR-2--5p, miR-30-5p, miR21-5p	Tamoxifen-resistant breast cancer	(Lin *et al.* 2018)
7	*Urtica dioica* extract	Downregulate: miR-21	Breast Cancer	(Mansoori *et al.* 2017)
8	*Ilex rotunda* extract (Caffeic acid)	Upregulate: miR-31-5p	Colitis associated cancer	(Chen *et al.* 2019)
9	*Coixla crymajobi* extract	Downregulation: miR-21	Lung Cancer	(Wu *et al.* 2018)
10	*Artemesino liveriana* extract	miR-192	Lung Cancer	(Fard *et al.* 2018)
11	Oleuropin	miRNA modulation	Glioblastoma	(Tezcan *et al.* 2019)

ROLE OF MIRNAS IN MODULATION OF OXIDATIVE STRESS AND ROS PRODUCTION

Oxidative stress is a physiological condition which may arise due to two reasons, first the overabundance of free radicals and second the imbalance of antioxidant defense system (Betteridge 2000). However, in most cases, both reasons collectively enhance oxidative stress in different diseases. These free radicals can also generated in large amounts as an unavoidable secondary product of many biochemical processes. Immune cells also generate free radicals in order to kill or neutralize alien cells and antigens. Environmental electromagnetic radiations are another cause for the generation of free radicals.

These free radicals are of diverse nature chemical species that contain singlet/unpaired electrons in their valance shell. These unpaired electrons are very reactive and can donate their free electron to other molecules and ultimately make them more unstable. These free radicals include hydroxyl radicals ($^{\cdot}OH$), superoxide anions ($O_2^{\cdot-}$), transition metals, nitric oxide ($NO^{\cdot}$) and peroxynitrite ($ONOO^{-}$). These all contain oxygen atoms and hence also known as reactive oxygen species (ROS). The generation of ROS is regulated through homeostasis under normal physiological conditions but imbalance under certain circumstances lead to disease. Under homeostatic conditions, free radicals are produced by several biochemical processes including reduction of molecular oxygen during aerobic respiration, by-product of chemical reactions during metabolism, production of hypochlorous acid by activated phagocytes during an immune response, production of nitric oxide by vascular endothelium and many more. These radicals are captured by various enzymes and natural products known as antioxidants and convert them to more stable form in the microenvironment. Production of excessive ROS and insufficient antioxidant response can play a role in stroke, myocardial infarction, diabetic vasculopathy, atherosclerosis, heart failure, hypercholesterolemia, systematic and pulmonary hypertension, pulmonary fibrosis and cancer (Napoli *et al.* 2001, Madamanchi *et al.* 2005, Irani 2000, Giorgio *et al.* 2007).

Different stimuli including UV, H_2O_2, ionizing radiations, and anticancer drugs are believed to modulate the expression of micro RNA (miRNA) during oxidative stress (Simone *et al.* 2009, Magenta *et al.* 2011). These bind to 3'-UTR, 5'-UTR and exons of the mRNA target (Vishnoi *et al.* 2017, Ørom *et al.* 2008). The incomplete complementation suppresses the translation while complete complementation hydrolyzes the target mRNA (Drusco *et al.* 2017). miRNA regulates a number of biological processes under homeostatic conditions such as differentiation, cell division, migration and apoptosis. MiRNA-1 targets superoxide dismutase (SOD) for post-transcriptional repression which contributes to increased ROS levels and ultimately oxidative stress (Wang *et al.* 2015). miRNA-21 decreases the function of SOD-2 in angiogenic progenitor cell (APC) of patients with coronary artery disease (CAD) (Fleissner *et al.* 2010). Similarly, miRNA-141 and miRNA-200a targets p38α and enhance associated oxidative stress signature in the mouse model (Mateescu *et al.* 2011). miRNAs also act as tumor suppressors by inhibiting hypoxia-inducible factor-1α. miRNA-153 reduces the proliferation and angiogenesis in MDA-MB-231 cells *via* inhibition of HIF-1α (Nagpal *et al.* 2015). ROS induced miRNA-128a targets Bmi-1 oncogene responsible for mitochondrial function and homeostasis (Venkataraman *et al.* 2010). miRNA-212 targets SOD2 resulting in the upregulation of ROS production, which ultimately mask the epithelial to mesenchymal transition and metastasis in colorectal cells (Meng *et al.* 2013). By contrast, the knockout miRNA-212 cells with stand oxidative stress due to sufficient supply of SOD2 and hence poor prognosis and more aggressive tumor phenotype. Conclusively, in the last decade, redox-dependent regulation come-up with a central aspect of the regulation of homeostasis and the role of miRNA in this process. The interplay between the ROS production on miRNA regulation and the ROS action *via* miRNA expression is very important for the functioning of the cell. It regulates the ratio between the ROS production system and the antioxidant defense system. It is also important for the understanding of miRNA involvement in response to chemotherapeutic drugs.

CONCLUSION

In the recent past, various mechanisms, signaling pathways including various genes, enzymes and nucleotides involved in a different type of cancers have been explored extensively. Among the above, the small non-coding peptides *i.e.* miRNA has emerged as a key part in cancer progression/suppression. Different types of miRNA are involved in the cancer-associated pathways. Although, some of which upregulates the proliferation of cancerous cell and others may demonstrate the opposite effect. The altered expressions of miRNA lead to cancer cell death/proliferation by modulation of apoptosis, oxidative stress, and reactive oxygen species. Moreover, the phytoconstituents also play a major role in cancer progression/suppression *via* miRNA modulation. Hence, the more focused exploration of these miRNAs in the future can give the researchers a precise view of progression/suppression of cancer cells which in turn will be helpful in the treatment of cancer.

CONFLICT OF INTEREST

The authors declare that there are no conflicts of interest.

ACKNOWLEDGMENT

We are grateful to the DST-INSPIRE (Department of Science & Technology); dated (04/10/2018) and CSIR-JRF (Council of Scientific & Industrial Research); dated (01/01/2019) for providing fellowship and special thanks to the Department of Botanical and Environmental Sciences for providing necessary facilities and support.

CONSENT FOR PUBLICATION

None

REFERENCES

Asuthkar, S, Velpula, KK, Chetty, C, Gorantla, B & Rao, JS (2012) Epigenetic regulation of miRNA-211 by MMP-9 governs glioma cell apoptosis, chemosensitivity and radiosensitivity. *Oncotarget,* 3, 1439-54.
[http://dx.doi.org/10.18632/oncotarget.683] [PMID: 23183822]

Babashah, S & Soleimani, M (2011) The oncogenic and tumour suppressive roles of microRNAs in cancer and apoptosis. *Eur J Cancer,* 47, 1127-37.
[http://dx.doi.org/10.1016/j.ejca.2011.02.008] [PMID: 21402473]

Bandyopadhyay, S, Mitra, R, Maulik, U & Zhang, MQ (2010) Development of the human cancer microRNA network. *Silence,* 1, 6.
[http://dx.doi.org/10.1186/1758-907X-1-6] [PMID: 20226080]

Betteridge, DJ (2000) What is oxidative stress? *Metabolism,* 49 (Suppl. 1), 3-8.
[http://dx.doi.org/10.1016/S0026-0495(00)80077-3] [PMID: 10693912]

Bi, L, Yang, Q, Yuan, J, Miao, Q, Duan, L, Li, F & Wang, S (2016) MicroRNA-127-3p acts as a tumor suppressor in epithelial ovarian cancer by regulating the BAG5 gene. *Oncol Rep,* 36, 2563-70.

[http://dx.doi.org/10.3892/or.2016.5055] [PMID: 27571744]

Buscaglia, LE & Li, Y (2011) Apoptosis and the target genes of microRNA-21. *Chin J Cancer,* 30, 371-80.
[http://dx.doi.org/10.5732/cjc.30.0371] [PMID: 21627859]

Chang, S, Sun, L & Feng, G (2019) SP1-mediated long noncoding RNA POU3F3 accelerates the cervical cancer through miR-127-5p/FOXD1. *Biomed Pharmacother,* 117109133
[http://dx.doi.org/10.1016/j.biopha.2019.109133] [PMID: 31252264]

Chen, G, Han, Y, Feng, Y, Wang, A, Li, X, Deng, S, Zhang, L, Xiao, J, Li, Y & Li, N (2019) Extract of Ilex rotunda Thunb alleviates experimental colitis-associated cancer *via* suppressing inflammation-induced miR-31-5p/YAP overexpression. *Phytomedicine,* 62152941
[http://dx.doi.org/10.1016/j.phymed.2019.152941] [PMID: 31100679]

Chen, J, Wang, M, Guo, M, Xie, Y & Cong, YS (2013) miR-127 regulates cell proliferation and senescence by targeting BCL6. *PLoS One,* 8e80266
[http://dx.doi.org/10.1371/journal.pone.0080266] [PMID: 24282530]

Chen, L & Bourguignon, LY (2014) Hyaluronan-CD44 interaction promotes c-Jun signaling and miRNA21 expression leading to Bcl-2 expression and chemoresistance in breast cancer cells. *Mol Cancer,* 13, 52.
[http://dx.doi.org/10.1186/1476-4598-13-52] [PMID: 24606718]

Chen, L, Li, C, Zhang, R, Gao, X, Qu, X, Zhao, M, Qiao, C, Xu, J & Li, J (2011) miR-17-92 cluster microRNAs confers tumorigenicity in multiple myeloma. *Cancer Lett,* 309, 62-70.
[http://dx.doi.org/10.1016/j.canlet.2011.05.017] [PMID: 21664042]

Crawford, M, Brawner, E, Batte, K, Yu, L, Hunter, MG, Otterson, GA, Nuovo, G, Marsh, CB & Nana-Sinkam, SP (2008) MicroRNA-126 inhibits invasion in non-small cell lung carcinoma cell lines. *Biochem Biophys Res Commun,* 373, 607-12.
[http://dx.doi.org/10.1016/j.bbrc.2008.06.090] [PMID: 18602365]

Cuk, K, Zucknick, M, Madhavan, D, Schott, S, Golatta, M, Heil, J, Marmé, F, Turchinovich, A, Sinn, P, Sohn, C, Junkermann, H, Schneeweiss, A & Burwinkel, B (2013) Plasma microRNA panel for minimally invasive detection of breast cancer. *PLoS One,* 8e76729
[http://dx.doi.org/10.1371/journal.pone.0076729] [PMID: 24194846]

Davis-Dusenbery, BN & Hata, A (2010) MicroRNA in cancer: the involvement of aberrant microRNA biogenesis regulatory pathways. *Genes Cancer,* 1, 1100-14.
[http://dx.doi.org/10.1177/1947601910396213] [PMID: 21533017]

Drusco, A & Croce, CM (2017) *MicroRNAs and cancer: a long story for short RNAs*

Fang, H, Xie, J, Zhang, M, Zhao, Z, Wan, Y & Yao, Y (2017) miRNA-21 promotes proliferation and invasion of triple-negative breast cancer cells through targeting PTEN. *Am J Transl Res,* 9, 953-61.
[PMID: 28386324]

Fard, NN, Noorbazargan, H, Mirzaie, A, Hedayati Ch, M, Moghimiyan, Z & Rahimi, A (2018) Biogenic synthesis of AgNPs using Artemisia oliveriana extract and their biological activities for an effective treatment of lung cancer. *Artif Cells Nanomed Biotechnol,* 46, S1047-58.
[http://dx.doi.org/10.1080/21691401.2018.1528983] [PMID: 30479160]

Fellenberg, J, Sähr, H, Kunz, P, Zhao, Z, Liu, L, Tichy, D & Herr, I (2016) Restoration of miR-127-3p and miR-376a-3p counteracts the neoplastic phenotype of giant cell tumor of bone derived stromal cells by targeting COA1, GLE1 and PDIA6. *Cancer Lett,* 371, 134-41.
[http://dx.doi.org/10.1016/j.canlet.2015.10.039] [PMID: 26655997]

Feng, R, Chen, X, Yu, Y, Su, L, Yu, B, Li, J, Cai, Q, Yan, M, Liu, B & Zhu, Z (2010) miR-126 functions as a tumour suppressor in human gastric cancer. *Cancer Lett,* 298, 50-63.
[http://dx.doi.org/10.1016/j.canlet.2010.06.004] [PMID: 20619534]

Fleissner, F, Jazbutyte, V, Fiedler, J, Galuppo, P, Mayr, M, Ertl, G, Bauersachs, J & Thum, T (2010) The endogenous NO synthase inhibitor asymmetric dimethylarginine impairs angiogenic progenitor cell function in patients with coronary artery disease through a microRNA dependent mechanism. *Cardiovasc Res,* 87, 45-

88.

Fu, Q, Liu, X, Liu, Y, Yang, J, Lv, G & Dong, S (2015) MicroRNA-335 and -543 suppress bone metastasis in prostate cancer *via* targeting endothelial nitric oxide synthase. *Int J Mol Med,* 36, 1417-25.
[http://dx.doi.org/10.3892/ijmm.2015.2355] [PMID: 26647850]

Gao, X, Wang, X, Cai, K, Wang, W, Ju, Q, Yang, X, Wang, H & Wu, H (2016) MicroRNA-127 is a tumor suppressor in human esophageal squamous cell carcinoma through the regulation of oncogene FMNL3. *Eur J Pharmacol,* 791, 603-10.
[http://dx.doi.org/10.1016/j.ejphar.2016.09.025] [PMID: 27645894]

Giorgio, M, Trinei, M, Migliaccio, E & Pelicci, PG (2007) Hydrogen peroxide: a metabolic by-product or a common mediator of ageing signals? *Nat Rev Mol Cell Biol,* 8, 722-8.
[http://dx.doi.org/10.1038/nrm2240] [PMID: 17700625]

Guo, LH, Li, H, Wang, F, Yu, J & He, JS (2013) The tumor suppressor roles of miR-433 and miR-127 in gastric cancer. *Int J Mol Sci,* 14, 14171-84.
[http://dx.doi.org/10.3390/ijms140714171] [PMID: 23880861]

Hamada, S, Satoh, K, Fujibuchi, W, Hirota, M, Kanno, A, Unno, J, Masamune, A, Kikuta, K, Kume, K & Shimosegawa, T (2012) MiR-126 acts as a tumor suppressor in pancreatic cancer cells *via* the regulation of ADAM9. *Mol Cancer Res,* 10, 3-10.
[http://dx.doi.org/10.1158/1541-7786.MCR-11-0272] [PMID: 22064652]

Han, S, Yang, S, Cai, Z, Pan, D, Li, Z, Huang, Z, Zhang, P, Zhu, H, Lei, L & Wang, W (2015) Anti-Warburg effect of rosmarinic acid *via* miR-155 in gastric cancer cells. *Drug Des Devel Ther,* 9, 2695-703.
[PMID: 26056431]

Hata, A & Lieberman, J (2015) Dysregulation of microRNA biogenesis and gene silencing in cancer. *Sci Signal,* 8, re3.
[http://dx.doi.org/10.1126/scisignal.2005825] [PMID: 25783160]

Herr, I, Sähr, H, Zhao, Z, Yin, L, Omlor, G, Lehner, B & Fellenberg, J (2017) MiR-127 and miR-376a act as tumor suppressors by *in vivo* targeting of COA1 and PDIA6 in giant cell tumor of bone. *Cancer Lett,* 409, 49-55.
[http://dx.doi.org/10.1016/j.canlet.2017.08.029] [PMID: 28866093]

Hogg, DR & Harries, LW (2014) Human genetic variation and its effect on miRNA biogenesis, activity and function. *Biochem Soc Trans,* 42, 1184-9.
[http://dx.doi.org/10.1042/BST20140055] [PMID: 25110023]

Ihle, MA, Trautmann, M, Kuenstlinger, H, Huss, S, Heydt, C, Fassunke, J, Wardelmann, E, Bauer, S, Schildhaus, HU, Buettner, R & Merkelbach-Bruse, S (2015) miRNA-221 and miRNA-222 induce apoptosis *via* the KIT/AKT signalling pathway in gastrointestinal stromal tumours. *Mol Oncol,* 9, 1421-33.
[http://dx.doi.org/10.1016/j.molonc.2015.03.013] [PMID: 25898773]

Iorio, MV & Croce, CM (2012) MicroRNA dysregulation in cancer: diagnostics, monitoring and therapeutics. A comprehensive review. *EMBO Mol Med,* 4, 143-59.
[http://dx.doi.org/10.1002/emmm.201100209] [PMID: 22351564]

Irani, K (2000) Oxidant signaling in vascular cell growth, death, and survival : a review of the roles of reactive oxygen species in smooth muscle and endothelial cell mitogenic and apoptotic signaling. *Circ Res,* 87, 179-83.
[http://dx.doi.org/10.1161/01.RES.87.3.179] [PMID: 10926866]

Ito, M, Sferruzzi-Perri, AN, Edwards, CA, Adalsteinsson, BT, Allen, SE, Loo, TH, Kitazawa, M, Kaneko-Ishino, T, Ishino, F, Stewart, CL & Ferguson-Smith, AC (2015) A trans-homologue interaction between reciprocally imprinted miR-127 and Rtl1 regulates placenta development. *Development,* 142, 2425-30.
[http://dx.doi.org/10.1242/dev.121996] [PMID: 26138477]

Jansson, MD & Lund, AH (2012) MicroRNA and cancer. *Mol Oncol,* 6, 590-610.
[http://dx.doi.org/10.1016/j.molonc.2012.09.006] [PMID: 23102669]

Jiang, H, Jin, C, Liu, J, Hua, D, Zhou, F, Lou, X, Zhao, N, Lan, Q, Huang, Q, Yoon, JG, Zheng, S & Lin, B (2014) Next generation sequencing analysis of miRNAs: MiR-127-3p inhibits glioblastoma proliferation and activates TGF-β signaling by targeting SKI. *OMICS*, 18, 196-206.
[http://dx.doi.org/10.1089/omi.2013.0122] [PMID: 24517116]

Jiang, S, Zhang, HW, Lu, MH, He, XH, Li, Y, Gu, H, Liu, MF & Wang, ED (2010) MicroRNA-155 functions as an OncomiR in breast cancer by targeting the suppressor of cytokine signaling 1 gene. *Cancer Res*, 70, 3119-27.
[http://dx.doi.org/10.1158/0008-5472.CAN-09-4250] [PMID: 20354188]

Jiang, S, Zhang, LF, Zhang, HW, Hu, S, Lu, MH, Liang, S, Li, B, Li, Y, Li, D, Wang, ED & Liu, MF (2012) A novel miR-155/miR-143 cascade controls glycolysis by regulating hexokinase 2 in breast cancer cells. *EMBO J*, 31, 1985-98.
[http://dx.doi.org/10.1038/emboj.2012.45] [PMID: 22354042]

Kasinski, AL & Slack, FJ (2012) miRNA-34 prevents cancer initiation and progression in a therapeutically resistant K-ras and p53-induced mouse model of lung adenocarcinoma. *Cancer Res*, 72, 5576-87.
[http://dx.doi.org/10.1158/0008-5472.CAN-12-2001] [PMID: 22964582]

Kastl, L, Brown, I & Schofield, AC (2012) miRNA-34a is associated with docetaxel resistance in human breast cancer cells. *Breast Cancer Res Treat*, 131, 445-54.
[http://dx.doi.org/10.1007/s10549-011-1424-3] [PMID: 21399894]

Kavitha, N, Vijayarathna, S, Shanmugapriya, , Oon, CE, Chen, Y, Kanwar, JR, Punj, V & Sasidharan, S (2018) MicroRNA profiling in MDA-MB-231 human breast cancer cell exposed to the Phaleria macrocarpa (Boerl.) fruit ethyl acetate fraction (PMEAF) through Illumina Hi-Seq technologies and various in silico bioinformatics tools. *J Ethnopharmacol*, 213, 118-31.
[http://dx.doi.org/10.1016/j.jep.2017.11.009] [PMID: 29154802]

Kiani, S, Akhavan-Niaki, H, Fattahi, S, Kavoosian, S, Babaian Jelodar, N, Bagheri, N & Najafi Zarrini, H (2018) Purified sulforaphane from broccoli (Brassica oleracea var. italica) leads to alterations of CDX1 and CDX2 expression and changes in miR-9 and miR-326 levels in human gastric cancer cells. *Gene*, 678, 115-23.
[http://dx.doi.org/10.1016/j.gene.2018.08.026] [PMID: 30096452]

Kosaka, N, Iguchi, H & Ochiya, T (2010) Circulating microRNA in body fluid: a new potential biomarker for cancer diagnosis and prognosis. *Cancer Sci*, 101, 2087-92.
[http://dx.doi.org/10.1111/j.1349-7006.2010.01650.x] [PMID: 20624164]

Lao, G, Liu, P, Wu, Q, Zhang, W, Liu, Y, Yang, L & Ma, C (2014) Mir-155 promotes cervical cancer cell proliferation through suppression of its target gene LKB1. *Tumour Biol*, 35, 11933-8.
[http://dx.doi.org/10.1007/s13277-014-2479-7] [PMID: 25155037]

Li, J, Huang, J, Dai, L, Yu, D, Chen, Q, Zhang, X & Dai, K (2012) miR-146a, an IL-1β responsive miRNA, induces vascular endothelial growth factor and chondrocyte apoptosis by targeting Smad4. *Arthritis Res Ther*, 14, 1-3.
[http://dx.doi.org/10.1186/ar3798]

Lin, YS, Lin, YY, Yang, YH, Lin, CL, Kuan, FC, Lu, CN, Chang, GH, Tsai, MS, Hsu, CM, Yeh, RA, Yang, PR, Lee, IY, Shu, LH, Cheng, YC, Liu, HT, Lee, KD, Chang, DC & Wu, CY (2018) Antrodia cinnamomea extract inhibits the proliferation of tamoxifen-resistant breast cancer cells through apoptosis and skp2/microRNAs pathway. *BMC Complement Altern Med*, 18, 152.
[http://dx.doi.org/10.1186/s12906-018-2204-y] [PMID: 29743060]

Liu, G, Jiang, C, Li, D, Wang, R & Wang, W (2014) MiRNA-34a inhibits EGFR-signaling-dependent MMP7 activation in gastric cancer. *Tumour Biol*, 35, 9801-6.
[http://dx.doi.org/10.1007/s13277-014-2273-6] [PMID: 24981249]

Liu, J, Mao, Q, Liu, Y, Hao, X, Zhang, S & Zhang, J (2013) Analysis of miR-205 and miR-155 expression in the blood of breast cancer patients. *Chin J Cancer Res*, 25, 46-54.

[PMID: 23372341]

Liu, X, Wang, S, Xu, J, Kou, B, Chen, D, Wang, Y & Zhu, X (2018) Extract of Stellerachamaejasme L(ESC) inhibits growth and metastasis of human hepatocellular carcinoma *via* regulating microRNA expression. *BMC Complement Altern Med,* 18, 99.
[http://dx.doi.org/10.1186/s12906-018-2123-y] [PMID: 29554896]

Lowe, SW & Lin, AW (2000) Apoptosis in cancer. *Carcinogenesis,* 21, 485-95.
[http://dx.doi.org/10.1093/carcin/21.3.485] [PMID: 10688869]

Ma, J, Fang, B, Zeng, F, Pang, H, Ma, C & Xia, J (2015) Grape seed proanthocyanidins extract inhibits pancreatic cancer cell growth through down-regulation of miR-27a expression. Zhong nan da xue xue bao. Yi xue ban= Journal of Central South University. *Med Sci,* 40, 46-52.

Macfarlane, LA & Murphy, PR (2010) MicroRNA: biogenesis, function and role in cancer. *Curr Genomics,* 11, 537-61.
[http://dx.doi.org/10.2174/138920210793175895] [PMID: 21532838]

Madamanchi, NR, Vendrov, A & Runge, MS (2005) Oxidative stress and vascular disease. *Arterioscler Thromb Vasc Biol,* 25, 29-38.
[http://dx.doi.org/10.1161/01.ATV.0000150649.39934.13] [PMID: 15539615]

Magenta, A, Cencioni, C, Fasanaro, P, Zaccagnini, G, Greco, S, Sarra-Ferraris, G, Antonini, A, Martelli, F & Capogrossi, MC (2011) miR-200c is upregulated by oxidative stress and induces endothelial cell apoptosis and senescence *via* ZEB1 inhibition. *Cell Death Differ,* 18, 1628-39.
[http://dx.doi.org/10.1038/cdd.2011.42] [PMID: 21527937]

Mansoori, B, Mohammadi, A, Hashemzadeh, S, Shirjang, S, Baradaran, A, Asadi, M, Doustvandi, MA & Baradaran, B (2017) Urtica dioica extract suppresses miR-21 and metastasis-related genes in breast cancer. *Biomed Pharmacother,* 93, 95-102.
[http://dx.doi.org/10.1016/j.biopha.2017.06.021] [PMID: 28628833]

Mao, JT, Xue, B, Smoake, J, Lu, QY, Park, H, Henning, SM, Burns, W, Bernabei, A, Elashoff, D, Serio, KJ & Massie, L (2016) MicroRNA-19a/b mediates grape seed procyanidin extract-induced anti-neoplastic effects against lung cancer. *J Nutr Biochem,* 34, 118-25.
[http://dx.doi.org/10.1016/j.jnutbio.2016.05.003] [PMID: 27289489]

Martin, SL, Kala, R & Tollefsbol, TO (2018) Mechanisms for the inhibition of colon cancer cells by sulforaphane through epigenetic modulation of microRNA-21 and human telomerase reverse transcriptase (hTERT) down-regulation. *Curr Cancer Drug Targets,* 18, 97-106.
[http://dx.doi.org/10.2174/1568009617666170206104032] [PMID: 28176652]

Mateescu, B, Batista, L, Cardon, M, Gruosso, T, de Feraudy, Y, Mariani, O, Nicolas, A, Meyniel, JP, Cottu, P, Sastre-Garau, X & Mechta-Grigoriou, F (2011) miR-141 and miR-200a act on ovarian tumorigenesis by controlling oxidative stress response. *Nat Med,* 17, 1627-35.
[http://dx.doi.org/10.1038/nm.2512] [PMID: 22101765]

Meng, X, Wu, J, Pan, C, Wang, H, Ying, X, Zhou, Y, Yu, H, Zuo, Y, Pan, Z, Liu, RY & Huang, W (2013) Genetic and epigenetic down-regulation of microRNA-212 promotes colorectal tumor metastasis *via* dysregulation of MnSOD. *Gastroenterology,* 145, 426-36.e1, 6.
[http://dx.doi.org/10.1053/j.gastro.2013.04.004] [PMID: 23583431]

Mestdagh, P, Boström, AK, Impens, F, Fredlund, E, Van Peer, G, De Antonellis, P, von Stedingk, K, Ghesquière, B, Schulte, S, Dews, M, Thomas-Tikhonenko, A, Schulte, JH, Zollo, M, Schramm, A, Gevaert, K, Axelson, H, Speleman, F & Vandesompele, J (2010) The miR-17-92 microRNA cluster regulates multiple components of the TGF-β pathway in neuroblastoma. *Mol Cell,* 40, 762-73.
[http://dx.doi.org/10.1016/j.molcel.2010.11.038] [PMID: 21145484]

Nagpal, N, Ahmad, HM, Chameettachal, S, Sundar, D, Ghosh, S & Kulshreshtha, R (2015) HIF-inducible miR-191 promotes migration in breast cancer through complex regulation of TGFβ-signaling in hypoxic microenvironment. *Sci Rep,* 5, 1-4.

[http://dx.doi.org/10.1038/srep09650]

Napoli, C, de Nigris, F & Palinski, W (2001) Multiple role of reactive oxygen species in the arterial wall. *J Cell Biochem,* 82, 674-82.
[http://dx.doi.org/10.1002/jcb.1198] [PMID: 11500945]

Ørom, UA, Nielsen, FC & Lund, AH (2008) MicroRNA-10a binds the 5'UTR of ribosomal protein mRNAs and enhances their translation. *Mol Cell,* 30, 460-71.
[http://dx.doi.org/10.1016/j.molcel.2008.05.001] [PMID: 18498749]

Pan, C, Chen, H, Wang, L, Yang, S, Fu, H, Zheng, Y, Miao, M & Jiao, B (2012) Down-regulation of MiR-127 facilitates hepatocyte proliferation during rat liver regeneration. *PLoS One,* 7e39151
[http://dx.doi.org/10.1371/journal.pone.0039151] [PMID: 22720056]

Pan, X, Wang, ZX & Wang, R (2010) MicroRNA-21: a novel therapeutic target in human cancer. *Cancer Biol Ther,* 10, 1224-32.
[http://dx.doi.org/10.4161/cbt.10.12.14252] [PMID: 21139417]

Peng, HH, Zhang, YD, Gong, LS, Liu, WD & Zhang, Y (2013) Increased expression of microRNA-335 predicts a favorable prognosis in primary gallbladder carcinoma. *OncoTargets Ther,* 6, 1625-30.
[PMID: 24250228]

Peng, Y & Croce, CM (2016) The role of MicroRNAs in human cancer. *Signal Transduct Target Ther,* 1, 15004.
[http://dx.doi.org/10.1038/sigtrans.2015.4] [PMID: 29263891]

Reddy, KB (2015) MicroRNA (miRNA) in cancer. *Cancer Cell Int,* 15, 38.
[http://dx.doi.org/10.1186/s12935-015-0185-1] [PMID: 25960691]

Ross, SA & Davis, CD (2011) MicroRNA, nutrition, and cancer prevention. *Adv Nutr,* 2, 472-85.
[http://dx.doi.org/10.3945/an.111.001206] [PMID: 22332090]

Ryan, BM, Robles, AI & Harris, CC (2010) Genetic variation in microRNA networks: the implications for cancer research. *Nat Rev Cancer,* 10, 389-402.
[http://dx.doi.org/10.1038/nrc2867] [PMID: 20495573]

Shimizu, S, Takehara, T, Hikita, H, Kodama, T, Miyagi, T, Hosui, A, Tatsumi, T, Ishida, H, Noda, T, Nagano, H, Doki, Y, Mori, M & Hayashi, N (2010) The let-7 family of microRNAs inhibits Bcl-xL expression and potentiates sorafenib-induced apoptosis in human hepatocellular carcinoma. *J Hepatol,* 52, 698-704.
[http://dx.doi.org/10.1016/j.jhep.2009.12.024] [PMID: 20347499]

Simone, NL, Soule, BP, Ly, D, Saleh, AD, Savage, JE, Degraff, W, Cook, J, Harris, CC, Gius, D & Mitchell, JB (2009) Ionizing radiation-induced oxidative stress alters miRNA expression. *PLoS One,* 4e6377
[http://dx.doi.org/10.1371/journal.pone.0006377] [PMID: 19633716]

Sochor, M, Basova, P, Pesta, M, Dusilkova, N, Bartos, J, Burda, P, Pospisil, V & Stopka, T (2014) Oncogenic microRNAs: miR-155, miR-19a, miR-181b, and miR-24 enable monitoring of early breast cancer in serum. *BMC Cancer,* 14, 448.
[http://dx.doi.org/10.1186/1471-2407-14-448] [PMID: 24938880]

Sophia, J, Kowshik, J, Dwivedi, A, Bhutia, SK, Manavathi, B, Mishra, R & Nagini, S (2018) Nimbolide, a neem limonoid inhibits cytoprotective autophagy to activate apoptosis *via* modulation of the PI3K/Akt/GSK-3β signalling pathway in oral cancer. *Cell Death Dis,* 9, 1087.
[http://dx.doi.org/10.1038/s41419-018-1126-4] [PMID: 30352996]

Strasser, A, O'Connor, L & Dixit, VM (2000) Apoptosis signaling. *Annu Rev Biochem,* 69, 217-45.
[http://dx.doi.org/10.1146/annurev.biochem.69.1.217] [PMID: 10966458]

Subramaniam, D, Ponnurangam, S, Ramamoorthy, P, Standing, D, Battafarano, RJ, Anant, S & Sharma, P (2012) Curcumin induces cell death in esophageal cancer cells through modulating Notch signaling. *PLoS One,* 7e30590

[http://dx.doi.org/10.1371/journal.pone.0030590] [PMID: 22363450]

Sun, Y, Wang, M, Lin, G, Sun, S, Li, X, Qi, J & Li, J (2012) Serum microRNA-155 as a potential biomarker to track disease in breast cancer. *PLoS One,* 7e47003
[http://dx.doi.org/10.1371/journal.pone.0047003] [PMID: 23071695]

Sun, Z, Zhang, Z, Liu, Z, Qiu, B, Liu, K & Dong, G (2014) MicroRNA-335 inhibits invasion and metastasis of colorectal cancer by targeting ZEB2. *Med Oncol,* 31, 982.
[http://dx.doi.org/10.1007/s12032-014-0982-8] [PMID: 24829139]

Suzuki, H, Maruyama, R, Yamamoto, E & Kai, M (2012) DNA methylation and microRNA dysregulation in cancer. *Mol Oncol,* 6, 567-78.
[http://dx.doi.org/10.1016/j.molonc.2012.07.007] [PMID: 22902148]

Suzuki, H, Maruyama, R, Yamamoto, E & Kai, M (2013) Epigenetic alteration and microRNA dysregulation in cancer. *Front Genet,* 4, 258.
[http://dx.doi.org/10.3389/fgene.2013.00258] [PMID: 24348513]

Tezcan, G, Aksoy, SA, Tunca, B, Bekar, A, Mutlu, M, Cecener, G, Egeli, U, Kocaeli, H, Demirci, H & Taskapilioglu, MO (2019) Oleuropein modulates glioblastoma miRNA pattern different from *Olea europaea* leaf extract. *Hum Exp Toxicol,* 38, 1102-10.
[http://dx.doi.org/10.1177/0960327119855123] [PMID: 31169033]

Tryndyak, VP, Ross, SA, Beland, FA & Pogribny, IP (2009) *Down-regulation of the microRNAs miR-34a, miR-127, and miR-200b in rat liver during hepatocarcinogenesis induced by a methyl-deficient diet* Molecular Carcinogenesis, Published in cooperation with the University of Texas MD Anderson Cancer Center 87-479.

Tsuchida, A, Ohno, S, Wu, W, Borjigin, N, Fujita, K, Aoki, T, Ueda, S, Takanashi, M & Kuroda, M (2011) miR-92 is a key oncogenic component of the miR-17-92 cluster in colon cancer. *Cancer Sci,* 102, 2264-71.
[http://dx.doi.org/10.1111/j.1349-7006.2011.02081.x] [PMID: 21883694]

Venkataraman, S, Alimova, I, Fan, R, Harris, P, Foreman, N & Vibhakar, R (2010) MicroRNA 128a increases intracellular ROS level by targeting Bmi-1 and inhibits medulloblastoma cancer cell growth by promoting senescence. *PLoS One,* 5e10748
[http://dx.doi.org/10.1371/journal.pone.0010748] [PMID: 20574517]

Vishnoi, A & Rani, S (2017) *MiRNA biogenesis and regulation of diseases: an overview*

Wang, L, Yuan, Y, Li, J, Ren, H, Cai, Q, Chen, X, Liang, H, Shan, H, Fu, ZD, Gao, X, Lv, Y, Yang, B & Zhang, Y (2015) MicroRNA-1 aggravates cardiac oxidative stress by post-transcriptional modification of the antioxidant network. *Cell Stress Chaperones,* 20, 411-20.
[http://dx.doi.org/10.1007/s12192-014-0565-9] [PMID: 25583113]

Wang, S, Li, H, Wang, J, Wang, D, Yao, A & Li, Q (2014) Prognostic and biological significance of microRNA-127 expression in human breast cancer. *Dis Markers,* 2014401986
[http://dx.doi.org/10.1155/2014/401986] [PMID: 25477702]

Wang, Y & Kong, D (2018) Knockdown of lncRNA MEG3 inhibits viability, migration, and invasion and promotes apoptosis by sponging miR-127 in osteosarcoma cell. *J Cell Biochem,* 119, 669-79.
[http://dx.doi.org/10.1002/jcb.26230] [PMID: 28636101]

Wiggins, JF, Ruffino, L, Kelnar, K, Omotola, M, Patrawala, L, Brown, D & Bader, AG (2010) Development of a lung cancer therapeutic based on the tumor suppressor microRNA-34. *Cancer Res,* 70, 5923-30.
[http://dx.doi.org/10.1158/0008-5472.CAN-10-0655] [PMID: 20570894]

Willers, IM, Martínez-Reyes, I, Martínez-Diez, M & Cuezva, JM (2012) miR-127-5p targets the 3'UTR of human β-F1-ATPase mRNA and inhibits its translation. *Biochim Biophys Acta,* 1817, 838-48.
[http://dx.doi.org/10.1016/j.bbabio.2012.03.005] [PMID: 22433606]

Wu, Y, Zhang, J, Hong, Y & Wang, X (2018) Effects of Kanglaite injection on serum miRNA-21 in patients with advanced lung cancer. *Med Sci Monit,* 24, 2901-6.

[http://dx.doi.org/10.12659/MSM.909719] [PMID: 29735968]

Xiong, SW, Lin, TX, Xu, KW, Dong, W, Ling, XH, Jiang, FN, Chen, G, Zhong, WD & Huang, J (2013) MicroRNA-335 acts as a candidate tumor suppressor in prostate cancer. *Pathol Oncol Res,* 19, 529-37.
[http://dx.doi.org/10.1007/s12253-013-9613-5] [PMID: 23456549]

Xu, Y, Luo, S, Liu, Y, Li, J, Lu, Y, Jia, Z, Zhao, Q, Ma, X, Yang, M, Zhao, Y & Chen, P (2015) Retraction note: Integrated gene network analysis and text mining revealing PIK3R1 regulated by miR-127 in human bladder cancer. *Eur J Med Res,* 20, 43.
[http://dx.doi.org/10.1186/s40001-015-0119-3] [PMID: 25889830]

Yang, M, Shen, H, Qiu, C, Ni, Y, Wang, L, Dong, W, Liao, Y & Du, J (2013) High expression of miR-21 and miR-155 predicts recurrence and unfavourable survival in non-small cell lung cancer. *Eur J Cancer,* 49, 604-15.
[http://dx.doi.org/10.1016/j.ejca.2012.09.031] [PMID: 23099007]

Yang, R, Dick, M, Marme, F, Schneeweiss, A, Langheinz, A, Hemminki, K, Sutter, C, Bugert, P, Wappenschmidt, B, Varon, R, Schott, S, Weber, BH, Niederacher, D, Arnold, N, Meindl, A, Bartram, CR, Schmutzler, RK, Müller, H, Arndt, V, Brenner, H, Sohn, C & Burwinkel, B (2011) Genetic variants within miR-126 and miR-335 are not associated with breast cancer risk. *Breast Cancer Res Treat,* 127, 549-54.
[http://dx.doi.org/10.1007/s10549-010-1244-x] [PMID: 21046227]

Yang, Z, Zhang, Y & Wang, L (2013) A feedback inhibition between miRNA-127 and TGFβ/c-Jun cascade in HCC cell migration *via* MMP13. *PLoS One,* 8, 1-9.
[http://dx.doi.org/10.1371/journal.pone.0065256]

You, W, Wang, Y & Zheng, J (2015) Plasma miR-127 and miR-218 might serve as potential biomarkers for cervical cancer. *Reprod Sci,* 22, 1037-41.
[http://dx.doi.org/10.1177/1933719115570902] [PMID: 25701838]

Yu, Y, Liu, L, Ma, R, Gong, H, Xu, P & Wang, C (2016) MicroRNA-127 is aberrantly downregulated and acted as a functional tumor suppressor in human pancreatic cancer. *Tumour Biol,* 37, 14249-57.
[http://dx.doi.org/10.1007/s13277-016-5270-0] [PMID: 27571739]

Zaman, MS, Shahryari, V, Deng, G, Thamminana, S, Saini, S, Majid, S, Chang, I, Hirata, H, Ueno, K, Yamamura, S, Singh, K, Tanaka, Y, Tabatabai, ZL & Dahiya, R (2012) Up-regulation of microRNA-21 correlates with lower kidney cancer survival. *PLoS One,* 7e31060
[http://dx.doi.org/10.1371/journal.pone.0031060] [PMID: 22347428]

Zhang, J, Du, YY, Lin, YF, Chen, YT, Yang, L, Wang, HJ & Ma, D (2008) The cell growth suppressor, mir-126, targets IRS-1. *Biochem Biophys Res Commun,* 377, 136-40.
[http://dx.doi.org/10.1016/j.bbrc.2008.09.089] [PMID: 18834857]

Zhang, L, Fang, Y, Feng, JY, Cai, QY, Wei, LH, Lin, S & Peng, J (2017) Chloroform fraction of Scutellaria barbata D. Don inhibits the growth of colorectal cancer cells by activating miR-34a. *Oncol Rep,* 37, 3695-701.
[http://dx.doi.org/10.3892/or.2017.5625] [PMID: 28498458]

Zhang, Y, Wang, X, Xu, B, Wang, B, Wang, Z, Liang, Y, Zhou, J, Hu, J & Jiang, B (2013) Epigenetic silencing of miR-126 contributes to tumor invasion and angiogenesis in colorectal cancer. *Oncol Rep,* 30, 1976-84.
[http://dx.doi.org/10.3892/or.2013.2633] [PMID: 23900443]

Zhou, Y, Feng, X, Liu, YL, Ye, SC, Wang, H, Tan, WK, Tian, T, Qiu, YM & Luo, HS (2013) Down-regulation of miR-126 is associated with colorectal cancer cells proliferation, migration and invasion by targeting IRS-1 *via* the AKT and ERK1/2 signaling pathways. *PLoS One,* 8e81203
[http://dx.doi.org/10.1371/journal.pone.0081203] [PMID: 24312276]

Zhu, H, Han, C, Lu, D & Wu, T (2014) miR-17-92 cluster promotes cholangiocarcinoma growth: evidence for PTEN as downstream target and IL-6/Stat3 as upstream activator. *Am J Pathol,* 184, 2828-39.
[http://dx.doi.org/10.1016/j.ajpath.2014.06.024] [PMID: 25239565]

CHAPTER 12

Antioxidant and Anti-Inflammatory Action of Phytobioactive Compounds in Cardiovascular Disorders

Hiral K. Mistry[1], **Ginpreet Kaur**[1,*], **Saraswathy Nagendran**[1] and **Harpal S. Buttar**[2]

[1] *Shobhaben Pratapbhai Patel School of Pharmacy and Technology Management, SVKM'S NMIMS, Mumbai-56, Maharashtra, India*

[2] *Department of Pathology and Laboratory Medicine, University of Ottawa, School of Medicine, Ottawa, Canada*

Abstract: Oxidative stress distorts the mitochondrial function and triggers deleterious effects in the cardiovascular system. Further, oxidative stress-induced overproduction of highly reactive oxygen/nitrogen species (RONS) is amplified in patients exposed to radiation, excessive consumption of alcohol and tobacco, environmental pollutants, exposure to agrochemicals like fertilizers, pesticides or endocrine disrupters. In modern times, oxidative stress-induced cardiovascular diseases (CVDs) have escalated globally. Synthetic medicines prescribed for the amelioration of CVDs are expensive and can cause life-time dependency in some patients, thus escalating the treatment cost. Sometimes, long-term use of synthetic medicines or drug polytherapy for co-morbid conditions can cause undesirable side-effects. Quite often, these therapeutic strategies do not succeed in attenuating the oxidative stress related CVDs. Therefore, researchers are exploring alternative and cost-effective phytobioactive therapies which have strong antioxidant and anti-inflammation properties, and can act as scavengers of RONS. Phytobioactive compounds, nutraceuticals and probiotics prepared from plant/animal origin are potential therapeutic substances for the promotion of health and well-being. Several plant-derived phytotherapies have demonstrated strong antioxidant, anti-inflammatory, cardio-protective effects, inhibition of ischemic injury as well as alleviation in the pathological cardiac biomarkers and cardiac apoptotic proteins. In this review, we have described the therapeutic functions of various phytobioactive compounds and their purported mechanism of action at the genetic, epigenetic, cellular and molecular level with respect to their antioxidant and anti-inflammatory actions for the prevention and treatment of cardiovascular disorders.

* **Corresponding author Ginpreet Kaur:** Shobhaben Pratapbhai Patel School of Pharmacy and Technology Management, SVKM'S NMIMS, Mumbai-56, Maharashtra, India. E-mail: Ginpreet.kaur @nmims.edu

Keywords: Anti-inflammation, Antioxidants, Cardiovascular diseases, Myocardial infarction, Nutraceuticals, Oxidative stress, Phytobioactive compounds, Probiotics.

INTRODUCTION

Cardiovascular diseases (CVDs) comprise collective disorders of the coronary blood vessels, heart, and stroke, which are one of the major causes of deaths in developed and developing countries. CVDs not only pose a major threat to an individual's health but also cause a tremendous economic burden on the healthcare systems globally. The major type of CVDs are caused by oxidative stress that triggers atherosclerosis, coronary artery disease, hypertension, cerebrovascular disease, disorders of the major arteries, and peripheral vascular disorders. Further, congenital heart disease, rheumatic heart disorders, congenital cardiomyopathies, arrhythmias, *etc.*, are other types of CVDs (Murabito *et al.* 1993, Riccioni *et al.* 2007). Over 17.3 million deaths are caused annually due to CVDs worldwide (World Health Organization 2011). Deaths due to various types of CVDs in men and women are shown in Fig. (**1**) as below:

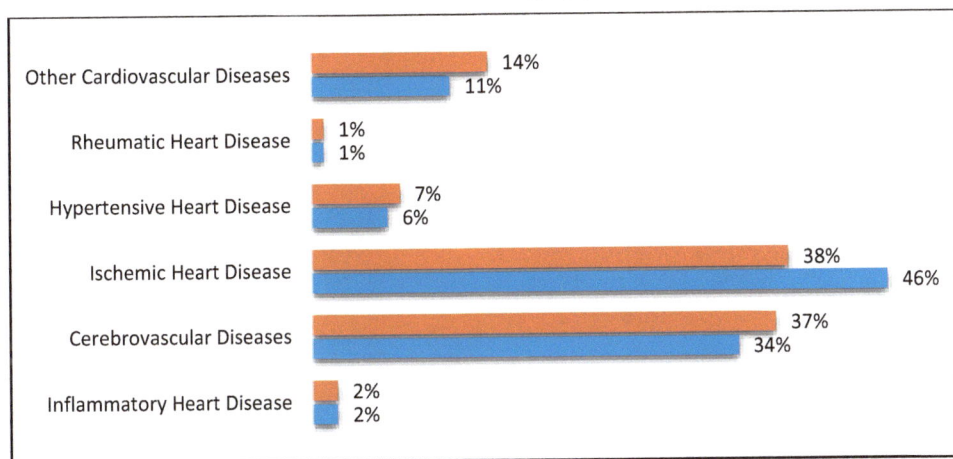

Fig. (1). Distribution of CVD deaths in males and females.

One of the major underlying pathophysiological processes that lead to various types of CVDs is atherosclerosis. Atherosclerosis is caused due to inflammation affecting the lining of blood vessels of the entire cardiovascular system. On exposure to increased levels of LDL cholesterol and further components such as cytokines, hormones and oxidative species on the lining of the blood vessels; the endothelium becomes permeable to certain inflammatory mediators leading to the formation of plaque. A development of cholesterol plaque on the inner side of the artery's walls causes a blockage in the blood flow. The rupture of the plaque may lead to heart attack or stroke because of acute blockage of the artery by the blood clot.

A number of pharmacological and non-pharmacological approaches have been made to combat CVDs. The non-pharmacological approaches include certain lifestyle changes such as smoking cessation, weight control, regular exercising, maintaining a healthy diet and antioxidant therapy (Wilson *et al.* 1998). Our major focus in this chapter is on the role of phytobioactive antioxidants and anti-inflammatory agents to prevent and treat cardiovascular diseases (Nuttall *et al.* 1999).

OXIDATIVE DAMAGE IN CARDIOVASCULAR DISEASES

A large number of reactive oxygen species (ROS) are constantly produced in cells. These reactive oxygen species (ROS) expedite the irreversible oxidation of carbohydrates, proteins, lipids and nucleic acids, which are some of the essential biological macromolecules (Fig. **3**). The development of atherosclerosis is majorly because of the oxidative modification of circulating lipoproteins by free radicals, particularly low-density lipoproteins (LDL). In the early stage of atherogenesis (the first step to the formation of plaque), LDLs are oxidized. Once these Ox-LDLs begin to accumulate, an immune response is stimulated. These immune responses lead to progression of atherosclerosis by releasing reactive oxygen species and pro-inflammatory cytokines which promote the formation and accumulation of oxidized LDLs (Mann 2015). Oxidative stress occurring in the mitochondria in cardiovascular diseases due to increased production of reactive oxygen species (ROS) and reactive nitrogen species (RNS) lead to free radical formation, which promotes inflammation in the vascular wall and may be the underlying cause of stroke and coronary heart disease. Fig. (**2**) explains the process of oxidative damage in CVDs (Bo *et al.* 2013).

LINK BETWEEN INFLAMMATION AND CVD

Even though inflammation is a part of the natural biological response of body tissues developed by the organisms to get rid of harmful stimuli, persistent increase in certain pro-inflammatory biomarkers leads to chronic low-grade inflammation, which is the key component in the development of cardiovascular disease (Hennekens *et al.* 1996). C-reactive protein (CRP), a predictor of endothelial function and an active mediator in the pathogenesis of vascular disease, is a preliminary example of a reversible atherosclerosis precursor (Gajendragadkar *et al.* 2014). CRP induces vascular remodeling, by producing reactive oxygen species and upregulating angiotensin type 1 enzyme. It also enhances the release of tumor necrosis factor-α (TNF-α), interleukin 1β (IL-1β) and interleukin-6 (IL-6), the pro-inflammatory cytokines, through foam cells in the neointima and macrophages, promoting angiogenesis and are considered as pivotal factors which lead to cardiovascular diseases (Kosmas *et al.* 2019).

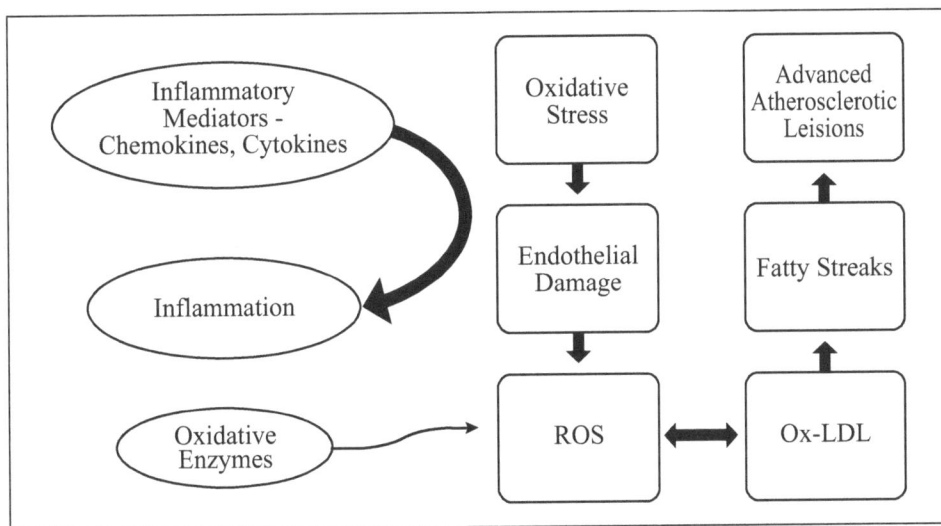

Fig. (2). Diagrammatic representation of oxidative stress in the pathogenesis of CVDs.

ROLE OF ANTIOXIDANTS AND ANTI-INFLAMMATORY AGENTS IN CVDS

Every individual can benefit from healthy-heart practices and fortunately there are various choices available for people who are considering to be proactive. The voyage to CVD can begin in infanthood itself, and as per the latest report from the American Heart Association, there are a few children who can meet all the criteria for ideal heart health. Phytobioactive nutrients contain antioxidants that are inherently present in herbs and spices and are gaining wide acceptance these days. They are helpful in preventing and also managing a variety of cardiovascular health issues. An imbalance in the production and elimination of free radicals in the biological system leads to the formation of oxidative stress. Reactive oxygen species are potentially harmful agents and contradictorily, they are also helpful for constructive regulatory functions. They play a role in cellular signaling processes like the generation of ROS in the mitochondria which acts as a component of TNF – signal transduction pathway during apoptosis (Fig. **3**) (Adams *et al.* 1999). They might also hinder the process of gene expression and may have an impact on phosphorylation of proteins (Alves *et al.* 2019, Rimm *et al.* 1993). Sometimes, reactive oxygen species show a positive impact on inflammation and are thus regarded as "protective molecules" (Nikhra 2018, Vasanthi *et al.* 2012). An imbalance between the formation and detoxification of ROS leads to its overproduction, resulting in a range of abnormalities linked with chronic diseases such as cancer, diabetes, cardiovascular diseases or various types of inflammation. Therefore, compounds that help to regulate the concentration of ROS and prevent its excessive formation are very vital for an individual's health (Cherubini *et al.* 2005).

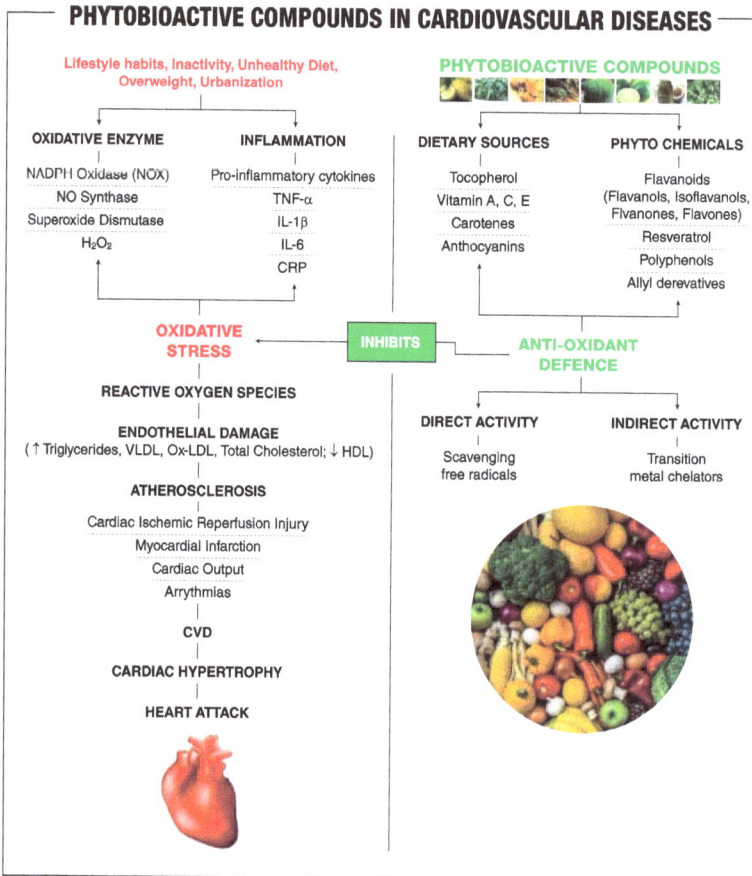

Fig. (3). Diagrammatic representation of the antioxidant and anti-inflammation action of phytobioactive compounds and their mechanism of action in the prevention of atherosclerosis and CVDs.

Antioxidants are molecules that obstruct the formation and progression of free radicals, and thus support by delaying or inhibiting cellular injury. The oxidative stress state can be reversed by both endogenous antioxidants (glutathione, L-cysteine, superoxide dismutase, catalase), and exogenous micronutrients (vitamin C and E, Zn and Cu), and flavonoids, polyphenolic compounds, and carotenoids. Antioxidants such as superoxide dismutase, catalase and glutathione peroxidase; help neutralize the effect of free radicals by donating electrons. They scavenge the free radicals in the circulation that protect lipoproteins from oxidative modification in the extracellular fluid by acting within the intracellular compartments.

Several nutraceutical and natural products act against the pathologies causing CVDs through their anti-oxidant and anti-inflammatory abilities. Phytobioactive compounds obtained from natural origin are very good sources of anti-oxidants. Majority of these natural antioxidants which include vegetables, fruits and extracts of plants, are integrated into dietary supplements and foodstuff. With the increasing awareness of the benefits of antioxidants, further, they have entered the cosmeceutical world as well. These nutrients play a crucial role in the battle against oxidative stress, support immune function, promote cardiovascular health, and also the brain, joints and skin through various mechanisms.

1. Free Radical Scavenging Action

Antioxidants scavenge free radicals and reactive oxygen species produced during intermediary metabolic routes.

2. Preventing Lipid Peroxidation

The antioxidant enzymes prevent damage to cell membrane and DNA by reducing the levels of membrane phospholipids - lipid hydro-peroxide and hydrogen peroxide.

3. Quench Singlet Oxygen

The cell membrane lipids are protected from the harmful effects of oxidative degeneration through quenching of singlet oxygen and free radical scavenging activity.

To comprehend these mechanism of action of antioxidants, it is very important to understand how these free radicals are generated and their damaging reactions. This chapter highlights the potential of phytobioactive compounds for prevention and treatment of CVDs, the sources of these antioxidants, mechanism of action and the clinical and pre-clinical studies of these compounds.

PHYTOBIOACTIVE COMPOUNDS FOR CVDS

The role of medicinal plants for treatment of human diseases has been known since centuries. Thus it is especially important to include sufficient vegetables and food in the diet (Bruckdorfer 2008). Using conventional drugs for CVDs has been proved effective, but it comes along with additional side effects, making their use limited. The cardio-protective activity of medicinal plants by providing nutritional substances, mainly phytochemicals with potential of restoring normal body functions, are considered safe and are gaining attention these days. Phytobioactive nutrients are natural compounds established in various therapeutic and aromatic plants, and act as a defense mechanism against various diseases. Majority of these compounds act as antioxidants, reduce cholesterol, angina, ischemia, platelet aggregation, and fight against inflammation, thus demonstrating their cardioprotective activity (de Andrade *et al.* 2017). They are obtained from natural products such as polyphenols, flavonoids, isoflavones, diosgenin, resveratrol, quercetin, catechin, sulforaphane, tocotrienols and carotenoids (Nimse and Pal 2015). Table **1** depicts specific illustrations of phyto-bioactive antioxidants along with their dietary sources and primary structures:

Table 1. Dietary and chemical sources of phytobioactive antioxidants.

Antioxidant	Food Source	Basic Structure	Reference
B-Carotene	Mangoes, Carrot, Apricot, Red pepper, Kale, Spinach, Broccoli		(Adams *et al.* 1999, Frei 1994)
Lycopene	Tomatoes, Guavas, Pink grapefruit, Watermelon		(Al-Khudairy *et al.* 2017, Frei 1994)
Vitamin C (Ascorbic acid)	Citrus fruits, Straw berries, Cantaloupe, Tomatoes, Cabbage, Green leafy vegetables		(Stephens *et al.* 1996)
Vitamin E (Alpha-Tocopherol)	Seed oils, Wheat germ, Meat, Fish, Fruits, Vegetables		(Frei 1994, Voutilainen *et al.* 2006)

(Table 1) cont.....

Antioxidant	Food Source	Basic Structure	Reference
Resveratrol	Roots of P. *cuspidatum,* Grapes, Peanuts, Pine trees, *Cassia*		(Lakhanpal 2008)
Flavanoids	Red wine, Tea, Onions		(Reis *et al.* 2016)
Anthocyanins	Berries, Red onions, Kidney Beans, Pomegranates, Grapes, Tomatoes, Acai, Bilberry, Chokeberry, Elderberry, Tart cherries		(Ak and Gulcin 2008)
Curcumin	Turmeric (*Curcuma longa*)		(Zordoky *et al.* 2015)
Allyl Cysteine, Alliin, Allicin Allyl Disulphide	Garlic (*Allium sativum*)		(World Health Organization 2011)

CLINICAL AND PRE-CLINICAL STUDIES OF PHYTOBIOACTIVE COMPOUNDS

Several large-scale pre-clinical and clinical studies are being conducted that interpret the effectiveness of phytobioactive compounds in CVDs (Knekt *et al.* 1994, Marchioli *et al.* 2001). Various parameters related to the diet and lifestyle of individuals have also been taken into consideration in these studies.

Table 2. Pre-clinical and clinical CVD studies of phytobioactive compounds.

Phytobioactive Compound	Test Organism	Study Duration	Study Design	Results	Reference
β-Carotene	Adult male rats	4 weeks	High fat diet induced	↓ Oxidative stress and inflammation at low doses of beta carotene	(Csepanyi *et al.* 2015)
β-Carotene	22071 male humans, 40-84 years age	12 years	Double-blind randomized, placebo-controlled trial	CVD mortality in the β-carotene–supplemented group not found	(Hennekens *et al.* 1996)
Lycopene	40 adult male rabbits	8 weeks	High fat diet induced	↓ Atherosclerotic plaque formation, ↓ total cholesterol, serum triglycerides, LDL, interleukin-1 ↑ Nitric Oxide	(Hu *et al.* 2008)
Lycopene	36 CVD patients	2 months	Double-blind randomized, placebo-controlled, parallel group study	Improved endothelial function in CVD patients	(Gajendragadkar *et al.* 2014)
Resveratrol	C57Bl mice	8 weeks	High fat diet-fed	↓LDL and total Cholesterol; ↑HDL; no effect on triglycerides	(Ahn *et al.* 2008)
Resveratrol	50 adult smokers	30 days	Double-blind randomized, cross-over clinical trial	↓ROS, CRP and TG	(Bo *et al.* 2013)
Quercetin	Wistar rats	30 days	Isoproterenol treated rats	↓ LDL ↑ Nitric oxide	(Liu *et al.* 2012)
Quercetin	72 women	10 weeks	Double-blind randomized clinical trial	↓ Systolic blood pressure No effect on other cardiovascular risk factors and inflammatory biomarkers	(Zahedi *et al.* 2013)
Anthocyanin	Male Fischer 344 rats	10 weeks	High-fat diet induced	Changes in plasma fatty acids, ↓ Serum cholesterol, leptin, and resistin concentrations	(Graf *et al.* 2013)
Anthocyanin	Healthy volunteers	1 month	Double-blind randomized, placebo-controlled trial	↓ Cholesterol, LDL and triglycerides	(Alvarez-Suarez *et al.* 2014)

(Table 2) cont.....

Phytobioactive Compound	Test Organism	Study Duration	Study Design	Results	Reference
Curcumin	33 CAD patients	2 months	Double-blind randomized, placebo-controlled trial	↓ Serum Cholesterol, LDL, VLDL and triglycerides	(Mirzabeigi *et al.* 2015)

β-Carotene

β-Carotene, the red colouration of plants and fruits, exhibit potential cardio-protective activity. It is a precursor of vitamin A and is carried in plasma and LDL. As an anti-oxidant, it helps to reduce the oxidized LDL uptake, thus preventing cellular lipid damage by cholesterol but doesn't prevent LDL oxidation (Adams *et al.* 1999). Various studies have shown that people with intake of higher dietary levels of beta carotene containing fruits and vegetables are at less risk of CVDs. Yellow to orange colored vegetables and fruits such as sweet potatoes, carrots, *etc.*, and green vegetables like broccoli and spinach are some of the major sources of beta carotenoids (D'Odorico *et al.* 2000, Daviglus *et al.* 1997).

Pre-clinical Study

Various studies are conducted to monitor the effects of beta carotene on myocardial tissue and organ functions so as to develop novel strategies to manage CVDs (Klipstein-Grobusch *et al.* 1999). A pre-clinical trial to study the effects of beta carotene was performed by Csepanyi *et al.* (2015) in a rat model, wherein adult male rats weighing between 350 to 400 g, were gavage-fed beta-carotene for 4 weeks at dosages 30 and 150 mg/kg/day. Cardiac functions such as the infarct size, the myocardial anti-oxidant property, *etc.*, were evaluated (Table **2**). The study showed that beta carotene, at lower dose was effective in quenching the oxidative stress promoting-free radicals and pro-oxidant compounds produced by the cardiac tissues because of the inflammatory reactions triggered by ischemia and reperfusion induced injury or the counter-acting unfavorable effects of these metabolites. Increasing the dose of beta carotene failed to exhibit any significant effect. Thus, the concentration of beta carotene plays a significant role in determining its effectiveness in cardiovascular functions (Csepanyi *et al.* 2015).

Clinical Study

β-Carotene, the organic red-orange colored pigment is profusely found in plants, fruits and fungi. People with a diet intake rich in beta carotene containing vegetables and fruits are less prone to chronic diseases such as cancer and CVDs (Greenberg *et al.* 1990). To verify the efficacy of beta carotene rich supplementation in CVDs, a double blind, randomized trial was conducted by Hennekens *et al.* (1996), where 50 mg β-carotene was given to 22,071 individuals (males) aged between 40 to 84 years on alternate days. 11% of these members were existing smokers and 39% were former smokers at the start of the study. The trial was piloted for a period of 12 years, as the efficacy of beta carotene in prevention of CVDs can be directly tested through such large, long term, randomized trials. Various parameters relating to the myocardial activity, infarction, stroke, and other cardiac measures were observed (Table **2**). The study concluded that beta carotene intake led to no significant damage or benefit in the occurrence of CVD, cancer or death from all reasons.

Lycopene

Lycopene is a fat-soluble pigment which gives red color to tomatoes, guavas, pink grapefruit, watermelon and some other foods. It is a type of carotenoid that has proven effects in preventing prostate cancer and cardiovascular diseases in humans. Among majority of the carotenoids, lycopene is one of the most powerful antioxidant with cardiovascular benefits which include effects on cardiac, endothelial and vascular functions. Its anti-oxidative mechanisms root from the ability of the molecule to scavenge free radicals by removing the singlet oxygen 10 times more effectively than alpha tocopherol and 2 times higher than beta carotene (Przybylska 2019). The singlet oxygen quenching property of lycopene is due to the increased number of double bonds present in the lycopene molecule, thus making it a potentially powerful antioxidant (Adams *et al.* 1999). It has also shown to modulate the action of NADPH oxidase, COX-2, NOS and 5-lipoxygenase, the enzymes responsible for the formation of free radicals. Lycopene, when consumed through food, is absorbed from the GIT and transported into the liver through the sub-epithelial lymphatic vessels leading to formation of lipoprotein LDL and VLDL complexes (Arab and Steck 2000). These complexes transfer lycopene to various organs and tissues through the blood circulation, where it gets absorbed *via* the LDL receptors present on these organs. The consumption of lycopene prevents lipid formation, LDL lipoprotein segmentation, protein and DNA oxidation, thus protecting the system against myocardial infarction, coronary insufficiency and angina pectoris (Muller *et al.* 2016). It has been concluded from various studies that the increased serum lycopene concentration as a result of higher dietary intake of lycopene has considerably reduced the risk of major cardiovascular disorders (Table **2**) (Przybylska 2019, Bansal *et al.* 2006). Human beings are unable to produce lycopene naturally, because of which we need to increase our dietary consumption of lycopene.

Pre-clinical Study

Lycopene acts by curbing the oxidation of LDL cholesterol which leads to the formation of atherosclerotic plaque. In 2008, Hu *et al.* assessed the anti-atherogenic effect through intra-gastric supplementation of lycopene (4 to 12 mg/day for 4 and 8 weeks) in rabbits that were fed a high-fat diet. The study showed a marked decrease in the atherosclerotic plaque formation in the aorta of these rabbits. It also resulted in the reduction of LDL cholesterol, total cholesterol, triglycerides, ox-LDL and IL-1, and a spike in the nitric oxide and antioxidant capacity. Similar studies were conducted with fulvastatin (a synthetic lipid-lowering agent) in the same animal model, and surprisingly, the effects of diet induced lycopene were more remarkable than those obtained by fulvastatin (Hu *et al.* 2008).

Clinical Study

To investigate effects of lycopene on the vasculature of CVD patients, Gajendragadkar *et al.* (2014) conducted a prospective, double blind, randomized, placebo controlled group study in 36 patients with CVD and 36 healthy volunteers. They were administered 7 mg of lycopene on daily basis for 2 months. The effects on the vascular system, blood pressure, arterial stiffness, lipid profile and inflammatory factors were monitored closely. All of the above tests and post-therapy observations suggest that lycopene supplementation was effective in improving the endothelial function in CVD patients. This shows that a diet rich in lycopene is necessary for supplementing endothelial activities in people prone to CVD in spite of the available therapeutic medications. Nonetheless, further reports are necessary to identify the various cardiovascular outcomes through lycopene supplementation in high risk populations (Gajendragadkar *et al.* 2014).

Resveratrol

Resveratrol, a naturally occurring polyphenolic compound, contains a unique stilbene structure (Table **1**) having the ability to upregulate NOS thus favoring vasodilation. Resveratrol has greater importance amongst the foods wielding anti-oxidant properties. It works *via* 3 separate mechanism of actions: (1) quenching free radicals; (2) increasing the free radical metabolizing enzyme activity; (3) inhibiting enzymatic ROS production. The neutralization of free radicals thus prevents mitochondrial biogenesis averting various chronic disorders including CVD. Resveratrol can be found in a variety of fruits and plants such as, the roots of *P. cuspidium* (which produces 98% pure trans-resveratrol), grapes, peanuts, pine trees, *cassia* and other plants (Carrizzo *et al.* 2013, Ghanim *et al.* 2010). Due to the importance of resveratrol in anti-oxidant, anti-inflammatory, anti-aging, cardioprotective and neuroprotective activities, a significant interest for this molecule has been developed by researchers across the globe.

Pre-clinical Study

Hypercholesterolemia, an increase in the serum concentration of LDL is a chief risk factor of atherosclerosis resulting in CVD. The liver degrades cholesterol with the help of enzyme CYP7A1 and converts it into bile acids, and is the only organ to perform this function. The enzyme hepatic cholesterol 7α-hydroxylase (CYP7A1) has a very vital role in the regulation of metabolism of cholesterol in the entire system. A deficiency of CYP7A1 may significantly elevate the level of LDL-C and total cholesterol, and enhance coronary and peripheral vascular disease. A trial conducted by Chen *et al.* (2012) demonstrated the activity of resveratrol on the accumulation of serum and hepatic cholesterol in mice model, fed with high fat diet. Pharmacological properties of resveratrol related to increased endothelial NOS activation, reduction in aggregation of platelets, oxidation of LDL-C, and prostaglandin synthesis were observed. Reduction in blood cholesterol levels by resveratrol supplementation, through the activation of bile acid synthetic pathways by CYP7A1 was seen. This concluded that dietary resveratrol increased CYP7A1 expression and resulted in significant reduction in blood cholesterol and LDL-C concentrations.

Clinical Study

Low grade systemic inflammation is a common trait observed in smokers, causing oxidative stress which accelerates or leads to various cardiovascular diseases. A randomized, cross over, double-blind trial was performed by Bo *et al.* (2013) on 50 healthy adult smokers with a dose of 500 mg resveratrol per day for a period of 30 days. Resveratrol showed significant drop in the levels of C-reactive protein (CRP) and triglycerides, and presented a spike in total antioxidant status (TAS) values. Other parameters such as cholesterol, blood glucose, uric acid, insulin, concentrations of liver enzyme, BMR and blood pressure were observed and didn't show significant difference post supplementation of resveratrol. C-reactive protein (CRP) help in predicting the endothelial activity and play an important role in the pathogenesis of vascular diseases. The study revealed that reduction in CRP and triglyceride levels along with the antioxidant, anti-inflammatory and hypotriglyceridemic effects would significantly improve the endothelial activity, thus prevent or reduce the intensity of CVDs.

Flavonoids

Flavonoids, a widely distributed group of natural benzopyran derivatives found in fruits and vegetables, possess strong antioxidant properties and employ several mechanisms which involve free radical scavenging activity. The cardiovascular protective mechanism of flavonoids includes the metal ion chelating property complexed along with copper/iron to prevent the generation of the ROS (Nuttall *et al.* 1999). Major role of flavonoids as radical scavenging activity are dependent on the different moieties that are attached to it, such as presence of catechol group in benzene ring and 2,3 double bond in conjugation with 4-oxo group which is responsible for electron delocalization thus, has a better electron donating property (Adams *et al.* 1999, Lovegrove *et al.* 2017) (Table **1**).

In addition to this, flavonoids also have beneficial effects on lipid profile by inhibiting platelet aggregation, modulating generation of inflammatory cells and enhance nitric oxide synthesis. Different flavonoids used for CVD are flavonols (quercetin, kaempferol), isoflavones (genistein, daidzein), flavones (luteolin), flavanones (hesperidin) and flavanols (catechin, epicatechin, gallocatechin). Natural sources of flavonoids include cocoa, red wine or grape, tea and onions which may have measurable effect in CVD including reduction in blood pressure (Erdman *et al.* 2007).

Quercetin is an opulent flavonol in our diet that possesses anti-oxidative, anti-carcinogenic and enzyme-inhibiting activities. Quercetin has been distributed in a variety of foods such as onions, apples, and tea (Baghel 2012).

Pre-clinical Study

Ischemia (insufficient blood supply), the underlying cause for many chronic diseases such as myocardial infarction, angina pectoris, thrombotic stroke, *etc.*, can be reversed by allowing rapid return of blood flow to the ischemic zone of myocardium, also known as reperfusion that leads to the reduction in mortality by almost half (Arumugam *et al.* 2012, Dong *et al.* 2018). A trial by Liu *et al.* (2012) helped to study the effects of quercetin on myocardial oxidative stress and weakening of immunity stimulated by isoproterenol in rats for a period of 30 days. Isoproterenol 70 mg/kg was subcutaneously injected in Wistar rats in order to induce myocardial ischemia. Reperfusion and myocardial ischemia can trigger an intense inflammatory response and generation of free radicals that react with tissue components leading to production of metabolites, which can be used for estimating oxidative stress. Evaluation of blood-immunity index, cardiac marker enzymes and antioxidative parameters in hearts revealed that the concentration of blood AST, nitric oxide, inflammatory markers such as creatine kinase, IL-10, IL-1, IL-8 and lactate dehydrogenase were significantly increased. Dietary intake of quercetin substantially improved myocardial damage due to ischemia and weakened immune function stimulated by isoproterenol. The study concluded that quercetin demonstrated its cardio-protective activity by effectively increasing plasma antioxidant capacity and provided protection against ischemia–reperfusion injury significantly in rats (Liu *et al.* 2012).

Clinical Study

Some of its cardio-protective effects are shown *viain-vitro* studies, but are not proven in human studies. Diabetes, a major risk factor for cardiovascular diseases (CVDs) occurs because of accelerated atherosclerosis among such individuals. A trial on the effect of quercetin on various risk factors and inflammatory biomarkers in CVD was conducted by Zahedi *et al.* (2013) in 72 women with type 2 diabetes for a period of 10 weeks. Quercetin was given to participants at a dose of 500 mg capsule per day. Biochemical variables were measured at baseline and at the end of the study, and changes were compared using appropriate statistical methods. Parameters such as blood pressure, HDL-C, LDL-C, triglycerides were measured along with the serum concentrations of tumor necrosis factor-α (TNF-α) and interleukin-6 (IL-6). Results demonstrated that quercetin supplementation helped reduce systolic blood pressure significantly but was ineffective on other cardiovascular risk factors and inflammatory biomarkers. Taking into consideration the *in-vitro* effects of quercetin, there is scope for more studies to be conducted with varied doses of quercetin (Hertog *et al.* 1993, Malishevskaia *et al.* 2013).

Anthocyanins

Anthocyanins are aqueous pigments of the flavonoid group, responsible for colouration of plants including vegetables/fruits like strawberry, chokeberry, *etc* (Ak and Gulcin 2008). They exert antioxidant property by inhibiting lipid oxidation through their metal-ion chelating activity for transitional elements such as copper or by free radical scavenging activity. Several studies have proved the benefits of anthocyanin in preventing and treating cardiovascular diseases by various mechanisms, *e.g.,* xanthine oxidase inhibition (by structuralmodification of –OH group leading to obstruction of XO pathways), chelation of metal ions, and suppression of nitric oxide production, inflammatory processes, and endothelial dysfunction. Their dietary sources include berries, red onions, kidney beans, pomegranates, grapes (including wine), tomatoes, acai, bilberry, chokeberry, elderberry, and tart cherries, *etc.*

Pre-clinical Study

Several anti-diabetic and cardio-protective properties have been discussed about anthocyanins. Animal models have provided positive results in authenticating theories of anthocyanins efficacy associated with human trials. The effect of grape bilberry on atherogenesis was demonstrated by Graf *et al.* (2013) on rat model. It was seen that grape bilberry juice enriched with 1551 mg/l anthocyanins reduced the total cholesterol and triglyceride levels. Further investigation on the plasma distribution of fatty acids revealed reduction in the saturated fatty acids and increase in the long-chain n3-polyunsaturated fatty acids (PUFA). Prominent changes were observed with significant reduction in the plasma fatty acids, serum cholesterol, resistin and leptin levels. This concluded that the anthocyanin-rich juice intake was constructive in preventing atherosclerosis by improving endothelial function and moderating the serum lipid concentration thus, having a preventive potential for obesity-associated diseases such as CVD or type 2 diabetes.

Clinical Study

Strawberries are a vital fruit in the Mediterranean diet, which exert beneficial effects on human health due to elevated contents of essential nutrients and useful phytochemicals. Alvarez-Suarez *et al.* (2014) supplemented healthy human volunteers with strawberry, fresh fruit rich in anthocyanin, for a period of 1 month. If the participants had previously consumed strawberry, they were advised to avoid it along with other polyphenols for a duration of 10 days. Post 30 days of strawberry consumption, factors such as plasma lipid profile, antioxidant status, platelet functioning and oxidative stress were evaluated. The results demonstrated that the patients presented a reduction in the levels of LDL cholesterol and triglyceride after strawberry supplementation. Another study also showed decrease in levels of spontaneous and oxidative hemolysis hence proving that strawberry rich diet could help in the prevention against CVDs (Adegbola *et al.* 2017).

Curcumin

Curcumin is a polyphenolic yellow pigment of *Curcuma longa*. The antioxidant activity of curcumin is observed through the inhibition of the mitogen- activated protein kinase which is responsible for the atherosclerosis and atrial arrhythmias due to blood vessel inflammation (Adams *et al.* 1999). Curcumin has the ability to scavenge ROS, thus reducing the oxidative stress and inflammatory damage. Long term ingestion of curcumin has shown to modify genetic expressions involved in cholesterol homeostasis by decreasing serum lipid peroxidase and total serum cholesterol. Also, because of the membrane stabilizing effect of curcuminoids, the compound is proved to be effective in myocardial ischemia, cardiac hypertrophy and heart failure. Recent studies showed that curcumin in combination with bioperine enhances its bioavailability, leading to significant reductions in inflammatory cytokines that mediate in the action of chronic inflammation. It improves HDL-C and has a lipid modifying effect that influences all pathways through which cholesterol reaches the bloodstream (Vasanthi *et al.* 2012).

Clinical Study

A double blind, randomized, placebo controlled clinical trial on human subjects with coronary artery disease (CAD) exhibited promising results in reducing the serum levels of triglycerides, LDL and VLDL cholesterol (Table **2**). In this 8 week study by Mirzabeigi *et al.* (2015) 33 subjects with coronary artery disease were administered 500 mg/day (4 capsules) of Curcumin-C3 complex for a period of two months along with the conventional therapies. A significant reduction in the serum LDL, VLDL and triglyceride levels was observed when compared to the baseline. Thus, in conclusion, curcumin showed potential effects against cholesterol and triglyceride levels. The results of the present studies requisite a larger scale of clinical trials evaluating the anti-oxidant and anti-inflammatory effects of Curcumin supplementation for CVD patients (Moloughney 2017).

Allyl cysteine, Alliin, Allicin and Allyl disulphide

Garlic (*Allium Sativum*) is used worldwide for its therapeutic properties. Allicin (diallyl thiosulfinate), the biologically active compound in garlic, plays a role in the cardiovascular health benefits of an individual. This compound is also known to acquire various other activities such as anti-biotic, anti-fungal, and carcinogenic inhibitory activity. It has been identified to decrease triglyceride and serum cholesterol levels and decrease formation of atherosclerotic plaque and platelet aggregation. The cellular assembly of garlic, when damaged, C-S-lyase (alliinase) acts on alliin (S-allyl-L-Cysteine sulfoxide) and gets converted to allicin (allylthiosulfinate). Allicin forms several sulfides by non-enzymatic reaction as diallyl sulfide, diallyl disulfide (DADs), diallyl trisulfide (DATS), or methyl allyl trisulfide (MATS) all of which possess potent anti-platelet activity (Vasanthi *et al.* 2012).

Vitamin C (Ascorbic acid)

It is a hydrophilic antioxidant found as ascorbic acid and dehydro-ascorbic acid, its two biologically active forms. Its major role is related to its property wherein ascorbate is readily oxidized to its dehydroascorbate form, which donates hydrogen to reverse oxidation, thus inactivating free radicals preventing lipid damage (Murabito *et al.* 1993). Vitamin C improves endothelium-dependent vasodilation and reduces monocyte adhesion. Dietary vitamin C is mostly found in citrus fruits, strawberries, cantaloupe, tomatoes, cabbage, and green leafy vegetables. The recommended daily allowance (RDA) for intake of vitamin C is

60 mg. Consumption of high levels of vitamin C is recommended for smokers, patients and lactating mothers to prevent CVD.

Vitamin E (Alpha-Tocopherol)

It is a hydrophobic antioxidant, playing an essential role in protection against free radical damage. Vitamin E is comprised of tocopherols and tocotrienols, in the alpha, beta and delta isomeric forms. The alpha-tocopherol form accounts for 90% vitamin activity in the tissue (Murabito *et al.* 1993). It acts as a chain breaker during lipid peroxidation in cell membranes. The chemical structure of tocopherols makes them good hydrogen donors, because of which Vitamin E is oxidized, thus preventing polyunsaturated fatty acid oxidation on the cell membrane (Adams *et al.* 1999). Vitamin E is the most fat-soluble vitamin, and is incorporated into lipoproteins and cell membranes, thus limiting LDL oxidation (Jha *et al.* 1995, Kushi *et al.* 1996). Major dietary sources of Vitamin E include vegetables and seed oils, wheat germ, whereas, small quantities are found in meat, fish and fruits. The RDA of Vitamin E is 30 IU (equivalent to 30 mg/day) and varies according to the dietary intake of PUFA.

CONCLUSION

Heart disease remains the foremost cause of mortality around the world, and our aging populations are increasingly aware of its health risks *via* various public education campaigns, physicians and nutritionist's recommendation, and intermittent scientific news. Multiple medical complications and issues related to life-style increases the risk of heart disease, including diabetes, obesity, poor diet, and physical inactivity, which are all very common in modern world (Jayathilake *et al.* 2016). The market for heart health supplements is thriving. This chapter abridges the findings of recent studies on selected phytochemicals as prophylactic and therapeutic agents for the prevention and treatment of various cardiovascular diseases (ClinicalTrials.gov 2020, Madjid *et al.* 2020). A limited number of clinical studies on phytobioactive nutrients have proved optimistic results for encouraging health and well-being including reduction of CVDs in humans. Some phyto-nutrients which are discussed in this review such as carotenoids, vitamin C, vitamin E, flavonoids, resveratrol, anthocyanins, curcumin, *etc.* have played a vital role in reduction of CVDs and balancing the quality of life of individuals (Jain *et al.* 2018). Prevention of CVDs with anti-inflammatory and anti-oxidant agents has been a challenging to us for decades. Presently, CVDs are leading among the health-related issues and are considered the primary cause of mortality and morbidity around the globe. Thus, the findings of this literature revealed the enormous potential of various phytobioactive compounds to prevent and treat CVDs with less side-effects and thus decreasing the mortality rate in CVD.

LIST OF ABBREVIATIONS

HDL	High Density Lipoprotein
LDL	Low Density Lipoprotein
TC	Total Cholesterol
TAG	Triacylglyceride
NO	Nitric Oxide
ROS	Reactive Oxygen Species
RNS	Reactive Nitrogen Species
HCD	High Cholesterol Diet
TNF-α	Tumor Necrosis Factor Alpha
IL-1	Interleukin-1
IL-6	Interleukin-6
CRP	C-Reactive Protein
MI	Myocardial infarction

CONFLICT OF INTEREST

The authors declare no conflict of interest, financial or otherwise.

ACKNOWLEDGEMENTS

We would like to thank SPPSPTM, SVKM's NMIMS University, Mumbai, for the encouragement and moral support in writing this chapter.

CONSENT FOR PUBLICATION

None

REFERENCES

Adams, AK, Wermuth, EO & McBride, PE (1999) Antioxidant vitamins and the prevention of coronary heart disease. *Am Fam Physician,* 60, 895-904.
[PMID: 10498115]

Adegbola, P, Aderibigbe, I, Hammed, W & Omotayo, T (2017) Antioxidant and anti-inflammatory medicinal plants have potential role in the treatment of cardiovascular disease: a review. *Am J Cardiovasc Dis,* 7, 19-32.
[PMID: 28533927]

Ahn, J, Cho, I, Kim, S, Kwon, D & Ha, T (2008) Dietary resveratrol alters lipid metabolism-related gene expression of mice on an atherogenic diet. *J Hepatol,* 49, 1019-28.
[http://dx.doi.org/10.1016/j.jhep.2008.08.012] [PMID: 18930334]

Ak, T & Gülçin, I (2008) Antioxidant and radical scavenging properties of curcumin. *Chem Biol Interact,* 174, 27-37.
[http://dx.doi.org/10.1016/j.cbi.2008.05.003] [PMID: 18547552]

Al-Khudairy, L, Flowers, N, Wheelhouse, R, Ghannam, O, Hartley, L, Stranges, S & Rees, K (2017) Vitamin

C supplementation for the primary prevention of cardiovascular disease. *Cochrane Database Syst Rev,* 3CD011114
[http://dx.doi.org/10.1002/14651858.CD011114.pub2] [PMID: 28301692]

Alpha-Tocopherol, BCCPSG (1994) The effect of vitamin E and beta carotene on the incidence of lung cancer and other cancers in male smokers. *N Engl J Med,* 330, 1029-35.
[http://dx.doi.org/10.1056/NEJM199404143301501] [PMID: 8127329]

Alvarez-Suarez, JM, Giampieri, F, Tulipani, S, Casoli, T, Di Stefano, G, González-Paramás, AM, Santos-Buelga, C, Busco, F, Quiles, JL, Cordero, MD, Bompadre, S, Mezzetti, B & Battino, M (2014) One-month strawberry-rich anthocyanin supplementation ameliorates cardiovascular risk, oxidative stress markers and platelet activation in humans. *J Nutr Biochem,* 25, 289-94.
[http://dx.doi.org/10.1016/j.jnutbio.2013.11.002] [PMID: 24406274]

Alves, QL & Camargo, SB (2019) Role of Nutraceuticals in the Prevention and Treatment of Hypertension and Cardiovascular Diseases. *J Hypertens Manag Journal of Hypertension and Management,* 5

Arab, L & Steck, S (2000) Lycopene and cardiovascular disease. *Am J Clin Nutr,* 71 (Suppl.), 1691S-5S.
[http://dx.doi.org/10.1093/ajcn/71.6.1691S] [PMID: 10837319]

Arumugam, S, Thandavarayan, RA, Arozal, W, Sari, FR, Giridharan, VV, Soetikno, V, Palaniyandi, SS, Harima, M, Suzuki, K, Nagata, M, Tagaki, R, Kodama, M & Watanabe, K (2012) Quercetin offers cardioprotection against progression of experimental autoimmune myocarditis by suppression of oxidative and endoplasmic reticulum stress *via* endothelin-1/MAPK signalling. *Free Radic Res,* 46, 154-63.
[http://dx.doi.org/10.3109/10715762.2011.647010] [PMID: 22145946]

Baghel, SSS (2012) A review of quercetin: antioxidant and anticancer properties. *World J Pharm Pharm Sci,* 1, 146-50.

Bansal, P, Gupta, SK, Ojha, SK, Nandave, M, Mittal, R, Kumari, S & Arya, DS (2006) Cardioprotective effect of lycopene in the experimental model of myocardial ischemia-reperfusion injury. *Mol Cell Biochem,* 289, 1-9.
[http://dx.doi.org/10.1007/s11010-006-9141-7] [PMID: 16601921]

Bo, S, Ciccone, G, Castiglione, A, Gambino, R, De Michieli, F, Villois, P, Durazzo, M, Cavallo-Perin, P & Cassader, M (2013) Anti-inflammatory and antioxidant effects of resveratrol in healthy smokers a randomized, double-blind, placebo-controlled, cross-over trial. *Curr Med Chem,* 20, 1323-31.
[http://dx.doi.org/10.2174/0929867311320100009] [PMID: 23298135]

Bruckdorfer, KR (2008) Antioxidants and CVD. *Proc Nutr Soc,* 67, 214-22.
[http://dx.doi.org/10.1017/S0029665108007052] [PMID: 18412995]

Carrizzo, A, Forte, M, Damato, A, Trimarco, V, Salzano, F, Bartolo, M, Maciag, A, Puca, AA & Vecchione, C (2013) Antioxidant effects of resveratrol in cardiovascular, cerebral and metabolic diseases. *Food Chem Toxicol,* 61, 215-26.
[http://dx.doi.org/10.1016/j.fct.2013.07.021] [PMID: 23872128]

Chen, Q, Wang, E, Ma, L & Zhai, P (2012) Dietary resveratrol increases the expression of hepatic 7α-hydroxylase and ameliorates hypercholesterolemia in high-fat fed C57BL/6J mice. *Lipids Health Dis,* 11, 56.
[http://dx.doi.org/10.1186/1476-511X-11-56] [PMID: 22607622]

Cherubini, A, Vigna, GB, Zuliani, G, Ruggiero, C, Senin, U & Fellin, R (2005) Role of antioxidants in atherosclerosis: epidemiological and clinical update. *Curr Pharm Des,* 11, 2017-32.
[http://dx.doi.org/10.2174/1381612054065783] [PMID: 15974956]

(2020) https://ClinicalTrials.gov/show/NCT04323228

Csepanyi, E, Czompa, A, Haines, D, Lekli, I, Bakondi, E, Balla, G, Tosaki, A & Bak, I (2015) Cardiovascular effects of low *versus* high-dose beta-carotene in a rat model. *Pharmacol Res,* 100, 148-56.
[http://dx.doi.org/10.1016/j.phrs.2015.07.021] [PMID: 26225824]

D'Odorico, A, Martines, D, Kiechl, S, Egger, G, Oberhollenzer, F, Bonvicini, P, Sturniolo, GC, Naccarato, R & Willeit, J (2000) High plasma levels of alpha- and beta-carotene are associated with a lower risk of

atherosclerosis: results from the Bruneck study. *Atherosclerosis,* 153, 231-9.
[http://dx.doi.org/10.1016/S0021-9150(00)00403-2] [PMID: 11058719]

Daviglus, ML, Orencia, AJ, Dyer, AR, Liu, K, Morris, DK, Persky, V, Chavez, N, Goldberg, J, Drum, M, Shekelle, RB & Stamler, J (1997) Dietary vitamin C, beta-carotene and 30-year risk of stroke: results from the Western Electric Study. *Neuroepidemiology,* 16, 69-77.
[http://dx.doi.org/10.1159/000109673] [PMID: 9057168]

de Andrade, TU, Brasil, GA, Endringer, DC, da Nóbrega, FR & de Sousa, DP (2017) Cardiovascular Activity of the Chemical Constituents of Essential Oils. *Molecules,* 22, 22.
[http://dx.doi.org/10.3390/molecules22091539] [PMID: 28926969]

Dong, LY, Chen, F, Xu, M, Yao, LP, Zhang, YJ & Zhuang, Y (2018) Quercetin attenuates myocardial ischemia-reperfusion injury *via* downregulation of the HMGB1-TLR4-NF-κB signaling pathway. *Am J Transl Res,* 10, 1273-83.
[PMID: 29887944]

Erdman, JW, Jr, Balentine, D, Arab, L, Beecher, G, Dwyer, JT, Folts, J, Harnly, J, Hollman, P, Keen, CL, Mazza, G, Messina, M, Scalbert, A, Vita, J, Williamson, G & Burrowes, J (2007) Flavonoids and heart health: proceedings of the ILSI North America Flavonoids Workshop, May 31-June 1, 2005, Washington, DC. *J Nutr,* 137 (Suppl. 1), 718S-37S.
[http://dx.doi.org/10.1093/jn/137.3.718S] [PMID: 17311968]

Frei, B (1994) Reactive oxygen species and antioxidant vitamins: mechanisms of action. *Am J Med,* 97, 5S-13S.
[http://dx.doi.org/10.1016/0002-9343(94)90292-5] [PMID: 8085584]

Gajendragadkar, PR, Hubsch, A, Mäki-Petäjä, KM, Serg, M, Wilkinson, IB & Cheriyan, J (2014) Effects of oral lycopene supplementation on vascular function in patients with cardiovascular disease and healthy volunteers: a randomised controlled trial. *PLoS One,* 9e99070
[http://dx.doi.org/10.1371/journal.pone.0099070] [PMID: 24911964]

Ghanim, H, Sia, CL, Abuaysheh, S, Korzeniewski, K, Patnaik, P, Marumganti, A, Chaudhuri, A & Dandona, P (2010) An antiinflammatory and reactive oxygen species suppressive effects of an extract of Polygonum cuspidatum containing resveratrol. *J Clin Endocrinol Metab,* 95, E1-8.
[http://dx.doi.org/10.1210/jc.2010-0482] [PMID: 20534755]

Graf, D, Seifert, S, Jaudszus, A, Bub, A & Watzl, B (2013) Anthocyanin-Rich Juice Lowers Serum Cholesterol, Leptin, and Resistin and Improves Plasma Fatty Acid Composition in Fischer Rats. *PLoS One,* 8e66690
[http://dx.doi.org/10.1371/journal.pone.0066690] [PMID: 23825152]

Greenberg, ER, Baron, JA, Stukel, TA, Stevens, MM, Mandel, JS, Spencer, SK, Elias, PM, Lowe, N, Nierenberg, DW & Bayrd, G (1990) A clinical trial of beta carotene to prevent basal-cell and squamous-cell cancers of the skin. *N Engl J Med,* 323, 789-95.
[http://dx.doi.org/10.1056/NEJM199009203231204] [PMID: 2202901]

Hennekens, CH, Buring, JE, Manson, JE, Stampfer, M, Rosner, B, Cook, NR, Belanger, C, LaMotte, F, Gaziano, JM, Ridker, PM, Willett, W & Peto, R (1996) Lack of effect of long-term supplementation with beta carotene on the incidence of malignant neoplasms and cardiovascular disease. *N Engl J Med,* 334, 1145-9.
[http://dx.doi.org/10.1056/NEJM199605023341801] [PMID: 8602179]

Hertog, MG, Feskens, EJ, Hollman, PC, Katan, MB & Kromhout, D (1993) Dietary antioxidant flavonoids and risk of coronary heart disease: the Zutphen Elderly Study. *Lancet,* 342, 1007-11.
[http://dx.doi.org/10.1016/0140-6736(93)92876-U] [PMID: 8105262]

Hu, MY, Li, YL, Jiang, CH, Liu, ZQ, Qu, SL & Huang, YM (2008) Comparison of lycopene and fluvastatin effects on atherosclerosis induced by a high-fat diet in rabbits. *Nutrition,* 24, 1030-8.
[http://dx.doi.org/10.1016/j.nut.2008.05.006] [PMID: 18585898]

Jain, S, Buttar, HS, Chintameneni, M & Kaur, G (2018) Prevention of Cardiovascular Diseases with Anti-

Inflammatory and Anti- Oxidant Nutraceuticals and Herbal Products: An Overview of Pre-Clinical and Clinical Studies. *Recent Pat Inflamm Allergy Drug Discov,* 12, 145-57.
[http://dx.doi.org/10.2174/1872213X12666180815144803] [PMID: 30109827]

Jayathilake, C, Rizliya, V & Liyanage, R (2016) Antioxidant and Free Radical Scavenging Capacity of Extensively Used Medicinal Plants in Sri Lanka. *Procedia Food Sci,* 6, 123-6.
[http://dx.doi.org/10.1016/j.profoo.2016.02.028]

Jha, P, Flather, M, Lonn, E, Farkouh, M & Yusuf, S (1995) The antioxidant vitamins and cardiovascular disease. A critical review of epidemiologic and clinical trial data. *Ann Intern Med,* 123, 860-72.
[http://dx.doi.org/10.7326/0003-4819-123-11-199512010-00009] [PMID: 7486470]

Klipstein-Grobusch, K, Geleijnse, JM, den Breeijen, JH, Boeing, H, Hofman, A, Grobbee, DE & Witteman, JC (1999) Dietary antioxidants and risk of myocardial infarction in the elderly: the Rotterdam Study. *Am J Clin Nutr,* 69, 261-6.
[http://dx.doi.org/10.1093/ajcn/69.2.261] [PMID: 9989690]

Knekt, P, Reunanen, A, Järvinen, R, Seppänen, R, Heliövaara, M & Aromaa, A (1994) Antioxidant vitamin intake and coronary mortality in a longitudinal population study. *Am J Epidemiol,* 139, 1180-9.
[http://dx.doi.org/10.1093/oxfordjournals.aje.a116964] [PMID: 8209876]

Kosmas, CE, Silverio, D, Sourlas, A, Montan, PD, Guzman, E & Garcia, MJ (2019) Anti-inflammatory therapy for cardiovascular disease. *Ann Transl Med,* 7, 147.
[http://dx.doi.org/10.21037/atm.2019.02.34] [PMID: 31157268]

Kushi, LH, Folsom, AR, Prineas, RJ, Mink, PJ, Wu, Y & Bostick, RM (1996) Dietary antioxidant vitamins and death from coronary heart disease in postmenopausal women. *N Engl J Med,* 334, 1156-62.
[http://dx.doi.org/10.1056/NEJM199605023341803] [PMID: 8602181]

Lakhanpal, PR (2008) Role of quercetin in cardiovascular diseases. *Internet Journal of Medical Update,* 3, 31-49.

Liu, H, Zhang, L & Lu, S (2012) Evaluation of antioxidant and immunity activities of quercetin in isoproterenol-treated rats. *Molecules,* 17, 4281-91.
[http://dx.doi.org/10.3390/molecules17044281] [PMID: 22491677]

Lovegrove, JA, Stainer, A & Hobbs, DA (2017) Role of flavonoids and nitrates in cardiovascular health. *Proc Nutr Soc,* 1-13.
[http://dx.doi.org/10.1017/S0029665116002871] [PMID: 28100284]

Madjid, M, Safavi-Naeini, P, Solomon, SD & Vardeny, O (2020) Potential Effects of Coronaviruses on the Cardiovascular System: A Review. *JAMA Cardiol,* 5, 831-40.
[http://dx.doi.org/10.1001/jamacardio.2020.1286] [PMID: 32219363]

Malishevskaia, IV, Ilashchuk, TA & Okipniak, IV (2013) [Therapeutic efficacy of quercetin in patients with is ischemic heart disease with underlying metabolic syndrome]. *Georgian Med News,* 67-71. [Therapeutic efficacy of quercetin in patients with is ischemic heart disease with underlying metabolic syndrome].
[PMID: 24423679]

Mann, DL (2015) Innate immunity and the failing heart: the cytokine hypothesis revisited. *Circ Res,* 116, 1254-68.
[http://dx.doi.org/10.1161/CIRCRESAHA.116.302317] [PMID: 25814686]

Marchioli, R, Schweiger, C, Levantesi, G, Tavazzi, L & Valagussa, F (2001) *Antioxidant vitamins and prevention of cardiovascular disease: epidemiological and clinical trial data*
[http://dx.doi.org/10.1007/s11745-001-0683-y]

Mirzabeigi, P, Mohammadpour, AH, Salarifar, M, Gholami, K, Mojtahedzadeh, M & Javadi, MR (2015) The Effect of Curcumin on some of Traditional and Non-traditional Cardiovascular Risk Factors: A Pilot Randomized, Double-blind, Placebo-controlled Trial. *Iran J Pharm Res,* 14, 479-86.
[PMID: 25901155]

Moloughney, S (2017) https://www.nutraceuticalsworld.com/issues/2017-04/view_features/getting-to--

he-heart-of-cardiovascular-health/ [Accessed]

Müller, L, Caris-Veyrat, C, Lowe, G & Böhm, V (2016) Lycopene and Its Antioxidant Role in the Prevention of Cardiovascular Diseases-A Critical Review. *Crit Rev Food Sci Nutr,* 56, 1868-79.
[http://dx.doi.org/10.1080/10408398.2013.801827] [PMID: 25675359]

Murabito, JM, Evans, JC, Larson, MG & Levy, D (1993) Prognosis after the onset of coronary heart disease. An investigation of differences in outcome between the sexes according to initial coronary disease presentation. *Circulation,* 88, 2548-55.
[http://dx.doi.org/10.1161/01.CIR.88.6.2548] [PMID: 8252666]

Nikhra, V (2018) Nutraceuticals for Improving cardiovascular health and prognosis in cardiovascular diseases. *Journal of Nutritional Dietetics & Probiotics,* 1, 1-13.

Nimse, SB & Pal, D (2015) Free radicals, natural antioxidants, and their reaction mechanisms. *RSC Advances,* 5, 27986-8006.
[http://dx.doi.org/10.1039/C4RA13315C]

Nuttall, SL, Kendall, MJ & Martin, U (1999) Antioxidant therapy for the prevention of cardiovascular disease. *QJM,* 92, 239-44.
[http://dx.doi.org/10.1093/qjmed/92.5.239] [PMID: 10615478]

Przybylska, S (2019) Lycopene – a bioactive carotenoid offering multiple health benefits: a review. *Int J Food Sci Technol,* 55, 11-32.
[http://dx.doi.org/10.1111/ijfs.14260]

Reis, JF, Monteiro, VV, de Souza Gomes, R, do Carmo, MM, da Costa, GV, Ribera, PC & Monteiro, MC (2016) Action mechanism and cardiovascular effect of anthocyanins: a systematic review of animal and human studies. *J Transl Med,* 14, 315.
[http://dx.doi.org/10.1186/s12967-016-1076-5] [PMID: 27846846]

Riccioni, G, Bucciarelli, T, Mancini, B, Corradi, F, Di Ilio, C, Mattei, PA & D'Orazio, N (2007) Antioxidant vitamin supplementation in cardiovascular diseases. *Ann Clin Lab Sci,* 37, 89-95.
[PMID: 17311876]

Rimm, EB, Stampfer, MJ, Ascherio, A, Giovannucci, E, Colditz, GA & Willett, WC (1993) Vitamin E consumption and the risk of coronary heart disease in men. *N Engl J Med,* 328, 1450-6.
[http://dx.doi.org/10.1056/NEJM199305203282004] [PMID: 8479464]

Stephens, NG, Parsons, A, Schofield, PM, Kelly, F, Cheeseman, K & Mitchinson, MJ (1996) Randomised controlled trial of vitamin E in patients with coronary disease: Cambridge Heart Antioxidant Study (CHAOS). *Lancet,* 347, 781-6.
[http://dx.doi.org/10.1016/S0140-6736(96)90866-1] [PMID: 8622332]

Vasanthi, HR, ShriShriMal, N & Das, DK (2012) Retraction Notice: Phytochemicals from plants to combat cardiovascular disease. *Curr Med Chem,* 19, 2242-51.
[http://dx.doi.org/10.2174/092986712800229078] [PMID: 22414106]

Voutilainen, S, Nurmi, T, Mursu, J & Rissanen, TH (2006) Carotenoids and cardiovascular health. *Am J Clin Nutr,* 83, 1265-71.
[http://dx.doi.org/10.1093/ajcn/83.6.1265] [PMID: 16762935]

Wilson, PW, D'Agostino, RB, Levy, D, Belanger, AM, Silbershatz, H & Kannel, WB (1998) Prediction of coronary heart disease using risk factor categories. *Circulation,* 97, 1837-47.
[http://dx.doi.org/10.1161/01.CIR.97.18.1837] [PMID: 9603539]

World Health Organization, WHO (2011) Causes of death 2008: data sources and methods, Geneva, World Health Organization.

Zahedi, M, Ghiasvand, R, Feizi, A, Asgari, G & Darvish, L (2013) Does Quercetin Improve Cardiovascular Risk factors and Inflammatory Biomarkers in Women with Type 2 Diabetes: A Double-blind Randomized Controlled Clinical Trial. *Int J Prev Med,* 4, 777-85.

[PMID: 24049596]

Zordoky, BN, Robertson, IM & Dyck, JR (2015) Preclinical and clinical evidence for the role of resveratrol in the treatment of cardiovascular diseases. *Biochim Biophys Acta,* 1852, 1155-77.
[http://dx.doi.org/10.1016/j.bbadis.2014.10.016] [PMID: 25451966]

CHAPTER 13

Therapeutic Potential of Phyto-Constituents for the Treatment of Alzheimer's Disease

Priyankshi Thakkar[1], Siddhi Bagwe-Parab[1], Ginpreet Kaur[1,*], Meena Chintamaneni[1] and Harpal S. Buttar[2]

[1] *Shobhaben Pratapbhai Patel School of Pharmacy and Technology Management, SVKM's NMIMS, Mumbai-56, Maharashtra, India*

[2] *Department of Pathology and Laboratory Medicine, University of Ottawa, School of Medicine, Ottawa, Canada*

Abstract: Alzheimer's disease (AD) is acknowledged as one of the most serious and progressive neurodegenerative disorder, and is the leading cause of dementia in late adult life having unknown etiological pathways. AD is characterized by the formation of intracellular neurofibrillary tangles leading to tau phosphorylation and extracellular amyloid deposits that develop into senile plaques. Amyloid beta (Aβ) plaques, the classic hallmarks of AD, in turn, cause the generation of free radical species of different metals (copper, iron) which modulate neuronal growth, differentiation, and progression of cell death through several signalling pathways. The conventional therapies recommended for the amelioration of AD are only restricted to treat the symptoms of AD and do not focus on the underlying causes of the disease. These allopathic medicines are non-economical and also have unwanted side-effects, which further decrease the quality of life (QOL) of the patients. Therefore, it is of utmost importance to explore alternatives to decrease the expression of neurodegeneration. Antioxidant and anti-inflammatory phytoconstituents play a crucial role in preventing the onset of neurodegenerative diseases and exert neuroprotection. Numerous antioxidant phytonutrients, herbal remedies, and food supplements have been reported for the prevention of cognitive decline and management of AD. The neuroprotective potential of phytotherapies has been demonstrated in numerous *in vitro* and *in vivo* studies. The purpose of this review is to describe phytoconstituents based on their therapeutic effects on etiological pathways (microglia, inflammasome, CB2, NLRP3 and NFKβ) of AD and their underlying molecular mechanisms of action involved in neuroprotection and prevention of AD.

Keywords: Alzheimer's disease, Antioxidants, Cognition enhancement, Cognitive decline, Dementia, Dietary phytoconstituents, Microglial cell activation, Neuroinflammation, Neuronal cell injury, Reactive metal ion species.

* **Corresponding author Ginpreet Kaur:** Shobhaben Pratapbhai Patel School of Pharmacy and Technology Management, SVKM's NMIMS, Mumbai-56, Maharashtra, India. E-mail: Ginpreet.kaur@nmims.edu

INTRODUCTION

Alzheimer's disease (AD) is a chronic neurodegenerative disease that occurs in old age and worsens with time. According to the Alzheimer's Association report (2020), by 2050, people with age above 65 years suffering from AD and dementia are projected to reach 13.8 million. It is also estimated that by the end of the year 2020, 70% of the world's population above the age of 60 will be suffering from AD, 14.2% from India itself (Mathuranath *et al.* 2010). Between 2000 and 2017, the number of deaths due to AD have increased by 145%, as per Alzheimer's Association report (2019). There are several discoveries made with respect to the pathogenesis of AD, but the major hallmark has been the discovery of the amyloid beta (Aß) of senile plaques. Oligomeric forms of this peptide are the main causative agents in the development of AD.

Oxidative stress is a major cause of various age-related disorders like AD. Major pathophysiology arises due to the occurrence of oxidative stress. It has been proved that an increase in oxidative stress causes a modification in the protein side-chain due to the presence of reactive oxygen species (ROS) or reactive nitrogen species (RNS), thus resulting in tau hyperphosphorylation. Overproduction of ROS results in major oxidative stress, an important mediator of damage to cell structures and leads to lipid peroxidation, mitochondrial dysfunction, protein damage, DNA damage, lysosomal dysfunction causing various age-related disorders including AD (Singh *et al.* 2016, Venkatesan *et al.* 2015). Aß secretion due to the stressed and degenerated neurons leads to the formation of Aß aggregates, in turn causing major degenerative events in the cells like neurons, macrophages, and microglia (Bayer *et al.* 2001). The pathophysiology of AD is mainly related to the neuropathological features *i.e.,* hyperphosphorylated neurofibrillary tangles (NFTs) and amyloid plaques.

Currently, there is no reliable therapy for the treatment of neurodegenerative disorders. However, there has been evidence regarding the use of phytoconstituents for the prevention and treatment of disorders including AD. Phytoconstituents present in dietary supplements help reduce the occurrence and risk associated with several non-communicable diseases such as cardiovascular, cancer and neurodegenerative disorders. People consuming antioxidant and anti-inflammatory dietary supplements are at a lower risk of neuronal dysfunction (Kumar and Khanum 2012). Intake of phytoconstituents containing flavonoids and retinoids have shown beneficial effects on the overall health and well-being as well as helped in improving mental and physical performance by boosting the body's antioxidant systems (Venkatesan *et al.* 2015). The purpose of this review is to highlight how phytoconstituents such as crocin, curcumin, cinnamaldehyde, withaferin, *etc.,* present in dietary supplements like turmeric, cinnamon, ashwagandha, *etc.,* exert useful actions in treating neurodegenerative disorders either as a single entity or in combination with other dietary supplements. Various pathways involved in causing AD, including microglia, NLRP3, NFKB, and CB2, as well as mitochondrial dysfunction pathway and sirtuin SIRT1 are also discussed. It has been reported that various phytoconstituents act on these pathways. Therefore, the overall focus of this review is on the influence of phytoconstituents used for curing AD and other CNS disorders.

LINK BETWEEN OXIDATIVE STRESS, NEURONAL INFLAMMATION AND ALZHEIMER'S DISEASE

AD is characterized by neuronal dysfunction and shrinkage of brain tissue. The two most known hallmarks of AD are amyloid plaques (Aß) and neurofibrillary tangles. These hallmarks are the predisposing factors for causing neuroinflammation. An Alzheimer's associated brain results in atrophy of the cerebral cortex and hippocampus. Also, the gyri are narrowed, the sulci are expanded and cerebrospinal fluid (CSF) in the ventricles is increased. These changes in the brain take place due to neurodegeneration which is associated with the formation of extracellular senile plaques and intracellular neurofibrillary tangles (NFTs). NFTs are intracellular aggregates, in the form of fibrils of the associated tau proteins which show oxidative changes as well as hyperphosphorylation. These tangles and plaques are involved in learning, memory and emotional behavior in regions such as the hippocampus, basal forebrain, and amygdala (Mizuno *et al.* 2012, Morales *et al.* 2014). Oxidative imbalance and neuronal damage play an important role in the progression of AD. The accumulation of Aß increases oxidative stress, elevates mitochondrial dysfunction, increases the phosphorylation of tau protein which induces pathogenesis of AD (Kim *et al.* 2015, Zhao and Zhao 2013). Another important parameter involved in the pathogenesis of AD is the formation of free radicals. Radical species production takes place due to the presence of amyloid beta peptide of 42 residues (Aß42). The amyloid beta peptides bind to metal ions like copper ions (Cu^{2+}) which are present in abundance in the brains of AD patients. Cu^{2+} leads to the formation of H_2O_2, a reactive oxygen species (ROS) leading to oxidative stress and thus induces AD (Rosales Hernández *et al.* 2016). The presence of bound Fe^{3+} to Aß is also observed in AD, which when reduced to Fe^{2+} escalates the production of ROS (Peters *et al.* 2015). Also, there are many genetic and environmental factors that are responsible for AD. As mentioned, the pathophysiology of AD is shown in Fig. (**1**).

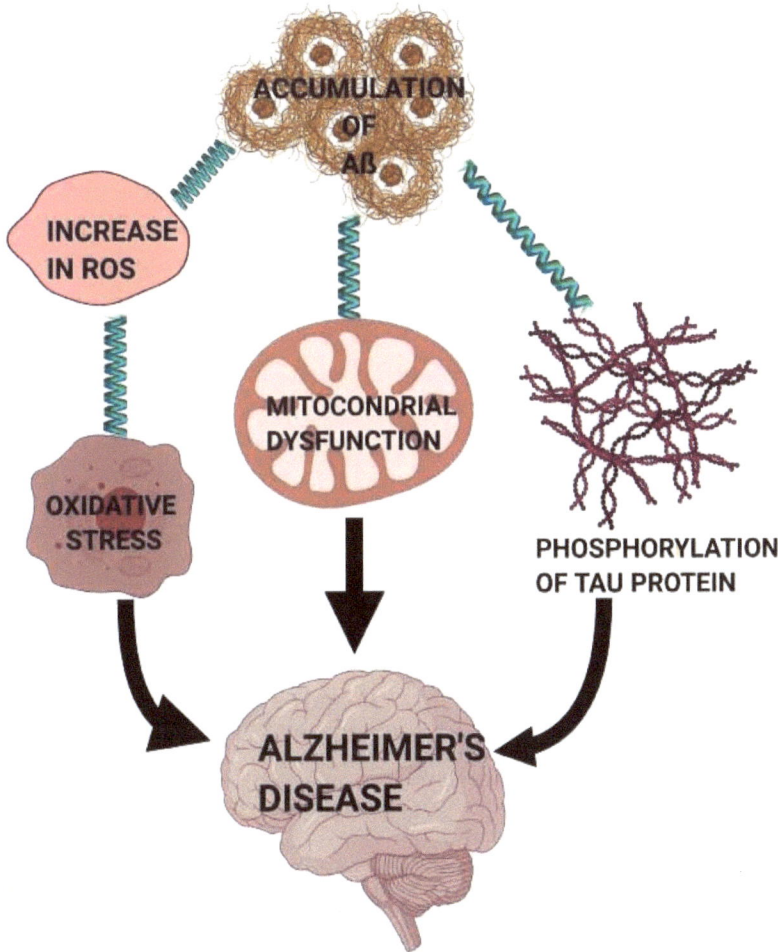

Fig. (1). Diagrammatic representation of the pathophysiology of Alzheimer's disease.

Microglial and Beta-Amyloid Aggregation

Microglia are one of the key promoters of neuroinflammation. Microglial inflammation takes place not only in Alzheimer's disease but also in Parkinson's disease, cerebral ischemia, traumatic brain injury, and many other neurodegenerative diseases. Microglia are forms of macrophages that mediate the neuroinflammatory cytokines. Aggregate proteins such as Aß release pro-inflammatory cytokines like TNF-α, interleukin-1ß (IL-1ß), IL-16, and reactive oxygen species. These aggregate proteins activate the microglia (Tang *et al.* 2018).

The function of the microglia and macrophages are controlled by signals produced at the site of tissue injury, which induce either a pro-inflammatory M1 phenotype or an inhibitory M2 phenotype activation (Gupta and Kaur 2016). Activation of M1 phenotype like interferon-γ (IFN-γ) and tumor necrosis factor (TNF-α) leads to the production of cytokines and proteases in microglia as a defense mechanism. The M1 phenotypes also include the cyclooxygenase-2 and nitric oxides (NOs). M2 phenotype comprises activation of anti-inflammatory cytokines which include IL-4, IL-10, IL-13, and tumor growth factor-ß (TGF-ß). These are important for the demyelination repair, and mainly for wound healing, thus reducing neuroinflammation. It is proved that not only the help of Th2 cytokines is required in the conversion of M1 to M2 but also that of cyclic AMP. Cyclic AMP suppresses the M1 activating the inhibitory M2 phenotypes, thus helping in reducing neuroinflammation (Ghosh *et al.* 2016).

NFkß Pathway

NFkß is a part of the inflammatory responses which are expressed in the brains of patients suffering from Alzheimer's disease. The activity is increased by the presence of Aß. There are two major pathways for NFkß activation, canonical and non-canonical pathways. The canonical pathway is dependent on phosphorylation of the inhibitors of NFkß and its signals are received from receptors like the Toll-like receptors (TLRs), interleukin receptors, and the TNF-α receptors. In the canonical pathway, there is mainly a degradation of the Ikß kinase, and thus the NFkß particles are released. The TLRs cause the activation of the NFkß which lead to the formation of many inflammatory cytokine genes.

The binding of Aß to the TLR causes nuclear translocation of NF-kB p65, which increases the mediators such as IL-1ß and TNF-α (Kawai and Akira 2007). Lipopolysaccharides (LPS) stimulate the immune system of many organisms. LPS leads to an inflammatory progression which causes a severe effect on the brain and many other organs in the body. The immune responses are generated by the TLR-4. LPS recognized by the TLR-4 receptor is expressed in the microglia of the CNS. The down streaming signal transduction stimulates the NFkß pathway, thus releasing the pro-inflammatory cytokines that initiate inflammation and cause neuronal damage (Zhang and Xu 2018). NFkß inhibitors help in reducing neuronal damage as well as oxidative stress. It has been suggested that the NFkß inhibitors and phytochemicals help in the treatment of Alzheimer's disease (Seo *et al.* 2018).

NLRP3 and Inflammasome Pathway

The NLRP3 influx is detected and activated *via* bacterial RNA species. The activation of inflammasomes is also induced by bacterial RNA and ssRNA mediated by caspase 1, NLRP3, and ASC. Phagocytosis and mitochondrial generated reactive oxygen species (ROS) also lead to the formation of NLRP3 inflammasome (Sha *et al.* 2014).

The deposition of β-amyloid leads to AD. Aβ causes the release of IL-1β by being activated through NLRP3 inflammasome in the microglia. This inflammasome is said to be stimulated by bacterial toxins and their phagocytosis is needed for the activation of NLRP3 inflammasome. An experiment was performed where microbial cells incubated with cytochalasin D (acts as an inhibitor for phagocytosis) indicated that phagocytosis was needed for the activation of IL-1β by Aβ (Song *et al.* 2017).

The innate immune system helps in recognizing and potentially destroying harmful microorganisms. The innate immune system discriminates microbes from self by recognizing several microbial structures called pathogen-associated molecular patterns (PAMPs) such as peptidoglycan (PGN), lipopolysaccharides (LPS) and flagellin and damage associated molecular patterns (DAMPs) such as uric acid, misfolded proteins, and cholesterol crystals (Halle *et al.* 2008). There are two signals generated for full inflammasome activation along with cytokine secretion. First is priming signal which is required for gene transcription and second is activation signal that causes the formation of the inflammasome complex, leading to cleavage of caspase-1 into enzymatically active heterodimers. Toll-like receptor signaling serves as signal 1 and causes gene transcription of NLRP3, procaspase-1, pro-IL-1β, pro-IL-18 providing an abundance of protein for downstream activation. Signal 2 generates an NLRP3 response leading to inflammasome activity (Saco *et al.* 2014).

Inflammasomes are platforms that lead to the formation and secretion of the pro-inflammatory cytokines IL-1β and IL-18. Inflammasome leads to the activation of caspase-1 containing 20 complexes. Caspases have been studied in apoptosis where they play a role in the activation of cellular demise. An active form of caspase 1 assists in the cleavage of pro-IL-1β and pro-IL-18 into their active forms. In AD, the NLRP3 has a role in increasing the caspase 1 level. An increased level of IL-1β and IL-18 is seen in the cerebrospinal fluid of patients suffering from dementia and AD (Olsen and Singhrao 2016).

The inflammasome is a macromolecule with apoptosis associated speck like protein and a caspase-activation recruitment domain (ASC) which comprises of a carboxy terminal CARD-like domain and a N-terminal pyrin only domain (PYD). It also has a central nucleotide-binding domain (NACHT) and a C-terminus leucine-rich receptor (LRR) that recognizes the pathogens. ASC interacts with procaspase 1 which mediates the formation of caspase 1, and the conversion of the proenzyme to its active form. This active form leads to the formation of IL-1β and IL-18, the pro-inflammatory cytokines (Zheng *et al.* 2016).

IL-1ß activates the microglia cells which generates pro-inflammatory factors like IL-16 and TNF-α and also causes initiation of inflammatory reactions in the CNS and thus affects the blood-brain barrier, which causes infiltration of immune cells in the CNS (Halle *et al.* 2008). IL-18 stimulates the production of pro-inflammatory cytokines and chemokine, ß-cells through the T-helper cells present in the immune system. IL-18 activates pathways that lead to increased production of caspase-1 and inflammatory cytokines (Franchi *et al.* 2009).

Cannabinoid Receptor Type-2 Pathway

The cannabinoid receptor type 2, abbreviated as CB2, is a G protein-coupled receptor from the cannabinoid receptor family that in humans is encoded by the CNR2 gene. There are a couple of studies on the examination of CB2, substance in AD mind, yet, every one of them has brought about comparable discoveries. A huge increment in CB2 receptor levels has been found in postmortem AD minds that principally expressed in microglia encompassing feeble plaques (Benito *et al.* 2003). The presence of CB2 receptors in influenced microglia is very helpful since it would allow their specific action in harmed tissues, in this manner limiting the likelihood of injurious symptoms. Although CB2 receptors in AD cerebrum are nitrosylated, likely as an outcome of microglial enactment and peroxynitrite radical development, and this may add to the coupling of these receptors to downstream effector flagging atoms (Ramirez *et al.* 2005).

Sirtuin SIRT1 Pathway

Resveratrol has been found in more than 70 plant species, which promotes a reduction in neuronal damage and the non-amyloidogenic cleavage of amyloid beta-peptides. It is the first polyphenolic compound, which has been shown to activate SIRT1 (Baur *et al.* 2012). SIRT1 plays an essential role in the ability of moderate doses of resveratrol to stimulate AMPK and improve mitochondrial function both *in vitro* and *in vivo* settings. A reduction of reactive oxygen species (ROS) production in PC12 cells was seen with resveratrol followed by reversing rotenone-induced neurotoxicity through activation of the SIRT/Akt1 signaling pathway (Tang *et al.* 2018).

PLANT-DERIVED BIOACTIVE CONSTITUENTS

The dietary supplements targeted for the treatment of Alzheimer's disease are shown in Table **1**.

Almonds

Almonds (*Amygdalus communis* or *Prunus dulcis*) belong to family *Rosaceae* (Safarian *et al.* 2016), and occur in bitter or sweet forms, comprising of fixed oils as well as glycerides such as oleic acid (80%), linoleic acid (15%) and palmitic acid (5%) (Kulkarni *et al.* 2010). A preclinical study was conducted in scopolamine-induced male albino Wistar strain amnesic rats, where paste of almond 150, 300, 600 mg/kg p.o. for 14 days showed a reduction in the rat brain cholinesterase, along with an increase in the glucose levels and a significant decrease in glycerides and cholesterol (Safarian *et al.* 2016).

Another preclinical study was conducted in locally bred male Albino Wistar rats where a paste of 80 mg crushed almonds was orally administered for 28 days with a feeding tube. The improvement in cognitive functioning in the rats was assessed by elevated plus maze (EPM) and radial arm maze (RAM). Almonds helped to improve the memory as well as enhanced the brain tryptophan (TRP) levels. This showed that almonds have a significant hypophagic and nootropic effect (Haider *et al.* 2012).

Almond contains both acetyl-L-carnitine and riboflavin which helps improve brain health. Acetyl-L-carnitine is structurally related to acetylcholine and it acts upon neural transmission and also affects neuronal metabolism. A randomized, placebo-controlled, double-blind clinical study was conducted in 36 patients (10 males and 26 females) for 24 weeks, out of which only 20 completed the study. A dose of 1.0 g was given twice daily or a placebo. At the end of the trial, it was found that acetyl-L-carnitine has a significant effect on the clinical features of dementia of the Alzheimer's disease, mainly the dementia associated with short-term memory (Rai *et al.* 1990).

Hazelnut

Hazelnut (*Corylus avellana)* belongs to the Birch family (Martins *et al.* 2013). The total oil content of hazelnuts ranges from 54.6-63.2%, but the crude protein and dietary fibre is only 14.3-18.2% and 9.8-13.2% respectively (Savage and McNeil 1998). The hazelnut oil is highly rich in triacylglycerols, unsaturated fatty acids, palmitic acid, stearic acid, and linoleic acid (Dobhal *et al.* 2018).

A preclinical study was conducted on amyloid-ß injected male albino Wistar rats where they were fed an oral suspension of hazelnut kernel (without skin) for 16 consecutive days with a dose of 800 mg/kg/day and the effect on the memory, anxiety, as well as neuroinflammation, was recorded. The results showed improvement in memory and reduced anxiety, using an elevated plus maze Method. The treatment improved spatial working memory and decreased anxiety-like behaviour, along with decrease in TNF-α, COX-2, and IL-1β in the hippocampus of Aβ-injected rats (Bahaeddin *et al.* 2017).

Table 1. Various dietary supplements targeted for the treatment of Alzheimer's disease.

Dietary Supplements	Scientific Name	Preclinical/ Clinical Study	Pathways/ Cause	Dose	Formulation Route of Administration	Phyto-constituents	Citations
Almond	*Amygdalus communis*	Preclinical studies in male albino Wistar rats. Preclinical studies in male albino Wistar rats. Clinical study	Beta-amyloid aggregation Beta-amyloid aggregation Beta-amyloid aggregation	150,300 600 mg/kg 400 mg/kg/day 1 gm/day	Powder, oral route Suspension, oral route Oral	Oleic acid, Linoleic acid, Palmitic acid. L- acetyl carnitine	(Safarian *et al.* 2016) (Haider *et al.* 2012) (Rai *et al.* 1990)
Hazelnut	*Corylus avellana*	Preclinical studies on male albino wistar rats	Beta-amyloid aggregation Aß 25-35	800 mg/kg/ Day	Suspension, Oral route	Triacylglycerols, unsaturated fatty acids, palmitic acid, stearic acid, linoleic acid	(Martins *et al.* 2013) (Savage and McNeil 1998) (Dobhal *et al.* 2018) (Bahaeddin *et al.* 2017)
Walnut	*Juglans regis*	Preclinical study on male Kunming mice	Beta-amyloid aggregation.	200, 400 800 mg/kg	Walnut + Distilled water, Oral route	Ash, lignin, cellulose and hemicellulose	(Delaviz *et al.* 2017) (Jahanban-Esfahlan *et al.* 2019) (Zou *et al.* 2016)
Ashwagandha	*Withania somnifera*	Preclinical study on transgenic mice along with APPS J20 Mice	Beta-amyloid aggregation	1 g/kg/ body weight	Suspension, oral route	Withaferin A	(Rao *et al.* 2012) (Tiwari *et al.* 2018) (Sehgal *et al.* 2012)
Lychee	*Litchi chinensis*	Preclinical studies in the lateral ventricle of male rats	Beta-amyloid aggregation Injecting Aß(25-35)	120, 240, 480 mg/kg	Intragastric route	Polyphenols and Anthocyanins	(Wang *et al.* 2017)
Saffron	*Crocus sativus* L.	Preclinical studies on rats Clinical study	Beta-amyloid aggregation Beta-amyloid aggregation	100 mg/kg 2 groups Group A: 30 mg/day Group B- 2 capsules a day	Oral route Capsule, Oral route	Crocin Crocetin, Crocin and Di-methyl crocetin	(Farkhondeh *et al.* 2018) (Razavi *et al.* 2018) (Akhondzadeh *et al.* 2010)
Curcumin	*Curcuma longa*	Preclinical Study Clinical study	Beta-amyloid aggregation Beta-amyloid aggregation	1% curcumin dose 4 gm/day or placebo 2 gm/day	Oral route Powder, Oral route	Curcumin Curcumin	(Hewlings and Kalman 2017) (Mirmosayyeb *et al.* 2017) (Shivanoor and David 2016) (Ringman *et al.* 2012)

(Table 1) cont.....

Dietary Supplements	Scientific Name	Preclinical/ Clinical Study	Pathways/ Cause	Dose	Formulation Route of Administration	Phyto-constituents	Citations
Gotu kola	*Centella asiatica*	Preclinical studies on PSAPP mice	Beta-amyloid levels are affected	2.5 g/kg/ day	Powder, Oral route	Asiaticoside, asiatic acid, centallose and centelloside	(Gohil *et al.* 2010) (Dhanasekaran *et al.* 2009)
Cinnamon	*Cinnamomum zeylanicum* and *Cinnamomum cassia*	Preclinical study on *Drosophila melanogaster* models of AD	Beta amyloid pathway - overexpressing the Tau protein	No dose Performed on *Drosophila melanogaster* models	Liquid	Cinnam-aldehyde	(Rao *et al.* 2012) (Ranasinghe *et al.* 2013) (Pham *et al.* 2018)
Green tea	*Camellia sinensis*	Preclinical study with transgenic mice	Beta amyloid pathway	50 mg/kg	Oral	Epigallocatechin-3-gallate, vitamin E and vitamin C	(Tao *et al.* 2014) (Rezai-Zadeh *et al.* 2008)
Clover	*Melitotus officinalis*	Preclinical study on male wistar rats	NFkß pathway	3 mg/kg	ICV injection	Eugenol	(Luo *et al.* 2016) (Bazazzadegan *et al.* 2017)
Lycopene	*Solanum lycopersicum*	Preclinical study on adult male wistar rats	NFkß pathway	Lycopene 1,2,4 mg/kg Rivastigmine 2 mg/kg	Oral dose	Lycopene	(Garcia *et al.* 2015) (Seo *et al.* 2018) (Sachdeva and Chopra 2015)
Ginger	*Zingiber officinale*	Preclinical study on BV2 cells	NFkß pathway	No dose, powdered ginger extract on BV2 cells	Powder dose	Gingerols and paradols	(Prasad and Tyagi 2015) (Srinivasan 2017) (Jung *et al.* 2009)
Virgin coconut oil	*Cocus nucifera*	Preclinical study on male wistar rats.	Inflammasome pathway	2-3.5 table spoons	Liquid, oral dose	Polyphenols, vitamins and minerals	(Dayrit *et al.* 2011) (Mirzaei *et al.* 2018)
Omega 3- unsaturated fats	-	Clinical study	CB2 pathway	39 participants	Oral dose	α-Linolenic acid, eicosapentaenoic acid and docosahexaenoic acid	(Hooijmans *et al.* 2012) (Shinto *et al.* 2014)
Caryophyllum	*Syzygium aromaticum* L.	Preclinical study in male double transgenic APP/PS1 mice	Prevents neuronal degeneration	16, 48, or 144 mg/kg	Oral dose	Triterpenes, alkaloids, coumarins, cyanogenic glycoside and cyanidin	(Al-Snafi 2017) (Viveros-Paredes *et al.* 2017) (Cheng *et al.* 2014)

Walnut

Walnut originally comes from a Persian tree (*Juglans regia*) belonging to the family *Juglandaceae*. Walnuts contain water (4%), protein (15%), fat (65%) and carbohydrates (14%). They comprise of polyphenols as well as ellagitannins (Delaviz *et al.* 2017). The chemical composition of walnut shell fibers comprises ash, lignin, cellulose and hemicellulose (Jahanban-Esfahlan *et al.* 2019).

A preclinical study was conducted to test the effect against neurotoxicity induced by Aß(25-35) into the bilateral hippocampus of male Kunming mice, Aß(25-35) was injected for 5 weeks. Walnuts were given in doses of 200, 400 and 800 mg/kg in distilled water by the oral route. The methods used were the Morris water maze test, step down avoidance test as well as the level of tumor necrosis factor, interleukin 1ß and IL-6 were measured using the ELISA technique. The primary outcomes resulted in reduced levels of AChE and nitric oxide in the hippocampus of the mice. These studies indicated the use of walnut to reduce neuroinflammation in Alzheimer's disease (Zou *et al.* 2016).

Ashwagandha

Ashwagandha (*Withania somnifera*), a member of the *Solanaceae* family is a nervine tonic, aphrodisiac and an adaptogen, which helps the body to adapt during stress conditions. Ashwagandha has the ability to support the immune system and causes a calming effect on the central nervous system (Rao *et al.* 2012, Kaur *et al.* 2017).

The major phytoconstituent in Ashwagandha (*Withania Somnifera*) is withaferin A, which is isolated from the root extract of this medicinal plant and has the potential to reverse β amyloid peptide 1-42 (Aβ42) induced toxicity in neuronal cells in humans (Tiwari *et al.* 2018). A study on transgenic mice revealed that, administration of *Withania Somnifera* (WS) root extract reduced the brain Aβ42 levels in 3 weeks through a single oral dose of 1 g/kg body weight suspended in ethanol, administered for 7-30 days. The WS root extract comprised withanolides (75%) and withanosides (20%). The decrease in plasma brain Aβ monomer levels was observed *via*upregulation of liver low-density lipoprotein receptor-related protein (LRP) and reversing the pathology of AD (Sehgal *et al.* 2012).

Lychee

Lychee (*Litchi chinensis*) is a member of family *Sapindaceae* belonging to the genus *Litchi*. Lychee has a moderate amount of polyphenols with flavan-3-ol monomers and dimers comprising 87% of the total polyphenols present. Along with polyphenols, anthocyanins (cyanidin-3-glucoside (92%)) are also present. Lychee has been used in traditional Chinese medicine and utilized as an antioxidant in protection against viruses and tumors (Wang *et al.* 2017).

A preclinical study was conducted by injecting Aß(25-35) in the lateral ventricle of male rats treated with normal saline (NS), 0.42 mg/kg donepezil and 120, 240 and 480 mg/kg lychee seed saponins (LSS) by intragastric route of administration (IG) once daily for 28 consecutive days. The method for evaluation was Morris water maze. Neuronal apoptosis was analyzed by hematoxylin and eosin stain and the m-RNA expression on caspase-3 and protein expression by reverse transcription-polymerase chain reaction were evaluated. The lychee seed saponins (LSS) showed an improved cognitive function and a deficiency in the neuronal injury by inhibiting apoptosis in the AD rats, thus proving that LSS can be used as a nutritional supplement for the treatment and prevention of AD (Wang *et al.* 2017).

Saffron

Saffron, known as *Crocus sativus* L., belongs to the *Iridaceae* family. The chemical constituents present in saffron are crocetin, crocin, di-methyl crocetin as well as many carotenoids. Many clinical studies on humans as well as pre-clinical studies on rats have been conducted to prove the effect of saffron in neuroinflammation (Farkhondeh *et al.* 2018).

A preclinical study was conducted on adult male Wistar rats where the effect of crocin was seen on intracerebroventricular (ICV) injection of streptozotocin (STZ) induced cognitive impairment in rats. Crocin (100 mg/kg, p.o.) was given for 21 days consecutively. The method used was Morris water maze task and the results proved that crocin had improved cognitive performance which resulted in a decrease in the malondialdehyde levels and an increase in the thiol levels. Thus proves that crocin helps in the treatment of neurodegenerative diseases such as AD (Naghizadeh *et al.* 2013).

A placebo- controlled, double blind study was conducted in 46 patients for 16 weeks with patients suffering from mild or moderate AD. There were 2 groups, group A was to consume saffron (30 mg/day-15 mg two times a day) whereas group B was to consume a placebo capsule (2 capsules a day). It was proven that saffron had a better result in terms of cognitive functioning without any adverse effects. Thus proving that saffron helps in reducing the amyloid properties during AD (Akhondzadeh *et al.* 2010).

Turmeric

Turmeric (*Curcuma longa*) belongs to the family *Zingiberaceae,* and curcumin is its major phytoconstituent. It has been used for medicinal properties in the Indian Ayurveda system as well as other traditional medicinal systems of the middle east and southeast Asian countries (Hewlings and Kalman 2017). Curcumin, a diarylheptanoid, is a natural phenol responsible for the yellow color of turmeric (Mirmosayyeb *et al.* 2017).

A preclinical study was conducted on Wistar albino rats, with therapeutic dose of 1% turmeric diet for 48 days, to prove the protective effect of turmeric against neural oxidative damage caused by deltamethrin (DLM). Fourier transform infrared (FT-IR) spectroscopy was mainly used for analysis. It was proved that curcumin plays an important role in neuroprotection and reduced amyloid pathology in AD and overall helps in the reduction of oxidative stress in neural tissues in animals (Shivanoor and David 2016).

A double-blind placebo-controlled study conducted for 24 weeks showed a reduction in Aß aggregation after treating with curcumin (turmeric). The primary outcome measures of the study include Alzheimer's disease assessment scale - cognitive subscale and the secondary outcomes include Alzheimer's Disease Cooperative Study - Activities of Daily Living. It was observed that levels of Aß40 and Aß42 were significantly improved. Therefore, curcumin can be applied in the treatment of AD (Ringman *et al.* 2012).

Gotu kola

Gotu kola (*Centella asiatica*) belongs to the family *Apiaceae,* is an important dietary supplement that is capable of increasing memory as well as intelligence. It has chemical constituents such as triterpenoids including asiaticoside, asiatic acid, centallose, and centelloside. A study proved that asiaticoside derivatives show a reduction in the hydrogen peroxide, as well as, Aß induced cell death *in-vitro* thus, helping in the treatment as well as the prevention of AD (Gohil *et al.* 2010).

A preclinical study was conducted on heterogeneous PSAPP mice to show the effect of *Centella asiatica* (CaE) extract to alter the amyloid beta levels. A dose of 2.5 to 5 mg/kg/day of CaE was orally administered for 2 months (60 days) and 8 months (240 days). The results showed a significant reduction in the Aß40 and Aß42 with 8 months study, therefore gotu kola can be applied in the treatment of AD (Dhanasekaran *et al.* 2009).

Cinnamon

Cinnamon is a common spice that is derived from the inner bark of trees of *Cinnamomum zeylanicum* (CZ) and *Cinnamomum cassia* belonging to the family *Lauraceae* (Rao *et al.* 2012). As per its medicinal properties, cinnamon is beneficial in respiratory, digestive as well as gynecological ailments. Different parts of the plant comprise hydrocarbons having cinnamaldehyde, eugenol, and camphor as its primary constituents. Cinnamaldehyde is one of the major components in the CZ extracts having both antimicrobial and antioxidant activity (Ranasinghe *et al.* 2013).

A preclinical study was conducted on *Drosophila melanogaster* models for AD, where the use of cinnamaldehyde showed improvement in the short term memory of male AD flies. To evaluate the impact of cinnamaldehyde on fly directionality and climbing ability, a rapid iterative negative geotaxis (RING) assay was performed on 20 flies to measure the locomotor ability. The primary outcomes resulted in increased climbing ability and improved short term memory in male AD flies overexpressing Tau proteins. The positive effects of this compound could be due to inhibition of the Tau aggregation (Pham *et al.* 2018).

Green Tea

The most abundant polyphenol derived from green tea is Epigallocatechin-3-gallate (EGCG). A typical cup of green tea (2.5 g of tea leaves in 250 ml of hot water) contains approximately 177 mg EGCG (Tao *et al.* 2014). EGCG produces several potent health-promoting effects, including antioxidant, anti-inflammatory, anti-aging and anti-cancer activities. Aβ deposition induces endoplasmic reticulum (ER) stress which is thought to be an important mechanism for neuronal apoptosis in AD.

A preclinical study was conducted in transgenic mice by administering 50 mg/kg of EGCG with water for 6 months. The primary outcomes of the EGCG oral treatment revealed the decrease in both soluble or insoluble forms of Aβ(1–40) and Aβ(1–42), with an effect on tau pathology and cognition in transgenic mice. Thus, ECGC can be used as a dietary supplement with potentially safe and effective prophylaxis of AD (Rezai-Zadeh *et al.* 2008).

Clover

Clover (*Melitotus officinalis*) is a legume belonging to family *Fabaceae*. Clover acts as in anti-inflammatory as well as an antioxidant. The major phytoconstituent present in clover is eugenol (Luo *et al.* 2016).

A preclinical study was conducted in the hippocampus of thirty-six males for genes of the death-domain associated protein (DAXX), NFkß, and the vascular endothelial growth factor (VEGF), to show the role of apoptosis, inflammation, and angiogenesis in AD. The group was given a bilateral intracerebroventricular (ICV) injection dose of 3 mg/kg streptozotocin. To measure the therapeutic levels of clover, the Morris water maze test was used and the hippocampus levels of the rats were compared using quantitative polymerase chain reaction (qPCR). The primary outcomes revealed a decrease in the expression of DAXX, NFkß and VEGF genes in the rats and in terms of memory level, there wasn't a significant change. Thus, the study concluded that clover has an effect on genes expression and behavior but not at the clinical level (Bazazzadegan *et al.* 2017).

Lycopene

Lycopene is a bright red carotenoid pigment found mainly in tomatoes (*Solanum lycopersicum*), some red fruits and vegetables like carrots, papayas, *etc.,* (Garcia *et al.* 2015). Lycopene has a strong antioxidant quality with a high singlet oxygen quenching capacity. It also precedes the effect of pro-inflammatory chemokine in macrophages (Seo *et al.* 2018).

A study was conducted on the Aß42 injected (intracerebroventricularly) adult male Wistar rats to prove the effect of lycopene in inhibition of NFkß activity and reduction of the neuroinflammatory cytokines such as TNF-α and TGF-ß. The lycopene and rivastigmine were administered at doses 1 mg/kg, 2 mg/kg, 4 mg/kg and 2 mg/kg respectively by oral gavage daily for 14 days. The levels of TNF-α, TGF-ß, NFKß, and caspase-3 were measured as well as Morris water maze and elevated plus maze tests were performed to check the memory levels. It was observed that lycopene inhibited the NFkß activity and downregulated neuroinflammatory cytokines expression. Thus, lycopene can be a potential candidate in the treatment of AD (Sachdeva and Chopra 2015).

Ginger

Ginger (*Zingiber officinale*), belongs to the family *Zingiberaceae*, has anti-obesity and anti-inflammatory actions and acts as a stimulant in protection of the gastrointestinal tract (Prasad and Tyagi 2015). The phytoconstituents present in ginger are gingerols and paradols and have health beneficial potential. These constituents act *via*inhibiting the production of nitric oxides, prostaglandins, and cytokinins such as IL-1ß and TNF-α. TNF-α, which causes microglia inflammation in neurodegenerative diseases (Srinivasan 2017).

A study was conducted to prove the effectiveness of the rhizome extract of *Zingiber officinale* against microglia inflammation. A powdered extract of ginger was used to evaluate its effect oo BV2 cells at different concentrations. The ginger extract inhibited the excessive production of NO, prostaglandins TNF-α cytokines, and COX-2. Thus the study proved that extract has an anti-inflammatory property *via*suppression of the genes through MAPK and NFKß pathways, thereby reducing the progress of neurodegenerative diseases (Jung *et al.* 2009).

Virgin Coconut Oil (VCO)

VCO is produced from coconuts (*Cocus nucifera)* which belongs to the family *Arecaceae*. VCO differs from regular coconut oil with respect to its source, method of extraction as well as its benefits. It acts as an antioxidant with a good fragrance and taste. Virgin coconut oil is comprised of many polyphenols, vitamins, and minerals. It is free from trans-fatty acids and has good cholesterol (Dayrit *et al.* 2011).

A study was conducted on male Wistar rats to prove the neuroprotective effect of Virgin Coconut Oil (VCO). Amyloid ß toxicity was induced in rats VCO effect was observed on inflammasome and oxidative stress in AD. VCO was administered with a dose of 2-3.5 tablespoons a day for 8 weeks. Memory and learning tests were conducted. The Aß was significantly decreased by the activation of NLRP3, inflammasome and oxidative stress. The study results stated that VCO improved the hippocampus histological changes and reduced Aß and tau phosphorylation, which is the major causes of AD, thus being a potential source for the treatment of AD and having a neuroprotective effect (Mirzaei *et al.* 2018).

Omega-3 Polyunsaturated Fatty Acid (PUFA)

To date, just a few randomized clinical preliminaries (RCTs) have explored the impacts of omega-3 unsaturated fats (ω-3) on Alzheimer's illness. ω-3 supplementation additionally enhance the psychological capacity. This effect seemed bigger in mice as compared to rats and even higher in females next to males with declined neuronal loss. The after effects of this compound demonstrate that it may be advantageous to perform new clinical tests with long haul omega-3 FA supplementation in Alzheimer's patients (Hooijmans *et al.* 2012).

A pilot study was conducted to evaluate the effects of supplementation of omega-3 fatty acid (ω-3) alone and omega-3 fatty acid with α-lipoic acid (ω-3+LA) and compared to placebo on 39 subjects for 12 months to show its effect on oxidative stress biomarkers in AD. The combination ω-3+LA showed a cognitive and functional decline in AD over this period (Shinto *et al.* 2014).

Caryophyllum

Caryophyllum (*Syzygium aromaticum* L.) is a medicinal herb used for the treatment of AD. The major phytoconstituents are triterpenes, alkaloids, coumarins, cyanogenic glycoside and cyanidin (Al-Snafi 2017).

A preclinical study was conducted on male double transgenic APP/PS1 mice to check the anti-inflammatory effect of β-caryophyllene. Oral dose of 16, 48, or 144 mg/kg β-caryophyllene was administered every morning for 10 weeks. β-caryophyllene prevented cognitive impairment in the mice and reduced the β-amyloid aggregation in both the cerebral cortex and hippocampus. These results show that β-caryophyllene sesquiterpene shows an anti-inflammatory effect involving CB2 receptor activation and the PPARγ pathway, and suggest that β-caryophyllene seems to be an attractive molecule with therapeutic potential for treatment in AD (Cheng *et al.* 2014).

CONCLUSION

Since hundreds of centuries, humans are exploring herbal medicines for ameliorating various acute and chronic disorders. In Indian traditional medicine systems like Ayurveda, Siddha, Unani and Homeopathy there are dedicated sections for the applicability of herbal medicines in the treatment of neurodegenerative disorders. Medicinal herbs and their active constituents enhance the cognition and intellect functions. Many physicians have tried a wide variety of pharmacological drugs to help patients suffering from neurodegenerative disorders to manage symptoms, however not all patients respond well to such therapies. Patients whose symptoms improve with pharmacological treatment generally experience major side effects. Thus, there is a need for developing alternative safe therapies for the treatment of neurological disorders. Dietary supplements have been proven effective in the management of neurodegenerative disorders. Many phytoconstituents possess antioxidant, anti-inflammatory, and metal chelation properties which make them eligible to target the promoters of neurological damage. Reduction in oxidative stress also reduce the load of Aß senile plaques in AD. Novel phytoconstituent formulations may prevent or delay the onset of neurodegenerative disorders. However, more clinical trials are needed to prove theirimportance in the treatment of neurodegenerative disorders. Based on the literature search, several pharmacological studies suggest that naturally occurring phytoconstituents can be used for the treatment and prevention of neurodegenerative disorders like AD. This chapter provides a comprehensive discussion of the literature regarding the pathways causing AD and the role of their phytocontituents in offering a safe approach to protect against neuronal damage and oxidative stress caused by neurodegenerative disorders.

ABBREVIATIONS

Aß	Amyloid Beta
AchE	Acetlycholinesterase
AD	Alzheimer's disease
AMPK	AMP-activated protein kinase
ASC	Apoptosis-associated speck-like protein containing a CARD
CaE	*Centella asiatica*
CNR2	Cannabinoid Receptor 2
CNS	Central nervous system
COX-2	Cyclooxygenase-2
Cyclic AMP	Cyclic adenosine monophosphate
DAXX	death-domain associated protein
DLM 1	Deltamethrin 1

DNA	Deoxyribonucleic acid
EGCG	Epigallocatechin-3-gallate
EPM	Elevated plus maze
FTIR	Fourier transform infrared spectroscopy
Ikß	I kappa ß kinase
LPS	Lipopolysaccardies
LRR	Leucine rich receptor
LSS	Lychee seed saponin
NFkß	Nuclear factor kappa-light-chain-enhancer of activated B cells
NFT	Neurofibrillary tangles
NLRP3	Nucleotide-binding domain (NOD)-like receptor protein 3
PC12	Pheochromocytoma
PYD	Pyrin only domain
PPARs	Peroxisome proliferator-activated receptors
PS2 transgenic mice	Presenilin 2 transgenic mice
QOL	Quality of life
RAM	Radical arm maze
RING	Rapid iterative negative geotaxis
RNA	Ribonucleic acid
TGF	Tumor growth factor
TLR	Toll like receptor
TNF	Tumor necrosis factor
TRP	Tryptophan levels
VCO	Virgin coconut oil
VEGF	Vascular endothelial growth factor
WA	Withaferin A

CONFLICT OF INTEREST

There is no conflict of interest regarding the publication of this article.

ACKNOWLEDGMENTS

We would like to thank SPPSPTM, SVKM's NMIMS University, Mumbai, for the encouragement and moral support in writing this chapter.

CONSENT FOR PUBLICATION

None

REFERENCES

Al-Snafi, PDAE (2017) Chemical contents and medical importance of Dianthus caryophyllus- A review. *IOSR J Pharm,* 07, 61-71. [IOSRPHR].
[http://dx.doi.org/10.9790/3013-0703016171]

Bahaeddin, Z, Yans, A, Khodagholi, F, Hajimehdipoor, H & Sahranavard, S (2017) Hazelnut and neuroprotection: Improved memory and hindered anxiety in response to intra-hippocampal Aβ injection. *Nutr Neurosci,* 20, 317-26.
[http://dx.doi.org/10.1080/1028415X.2015.1126954] [PMID: 26808646]

Baur, JA, Ungvari, Z, Minor, RK, Le Couteur, DG & de Cabo, R (2012) Are sirtuins viable targets for improving healthspan and lifespan? *Nat Rev Drug Discov,* 11, 443-61.
[http://dx.doi.org/10.1038/nrd3738] [PMID: 22653216]

Bayer, TA, Wirths, O, Majtényi, K, Hartmann, T, Multhaup, G, Beyreuther, K & Czech, C (2001) Key factors in Alzheimer's disease: beta-amyloid precursor protein processing, metabolism and intraneuronal transport. *Brain Pathol,* 11, 1-11.
[http://dx.doi.org/10.1111/j.1750-3639.2001.tb00376.x] [PMID: 11145195]

Bazazzadegan, N, Dehghan Shasaltaneh, M, Saliminejad, K, Kamali, K, Banan, M & Khorram Khorshid, HR (2017) The Effects of *Melilotus officinalis* Extract on Expression of *Daxx, Nfkb and Vegf* Genes in the Streptozotocin-Induced Rat Model of Sporadic Alzheimer's Disease. *Avicenna J Med Biotechnol,* 9, 133-7.
[PMID: 28706608]

Benito, C, Núñez, E, Tolón, RM, Carrier, EJ, Rábano, A, Hillard, CJ & Romero, J (2003) Cannabinoid CB2 receptors and fatty acid amide hydrolase are selectively overexpressed in neuritic plaque-associated glia in Alzheimer's disease brains. *J Neurosci,* 23, 11136-41.
[http://dx.doi.org/10.1523/JNEUROSCI.23-35-11136.2003] [PMID: 14657172]

Cheng, Y, Dong, Z & Liu, S (2014) β-Caryophyllene ameliorates the Alzheimer-like phenotype in APP/PS1 Mice through CB2 receptor activation and the PPARγ pathway. *Pharmacology,* 94, 1-12.
[http://dx.doi.org/10.1159/000362689] [PMID: 25171128]

Dayrit, FM, Dimzon, IKD, Valde, MF, Santos, JER, Garrovillas, MJM & Villarino, BJ (2011) Quality characteristics of virgin coconut oil: Comparisons with refined coconut oil. *Pure Appl Chem,* 83, 1789-99.
[http://dx.doi.org/10.1351/PAC-CON-11-04-01]

Delaviz, H, Mohammadi, J, Ghalamfarsa, G, Mohammadi, B & Farhadi, N (2017) A Review Study on Phytochemistry and Pharmacology Applications of *Juglans Regia* Plant. *Pharmacogn Rev,* 11, 145-52.
[http://dx.doi.org/10.4103/phrev.phrev_10_17] [PMID: 28989250]

Dhanasekaran, M, Holcomb, LA, Hitt, AR, Tharakan, B, Porter, JW, Young, KA & Manyam, BV (2009) Centella asiatica extract selectively decreases amyloid beta levels in hippocampus of Alzheimer's disease animal model. *Phytother Res,* 23, 14-9.
[http://dx.doi.org/10.1002/ptr.2405] [PMID: 19048607]

Dobhal, K, Singh, N, Semwal, A & Negi, A (2018) A brief review on: hazelnuts. *Int J Recent Sci Res,* 9, 23680-4.

Farkhondeh, T, Samarghandian, S, Shaterzadeh Yazdi, H & Samini, F (2018) The protective effects of crocin in the management of neurodegenerative diseases: a review. *Am J Neurodegener Dis,* 7, 1-10.
[PMID: 29531865]

Franchi, L, Eigenbrod, T, Muñoz-Planillo, R & Nuñez, G (2009) The inflammasome: a caspase-1-activation platform that regulates immune responses and disease pathogenesis. *Nat Immunol,* 10, 241-7.
[http://dx.doi.org/10.1038/ni.1703] [PMID: 19221555]

Garcia, D, Narváez-Vásquez, J & Orozco-Cárdenas, ML (2015) Tomato (Solanum lycopersicum). *Methods Mol Biol,* 1223, 349-61.
[http://dx.doi.org/10.1007/978-1-4939-1695-5_28] [PMID: 25300854]

Ghosh, M, Xu, Y & Pearse, DD (2016) Cyclic AMP is a key regulator of M1 to M2a phenotypic conversion

of microglia in the presence of Th2 cytokines. *J Neuroinflammation,* 13, 9.
[http://dx.doi.org/10.1186/s12974-015-0463-9] [PMID: 26757726]

Gohil, KJ, Patel, JA & Gajjar, AK (2010) Pharmacological Review on Centella asiatica: A Potential Herbal Cure-all. *Indian J Pharm Sci,* 72, 546-56.
[http://dx.doi.org/10.4103/0250-474X.78519] [PMID: 21694984]

Gupta, M & Kaur, G (2016) Aqueous extract from the Withania somnifera leaves as a potential anti-neuroinflammatory agent: a mechanistic study. *J Neuroinflammation,* 13, 193.
[http://dx.doi.org/10.1186/s12974-016-0650-3] [PMID: 27550017]

Haider, S, Batool, Z & Haleem, DJ (2012) Nootropic and hypophagic effects following long term intake of almonds (Prunus amygdalus) in rats. *Nutr Hosp,* 27, 2109-15.
[PMID: 23588464]

Halle, A, Hornung, V, Petzold, GC, Stewart, CR, Monks, BG, Reinheckel, T, Fitzgerald, KA, Latz, E, Moore, KJ & Golenbock, DT (2008) The NALP3 inflammasome is involved in the innate immune response to amyloid-beta. *Nat Immunol,* 9, 857-65.
[http://dx.doi.org/10.1038/ni.1636] [PMID: 18604209]

Hewlings, SJ & Kalman, DS (2017) Curcumin: A Review of Its Effects on Human Health. *Foods,* 6, 92-2.
[http://dx.doi.org/10.3390/foods6100092] [PMID: 29065496]

Hooijmans, CR, Pasker-de Jong, PC, de Vries, RB & Ritskes-Hoitinga, M (2012) The effects of long-term omega-3 fatty acid supplementation on cognition and Alzheimer's pathology in animal models of Alzheimer's disease: a systematic review and meta-analysis. *J Alzheimers Dis,* 28, 191-209.
[http://dx.doi.org/10.3233/JAD-2011-111217] [PMID: 22002791]

Jahanban-Esfahlan, A, Ostadrahimi, A, Tabibiazar, M & Amarowicz, R (2019) A Comprehensive Review on the Chemical Constituents and Functional Uses of Walnut (*Juglans* spp.) Husk. *Int J Mol Sci,* 20, 20.
[http://dx.doi.org/10.3390/ijms20163920] [PMID: 31409014]

Jung, HW, Yoon, CH, Park, KM, Han, HS & Park, YK (2009) Hexane fraction of Zingiberis Rhizoma Crudus extract inhibits the production of nitric oxide and proinflammatory cytokines in LPS-stimulated BV2 microglial cells *via*the NF-kappaB pathway. *Food Chem Toxicol,* 47, 1190-7.
[http://dx.doi.org/10.1016/j.fct.2009.02.012] [PMID: 19233241]

Kawai, T & Akira, S (2007) Signaling to NF-kappaB by Toll-like receptors. *Trends Mol Med,* 13, 460-9.
[http://dx.doi.org/10.1016/j.molmed.2007.09.002] [PMID: 18029230]

Kaur, P, Robin, , Makanjuola, VO, Arora, R, Singh, B & Arora, S (2017) Immunopotentiating significance of conventionally used plant adaptogens as modulators in biochemical and molecular signalling pathways in cell mediated processes. *Biomed Pharmacother,* 95, 1815-29.
[http://dx.doi.org/10.1016/j.biopha.2017.09.081] [PMID: 28968926]

Kim, GH, Kim, JE, Rhie, SJ & Yoon, S (2015) The Role of Oxidative Stress in Neurodegenerative Diseases. *Exp Neurobiol,* 24, 325-40.
[http://dx.doi.org/10.5607/en.2015.24.4.325] [PMID: 26713080]

Kulkarni, KS, Kasture, SB & Mengi, SA (2010) Efficacy study of Prunus amygdalus (almond) nuts in scopolamine-induced amnesia in rats. *Indian J Pharmacol,* 42, 168-73.
[http://dx.doi.org/10.4103/0253-7613.66841] [PMID: 20871769]

Kumar, GP & Khanum, F (2012) Neuroprotective potential of phytochemicals. *Pharmacogn Rev,* 6, 81-90.
[http://dx.doi.org/10.4103/0973-7847.99898] [PMID: 23055633]

Luo, K, Jahufer, MZ, Wu, F, Di, H, Zhang, D, Meng, X, Zhang, J & Wang, Y (2016) Genotypic Variation in a Breeding Population of Yellow Sweet Clover (Melilotus officinalis). *Front Plant Sci,* 7, 972.
[http://dx.doi.org/10.3389/fpls.2016.00972] [PMID: 27462321]

Martins, S, Simões, F, Matos, J, Silva, AP & Carnide, V (2013) Genetic relationship among wild, landraces and cultivars of hazelnut (Corylus avellana) from Portugal revealed through ISSR and AFLP markers. *Plant Syst Evol,* 300, 1035-46.

[http://dx.doi.org/10.1007/s00606-013-0942-3]

Mathuranath, PS, Cherian, PJ, Mathew, R, Kumar, S, George, A, Alexander, A, Ranjith, N & Sarma, PS (2010) Dementia in Kerala, South India: prevalence and influence of age, education and gender. *Int J Geriatr Psychiatry,* 25, 290-7.
[http://dx.doi.org/10.1002/gps.2338] [PMID: 19621355]

Mirmosayyeb, O, Tanhaei, A, Sohrabi, HR, Martins, RN, Tanhaei, M, Najafi, MA, Safaei, A & Meamar, R (2017) Possible Role of Common Spices as a Preventive and Therapeutic Agent for Alzheimer's Disease. *Int J Prev Med,* 8, 5.
[http://dx.doi.org/10.4103/2008-7802.199640] [PMID: 28250905]

Mirzaei, F, Khazaei, M, Komaki, A, Amiri, I & Jalili, C (2018) Virgin coconut oil (VCO) by normalizing NLRP3 inflammasome showed potential neuroprotective effects in Amyloid-β induced toxicity and high-fat diet fed rat. *Food Chem Toxicol,* 118, 68-83.
[http://dx.doi.org/10.1016/j.fct.2018.04.064] [PMID: 29729307]

Mizuno, S, Iijima, R, Ogishima, S, Kikuchi, M, Matsuoka, Y, Ghosh, S, Miyamoto, T, Miyashita, A, Kuwano, R & Tanaka, H (2012) AlzPathway: a comprehensive map of signaling pathways of Alzheimer's disease. *BMC Syst Biol,* 6, 52.
[http://dx.doi.org/10.1186/1752-0509-6-52] [PMID: 22647208]

Morales, I, Guzmán-Martínez, L, Cerda-Troncoso, C, Farías, GA & Maccioni, RB (2014) Neuroinflammation in the pathogenesis of Alzheimer's disease. A rational framework for the search of novel therapeutic approaches. *Front Cell Neurosci,* 8, 112.
[http://dx.doi.org/10.3389/fncel.2014.00112] [PMID: 24795567]

Olsen, I & Singhrao, SK (2016) Inflammasome Involvement in Alzheimer's Disease. *J Alzheimers Dis,* 54, 45-53.
[http://dx.doi.org/10.3233/JAD-160197] [PMID: 27314526]

Peters, DG, Connor, JR & Meadowcroft, MD (2015) The relationship between iron dyshomeostasis and amyloidogenesis in Alzheimer's disease: Two sides of the same coin. *Neurobiol Dis,* 81, 49-65.
[http://dx.doi.org/10.1016/j.nbd.2015.08.007] [PMID: 26303889]

Pham, HM, Xu, A, Schriner, SE, Sevrioukov, EA & Jafari, M (2018) Cinnamaldehyde Improves Lifespan and Healthspan in *Drosophila melanogaster* Models for Alzheimer's Disease. *BioMed Res Int,* 20183570830
[http://dx.doi.org/10.1155/2018/3570830] [PMID: 30228985]

Prasad, S & Tyagi, AK (2015) Ginger and its constituents: role in prevention and treatment of gastrointestinal cancer. *Gastroenterol Res Pract,* 2015142979
[http://dx.doi.org/10.1155/2015/142979] [PMID: 25838819]

Rai, G, Wright, G, Scott, L, Beston, B, Rest, J & Exton-Smith, AN (1990) Double-blind, placebo controlled study of acetyl-l-carnitine in patients with Alzheimer's dementia. *Curr Med Res Opin,* 11, 638-47.
[http://dx.doi.org/10.1185/03007999009112690] [PMID: 2178869]

Ramírez, BG, Blázquez, C, Gómez del Pulgar, T, Guzmán, M & de Ceballos, ML (2005) Prevention of Alzheimer's disease pathology by cannabinoids: neuroprotection mediated by blockade of microglial activation. *J Neurosci,* 25, 1904-13.
[http://dx.doi.org/10.1523/JNEUROSCI.4540-04.2005] [PMID: 15728830]

Ranasinghe, P, Pigera, S, Premakumara, GA, Galappaththy, P, Constantine, GR & Katulanda, P (2013) Medicinal properties of 'true' cinnamon (Cinnamomum zeylanicum): a systematic review. *BMC Complement Altern Med,* 13, 275.
[http://dx.doi.org/10.1186/1472-6882-13-275] [PMID: 24148965]

Rao, RV, Descamps, O, John, V & Bredesen, DE (2012) Ayurvedic medicinal plants for Alzheimer's disease: a review. *Alzheimers Res Ther,* 4, 22.
[http://dx.doi.org/10.1186/alzrt125] [PMID: 22747839]

Razavi, BM, Alyasin, A, Hosseinzadeh, H & Imenshahidi, M (2018) Saffron Induced Relaxation in Isolated

Rat Aorta *via*Endothelium Dependent and Independent Mechanisms. *Iran J Pharm Res,* 17, 1018-25. [PMID: 30127824]

Rezai-Zadeh, K, Arendash, GW, Hou, H, Fernandez, F, Jensen, M, Runfeldt, M, Shytle, RD & Tan, J (2008) Green tea epigallocatechin-3-gallate (EGCG) reduces beta-amyloid mediated cognitive impairment and modulates tau pathology in Alzheimer transgenic mice. *Brain Res,* 1214, 177-87. [http://dx.doi.org/10.1016/j.brainres.2008.02.107] [PMID: 18457818]

Ringman, JM, Frautschy, SA, Teng, E, Begum, AN, Bardens, J, Beigi, M, Gylys, KH, Badmaev, V, Heath, DD, Apostolova, LG, Porter, V, Vanek, Z, Marshall, GA, Hellemann, G, Sugar, C, Masterman, DL, Montine, TJ, Cummings, JL & Cole, GM (2012) Oral curcumin for Alzheimer's disease: tolerability and efficacy in a 24-week randomized, double blind, placebo-controlled study. *Alzheimers Res Ther,* 4, 43. [http://dx.doi.org/10.1186/alzrt146] [PMID: 23107780]

Rosales Hernández, MC, Hernández Rodríguez, M, Mendieta Wejebe, JE & Correa Basurto, J (2016) *Involvement of Free Radicals in the Development and Progression of Alzheimer's Disease Free Radicals and Diseases.*InTech.

Sachdeva, AK & Chopra, K (2015) Lycopene abrogates Aβ(1-42)-mediated neuroinflammatory cascade in an experimental model of Alzheimer's disease. *J Nutr Biochem,* 26, 736-44. [http://dx.doi.org/10.1016/j.jnutbio.2015.01.012] [PMID: 25869595]

Saco, T, Parthasarathy, PT, Cho, Y, Lockey, RF & Kolliputi, N (2014) Inflammasome: a new trigger of Alzheimer's disease. *Front Aging Neurosci,* 6, 80. [http://dx.doi.org/10.3389/fnagi.2014.00080] [PMID: 24834051]

Safarian, S, Azarmi, Y, Jahanban-Esfahlan, A & Jahanban-Esfahlan, H (2016) The beneficial effects of almond (Prunus amygdalus Batsch) hull on serum lipid profile and antioxidant capacity in male rats. *Turk J Med Sci,* 46, 1223-32. [http://dx.doi.org/10.3906/sag-1504-127] [PMID: 27513429]

Savage, GP & McNeil, DL (1998) Chemical composition of hazelnuts (Corylus avellana L.) grown in New Zealand. *Int J Food Sci Nutr,* 49, 199-203. [http://dx.doi.org/10.3109/09637489809086412] [PMID: 10616661]

Sehgal, N, Gupta, A, Valli, RK, Joshi, SD, Mills, JT, Hamel, E, Khanna, P, Jain, SC, Thakur, SS & Ravindranath, V (2012) Withania somnifera reverses Alzheimer's disease pathology by enhancing low-density lipoprotein receptor-related protein in liver. *Proc Natl Acad Sci USA,* 109, 3510-5. [http://dx.doi.org/10.1073/pnas.1112209109] [PMID: 22308347]

Seo, EJ, Fischer, N & Efferth, T (2018) Phytochemicals as inhibitors of NF-κB for treatment of Alzheimer's disease. *Pharmacol Res,* 129, 262-73. [http://dx.doi.org/10.1016/j.phrs.2017.11.030] [PMID: 29179999]

Sha, W, Mitoma, H, Hanabuchi, S, Bao, M, Weng, L, Sugimoto, N, Liu, Y, Zhang, Z, Zhong, J, Sun, B & Liu, YJ (2014) Human NLRP3 inflammasome senses multiple types of bacterial RNAs. *Proc Natl Acad Sci USA,* 111, 16059-64. [http://dx.doi.org/10.1073/pnas.1412487111] [PMID: 25355909]

Shinto, L, Quinn, J, Montine, T, Dodge, HH, Woodward, W, Baldauf-Wagner, S, Waichunas, D, Bumgarner, L, Bourdette, D, Silbert, L & Kaye, J (2014) A randomized placebo-controlled pilot trial of omega-3 fatty acids and alpha lipoic acid in Alzheimer's disease. *J Alzheimers Dis,* 38, 111-20. [http://dx.doi.org/10.3233/JAD-130722] [PMID: 24077434]

Shivanoor, SM & David, M (2016) Reversal of deltamethrin-induced oxidative damage in rat neural tissues by turmeric-diet: Fourier transform-infrared and biochemical investigation. *J Basic Appl Zool,* 77, 56-68. [http://dx.doi.org/10.1016/j.jobaz.2016.10.003]

Singh, SK, Srivastav, S, Yadav, AK, Srikrishna, S & Perry, G (2016) Overview of Alzheimer's Disease and Some Therapeutic Approaches Targeting Aβ by Using Several Synthetic and Herbal Compounds. *Oxid Med Cell Longev,* 20167361613

[http://dx.doi.org/10.1155/2016/7361613] [PMID: 27034741]

Song, L, Pei, L, Yao, S, Wu, Y & Shang, Y (2017) NLRP3 Inflammasome in Neurological Diseases, from Functions to Therapies. *Front Cell Neurosci,* 11, 63.
[http://dx.doi.org/10.3389/fncel.2017.00063] [PMID: 28337127]

Srinivasan, K (2017) Ginger rhizomes (Zingiber officinale): A spice with multiple health beneficial potentials. *PharmaNutrition,* 5, 18-28.
[http://dx.doi.org/10.1016/j.phanu.2017.01.001]

Tang, Y, Xiong, R, Wu, AG, Yu, CL, Zhao, Y, Qiu, WQ, Wang, XL, Teng, JF, Liu, J, Chen, HX, Wu, JM & Qin, DL (2018) Polyphenols Derived from Lychee Seed Suppress Aβ (1-42)-Induced Neuroinflammation. *Int J Mol Sci,* 19, 2109-9.
[http://dx.doi.org/10.3390/ijms19072109] [PMID: 30036972]

Tao, L, Forester, SC & Lambert, JD (2014) The role of the mitochondrial oxidative stress in the cytotoxic effects of the green tea catechin, (-)-epigallocatechin-3-gallate, in oral cells. *Mol Nutr Food Res,* 58, 665-76.
[http://dx.doi.org/10.1002/mnfr.201300427] [PMID: 24249144]

Tiwari, S, Atluri, VSR, Yndart Arias, A, Jayant, RD, Kaushik, A, Geiger, J & Nair, MN (2018) Withaferin A Suppresses Beta Amyloid in APP Expressing Cells: Studies for Tat and Cocaine Associated Neurological Dysfunctions. *Front Aging Neurosci,* 10, 291.
[http://dx.doi.org/10.3389/fnagi.2018.00291] [PMID: 30356847]

Venkatesan, R, Ji, E & Kim, SY (2015) Phytochemicals that regulate neurodegenerative disease by targeting neurotrophins: a comprehensive review. *BioMed Res Int,* 2015814068
[http://dx.doi.org/10.1155/2015/814068] [PMID: 26075266]

Viveros-Paredes, JM, González-Castañeda, RE, Gertsch, J, Chaparro-Huerta, V, López-Roa, RI, Vázquez-Valls, E, Beas-Zarate, C, Camins-Espuny, A & Flores-Soto, ME (2017) Neuroprotective Effects of β-Caryophyllene against Dopaminergic Neuron Injury in a Murine Model of Parkinson's Disease Induced by MPTP. *Pharmaceuticals (Basel),* 10, 10.
[http://dx.doi.org/10.3390/ph10030060] [PMID: 28684694]

Wang, X, Wu, J, Yu, C, Tang, Y, Liu, J, Chen, H, Jin, B, Mei, Q, Cao, S & Qin, D (2017) Lychee Seed Saponins Improve Cognitive Function and Prevent Neuronal Injury *via*Inhibiting Neuronal Apoptosis in a Rat Model of Alzheimer's Disease. *Nutrients,* 9, 9.
[http://dx.doi.org/10.3390/nu9020105] [PMID: 28165366]

Zhang, FX & Xu, RS (2018) Juglanin ameliorates LPS-induced neuroinflammation in animal models of Parkinson's disease and cell culture *via*inactivating TLR4/NF-κB pathway. *Biomed Pharmacother,* 97, 1011-9.
[http://dx.doi.org/10.1016/j.biopha.2017.08.132] [PMID: 29136779]

Zhao, Y & Zhao, B (2013) Oxidative stress and the pathogenesis of Alzheimer's disease. *Oxid Med Cell Longev,* 2013316523
[http://dx.doi.org/10.1155/2013/316523] [PMID: 23983897]

Zheng, C, Zhou, XW & Wang, JZ (2016) The dual roles of cytokines in Alzheimer's disease: update on interleukins, TNF-α, TGF-β and IFN-γ. *Transl Neurodegener,* 5, 7.
[http://dx.doi.org/10.1186/s40035-016-0054-4] [PMID: 27054030]

Zou, J, Cai, PS, Xiong, CM & Ruan, JL (2016) Neuroprotective effect of peptides extracted from walnut (Juglans Sigilata Dode) proteins on Aβ25-35-induced memory impairment in mice. *J Huazhong Univ Sci Technolog Med Sci,* 36, 21-30.
[http://dx.doi.org/10.1007/s11596-016-1536-4] [PMID: 26838735]

CHAPTER 14

Mechanisms of Anti-Glutamate Neurotoxicity of Botanicals and their Chemical Constituents

Tewin Tencomnao[1,*], Atsadang Theerasri[1] and Sakawrat Janpaijit[1]

[1] *Natural Products for Neuroprotection and Anti-ageing Research Unit, Department of Clinical Chemistry, Faculty of Allied Health Sciences, Chulalongkorn University, Bangkok 10330, Thailand.*

Abstract: In many countries, including Asian countries such as Japan, Singapore and Thailand, aging populations have been increasing, thus promoting a high risk for age-associated chronic diseases. One of the devastating chronic diseases in people with old age known to greatly impact the patients' quality of life is a group of neurodegenerative diseases such as Alzheimer's disease and Parkinson's disease. It has been evident that neurotoxicity is a significant risk of neurodegenerative disorders. One of the crucial contributing factors leading to neurotoxicity in humans is glutamate, the excitatory neurotransmitter. If it is accumulated in the brain, this neurotransmitter can result in neurotoxicity *via* either glutamate-dependent pathway or glutamate-independent pathway. Glutamate neurotoxicity (GNT) is characterized by rising damage of cell components leading to cell death. In the death process due to oxidative stress, reactive oxygen species (ROS) are generated, thus impairing a vast array of cellular functions in many organelles such as mitochondria and endoplasmic reticulum. GNT has been clearly observed in the brain tissue because of the accumulation of glutamate, not only from the endogenous source, but also the exogenous source such as monosodium glutamate. Fortunately, numerous plant extracts and their chemical constituents, particularly the ones with high anti-oxidant activity, have been found to exhibit anti-GNT in both *vitro* and *in vivo* models. Herein, mechanisms of anti-GNT of botanicals and their chemical constituents are presented and discussed in detail. Their anti-GNT mechanisms elucidated could shed light on the discovery and application of neutraceuticals, and the cell defense mechanisms of natural neuroprotectants could certainly be beneficial to improve both healthspan and lifespan in humans.

Keywords: Glutamate neurotoxicity, Natural products, Neuroprotectants, Neutraceuticals, Reactive oxygen species.

* **Corresponding author Tewin Tencomnao:** Natural Products for Neuroprotection and Anti-ageing Research Unit, Department of Clinical Chemistry, Faculty of Allied Health Sciences, Chulalongkorn University, Bangkok 10330, Thailand. E-mails: tewin.t@chula.ac.th and tewintencomnao@gmail.com

INTRODUCTION

Glutamate is a major excitatory neurotransmitter in the central nervous system which is indispensable in learning and memory formation (Fonnum 1984, Nakanishi 1992). Generally, extracellular glutamate levels are kept low and tightly regulated by glutamate transporters predominantly located on the glial membranes (Auld and Robitaille 2003). The blood-brain barrier functions as a border impermeable to glutamate elsewhere (Hertz *et al.* 1999). The physiological role of glutamatergic transmission is determined by the specific binding between glutamate and various types of glutamate receptors, mainly divided into the ionotropic and metabotropic types (Riedel *et al.* 2003, Willard and Koochekpour 2013b). Dysregulation in the glutamate system can cause an impact on a wide range of neurological disturbances which include psychiatric conditions, neurodevelopmental disorders, neurodegenerative disorders and stroke (Miladinovic *et al.* 2015).

Nowadays, it is evident that consumption of fruits and vegetables exerts numerous health benefits either by boosting the defensive system of the body or assisting in the recovery from diseases (Liu *et al.* 2016, Hu *et al.* 2014a, Hyson 2015). Phytochemicals present in many plants were reported to have strong activity against several diseases and this could be developed for therapeutic purposes. Herbal medicine or phytomedicine which rely on plants or plant products, have been recognized as an effective way to fight against diseases for a long time. There are abundant indigenous plants distributed in several regions of the world that have yet to be studied, which might be useful in terms of health benefits. It is well known, one of the potential characteristics of these plants is that they usually have strong antioxidant activity which contributes to the disease therapy. However, how these dietary antioxidants act in several diseases is elusive. In this regard, Lee and colleagues, did a comprehensive review of how dietary phytochemicals act against adaptive cellular stress responses in the central nervous system *via* several molecular mechanisms (Lee *et al.* 2014b).

Currently, a number of studies have investigated the underlying mechanisms of plants and phytochemicals in the attenuation of glutamate excitotoxicity which includes the over-production of ROS and increase of intracellular Ca^{2+} influx *via* cell surface glutamate receptor activation, leading to neuronal cell death. The proposed neuroprotective mechanisms against glutamate toxicity involve several signaling cascades such as BDNF/TrkB, MAPKs, Nrf2/HO-1 and PI3K/Akt/GSK-3β (Mattson 2008, Wang *et al.* 2007). These molecular mechanisms usually provide protective or survival effects against harmful agents such as toxic levels of glutamate. Interestingly, many plants or plant-derived compounds were found to possess beneficial effects against neurological disorders, including glutamate-related disorders which might be an effective candidate for further investigation and development for therapeutic use. In the present review, we highlight the summary of homeostasis of glutamate in the CNS and how glutamate is relevant to CNS disorders. We also provide a list of natural plants and/or their bioactive compounds with their neuroprotective effect against glutamate neurotoxicity in several glutamate-induced models.

GLUTAMATE METABOLISM AND NEUROTRANSMISSION

Glutamate is a major excitatory neurotransmitter present in the brain (Fonnum 1984). It is a precursor of γ-aminobutyric acid (GABA), an inhibitory neurotransmitter (Petroff 2002). The release of glutamate from presynaptic neurons into the synaptic cleft can be recognized by various types of glutamate receptors in the synapses, predominantly receptors on the postsynaptic membranes which initiate action potentials mediating various physiological functions, including memory and learning (McEntee and Crook 1993, Riedel *et al.* 2003). Glutamate homeostasis in the synaptic cleft is mainly mediated by glial cells *via* glutamate uptake which then converts the glutamate to glutamine and transports it back to the presynaptic neurons as a glutamate precursor (Popoli *et al.* 2011). Undoubtedly, the release and maintenance of synaptic levels of glutamate are well-regulated and the basal concentration level of glutamate is controlled *via* complicated neuronal mechanisms together with the help of glial cells (Auld and Robitaille 2003). However, in pathological conditions, the regulation of glutamate homeostasis and transmission is dysregulated and this can cause a large number of neurological disorders (Miladinovic *et al.* 2015).

Like other amino acids, glutamate is primarily synthesized from glucose which crosses the blood-brain barrier *via* astrocytic endfeet (Pellerin and Magistretti 2004). The α-ketoglutarate from the tricarboxylic acid (TCA) cycle as well as glutamine are the main precursors of glutamate (Tapiero *et al.* 2002). In astrocytes, glutamate is converted to glutamine by glutamine synthetase and is transported out of the cells, which is then taken up by neurons *via* Na^+-dependent uptake proteins (Yudkoff *et al.* 2000). The newly taken up glutamine is then converted back to glutamate *via* glutaminase which is then compartmentalized within the synaptic vesicles *via* vesicular glutamate transporters (vGluTs) (Takamori 2006). This corresponds to evidence suggesting that a high concentration of glutamate is mainly found in synaptic vesicles.

In response to stimuli, vesicular glutamate release is mediated by voltage-dependent calcium channels and soluble N-ethylmaleimide-sensitive factor attachment protein receptors (SNAREs) to fuse into the presynaptic membrane and release the glutamate into the synaptic cleft (Sudhof and Rothman 2009), resulting in the propagation of action potentials *via* binding of glutamate to glutamate receptors on the postsynaptic membrane, in which this response is called the excitatory post-synaptic potential (EPSP) (Taube and Schwartzkroin 1988, Meldrum 2000). A wide range of responses depends on the mode of those glutamate receptors which are divided into two main categories ionotropic and metabotropic glutamate receptors. The ionotropic glutamate receptors (iGluR) are ligand-gated ion channels which include *N*-methyl-D-aspartate receptors (NMDARs), α-amino-3-hydroxy-5-methyl-4-isoxazole propionic acid receptors (AMPARs), and kainite receptors. Notably, iGluRs are formed from the conglomeration of numerous protein subunits creating a wide range of receptor isoforms. In contrast to iGluRs, metabotropic glutamate receptors (mGluRs) are G-protein-coupled receptors with seven transmembrane spanning domains. To date, eight mGluRs (mGluR1-8) in 3 categories have been identified which include the group I, II, and III subfamilies. Group I mGluR consists of mGluR1 and mGluR5, in which activation of these receptors causes a variety of cellular modulations involving phospholipase C (PLC), inositol-1,4,5-triphosphate (IP3), and diacylglycerol (DAG). In contrast, group II (mGluR2 and 3) and III (mGluR4-8) mGluRs can reduce cyclic adenosine monophosphate (cAMP) *via* inhibition of adenylyl cyclase/protein kinase A through the inhibitory G-protein, Gi. The structure and function of both types of glutamate receptors as well as downstream signaling pathways were intensively reviewed by Willard and Koochekpour (2013b).

In addition to glutamate receptors, the level of glutamate in the synaptic cleft usually remains constant due to the uptake by glial cells or neurons *via* glutamate transporters or high-affinity amino acid transporters (EAATs). Up to now, five types of glutamate transporters have been identified (EAAT1-5). EAAT1 is found primarily in astrocytes and oligodendrocytes, EAAT2 is ubiquitously found in astrocytes in the CNS, EAAT3 and EAAT4 are found in hippocampal and Purkinje neurons, respectively, while EAAT5 is found specifically in the retina. Glutamate transporters, which are mainly expressed in glial cells, play a crucial role in glutamate clearance *via* buffering the glutamate concentration in the synaptic cleft. Dysregulation in glutamate transporters can result in prolonged activation of the glutamate receptors implicating excitotoxicity in several neurological disorders.

Furthermore, glial cells also usually express the cystine/glutamate antiporters (system x_c^-) which have a regulatory role in glutamate homeostasis. The system x_c^- can uptake one cystine in exchange for release of one glutamate. The taken-up cystine is then reduced to cysteine serving as a precursor in the production of glutathione (GSH), a major neutralizing agent against reactive oxygen species (ROS). On the other hand, excess glutamate in the synaptic clefts can force the release of cystine resulting in deprivation of GSH. Targeting system x_c^- might be a promising strategy for neurological disorders. The contribution of system x_c^- under normal and pathological glutamatergic signaling was comprehensively described by Bridges *et al.* (2012).

ROLE OF GLUTAMATE IN CENTRAL NERVOUS SYSTEM PATHOLOGIES

Notably, glutamatergic transmission requires numerous processes to synergistically regulate the normal condition. Dysregulation in any of those processes in different regions of the brain is associated with central nervous system pathologies, including neurodevelopmental disorders, psychiatric disorders, neurodegenerative disorders, gliomas as well as stroke and ischemia (Miladinovic *et al.* 2015). Glutamate receptors and transporters are the major factor in the dysregulation, as evidenced by several clinical studies and animal models, highlighting the importance of glutamate-targeted therapeutic strategies. Herein, we briefly describe how glutamate as well as its regulation is involved in neurological pathogenesis.

Psychiatric Disorders

Psychiatric disorders are commonly comorbid with other neurological disorders and increase the disease burden (Hesdorffer 2016). Well-known psychiatric disorders include major depressive disorder, bipolar disorder, anxiety disorder, post-traumatic stress disorder, and schizophrenia. In the pathological conditions, glutamate signaling which has multiple roles in the tuning of neuronal function is disrupted. These result in these psychiatric disorders (Ohgi *et al.* 2015).

Major depressive disorder (MDD) is the most common mood disorder. Even though the cause of MDD is still poorly understood, glutamatergic dysregulation in MDD was found by the observation of increased cerebrospinal fluid (CSF) glutamine (Levine *et al.* 2000) and plasma glutamate was also found to correlate with the severity of depression in depressed patients (Mitani *et al.* 2006). Moreover, in stress-induced depression animals, the release and accumulation of glutamate was found in the hippocampus (Abraham *et al.* 1998, Stein-Behrens *et al.* 1994) and the glutamate receptor antagonist, ketamine, was also found to exert an anti-depressant effect (Niciu *et al.* 2014), suggesting the potential role of glutamate-modulating compounds against glutamate system abnormalities.

Bipolar disorder (BPD) is a major mood disorder which is characterized by the inconsistency in the mania, hypomania, and depressed periods. Although long-term treatment with lithium was proven to effectively stabilize patients with BPD (Geddes *et al.* 2004), studies have shown that hippocampal NMDAR dysregulation may be involved in BPD (Scarr *et al.* 2003). Supporting the role of glutamatergic neurotransmission in BPD, brain glutamate levels measured by magnetic resonance spectroscopy were found to be increased in patients with BPD (Ehrlich *et al.* 2015, Gigante *et al.* 2012).

Anxiety disorder is amongst the most prevalent psychiatric disorders. The standard treatment is antidepressant drugs, including selective serotonin reuptake inhibitors (SSRIs), serotonin-norepinephrine reuptake inhibitors (SNRIs), tricyclic antidepressants, and monoamine oxidase inhibitors (Riaza Bermudo-Soriano *et al.* 2012). Growing evidence has suggested that glutamatergic neurotransmission may be involved in the molecular mechanism of anxiety-related disorders (Amiel and Mathew 2007). Since fear conditioning and fear extinction in anxiety disorder are mediated by glutamatergic system, glutamate-modulating compounds may be promising in the treatment of anxiety disorder (Felts *et al.* 2013, Riaza Bermudo-Soriano *et al.* 2012).

Post-traumatic stress disorder (PTSD) is a stress-related disorder directly affecting physical and mental health problems (Meyerhoff *et al.* 2014, Friedman 2013). People with PTSD have at least one of these symptoms; reliving the traumatic event, avoiding thoughts about the event, having bad feeling about themselves, or having trouble sleeping (Spoont 2015). Accumulated evidence has suggested the involvement of glutamatergic system dysfunction in PTSD and therapeutic compounds targeting the glutamatergic system might have potential against PTSD (Nishi *et al.* 2015).

Schizophrenia (SZ) is another psychiatric disorder, characterized by a set of positive and negative symptoms. The positive symptoms include delusion and hallucination, whereas the negative symptoms include deficits in motivation, social interaction, and cognition (Tandon 2013, van Os and Kapur 2009). Several studies have suggested that NMDAR hypofunction in GABAergic inhibitory neurons leads to dysfunction of the glutamatergic neurons, resulting in increased release of glutamate and excitotoxicity (Nakazawa *et al.* 2012, Plitman *et al.* 2014).

Neurodevelopmental Disorders

Neurodevelopmental disorders are characterized by impairments in cognition, communication, behavior and/or motor skills caused by abnormal brain development (Mullin *et al.* 2013). The neurodevelopmental disorders usually have an early onset in childhood and consecutively affect through adulthood in which commonly include autism spectrum disorder and attention-deficit/hyperactivity disorder (Jeste 2015). Increasing evidence has suggested the role of glutamatergic system in the pathogenesis which might be ameliorated by glutamate-targeting therapeutic strategies (Tebartz van Elst *et al.* 2014, Chiocchetti *et al.* 2014).

Autism spectrum disorder (ASD) is a neurodevelopmental disorder with an early onset in childhood. The common symptoms are deficits in social interaction and communication, together with repetitively restricted behaviors, interests, or activities (Grant and Nozyce 2013). Certain evidence from animal models of ASD has shown that mGluR5 is related to the pathogenesis of the disorder. Moreover, a study of ASD patients using NMR has generated supporting evidence for the excitatory and inhibitory imbalance hypothesis (Tebartz van Elst *et al.* 2014) suggesting that targeting the glutamate system may be a viable therapeutic strategy.

Attention-deficit/hyperactivity disorder (ADHD) is a childhood-onset and multifactorial neurodevelopmental disorder with an unknown definite cause. Children with ADHD are likely to have these characteristics; inattention, hyperactivity, and impulsivity (Thapar and Cooper 2016). Several studies have found a correlation between the glutamatergic system and ADHD, for example, hyperactivity in mouse model of ADHD was significantly reduced when animals were treated with a NR2B specific blocker suggesting the involvement of NMDAR in ADHD (Jensen *et al.* 2009).

Neurodegenerative Disorders

Neurodegenerative disorders are still incurable, and they are caused by the deterioration of the neurons in various parts of the brain resulting in a spectrum of deficits either in motor or mental functioning (Lau and Tymianski 2010). Glutamate excitotoxicity is hypothesized to be involved in every aspect of brain disorders, including neurodegenerative disorders such as Alzheimer's disease, Parkinson's disease, amyotrophic lateral sclerosis, and so on.

Alzheimer's disease (AD) is the most common form of dementia, and accounts for up to 70% neurodegenerative cases (Reiman 2014). AD is characterized by the accumulation of neuritic plaques and neurofibrillary tangles together with progressive loss of cognitive function (De-Paula *et al.* 2012). Glutamate excitotoxicity is involved when the glutamate receptors are overstimulated by the Aβ peptide, a plaque-formation molecule, causing the loss of synaptic function and neuronal death (Hynd *et al.* 2004). AD is still an incurable disease for which one of the most effective drugs is memantine, an NMDAR antagonist, and other drugs can only help in partial improvement of systematic symptoms (Danysz and Parsons 2012). Strikingly, numerous studies focusing on plants and plant-derived compounds have shown desirable outcomes, which might be candidates for therapeutic use against AD (Miroddi *et al.* 2014, Yang *et al.* 2014, Malar and Devi 2014).

Parkinson's disease (PD) is characterized by the loss of dopamine and dopaminergic neurons in the substantia nigra pars compacta (SNpc) causing regulatory changes in this region where the glutamatergic activation can be observed (Blandini *et al.* 1996a, Blandini *et al.* 1996b). Some evidence has shown that NMDAR agonists can induce motor neuron dysfunction aggravating Parkinsonian traits in monkeys (Spencer *et al.* 1987). On the other hand, blockage of the glutamate receptors ameliorates the manifestation of PD (Vallano *et al.* 2013). In addition to glutamate receptors, glutamate transporter regulation may play a role in the downregulation of EAAT1 and EAAT2 by 50% and 40%, respectively, in the striatum of PD suggesting the potential roles of these transporters in the pathogenesis of PD (Zhang *et al.* 2016).

Huntington's disease (HD) is a neurodegenerative disorder of movement, mood, and cognition, resulted from the polyglutamine repeats in the huntingtin (Htt) protein (Ross and Tabrizi 2011). From post-mortem studies of HD brains, it was found that there is a reduction in glutamate transporter EAAT2 mRNA in the neostriatum which correlate with the progression of this disease. Moreover, mutations in the *Htt* gene can also affect striatal excitatory synaptic activity by reduction of glutamate uptake and increase in NMDAR-mediated excitotoxicity (Sepers and Raymond 2014). Consequently, targeting of glutamate excitability might be a promising strategy for the treatment of HD.

Amyotrophic Lateral Sclerosis (ALS) is a neuromuscular degenerative disorder (Vucic *et al.* 2014). In superoxide dismutase-1 (SOD1) transgenic mice, it was found that there is a reduction in glutamate transporter EAAT2 (Bruijn *et al.* 1997). Moreover, in patients with ALS, elevated CSF glutamate is believed to be caused by the decrease of EAAT2 in the motor cortex and spinal cord (Rothstein *et al.* 1992) and is associated with excitotoxicity (Van Damme *et al.* 2005). Thus, glutamate transporters are increasingly believed to be involved in motor neuron loss (Blasco *et al.* 2014). Moreover, deletion of system x_c^- in ALS mice significantly slows down the progression of the disease which might be another target of the treatment (Mesci *et al.* 2015).

Epilepsy is broadly characterized by aberrant neuronal excitability involving the glutamate system (Barker-Haliski and White 2015) which can lead to seizures. The use of glutamate transporter knockout mice has helped to understand the roles of glutamatergic system in epilepsy (Petr *et al.* 2015, Wada 1998). In patients with epilepsy, glutamate transporter dysfunction can causes extracellular glutamate levels to increase which then activate the glutamate receptors and cause excitotoxicity eventually (Barker-Haliski and White 2015). Moreover, the role of glutamate in epilepsy may be caused by the dysregulation in GABA, an inhibitor of glutamatergic neurons (DiNuzzo *et al.* 2014), highlighting the therapeutic action of compounds targeting glutamate and related system.

Gliomas

Glutamatergic dysregulation in glial cells has been intensively studied and results suggest that the excitotoxic glutamate levels are caused by system x_c^-, and other glutamate transporter dysregulation (Robert and Sontheimer 2014, de Groot and Sontheimer 2011). Moreover, glutamate receptors (including both ionotropic and metabotropic types) are also associated with the pathogenesis of gliomas. The overexpression or overactivation of the glutamate receptors has been investigated in glioma cells (Castillo *et al.* 2010, Ramaswamy *et al.* 2014, Willard and Koochekpour 2013a) in which glutamate receptor-targeting strategies in gliomas have also been reported (de Groot *et al.* 2008, Ishiuchi *et al.* 2002, Speyer *et al.* 2014).

Ischemic Stroke and Trauma

Ischemic stroke, which results from the lack of blood flow, causes inhibition of the brain functions that can affect numerous processes, including perception, movement, speaking, vision, and cognition (Donnan *et al.* 2008). Several studies have emphasized the effects of hypoxia-induced stroke on the glutamatergic system (Arundine and Tymianski 2004). It was found that glutamate transporter expression is reversed after ischemia which results in extracellular glutamate increase, excitotoxicity, and neuronal cell death (Rossi *et al.* 2000, Torp *et al.* 1995). Moreover, low concentration of memantine significantly protected neurons and glia *via* excitotoxic signaling interruption (Trotman *et al.* 2015) suggesting the possibility of treating ischemic stroke *via* focusing on glutamate system.

Traumatic brain injury (TBI) is caused by an external force and traumatically injures the brain which may be mild (also called concussion) or severe injury (Zetterberg and Blennow 2015). It was suggested that as little as a single traumatic brain injury can cause long-term brain atrophy, precipitate or accelerate age-related neurodegeneration, moreover it can increase the risk of developing Alzheimer's disease, Parkinson's disease, and motor neuron disease (McKee and Robinson 2014). NMDA and AMPA receptors activation have been implicated in the neuronal cell death after the trauma (Wada *et al.* 1999), thus inhibition of these glutamate receptors may provide effective improvement in the symptoms (Arundine and Tymianski 2004).

MECHANISMS OF NEUROPROTECTION AGAINST GLUTAMATE TOXICITY

Modulation of ER Stress Pathway

Apparently, glutamate toxicity can induce the oxidative stress and calcium overload leading to endoplasmic reticulum stress (ER stress). ER is an organelle which plays an important role in calcium storage, including the regulation of folding of proteins (Verkhratsky 2005). Thus, changes in calcium homeostasis by glutamate toxicity and accumulation of unfolded proteins can affect the function of ER, resulting in ER stress. ER stress can cause the induction of chaperones, inhibition of protein translation and activation of ER-associated degradations. ER sensor proteins controlled by a chaperone, such as Bip can activate the release of PKR (RNA-dependent protein kinase)-like ER protein kinase (PERK) that specifically, phosphorylate the pancreatic eukaryotic translation initiation factor 2 subunit α (eIF2α), which play a role in several stress-response pathways (Ma *et al.* 2002, Harding *et al.* 1999, Lu *et al.* 2004). The transcription factor 4 (ATF4) is induced by the phosphorylation of eIF2α by PERK that regulates the integrated stress response (ISR) process, which is the protective process mediated by the ER stress response in cells (Ron 2002).

In addition, ER-stress can activate some other molecules involved in the promotion of mitochondrial apoptosis pathway such as C/EBP-homologous protein (CHOP) and calpain, which can lead to the release of calcium from ER (French *et al.* 2006), and caspase 12 activation (Jin *et al.* 2014b, Lin *et al.* 2017). Calpain is also involved in the cleavage of striatal-enriched tyrosine phosphatase (STEP) members, which regulate MAPK signaling pathway (Xu *et al.* 2009). The natural products that modulate ER-stress pathway are listed in Table **1**.

Cleistocalyx nervosum var. *paniala* berry fruit extracts, which consist of several phenolic compounds, including cyanidin-3-glucoside, can inhibit the neurotoxicity of glutamate in HT22 cell line through the attenuation of ER-stress by reduction of CHOP, calpain and cleaved caspase 12 protein expression (Sukprasansap *et al.* 2017, Sukprasansap *et al.* 2020).

Longistyline C is a natural stilbene which is isolated from the leaves of *Cajanus cajan* (L.) Millsp., showed the neuroprotective effects on glutamate-induced PC12 cells through the reduction of ER-associated proteins, including GRP78, CHOP/GADD153, XBP-1, caspase 9 and caspase 12 (Liu *et al.* 2017).

Astaxanthin is a phytochemical which can reduce the production of ROS and Ca^{2+} influx resulting in the attenuation of ER-stress in SH-SY5Y cell line by declining the expression of calpain, CHOP, ER molecular chaperone glucose-regulated protein (GRP78), and caspase 4 (Lin *et al.* 2017).

Table 1. Plants and their bioactive compounds modulating ER stress pathway.

Plant	Bioactive Compounds	*In vitro/In vivo* model	Molecular Mechanisms	Reference
Berry fruits	Cyanidin-3-glucoside	HT22	↓ CHOP, caspase-12, calpain	(Sukprasansap *et al.* 2020)
Cajanus cajan	Longistyline C	PC12	↓ GRP78, CHOP, caspase9, caspase-12	(Liu *et al.* 2017)
Carotenoid-containing plants	Astaxanthin	SH-SY5Y	↓ CHOP, calpain, caspase-4	(Lin *et al.* 2017)
Cleistocalyx nervosum var. *paniala*	-	HT22	↓ CHOP, calpain, caspase-12	(Sukprasansap *et al.* 2017)

BDNF/TrkB Signaling Pathway

Activation of tropomyosin receptor kinase B (TrkB) receptor by a neurotrophic factor, a brain-derived growth factor (BDNF) provides neuroprotection against glutamate-induced excitotoxicity in many cell lines and primary cells (Almeida *et al.* 2005, Nguyen *et al.* 2010). Generally, the neurotrophic factor functions as the response of neurons to the stress generated by excessive glutamate (Nguyen *et al.* 2009). Thus, compounds with a property in upregulation of BDNF production or activation of TrkB receptor might be neuroprotective to the glutamate-induced neurons (Moosavi *et al.* 2016). Natural products modulating BDNF/TrkB signaling pathway are shown in Table **2**.

3,3'-Diindolylmethane (DIM) is a metabolite of indole-3-carbinol and can be found in Brassicaceae vegetables. It exhibited neuroprotective effects on glutamate-induced HT-22 cells by enhancing the production of BDNF and antioxidant enzymes, such as heme-oxygenase-1 (HO-1) through TrkB/protein kinase B (Akt) pathway (Lee *et al.* 2019).

Emodin offers the neuroprotective effect by modulating expression of phosphorylated CREB and BDNF on glutamate-induced cell death in HT22 cell line *via* PI3K signaling pathway which is partly involved in BDNF/CREB signaling pathway (Ahn *et al.* 2016).

Huperzine A could induce neurotrophic factor signaling pathway through BDNF/TrkB pathway by modulation of BDNF and phosphorylated TrkB protein expression, which is a receptor of BDNF against glutamate-induced neuronal damage in HT22 cell line. Moreover, a previous study demonstrated that the neuroprotective effect of Huperzine A *via* BDNF/TrkB signaling pathway is involved in PI3K/Akt/mTOR pathway which is confirmed by blocking of TrkB resulting in the decrease of p-Akt and p-mTOR (Mao *et al.* 2016).

1-methoxyoctadecan-1-ol (MOD), isolated from *Uncaria sinensis*, was reported to enhance the expression level of mature BDNF together with phosphorylated CREB against glutamate-induced neuronal cell death in HT22 cell line (Ahn *et al.* 2014).

Table 2. Plants and their bioactive compounds modulating BDNF/TrkB signaling pathway.

Plant	Bioactive Compounds	*In vitro/In vivo* model	Molecular Mechanisms	Reference
Brassicaceae vegetables	3,30-Diindolylmethane	HT22	↑ BDNF, p-TrkB	(Lee *et al.* 2019)
Polygonum multiflorum	Emodin	HT22	↑ p-CREB, BDNF	(Ahn *et al.* 2016)
Huperzia serrata	Huperzine A	HT22	↑ BDNF, p-TrkB	(Mao *et al.* 2016)
Uncaria sinensis	1-methoxyoctadecan-1-ol	HT22	↑ p-CREB, BDNF	(Ahn *et al.* 2014)

ERK/JNK/p38 Signaling Pathway

MAPK signaling molecules, including p38, extracellular signal-regulated kinase (ERK) and c-JUN N-terminal kinase (JNK) are the serine-threonine kinases, which are stimulated in response to various stimuli, such as environmental stressors, cytokines, and growth factors to modulate the molecular processes of cell survival and cell death (Lee *et al.* 2014b). Similarly, in response to glutamate toxicity, p38 and JNK become active and mediate the action of apoptotic molecules leading to neuronal cell death by apoptosis and inhibition of p38 and JNK exert the neuroprotective effect against glutamate toxicity (Chen *et al.* 2007). In contrast, upon glutamate induction, ERK1/2, a pro-survival kinase, is inhibited, thus an ERK1/2 enhancer exhibits an increase in neuroprotective activity (Navon *et al.* 2012). Plants and natural products modulating ERK/JNK/p38 signaling pathway are listed in Table **3**.

Sanguiin H-11 (SH-11), isolated from *Sanguisorbae radix* and Procyanidin C1 (PC-1), isolated from grape seeds showed the neuroprotective effects on glutamate-induced HT-22 cells by inhibiting the accumulation of intracellular ROS and attenuating the phosphorylation of MAPKs, including JNK, ERK and p38 (Song *et al.* 2019a, Song *et al.* 2019b).

Ginsenoside Rb2, which is a ginsenoside derivative found in the roots of *Panax ginseng* can inhibit the production of intracellular ROS and transmembrane calcium influx *via* downregulation of the phosphorylation of MAPKs, including JNK, ERK and p38 in HT-22 cells (Kim *et al.* 2019).

Withanolide A was reported to inhibit the activation of MAPKs kinase in response to glutamate toxicity in differentiated Neuro2A cell line *via* the decline of phosphorylated JNK, ERK and p38 protein expression (Dar *et al.* 2017).

The methanolic extract of *Sigesbeckia pubescens* (SP) could attenuate glutamate-induced oxidative stress in HT22 cell line *via* MAPKs kinase signaling pathway by decreasing p-JNK, p-ERK and p-p38 protein expression (Akanda *et al.* 2017).

Isoliquiritigenin, which is an active compound of *Glycyrrhizae radix*, can inhibit glutamate-induced neuronal cell death *via* the attenuation of ROS generation and phosphorylation of JNK, ERK and p38 signaling pathway in HT-22 cell line (Yang *et al.* 2016).

T-006, the derivative of tetramethylpyrazine in *Ligusticum wallichii* Franchet has been demonstrated to mitigate the toxicity of glutamate in primary cerebellar granule neuron (CGN) *via* ERK1/2 signaling pathway by inhibition of phosphorylated ERK1/2 and its upstream, MEK1/2 protein expression resulting in the increasing Bcl-2/Bax ratio (Xu *et al.* 2016).

Astragaloside IV, which is the main saponin compound of *Astragalus membranaceus* Bunge, could inhibit the neurotoxicity of glutamate in PC12 cell line through the reduction of p-MEK, p-ERK1/2 and p-JNK in MAPKs kinase signaling pathway (Yue *et al.* 2015).

Osmotin, which is an adiponectin isolated from *Nicotiana tabacum* has been reported to inhibit the activation of p-JNK in response to the neurotoxicity of glutamate in hippocampus and cortex of postnatal rats (Shah *et al.* 2014).

α-iso-cubebene isolated from *Schisandra chinensis* could inhibit the phosphorylated ERK expression in glutamate-induced HT22 cell line (Park *et al.* 2015).

The ethanolic extract of *Arctium lappa* L. inhibits MAPKs signaling pathway by reduction of the phosphorylation of JNK, ERK1/2 and p38 expression in response to the toxic effects of glutamate in PC12 cell line (Tian *et al.* 2014).

1-methoxyoctadecan-1-ol, isolated from *Uncaria sinensis*, showed the neuroprotective effects against glutamate-induced cell death in HT22 cell line *via* the down-regulation of JNK, ERK1/2 and p38 phosphorylated expression (Ahn *et al.* 2014).

Glycyrrhizic acid, isolated from *Glycyrrhizae radix* could induce the phosphorylated ERK expression in response to glutamate-mediated neuronal cell death in PC12 cell line (Wang *et al.* 2014).

Gastrodia elata could protect glutamate-induced neuronal cell death in HT22, partially *via* the down-regulation of phosphorylated p38 signaling pathway (Han *et al.* 2014).

Liquiritigenin, isolated from *Glycyrrhizae radix,* could attenuate the neurotoxicity of glutamate-induced neuronal cell death in HT22 cell line *via* the down-regulation of MAPKs signaling pathway, including ERK, JNK and p38 (Yang *et al.* 2013b).

Schizandrin, which is found in *Schisandra chinensis*, could inhibit the toxicity of glutamate-induced neuronal cell death in primary cortical neuron *via* MAPKs signaling pathway by down-regulation of p-JNK, p-ERK and p-p38 protein expression resulting in the up-regulation of Bcl-2, Bcl-xl and down-regulation of Bax (Lee *et al.* 2012).

Obovatol and *honokiol*, isolated from the ethanolic extract of *Magnoliae officinalis* Cortex showed the neuroprotective effects against glutamate-induced neurotoxicity in HT22 cell line *via* the reduction of phosphorylated MAPKs expression (Yang *et al.* 2013a)

Table 3. Plants and bioactive compounds modulating MAPK signaling pathway.

Plant	Bioactive Compounds	*In vitro/In vivo* model	Molecular Mechanisms	Reference
Sanguisorbae radix	Sanguiin H-11	HT22	↓ p-p38, p-JNK, p-ERK1/2	(Song *et al.* 2019a)
Grape seeds	Procyanidin C1	HT22	↓ p-p38, p-ERK1/2	(Song *et al.* 2019b)
Panax ginseng	Ginsenoside derivatives Rb2	HT22	↓ p-p38, p-JNK, p-ERK	(Kim *et al.* 2019)
Panax notoginseng	Protopanaxatriol	PC12	↓ p-p38, p-JNK	(Zhang *et al.* 2019)
Salvia miltiorrhiza	Tanshinone IIA	SH-SY5Y	↓ p-p38, p-JNK	(Li *et al.* 2017)
Terminalia arjuna	Casuarinin	HT22	↓ p-p38, p-ERK1/2	(Song *et al.* 2017)

(Table 3) cont.....

Plant	Bioactive Compounds	*In vitro/In vivo* model	Molecular Mechanisms	Reference
Xanthophylls	Astaxanthin	PC12 SH-SY5Y	↓ p-ERK1/2, p-p38	(Lin *et al.* 2017, Zhang *et al.* 2015)
Withania somnifera	Withanolide-A	Neuro2a	↓ p-p38, p-JNK, p-ERK	(Dar *et al.* 2017)
Sigesbeckia pubescens	-	HT22	↓ p-p38, p-JNK, p-ERK	(Akanda *et al.* 2017)
Glycyrrhizae radix	Isoliquiritigenin	HT22	↓ p-p38, p-JNK, p-ERK	(Yang *et al.* 2016)
Ligusticum wallichii Franchet	T-006	Primary cerebellar granule neuron (CGN)	↓ p-ERK1/2, p-MEK1/2	(Xu *et al.* 2016)
Astragalus membranaceus	Astragaloside IV	PC12	↓ p-ERK1/2, p-MEK, p-JNK	(Yue *et al.* 2015)
Nicotiana tabacum	Osmotin	Postnatal rat brain	↓ p-JNK	(Shah *et al.* 2014)
Schisandra chinensis	α-iso-cubebene	HT22	↓ p-ERK	(Park *et al.* 2015)
Arctium lappa L.	-	PC12	↓ p-p38, p-JNK, p-ERK1/2	(Tian *et al.* 2014)
Uncaria sinensis	1-methoxyoctadecan-1-ol	HT22	↓ p-p38, p-JNK, p-ERK1/2	(Ahn *et al.* 2014)
Glycyrrhizae radix	Glycyrrhizic acid	PC12	↑ p-ERK	(Wang *et al.* 2014)
Gastrodia elata	-	HT22	↓ p-p38	(Han *et al.* 2014)
Glycyrrhizae radix	Liquiritigenin	HT22	↓ p-p38, p-JNK, p-ERK	(Yang *et al.* 2013b)
Schisandra chinensis	Schizandrin	Primary cortical neuron	↓ p-p38, p-JNK, p-ERK	(Lee *et al.* 2012)
Magnoliae officinalis Cortex	Obovatol and honokiol	HT22	↓ p-p38, p-JNK, p-ERK	(Yang *et al.* 2013a)

PI3K/Akt/GSK-3β Signaling Pathway

Phosphoinositide 3-kinase (PI3K) and its downstream protein kinase B (Akt) act as pro-survival kinases to defend the cells from neurotoxicity-mediated neuronal cell death. Glutamate toxicity can lead to the activation of anti-apoptotic markers such as Bcl-2, Bcl-xl (Zhang *et al.* 2006, Sen *et al.* 2003). Additionally, PI3K/Akt signaling pathway is also involved in another protein kinase, glycogen synthase kinase 3-beta (GSK-3β). GSK-3β regulates the survival pathway, including Nrf2/HO-1 signaling cascade, which plays a critical role in response to oxidative stress and cell death caused by glutamate-induced toxicity (Zhang *et al.* 2012). Moreover, activation of CREB, a transcription factor in cell survival, is mediated by BDNF and PI3K signaling pathway leading to neuroprotection (Hu *et al.* 2014b). Plants and natural products modulating PI3K/Akt/GSK-3β signaling pathway are shown in Table **4**.

Syringic acid (SA), which is isolated from black burry, *Morus nigra*, has the neuroprotective effect in oxidative stress and glutamate toxicity within brain slices of mice *via* upregulation of PI3K/Akt/ GSK-3β signaling pathway (Dalmagro *et al.* 2019).

Withanolide A, isolated from *Withania somnifera*, has an inhibitory effect against glutamate-induced ROS in differentiated Neuro2A cell line *via* PI3K/Akt signaling pathway by reduction of PI3K and phosphorylated Akt protein expression. Withanolide A can also inhibit neuronal cell death by decreasing Bax/Bcl-2 ratio, p53 and truncated Bid (Dar *et al.* 2017).

Sparassis crispa polysaccharides were found to have an inhibitory effect against glutamate-mediated neuronal cell death in differentiated PC12 cell line induced through the activation of the phosphorylated forms of both Akt and GSK-3β in Akt/GSK-3β signaling pathway together with the enhancement of anti-apoptotic, Bcl-2 and Bcl-xl, expression (Hu *et al.* 2016).

Huperzine A (HupA), isolated from *Huperzia serrate*, is a lycopodium alkaloid compound with the neuroprotective effect in oxidative damage and neuronal cell death by the stimulation of glutamate toxicity in HT22 cell line *via* PI3K/Akt/mTOR signaling pathway. Previous studies showed that HupA increases the phosphorylated expression of Akt and mTOR. However, the inhibitor of PI3K, LY294002 and wortmannin abrogate the effect of HupA treatment in response to glutamate toxicity. In addition, HupA also reduces neuronal cell death induced by mitochondrial apoptotic pathway *via* decreasing Bax and caspase-3, and increasing Bcl-2 (Mao *et al.* 2016).

A novel multifunctional derivative of *tetramethylpyrazine*, T-006, is an active compound isolated from *Ligusticum wallichii* Franchet. This compound showed the neuroprotective effect against glutamate-induced toxicity in primary cerebellar granule neuron (CGN) *via* the suppression of Akt and GSK-3β phosphorylated expression. However, this effect of T-006 was inhibited in the presence of PI3K inhibitor indicating that the neuroprotective effect of T-006 involves the PI3K/Akt/GSK-3β signaling pathway (Xu *et al.* 2016).

Osmotin is an adiponectin isolated from *Nicotiana tabacum*. It can activate the expression of phosphorylated forms of PI3K and Akt and can also reduce the expression of caspase-3 and PARP-1. These effects are abrogated in the presence of PI3K inhibitor indicating that the neuroprotective effect of osmotin against glutamate-induced neuronal cell death relates to PI3K/Akt signaling pathway (Shah *et al.* 2014).

Table 4. Plants and bioactive compounds modulating PI3K/Akt/GSK-3β signaling pathway.

Plant	Bioactive Compounds	*In vitro/In vivo* model	Molecular Mechanisms	Reference
Morus nigra	Syringic acid	Brain slices	↑ p-Akt, p-GSK-3β	(Dalmagro *et al.* 2019)
Ligusticum wallichii Franchet	Compound 22a	Primary cerebellar granule neuron (CGN)	↑ p-PI3K, p-Akt, p-GSK-3β	(Chen *et al.* 2018)
Withania somnifera	Withanolide-A	Neuro2a	↑ PI3k, p-Akt	(Dar *et al.* 2017)
Sparassis crispa	-	PC12	↑ p-Akt ↑ p-GSK-3β	(Hu *et al.* 2016)
Huperzia serrata	Huperzine A	HT22	↑ p-Akt ↑ p-mTOR	(Mao *et al.* 2016)
Ligusticum wallichii Franchet	T-006	Primary cerebellar granule neuron (CGN)	↑ p-Akt ↑ p-GSK-3β	(Xu *et al.* 2016)
Nicotiana tabacum	Osmotin	Postnatal rat brain	↑ p-PI3k, p-Akt	(Shah *et al.* 2014)
Uncaria sinensis	1-methoxyoctadecan-1-ol	HT22	↑ p-PI3k	(Ahn *et al.* 2014)

Nrf2/HO-1 Signaling Pathway

Glutamate-induced ROS production and oxidative stress can be attenuated *via* Nrf2/HO-1 signaling pathway. Nuclear factor-E2-related factor 2 (Nrf2) is a transcription factor which can translocate from cytoplasm to nucleus in response to neuroprotective agents to enhance the anti-oxidant enzyme expression such as heme oxygenase-1 (HO-1) and correlate with the increase of antioxidant response element (ARE) activity (Lee *et al.* 2010, Li *et al.* 2014). Plants and natural products modulating Nrf2/HO-1 signaling pathway are listed in Table **5**.

The ethanolic extract of *Salicornia herbacea* L., including its methylene chloride fraction can induce the activation of Nrf2 and subsequently induce antioxidant systems *via* HO-1 expression to inhibit glutamate-induced toxicity in HT22 cell line (Kim *et al.* 2017).

Gartanin, a bioactive xanthone compound, isolated from *Garcinia mangostana* L. showed the inhibitory effect against glutamate-induced oxidative stress and cell death in HT22 cell line *via* Nrf2-independent HO-1 signaling pathway. In addition, gartanin can also inhibit neuronal cell death *via* anti-apoptotic Bcl-2 expression increase (Gao *et al.* 2016).

The phenolic compounds, *anthocyanins,* are well-known antioxidant flavonoids. These compounds increase the level of glutathione which is involved in the Nrf2/HO-1 signaling pathway. For instance, the increase of Nrf2 and HO-1 expression was observed after anthocyanin treatment against the glutamate-induced toxicity in the hippocampus brain of Sprague-Dawley (SD) rat pups and SH-SY5Y cell line (Shah *et al.* 2016).

Neolignans, isolated from ethanolic extract of *Aristolochia fordiana*, increase the expression of Nrf2 and HO-1 in response to glutamate-mediated oxidative stress and apoptosis in HT-22 cell line. These compounds can also enhance the anti-apoptotic Bcl-2 expression (Tang *et al.* 2015).

α-Iso-cubebene, isolated from *Schisandra chinensis*, induces the activation of Nrf2 expression, which include ARE/CREB activity resulting in the enhancement of HO-1 expression against glutamate-induced neuronal cell death in HT22 cell line. It was also observed that siRNA inhibition of Nrf2 and CREB mitigate the neuroprotective effects of α-iso-cubebene (Park *et al.* 2015).

N-Acyl 5-Hydroxytryptamines with palmitoyl chain is the phenolic endocannabinoids which could increase the anti-oxidant enzymes including HO-1, GCLC, and NQO-1, which downstream the expression of Nrf2 against the glutamate toxicity in HT22 cell line (Jin *et al.* 2014a).

Table 5. Plants and bioactive compounds modulating Nrf2/HO-1 signaling pathway.

Plant	Bioactive Compound	*In vitro/In vivo* model	Molecular Mechanisms	Reference
Cnidium monnieri	Osthole	HT22	↑ Nrf2, HO-1, SOD-1	(Chu *et al.* 2020)
Mulberry leaf	Morachalcone D	HT22	↑ Nrf2, HO-1	(Wen *et al.* 2020)
-	Gastrodin	HT22	↑ Nrf2, HO-1, GPX4	(Jiang *et al.* 2020)

(Table 5) cont.....

Plant	Bioactive Compound	*In vitro/In vivo* model	Molecular Mechanisms	Reference
Rhizoma smilacis glabrae, Astragalus membranaceus	Isoastilbin	PC12	↑ Nrf2, HO-1, SOD-1, CAT	(Yu *et al.* 2019)
Grape seed	Procyanidin C-1	HT22	↑ Nrf2, HO-1	(Song *et al.* 2019b)
Stephania tetrandra	Fangchinoline	HT22	↑ Nrf2, HO-1	(Bao *et al.* 2019)
Rosmarinus officinalis, Salvia officinalis	Carnosic acid	SH-SY5Y cell line	Nrf2-dependent	(de Oliveira *et al.* 2019)
Soybeans	Glyceollins	HT22	↑ Nrf2, HO-1	(Seo *et al.* 2018)
Dalbergia odorifera T. Chen	4-Methoxydalbergione	HT22	↑ Nrf2, HO-1	(Kim *et al.* 2018)
Grewia tiliaefolia	Vitexin	Neuro-2a	↑ Nrf2, HO-1, NQO-1	(Malar *et al.* 2018)
Ligusticum wallichii Franchet	Compound 22a	Primary cerebellar granule neuron (CGN)	↑ Nrf2, HO-1	(Chen *et al.* 2018)
Salicornia herbacea L.	-	HT22	↑ Nrf2, HO-1	(Kim *et al.* 2017)
Garcinia mangostana L	Gartanin	HT22	HO-1-dependent	(Gao *et al.* 2016)
-	Anthocyanins	Sprague-Dawley (SD) rat pups and SH-SY5Y cell line	↑ Nrf2, HO-1	(Shah *et al.* 2016)
Aristolochia fordiana	Neolignans	HT22	↑ Nrf2, HO-1	(Tang *et al.* 2015)
Schisandra chinensis	α-Iso-cubebene	HT22	Nrf2-dependent	(Park *et al.* 2015)
-	Tacrine-3-caffeic Acid	HT22	↑ HO-1	(Chao *et al.* 2014)
-	N-Acyl 5-Hydroxytryptamines	HT22	↑ HO-1, GCLC, NQO-1	(Jin *et al.* 2014a)
Cudrania tricuspidata	Cudarflavone B	HT22	Nrf2-dependent	(Lee *et al.* 2014a)
Euphorbia lagascae	Piceatannol	HT22	HO-1-dependent	(Son *et al.* 2013)

Others

In addition to the aforementioned signaling pathways, more plants and natural products are listed in Table **6** in response to glutamate toxicity. For example, when the cells are exposed to glutamate, it results in mitochondrial dysfunction. Some defense mechanisms may induce the upregulation of peroxisome proliferator-activated receptor γ coactivator α (PGC-1α), a regulator of mitochondria biogenesis and cellular energy, which can help to ameliorate the toxicity (Cui *et al.* 2006). In addition, PGC-1α can protect the cells against glutamate toxicity by targeting silent information regulator 2 family of proteins (sirtuins), which are NAD-dependent deacetylases that mediate the regulation of survival and longevity (Grubisha *et al.* 2005).

Furthermore, previous studies have shown that glutamate induces neuroinflammation *via* the NF-κB signaling pathway by increasing the phosphorylated p65 leading to the nuclear translocation of p65, which subsequently enhances its downstream targets, including pro-inflammatory cytokines such as TNF-α, IL-1β and IL-6, COX-2 and iNOS (Caccamo *et al.* 2005, Scholzke *et al.* 2003). In addition, nitric oxide (NO) generated from NO synthase (NOS) isoforms, including inducible NOS (iNOS), endothelial NOS (eNOS), and neuronal NOS (nNOS) (Dawson *et al.* 1996, Almeida and Bolanos 2001), was reported to mediate glutamate excitotoxicity (Dawson *et al.* 1991, Kume *et al.* 1997). Plants or bioactive compounds reduce these pro-inflammatory cytokines and they may be promising candidates against the neurotoxicity from glutamate.

Interestingly, blocking of NMDA receptors can mitigate the toxic effect of excessive glutamate, which is mediated by the stimulation of AMPA receptor signaling transduction and show the antidepressant effects (Koike *et al.* 2011). These actions may be involved with the interaction between the A-kinase anchoring proteins (AKAPs) and protein kinase A (PKA), which can target the regulation of several biological processes, including the antidepressant mechanisms *via* the NMDA receptor. In the brain, a subunit of AKAP, AKAP79, has high affinity to bind with regulatory subunit of PKA and anchor PKA into the GluR1 subunit of AMPA receptor in postsynaptic membrane by interplaying with cytoskeleton actin and PSD-95 (Burgers *et al.* 2012). Glutamate toxicity could disrupt the interaction of the AKAP79-PKA complex, resulting in the loss of AKAP79 from the postsynaptic membrane, which can affect the phosphorylation of GluR1, and downstream signaling pathway of PI3K dependent activation of MAPKs (Smith *et al.* 2006, Perkinton *et al.* 1999).

In some disorders such as ischemia, glutamate can activate excessive autophagy which can cause ischemic injury (Shi *et al.* 2012). Thus, the inhibition of glutamate-mediated excessive autophagy might be an alternative target to attenuate glutamate excitotoxicity. Several signaling molecules, including those in the PI3K/Akt/mTOR pathway, Bcl-2, Beclin-1, and cytoplasmic p53 (Yang and Klionsky 2010, He and Klionsky 2009) have been reported to be involved in the inhibition of autophagy.

Moreover, the influx of Ca^{2+} resulting from toxic activation of glutamate receptors triggers calcium-dependent neuronal cell death *via* a protease called calpain and subsequently stimulate the cleavage of striatal-enriched tyrosine phosphatase (STEP) from STEP61 into the STEP33 form (Nishizawa 2001, Volbracht *et al.* 2005, Poddar *et al.* 2010). STEP33 molecule mediates glutamate toxicity by regulating the MAPK signaling pathway and the GluN2B subunit of NMDAR (Paul *et al.* 2003, Snyder *et al.* 2005).

Asiatic acid, a pentacyclic triterpene found in *Centella asiatica*, attenuates oxidative stress and glutamate induced neuronal cell injury by the activation of Sirt1 and PGC-1α expression (Xu *et al.* 2012).

Alicin, which is the main bioactive compound of *Allium sativum*, also known as garlic, can ameliorate the effects of glutamate-induced oxidative stress in a model of spinal cord injury. The neuroprotective effect of alicin is through the inducible nitric oxide synthase/Heat shock protein 70 (iNOS/HSP70) signaling pathway. It was found that treatment with alicin can reduce the expression of iNOS and increase the HSP70 expression in response to the glutamate toxicity (Liu *et al.* 2015).

Anthocyanins were reported to have anti-inflammatory effects *via* the NF-κB signaling pathway specifically by reducing NF-κB p65 activity. The phosphorylation of p65, the expression of COX-2, TNF-α and caspase-3, as well as glial cell activation are reduced after treatment with anthocyanins (Shah *et al.* 2016).

EGb 761, which is a extract of *Ginkgo biloba* leaves, can inhibit the up-regulation of tissue plasminogen activator (tPA), which is activated in response to glutamate excess *via* reduction in the level of tPA mRNA. In addition, EGb 761 can also decrease the nuclear translocation of c-FOS, a modulator of tPA expression, in the glutamate-induced condition (Cho *et al.* 2016).

Curcumin can reduce the influx of Ca^{2+}, resulting in the inhibition of the complex between AKAP79 and PKA from the membrane to cytoplasm and can also induce the interaction between AKAP79 and PKA in SH-SY5Y cells (Chen *et al.* 2015).

9-Hydroxy epinootkatol (9OHEN), isolated from *Alpinia oxyphylla* Miquel ethanolic extract, can mitigate neuronal injury of primary cortical neurons, by reducing ROS production and caspase-3-like activity, in response to glutamate toxicity. Moreover, 9OHEN can also diminish glutamate-induced NO activation and nNOS expression (Zhao *et al.* 2015).

The phenol glycoside, *salidroside*, isolated from *Rhodiola rosea*, can inhibit neuronal cell death *via* the reduction of autophagy, increasing the interaction between Bcl-2 and Beclin-1, and increasing cytoplasmic p53 expression in primary cortical neuron (Yin *et al.* 2016).

JGH43IA, a novel compound isolated from the hexanol extract of *Uncaria sinensis,* exerts a neuroprotective effect against glutamate-induced neuronal cell death in primary cortical neuron *via* down-regulation of the phosphorylated GluN2B receptor subunit and its active form calpain 1, leading to blocking the production STEP33, and upregulation of phosphorylated cAMP responsive element binding protein (CREB) (Kim *et al.* 2015).

Table 6. Plants and bioactive compounds with neuroprotective action against glutamate.

Plant	Bioactive Compounds	*In vitro*/*In vivo* model	Molecular Mechanisms	Reference
Centella asiatica	Asiatic acid	SH-SY5Y	↑ SIRT1	(Xu *et al.* 2012)
			↑ PGC-1α	
Allium sativum	Alicin	Primary spinal cord neuron	↓ iNOS	(Liu *et al.* 2015)
			↑ HSP70	
Ginkgo biloba	Egb 761	Primary cortical neuron	↓ c-FOS	(Cho *et al.* 2016)
-	Anthocyanins	Sprague-Dawley (SD) rat pups	↓ p-NF-κB	(Shah *et al.* 2016)
			↓ Cox-2	
			↓ Caspase 3	
		SH-SY5Y	↓ p-NF-κB	
			↓ Cox-2	
			↓ Caspase 3	
Garcinia mangostana L	Gartanin	HT22	↑ p-AMPK	(Gao *et al.* 2016)
-	Anthocyanins	SH-SY5Y	↓ p-AMPK	(Shah *et al.* 2016)
-	Curcumin	SH-SY5Y	↑ AKAP79-PKA	(Chen *et al.* 2015)

(Table 6) cont.....

Plant	Bioactive Compounds	*In vitro/In vivo* model	Molecular Mechanisms	Reference
Alpinia oxyphylla Miquel	9-Hydroxy epinootkatol (9OHEN)	Primary cortical neuron	↓ NO, nNOS	(Zhao *et al.* 2015)
-	Salidroside	Primary cortical neuron	↑ Bcl-2-Beclin-1 ↑ cytoplasmic p53	(Yin *et al.* 2016)
Uncaria sinensis	JGH43IA	Primary cortical neuron	↓ p-GluN2B ↓ Calpain 1 ↓ STEP33 ↑ CREB	(Kim *et al.* 2015)

CONCLUSION AND FUTURE PERSPECTIVES

Glutamatergic transmission *via* diverse glutamate receptors is an essential event in many aspects of brain function, including motor and cognitive functions. On the other hand, dysregulation in the glutamate system, including glutamate metabolism, glutamate homeostasis, glutamate receptors, glutamate transporters, and inhibitory molecules of glutamate can cause harm to the cells through several mechanisms, which mainly result in excitotoxicity and oxidative/ER stress leading to neuronal cell death.

The glutamate-induced model has served as a rationale model representing glutamate-related disorders. The excess glutamate can trigger the glutamate receptors, mainly, ionotropic and metabotropic glutamate receptors, resulting in increased intracellular calcium, a crucial secondary signaling molecule. Excessive activation of calcium is the major cause of mitochondrial dysfunction, ROS production and ER stress, followed by the release of apoptotic molecules leading to neuronal death. Moreover, excess glutamate can also be taken up by system x_c^-, a glutamate/cystine antiporter, releasing cystine which then causes deprivation of glutathione, a defense action against free radical species, in these cells. These destructive mechanisms are at least partially implicated in several neurological disorders, including psychiatric disorders, neurodevelopmental disorders, neurodegenerative disorders, brain tumors and so on.

This model has been diversely studied in a various cell types to explore how cells exposed to glutamate undergo cell death so that we can seek for compounds to disrupt the responsible underlying mechanisms (Kritis *et al.* 2015). So far, much work has been undertaken to understand how medicinal plants or compounds work against numerous disorders, and with the contribution of molecular medicine, we are now gaining knowledge about neuroprotective mechanisms, including BDNF/TrkB signaling pathway, modulation of ER stress, Nrf2/HO-1 signaling pathway, MAPK signaling pathway, PI3K/Akt/GSK-3β signaling pathway and so on. The health benefits of plants or plant-derived compounds are evident. However, toxicity assessment is still needed in every case, which can further improve their effectiveness against human diseases.

Conversely, growing studies have highlighted the possibility of synergistic effects rather than the effects of single bioactive compounds (Song *et al.* 2016, Long *et al.* 2015, Kaur *et al.* 2019). This is relevant to how we have used the traditional herbs in the past. However, it is important to know how every single compound behaves in the body when we consider to adopt those plants or plant-derived compounds for human use.

From this review, we hope that the plants or bioactive compounds which were studied in many aspects of neuroprotection against glutamate toxicity will be chosen for further investigation, at least in animal models and toxicity assessment before testing in clinical trials for glutamate-related disorders. Eventually, natural neuroprotectants could certainly be beneficial to improve both healthspan and lifespan in humans.

CONFLICT OF INTEREST

The authors declare no competing interest.

ACKNOWLEDGEMENT

We are grateful for the support by Natural Products for Neuroprotection and Anti-ageing Research Unit, Department of Clinical Chemistry, Faculty of Allied Health Sciences, Chulalongkorn University.

CONSENT FOR PUBLICATION

None

REFERENCES

Abrahám, I, Juhász, G, Kékesi, KA & Kovács, KJ (1998) Corticosterone peak is responsible for stress-induced elevation of glutamate in the hippocampus. *Stress*, 2, 171-81.
[http://dx.doi.org/10.3109/10253899809167281] [PMID: 9787265]

Ahn, SM, Kim, HN, Kim, YR, Choi, YW, Kim, CM, Shin, HK & Choi, BT (2016) Emodin from Polygonum multiflorum ameliorates oxidative toxicity in HT22 cells and deficits in photothrombotic ischemia. *J Ethnopharmacol*, 188, 13-20.
[http://dx.doi.org/10.1016/j.jep.2016.04.058] [PMID: 27151150]

Ahn, SM, Kim, HN, Kim, YR, Oh, EY, Choi, YW, Shin, HK & Choi, BT (2014) Neuroprotective effect of 1-methoxyoctadecan-1-ol from Uncaria sinensis on glutamate-induced hippocampal neuronal cell death. *J Ethnopharmacol*, 155, 293-9.
[http://dx.doi.org/10.1016/j.jep.2014.05.027] [PMID: 24877848]

Akanda, MR, Kim, MJ, Kim, IS, Ahn, D, Tae, HJ, Rahman, MM, Park, YG, Seol, JW, Nam, HH, Choo, BK & Park, BY (2017) Park, BY Neuroprotective Effects of Sigesbeckia pubescens Extract on Glutamate-Induced Oxidative Stress in HT22 Cells *via* Downregulation of MAPK/caspase-3 Pathways. *Cellular and Molecular Neurobiology.*

Almeida, A & Bolaños, JP (2001) A transient inhibition of mitochondrial ATP synthesis by nitric oxide synthase activation triggered apoptosis in primary cortical neurons. *J Neurochem,* 77, 676-90.
[http://dx.doi.org/10.1046/j.1471-4159.2001.00276.x] [PMID: 11299330]

Almeida, RD, Manadas, BJ, Melo, CV, Gomes, JR, Mendes, CS, Grãos, MM, Carvalho, RF, Carvalho, AP & Duarte, CB (2005) Neuroprotection by BDNF against glutamate-induced apoptotic cell death is mediated by ERK and PI3-kinase pathways. *Cell Death Differ,* 12, 1329-43.
[http://dx.doi.org/10.1038/sj.cdd.4401662] [PMID: 15905876]

Amiel, JM & Mathew, SJ (2007) Glutamate and anxiety disorders. *Curr Psychiatry Rep,* 9, 278-83.
[http://dx.doi.org/10.1007/s11920-007-0033-7] [PMID: 17880858]

Arundine, M & Tymianski, M (2004) Molecular mechanisms of glutamate-dependent neurodegeneration in ischemia and traumatic brain injury. *Cell Mol Life Sci,* 61, 657-68.
[http://dx.doi.org/10.1007/s00018-003-3319-x] [PMID: 15052409]

Auld, DS & Robitaille, R (2003) Glial cells and neurotransmission: an inclusive view of synaptic function. *Neuron,* 40, 389-400.
[http://dx.doi.org/10.1016/S0896-6273(03)00607-X] [PMID: 14556716]

Bao, F, Tao, L & Zhang, H (2019) Neuroprotective Effect of Natural Alkaloid Fangchinoline Against Oxidative Glutamate Toxicity: Involvement of Keap1-Nrf2 Axis Regulation. *Cell Mol Neurobiol,* 39, 1177-86.
[http://dx.doi.org/10.1007/s10571-019-00711-6] [PMID: 31270710]

Barker-Haliski, M & White, HS (2015) Glutamatergic Mechanisms Associated with Seizures and Epilepsy. *Cold Spring Harb Perspect Med,* 5a022863
[http://dx.doi.org/10.1101/cshperspect.a022863] [PMID: 26101204]

Blandini, F, Greenamyre, JT & Nappi, G (1996) The role of glutamate in the pathophysiology of Parkinson's disease. *Funct Neurol,* 11, 3-15. a
[PMID: 8936453]

Blandini, F, Porter, RH & Greenamyre, JT (1996) Glutamate and Parkinson's disease. *Mol Neurobiol,* 12, 73-94. b
[http://dx.doi.org/10.1007/BF02740748] [PMID: 8732541]

Blasco, H, Mavel, S, Corcia, P & Gordon, PH (2014) The glutamate hypothesis in ALS: pathophysiology and drug development. *Curr Med Chem,* 21, 3551-75.
[http://dx.doi.org/10.2174/0929867321666140916120118] [PMID: 25245510]

Bridges, R, Lutgen, V, Lobner, D & Baker, DA (2012) Thinking outside the cleft to understand synaptic activity: contribution of the cystine-glutamate antiporter (System xc-) to normal and pathological glutamatergic signaling. *Pharmacol Rev,* 64, 780-802.
[http://dx.doi.org/10.1124/pr.110.003889] [PMID: 22759795]

Bruijn, LI, Becher, MW, Lee, MK, Anderson, KL, Jenkins, NA, Copeland, NG, Sisodia, SS, Rothstein, JD, Borchelt, DR, Price, DL & Cleveland, DW (1997) ALS-linked SOD1 mutant G85R mediates damage to astrocytes and promotes rapidly progressive disease with SOD1-containing inclusions. *Neuron,* 18, 327-38.
[http://dx.doi.org/10.1016/S0896-6273(00)80272-X] [PMID: 9052802]

Burgers, PP, Ma, Y, Margarucci, L, Mackey, M, van der Heyden, MA, Ellisman, M, Scholten, A, Taylor, SS & Heck, AJ (2012) A small novel A-kinase anchoring protein (AKAP) that localizes specifically protein kinase A-regulatory subunit I (PKA-RI) to the plasma membrane. *J Biol Chem,* 287, 43789-97.
[http://dx.doi.org/10.1074/jbc.M112.395970] [PMID: 23115245]

Caccamo, D, Campisi, A, Marini, H, Adamo, EB, Li Volti, G, Squadrito, F & Ientile, R (2005) Glutamate

promotes NF-kappaB pathway in primary astrocytes: protective effects of IRFI 016, a synthetic vitamin E analogue. *Exp Neurol,* 193, 377-83.
[http://dx.doi.org/10.1016/j.expneurol.2005.01.014] [PMID: 15869940]

Castillo, CA, León, DA, Ballesteros-Yáñez, I, Iglesias, I, Martín, M & Albansz, JL (2010) Glutamate differently modulates metabotropic glutamate receptors in neuronal and glial cells. *Neurochem Res,* 35, 1050-63.
[http://dx.doi.org/10.1007/s11064-010-0154-y] [PMID: 20309728]

Chao, XJ, Chen, ZW, Liu, AM, He, XX, Wang, SG, Wang, YT, Liu, PQ, Ramassamy, C, Mak, SH, Cui, W, Kong, AN, Yu, ZL, Han, YF & Pi, RB (2014) Effect of tacrine-3-caffeic acid, a novel multifunctional anti-Alzheimer's dimer, against oxidative-stress-induced cell death in HT22 hippocampal neurons: involvement of Nrf2/HO-1 pathway. *CNS Neurosci Ther,* 20, 840-50.
[http://dx.doi.org/10.1111/cns.12286] [PMID: 24922524]

Chen, H, Cao, J, Zhu, Z, Zhang, G, Shan, L, Yu, P, Wang, Y, Sun, Y & Zhang, Z (2018) A Novel Tetramethylpyrazine Derivative Protects Against Glutamate-Induced Cytotoxicity Through PGC1α/Nrf2 and PI3K/Akt Signaling Pathways. *Front Neurosci,* 12, 567.
[http://dx.doi.org/10.3389/fnins.2018.00567] [PMID: 30158850]

Chen, K, An, Y, Tie, L, Pan, Y & Li, X (2015) Curcumin Protects Neurons from Glutamate-Induced Excitotoxicity by Membrane Anchored AKAP79-PKA Interaction Network. *Evid Based Complement Alternat Med,* 2015706207
[http://dx.doi.org/10.1155/2015/706207] [PMID: 26170881]

Chen, RW, Lu, XC, Yao, C, Liao, Z, Jiang, ZG, Wei, H, Ghanbari, HA, Tortella, FC & Dave, JR (2007) PAN-811 provides neuroprotection against glutamate toxicity by suppressing activation of JNK and p38 MAPK. *Neurosci Lett,* 422, 64-7.
[http://dx.doi.org/10.1016/j.neulet.2007.06.004] [PMID: 17600621]

Chiocchetti, AG, Bour, HS & Freitag, CM (2014) Glutamatergic candidate genes in autism spectrum disorder: an overview. *J Neural Transm (Vienna),* 121, 1081-106.
[http://dx.doi.org/10.1007/s00702-014-1161-y] [PMID: 24493018]

Cho, KS, Lee, IM, Sim, S, Lee, EJ, Gonzales, EL, Ryu, JH, Cheong, JH, Shin, CY, Kwon, KJ & Han, SH (2016) Ginkgo biloba Extract (EGb 761®) Inhibits Glutamate-induced Up-regulation of Tissue Plasminogen Activator Through Inhibition of c-Fos Translocation in Rat Primary Cortical Neurons. *Phytother Res,* 30, 58-65.
[http://dx.doi.org/10.1002/ptr.5500] [PMID: 26478151]

Chu, Q, Zhu, Y, Cao, T, Zhang, Y, Chang, Z, Liu, Y, Lu, J & Zhang, Y (2020) Studies on the Neuroprotection of Osthole on Glutamate-Induced Apoptotic Cells and an Alzheimer's Disease Mouse Model *via* Modulation Oxidative Stress. *Appl Biochem Biotechnol,* 190, 634-44.
[http://dx.doi.org/10.1007/s12010-019-03101-2] [PMID: 31407160]

Cui, L, Jeong, H, Borovecki, F, Parkhurst, CN, Tanese, N & Krainc, D (2006) Transcriptional repression of PGC-1alpha by mutant huntingtin leads to mitochondrial dysfunction and neurodegeneration. *Cell,* 127, 59-69.
[http://dx.doi.org/10.1016/j.cell.2006.09.015] [PMID: 17018277]

Dalmagro, AP, Camargo, A, Severo Rodrigues, AL & Zeni, ALB (2019) Involvement of PI3K/Akt/GSK-3β signaling pathway in the antidepressant-like and neuroprotective effects of Morus nigra and its major phenolic, syringic acid. *Chem Biol Interact,* 314108843
[http://dx.doi.org/10.1016/j.cbi.2019.108843] [PMID: 31586550]

Danysz, W & Parsons, CG (2012) Alzheimer's disease, β-amyloid, glutamate, NMDA receptors and memantine--searching for the connections. *Br J Pharmacol,* 167, 324-52.
[http://dx.doi.org/10.1111/j.1476-5381.2012.02057.x] [PMID: 22646481]

Dar, NJ, Satti, NK, Dutt, P, Hamid, A & Ahmad, M (2017) Attenuation of Glutamate-Induced Excitotoxicity by Withanolide-A in Neuron-Like Cells: Role for PI3K/Akt/MAPK Signaling Pathway. *Molecular*

Neurobiology.

Dawson, VL, Dawson, TM, London, ED, Bredt, DS & Snyder, SH (1991) Nitric oxide mediates glutamate neurotoxicity in primary cortical cultures. *Proc Natl Acad Sci USA,* 88, 6368-71.
[http://dx.doi.org/10.1073/pnas.88.14.6368] [PMID: 1648740]

Dawson, VL, Kizushi, VM, Huang, PL, Snyder, SH & Dawson, TM (1996) Resistance to neurotoxicity in cortical cultures from neuronal nitric oxide synthase-deficient mice. *J Neurosci,* 16, 2479-87.
[http://dx.doi.org/10.1523/JNEUROSCI.16-08-02479.1996] [PMID: 8786424]

De-Paula, VJ, Radanovic, M, Diniz, BS & Forlenza, OV (2012) Alzheimer's disease. *Subcell Biochem,* 65, 329-52.
[http://dx.doi.org/10.1007/978-94-007-5416-4_14] [PMID: 23225010]

de Groot, J & Sontheimer, H (2011) Glutamate and the biology of gliomas. *Glia,* 59, 1181-9.
[http://dx.doi.org/10.1002/glia.21113] [PMID: 21192095]

de Groot, JF, Piao, Y, Lu, L, Fuller, GN & Yung, WK (2008) Knockdown of GluR1 expression by RNA interference inhibits glioma proliferation. *J Neurooncol,* 88, 121-33.
[http://dx.doi.org/10.1007/s11060-008-9552-2] [PMID: 18317690]

de Oliveira, MR, Duarte, AR, Chenet, AL, de Almeida, FJS & Andrade, CMB (2019) Carnosic Acid Pretreatment Attenuates Mitochondrial Dysfunction in SH-SY5Y Cells in an Experimental Model of Glutamate-Induced Excitotoxicity. *Neurotox Res,* 36, 551-62.
[http://dx.doi.org/10.1007/s12640-019-00044-8] [PMID: 31016690]

DiNuzzo, M, Mangia, S, Maraviglia, B & Giove, F (2014) Physiological bases of the K+ and the glutamate/GABA hypotheses of epilepsy. *Epilepsy Res,* 108, 995-1012.
[http://dx.doi.org/10.1016/j.eplepsyres.2014.04.001] [PMID: 24818957]

Donnan, GA, Fisher, M, Macleod, M & Davis, SM (2008) Stroke. *Lancet,* 371, 1612-23.
[http://dx.doi.org/10.1016/S0140-6736(08)60694-7] [PMID: 18468545]

Ehrlich, A, Schubert, F, Pehrs, C & Gallinat, J (2015) Alterations of cerebral glutamate in the euthymic state of patients with bipolar disorder. *Psychiatry Res,* 233, 73-80.
[http://dx.doi.org/10.1016/j.pscychresns.2015.05.010] [PMID: 26050195]

Felts, AS, Rodriguez, AL, Morrison, RD, Venable, DF, Manka, JT, Bates, BS, Blobaum, AL, Byers, FW, Daniels, JS, Niswender, CM, Jones, CK, Conn, PJ, Lindsley, CW & Emmitte, KA (2013) Discovery of VU0409106: A negative allosteric modulator of mGlu5 with activity in a mouse model of anxiety. *Bioorg Med Chem Lett,* 23, 5779-85.
[http://dx.doi.org/10.1016/j.bmcl.2013.09.001] [PMID: 24074843]

Fonnum, F (1984) Glutamate: a neurotransmitter in mammalian brain. *J Neurochem,* 42, 1-11.
[http://dx.doi.org/10.1111/j.1471-4159.1984.tb09689.x] [PMID: 6139418]

French, JP, Quindry, JC, Falk, DJ, Staib, JL, Lee, Y, Wang, KK & Powers, SK (2006) Ischemia-reperfusio--induced calpain activation and SERCA2a degradation are attenuated by exercise training and calpain inhibition. *Am J Physiol Heart Circ Physiol,* 290, H128-36.
[http://dx.doi.org/10.1152/ajpheart.00739.2005] [PMID: 16155100]

Friedman, MJ (2013) Finalizing PTSD in DSM-5: getting here from there and where to go next. *J Trauma Stress,* 26, 548-56.
[http://dx.doi.org/10.1002/jts.21840] [PMID: 24151001]

Gao, XY, Wang, SN, Yang, XH, Lan, WJ, Chen, ZW, Chen, JK, Xie, JH, Han, YF, Pi, RB & Yang, XB (2016) Gartanin Protects Neurons against Glutamate-Induced Cell Death in HT22 Cells: Independence of Nrf-2 but Involvement of HO-1 and AMPK. *Neurochem Res,* 41, 2267-77.
[http://dx.doi.org/10.1007/s11064-016-1941-x] [PMID: 27161377]

Geddes, JR, Burgess, S, Hawton, K, Jamison, K & Goodwin, GM (2004) Long-term lithium therapy for bipolar disorder: systematic review and meta-analysis of randomized controlled trials. *Am J Psychiatry,* 161, 217-22.

[http://dx.doi.org/10.1176/appi.ajp.161.2.217] [PMID: 14754766]

Gigante, AD, Bond, DJ, Lafer, B, Lam, RW, Young, LT & Yatham, LN (2012) Brain glutamate levels measured by magnetic resonance spectroscopy in patients with bipolar disorder: a meta-analysis. *Bipolar Disord,* 14, 478-87.
[http://dx.doi.org/10.1111/j.1399-5618.2012.01033.x] [PMID: 22834460]

Grant, R & Nozyce, M (2013) Proposed changes to the American Psychiatric Association diagnostic criteria for autism spectrum disorder: implications for young children and their families. *Matern Child Health J,* 17, 586-92.
[http://dx.doi.org/10.1007/s10995-013-1250-9] [PMID: 23456348]

Grubisha, O, Smith, BC & Denu, JM (2005) Small molecule regulation of Sir2 protein deacetylases. *FEBS J,* 272, 4607-16.
[http://dx.doi.org/10.1111/j.1742-4658.2005.04862.x] [PMID: 16156783]

Han, YJ, Je, JH, Kim, SH, Ahn, SM, Kim, HN, Kim, YR, Choi, YW, Shin, HK & Choi, BT (2014) Gastrodia elata shows neuroprotective effects *via* activation of PI3K signaling against oxidative glutamate toxicity in HT22 cells. *Am J Chin Med,* 42, 1007-19.
[http://dx.doi.org/10.1142/S0192415X14500633] [PMID: 25004888]

Harding, HP, Zhang, Y & Ron, D (1999) Protein translation and folding are coupled by an endoplasmic-reticulum-resident kinase. *Nature,* 397, 271-4.
[http://dx.doi.org/10.1038/16729] [PMID: 9930704]

He, C & Klionsky, DJ (2009) Regulation mechanisms and signaling pathways of autophagy. *Annu Rev Genet,* 43, 67-93.
[http://dx.doi.org/10.1146/annurev-genet-102808-114910] [PMID: 19653858]

Hertz, L, Dringen, R, Schousboe, A & Robinson, SR (1999) Astrocytes: glutamate producers for neurons. *J Neurosci Res,* 57, 417-28.
[http://dx.doi.org/10.1002/(SICI)1097-4547(19990815)57:4<417::AID-JNR1>3.0.CO;2-N]   [PMID: 10440891]

Hesdorffer, DC (2016) Comorbidity between neurological illness and psychiatric disorders. *CNS Spectr,* 21, 230-8.
[http://dx.doi.org/10.1017/S1092852915000929] [PMID: 26898322]

Hu, D, Huang, J, Wang, Y, Zhang, D & Qu, Y (2014) Fruits and vegetables consumption and risk of stroke: a meta-analysis of prospective cohort studies. *Stroke,* 45, 1613-9. a
[http://dx.doi.org/10.1161/STROKEAHA.114.004836] [PMID: 24811336]

Hu, S, Wang, D, Zhang, J, Du, M, Cheng, Y, Liu, Y, Zhang, N, Wang, D & Wu, Y (2016) Mitochondria Related Pathway Is Essential for Polysaccharides Purified from Sparassis crispa Mediated Neuro-Protection against Glutamate-Induced Toxicity in Differentiated PC12 Cells. *Int J Mol Sci,* 17, 17.
[http://dx.doi.org/10.3390/ijms17020133] [PMID: 26821016]

Hu, Y, Liu, MY, Liu, P, Dong, X & Boran, AD (2014) Neuroprotective effects of 3,6′-disinapoyl sucrose through increased BDNF levels and CREB phosphorylation *via* the CaMKII and ERK1/2 pathway. *J Mol Neurosci,* 53, 600-7. b
[http://dx.doi.org/10.1007/s12031-013-0226-y] [PMID: 24488601]

Hynd, MR, Scott, HL & Dodd, PR (2004) Glutamate-mediated excitotoxicity and neurodegeneration in Alzheimer's disease. *Neurochem Int,* 45, 583-95.
[http://dx.doi.org/10.1016/j.neuint.2004.03.007] [PMID: 15234100]

Hyson, DA (2015) A review and critical analysis of the scientific literature related to 100% fruit juice and human health. *Adv Nutr,* 6, 37-51.
[http://dx.doi.org/10.3945/an.114.005728] [PMID: 25593142]

Ishiuchi, S, Tsuzuki, K, Yoshida, Y, Yamada, N, Hagimura, N, Okado, H, Miwa, A, Kurihara, H, Nakazato, Y, Tamura, M, Sasaki, T & Ozawa, S (2002) Blockage of Ca(2+)-permeable AMPA receptors suppresses

migration and induces apoptosis in human glioblastoma cells. *Nat Med,* 8, 971-8.
[http://dx.doi.org/10.1038/nm746] [PMID: 12172541]

Jensen, V, Rinholm, JE, Johansen, TJ, Medin, T, Storm-Mathisen, J, Sagvolden, T, Hvalby, O & Bergersen, LH (2009) N-methyl-D-aspartate receptor subunit dysfunction at hippocampal glutamatergic synapses in an animal model of attention-deficit/hyperactivity disorder. *Neuroscience,* 158, 353-64.
[http://dx.doi.org/10.1016/j.neuroscience.2008.05.016] [PMID: 18571865]

Jeste, SS (2015) Neurodevelopmental behavioral and cognitive disorders. *Continuum (Minneap Minn),* 21, 690-714.
[http://dx.doi.org/10.1212/01.CON.0000466661.89908.3c] [PMID: 26039849]

Jiang, T, Cheng, H, Su, J, Wang, X, Wang, Q, Chu, J & Li, Q (2020) Gastrodin protects against glutamate-induced ferroptosis in HT-22 cells through Nrf2/HO-1 signaling pathway. *Toxicol In Vitro,* 62104715
[http://dx.doi.org/10.1016/j.tiv.2019.104715] [PMID: 31698019]

Jin, MC, Yoo, JM, Sok, DE & Kim, MR (2014) Neuroprotective effect of N-acyl 5-hydroxytryptamines on glutamate-induced cytotoxicity in HT-22 cells. *Neurochem Res,* 39, 2440-51. a
[http://dx.doi.org/10.1007/s11064-014-1448-2] [PMID: 25307111]

Jin, ML, Park, SY, Kim, YH, Oh, JI, Lee, SJ & Park, G (2014) The neuroprotective effects of cordycepin inhibit glutamate-induced oxidative and ER stress-associated apoptosis in hippocampal HT22 cells. *Neurotoxicology,* 41, 102-11. b
[http://dx.doi.org/10.1016/j.neuro.2014.01.005] [PMID: 24486958]

Kaur, P, Robin, , Mehta, RG, Singh, B & Arora, S (2019) Development of aqueous-based multi-herbal combination using principal component analysis and its functional significance in HepG2 cells. *BMC Complement Altern Med,* 19, 18.
[http://dx.doi.org/10.1186/s12906-019-2432-9] [PMID: 30646883]

Kim, DC, Lee, DS, Ko, W, Kim, KW, Kim, HJ, Yoon, CS, Oh, H & Kim, YC (2018) Heme Oxygenase--Inducing Activity of 4-Methoxydalbergione and 4′-Hydroxy-4-methoxydalbergione from Dalbergia odorifera and Their Anti-inflammatory and Cytoprotective Effects in Murine Hippocampal and BV2 Microglial Cell Line and Primary Rat Microglial Cells. *Neurotox Res,* 33, 337-52.
[http://dx.doi.org/10.1007/s12640-017-9796-8] [PMID: 28836188]

Kim, DH, Kim, DW, Jung, BH, Lee, JH, Lee, H, Hwang, GS, Kang, KS & Lee, JW (2019) Ginsenoside Rb2 suppresses the glutamate-mediated oxidative stress and neuronal cell death in HT22 cells. *J Ginseng Res,* 43, 326-34.
[http://dx.doi.org/10.1016/j.jgr.2018.12.002] [PMID: 30976171]

Kim, HN, Jang, JY & Choi, BT (2015) A single fraction from Uncaria sinensis exerts neuroprotective effects against glutamate-induced neurotoxicity in primary cultured cortical neurons. *Anat Cell Biol,* 48, 95-103.
[http://dx.doi.org/10.5115/acb.2015.48.2.95] [PMID: 26140220]

Kim, MS, Seo, JY, Oh, J, Jang, YK, Lee, CH & Kim, JS (2017) Neuroprotective Effect of Halophyte Salicornia herbacea L. Is Mediated by Activation of Heme Oxygenase-1 in Mouse Hippocampal HT22 Cells. *J Med Food,* 20, 140-51.
[http://dx.doi.org/10.1089/jmf.2016.3829] [PMID: 28146411]

Koike, H, Iijima, M & Chaki, S (2011) Involvement of AMPA receptor in both the rapid and sustained antidepressant-like effects of ketamine in animal models of depression. *Behav Brain Res,* 224, 107-11.
[http://dx.doi.org/10.1016/j.bbr.2011.05.035] [PMID: 21669235]

Kritis, AA, Stamoula, EG, Paniskaki, KA & Vavilis, TD (2015) Researching glutamate - induced cytotoxicity in different cell lines: a comparative/collective analysis/study. *Front Cell Neurosci,* 9, 91.
[http://dx.doi.org/10.3389/fncel.2015.00091] [PMID: 25852482]

Kume, T, Kouchiyama, H, Kaneko, S, Maeda, T, Kaneko, S, Akaike, A, Shimohama, S, Kihara, T, Kimura, J, Wada, K & Koizumi, S (1997) BDNF prevents NO mediated glutamate cytotoxicity in cultured cortical neurons. *Brain Res,* 756, 200-4.

[http://dx.doi.org/10.1016/S0006-8993(97)00195-9] [PMID: 9187333]

Lau, A & Tymianski, M (2010) Glutamate receptors, neurotoxicity and neurodegeneration. *Pflugers Arch,* 460, 525-42.
[http://dx.doi.org/10.1007/s00424-010-0809-1] [PMID: 20229265]

Lee, BD, Yoo, JM, Baek, SY, Li, FY, Sok, DE & Kim, MR (2019) 3,3′-Diindolylmethane Promotes BDNF and Antioxidant Enzyme Formation *via* TrkB/Akt Pathway Activation for Neuroprotection against Oxidative Stress-Induced Apoptosis in Hippocampal Neuronal Cells. *Antioxidants,* 9, 9.
[http://dx.doi.org/10.3390/antiox9010003] [PMID: 31861353]

Lee, DS, Ko, W, Kim, DC, Kim, YC & Jeong, GS (2014) Cudarflavone B provides neuroprotection against glutamate-induced mouse hippocampal HT22 cell damage through the Nrf2 and PI3K/Akt signaling pathways. *Molecules,* 19, 10818-31. a
[http://dx.doi.org/10.3390/molecules190810818] [PMID: 25061726]

Lee, HG, Li, MH, Joung, EJ, Na, HK, Cha, YN & Surh, YJ (2010) Nrf2-Mediated heme oxygenase-1 upregulation as adaptive survival response to glucose deprivation-induced apoptosis in HepG2 cells. *Antioxid Redox Signal,* 13, 1639-48.
[http://dx.doi.org/10.1089/ars.2010.3226] [PMID: 20446774]

Lee, J, Jo, DG, Park, D, Chung, HY & Mattson, MP (2014) Adaptive cellular stress pathways as therapeutic targets of dietary phytochemicals: focus on the nervous system. *Pharmacol Rev,* 66, 815-68. b
[http://dx.doi.org/10.1124/pr.113.007757] [PMID: 24958636]

Lee, MS, Chao, J, Yen, JC, Lin, LW, Tsai, FS, Hsieh, MT, Peng, WH & Cheng, HY (2012) Schizandrin protects primary rat cortical cell cultures from glutamate-induced apoptosis by inhibiting activation of the MAPK family and the mitochondria dependent pathway. *Molecules,* 18, 354-72.
[http://dx.doi.org/10.3390/molecules18010354] [PMID: 23271470]

Levine, J, Panchalingam, K, Rapoport, A, Gershon, S, McClure, RJ & Pettegrew, JW (2000) Increased cerebrospinal fluid glutamine levels in depressed patients. *Biol Psychiatry,* 47, 586-93.
[http://dx.doi.org/10.1016/S0006-3223(99)00284-X] [PMID: 10745050]

Li, H, Han, W, Wang, H, Ding, F, Xiao, L, Shi, R, Ai, L & Huang, Z (2017) Tanshinone IIA Inhibits Glutamate-Induced Oxidative Toxicity through Prevention of Mitochondrial Dysfunction and Suppression of MAPK Activation in SH-SY5Y Human Neuroblastoma Cells. *Oxid Med Cell Longev,* 20174517486
[http://dx.doi.org/10.1155/2017/4517486] [PMID: 28690763]

Li, L, Dong, H, Song, E, Xu, X, Liu, L & Song, Y (2014) Nrf2/ARE pathway activation, HO-1 and NQO1 induction by polychlorinated biphenyl quinone is associated with reactive oxygen species and PI3K/AKT signaling. *Chem Biol Interact,* 209, 56-67.
[http://dx.doi.org/10.1016/j.cbi.2013.12.005] [PMID: 24361488]

Lin, X, Zhao, Y & Li, S (2017) Astaxanthin attenuates glutamate-induced apoptosis *via* inhibition of calcium influx and endoplasmic reticulum stress. *Eur J Pharmacol,* 806, 43-51.
[http://dx.doi.org/10.1016/j.ejphar.2017.04.008] [PMID: 28400209]

Liu, SG, Ren, PY, Wang, GY, Yao, SX & He, XJ (2015) Allicin protects spinal cord neurons from glutamate-induced oxidative stress through regulating the heat shock protein 70/inducible nitric oxide synthase pathway. *Food Funct,* 6, 321-30.
[http://dx.doi.org/10.1039/C4FO00761A] [PMID: 25473931]

Liu, X, Yan, Y, Li, F & Zhang, D (2016) Fruit and vegetable consumption and the risk of depression: A meta-analysis. *Nutrition,* 32, 296-302.
[http://dx.doi.org/10.1016/j.nut.2015.09.009] [PMID: 26691768]

Liu, Y, Zhao, N, Li, C, Chang, Q, Liu, X, Liao, Y & Pan, R (2017) Longistyline C acts antidepressant *in vivo* and neuroprotection *in vitro* against glutamate-induced cytotoxicity by regulating NMDAR/NR2B-ERK pathway in PC12 cells. *PLoS One,* 12e0183702
[http://dx.doi.org/10.1371/journal.pone.0183702] [PMID: 28873095]

Long, F, Yang, H, Xu, Y, Hao, H & Li, P (2015) A strategy for the identification of combinatorial bioactive compounds contributing to the holistic effect of herbal medicines. *Sci Rep,* 5, 12361.
[http://dx.doi.org/10.1038/srep12361] [PMID: 26198093]

Lu, PD, Harding, HP & Ron, D (2004) Translation reinitiation at alternative open reading frames regulates gene expression in an integrated stress response. *J Cell Biol,* 167, 27-33.
[http://dx.doi.org/10.1083/jcb.200408003] [PMID: 15479734]

Ma, K, Vattem, KM & Wek, RC (2002) Dimerization and release of molecular chaperone inhibition facilitate activation of eukaryotic initiation factor-2 kinase in response to endoplasmic reticulum stress. *J Biol Chem,* 277, 18728-35.
[http://dx.doi.org/10.1074/jbc.M200903200] [PMID: 11907036]

Malar, DS & Devi, KP (2014) Dietary polyphenols for treatment of Alzheimer's disease--future research and development. *Curr Pharm Biotechnol,* 15, 330-42.
[http://dx.doi.org/10.2174/13892010156661408 13122703] [PMID: 25312617]

Malar, DS, Prasanth, MI, Shafreen, RB, Balamurugan, K & Devi, KP (2018) Grewia tiliaefolia and its active compound vitexin regulate the expression of glutamate transporters and protect Neuro-2a cells from glutamate toxicity. *Life Sci,* 203, 233-41.
[http://dx.doi.org/10.1016/j.lfs.2018.04.047] [PMID: 29704481]

Mao, XY, Zhou, HH, Li, X & Liu, ZQ (2016) Huperzine A Alleviates Oxidative Glutamate Toxicity in Hippocampal HT22 Cells *via* Activating BDNF/TrkB-Dependent PI3K/Akt/mTOR Signaling Pathway. *Cell Mol Neurobiol,* 36, 915-25.
[http://dx.doi.org/10.1007/s10571-015-0276-5] [PMID: 26440805]

Mattson, MP (2008) Glutamate and neurotrophic factors in neuronal plasticity and disease. *Ann N Y Acad Sci,* 1144, 97-112.
[http://dx.doi.org/10.1196/annals.1418.005] [PMID: 19076369]

McEntee, WJ & Crook, TH (1993) Glutamate: its role in learning, memory, and the aging brain. *Psychopharmacology (Berl),* 111, 391-401.
[http://dx.doi.org/10.1007/BF02253527] [PMID: 7870979]

McKee, AC & Robinson, ME (2014) Military-related traumatic brain injury and neurodegeneration. *Alzheimers Dement,* 10 (Suppl.), S242-53.
[http://dx.doi.org/10.1016/j.jalz.2014.04.003] [PMID: 24924675]

Meldrum, BS (2000) Glutamate as a neurotransmitter in the brain: review of physiology and pathology. *J Nutr,* 130 (Suppl.), 1007S-15S.
[http://dx.doi.org/10.1093/jn/130.4.1007S] [PMID: 10736372]

Mesci, P, Zaïdi, S, Lobsiger, CS, Millecamps, S, Escartin, C, Seilhean, D, Sato, H, Mallat, M & Boillée, S (2015) System xC- is a mediator of microglial function and its deletion slows symptoms in amyotrophic lateral sclerosis mice. *Brain,* 138, 53-68.
[http://dx.doi.org/10.1093/brain/awu312] [PMID: 25384799]

Meyerhoff, DJ, Mon, A, Metzler, T & Neylan, TC (2014) Cortical gamma-aminobutyric acid and glutamate in posttraumatic stress disorder and their relationships to self-reported sleep quality. *Sleep,* 37, 893-900.
[http://dx.doi.org/10.5665/sleep.3654] [PMID: 24790267]

Miladinovic, T, Nashed, MG & Singh, G (2015) Overview of Glutamatergic Dysregulation in Central Pathologies. *Biomolecules,* 5, 3112-41.
[http://dx.doi.org/10.3390/biom5043112] [PMID: 26569330]

Miroddi, M, Navarra, M, Quattropani, MC, Calapai, F, Gangemi, S & Calapai, G (2014) Systematic review of clinical trials assessing pharmacological properties of Salvia species on memory, cognitive impairment and Alzheimer's disease. *CNS Neurosci Ther,* 20, 485-95.
[http://dx.doi.org/10.1111/cns.12270] [PMID: 24836739]

Mitani, H, Shirayama, Y, Yamada, T, Maeda, K, Ashby, CR, Jr & Kawahara, R (2006) Correlation between

plasma levels of glutamate, alanine and serine with severity of depression. *Prog Neuropsychopharmacol Biol Psychiatry,* 30, 1155-8.
[http://dx.doi.org/10.1016/j.pnpbp.2006.03.036] [PMID: 16707201]

Moosavi, F, Hosseini, R, Saso, L & Firuzi, O (2015) Modulation of neurotrophic signaling pathways by polyphenols. *Drug Des Devel Ther,* 10, 23-42.
[PMID: 26730179]

Mullin, AP, Gokhale, A, Moreno-De-Luca, A, Sanyal, S, Waddington, JL & Faundez, V (2013) Neurodevelopmental disorders: mechanisms and boundary definitions from genomes, interactomes and proteomes. *Transl Psychiatry,* 3e329
[http://dx.doi.org/10.1038/tp.2013.108] [PMID: 24301647]

Nakanishi, S (1992) Molecular diversity of glutamate receptors and implications for brain function. *Science,* 258, 597-603.
[http://dx.doi.org/10.1126/science.1329206] [PMID: 1329206]

Nakazawa, K, Zsiros, V, Jiang, Z, Nakao, K, Kolata, S, Zhang, S & Belforte, JE (2012) GABAergic interneuron origin of schizophrenia pathophysiology. *Neuropharmacology,* 62, 1574-83.
[http://dx.doi.org/10.1016/j.neuropharm.2011.01.022] [PMID: 21277876]

Navon, H, Bromberg, Y, Sperling, O & Shani, E (2012) Neuroprotection by NMDA preconditioning against glutamate cytotoxicity is mediated through activation of ERK 1/2, inactivation of JNK, and by prevention of glutamate-induced CREB inactivation. *J Mol Neurosci,* 46, 100-8.
[http://dx.doi.org/10.1007/s12031-011-9532-4] [PMID: 21556733]

Nguyen, N, Lee, SB, Lee, YS, Lee, KH & Ahn, JY (2009) Neuroprotection by NGF and BDNF against neurotoxin-exerted apoptotic death in neural stem cells are mediated through Trk receptors, activating PI3-kinase and MAPK pathways. *Neurochem Res,* 34, 942-51.
[http://dx.doi.org/10.1007/s11064-008-9848-9] [PMID: 18846424]

Nguyen, TL, Kim, CK, Cho, JH, Lee, KH & Ahn, JY (2010) Neuroprotection signaling pathway of nerve growth factor and brain-derived neurotrophic factor against staurosporine induced apoptosis in hippocampal H19-7/IGF-IR [corrected]. *Exp Mol Med,* 42, 583-95. [corrected].
[http://dx.doi.org/10.3858/emm.2010.42.8.060] [PMID: 20644345]

Niciu, MJ, Ionescu, DF, Richards, EM & Zarate, CA, Jr (2014) Glutamate and its receptors in the pathophysiology and treatment of major depressive disorder. *J Neural Transm (Vienna),* 121, 907-24.
[http://dx.doi.org/10.1007/s00702-013-1130-x] [PMID: 24318540]

Nishi, D, Hashimoto, K, Noguchi, H, Hamazaki, K, Hamazaki, T & Matsuoka, Y (2015) Glutamatergic system abnormalities in posttraumatic stress disorder. *Psychopharmacology (Berl),* 232, 4261-8.
[http://dx.doi.org/10.1007/s00213-015-4052-5] [PMID: 26292802]

Nishizawa, Y (2001) Glutamate release and neuronal damage in ischemia. *Life Sci,* 69, 369-81.
[http://dx.doi.org/10.1016/S0024-3205(01)01142-0] [PMID: 11459428]

Ohgi, Y, Futamura, T & Hashimoto, K (2015) Glutamate Signaling in Synaptogenesis and NMDA Receptors as Potential Therapeutic Targets for Psychiatric Disorders. *Curr Mol Med,* 15, 206-21.
[http://dx.doi.org/10.2174/1566524015666150330143008] [PMID: 25817855]

Park, SY, Jung, WJ, Kang, JS, Kim, CM, Park, G & Choi, YW (2015) Neuroprotective effects of α-is--cubebene against glutamate-induced damage in the HT22 hippocampal neuronal cell line. *Int J Mol Med,* 35, 525-32.
[http://dx.doi.org/10.3892/ijmm.2014.2031] [PMID: 25503787]

Paul, S, Nairn, AC, Wang, P & Lombroso, PJ (2003) NMDA-mediated activation of the tyrosine phosphatase STEP regulates the duration of ERK signaling. *Nat Neurosci,* 6, 34-42.
[http://dx.doi.org/10.1038/nn989] [PMID: 12483215]

Pellerin, L & Magistretti, PJ (2004) Neuroenergetics: calling upon astrocytes to satisfy hungry neurons. *Neuroscientist,* 10, 53-62.

[http://dx.doi.org/10.1177/1073858403260159] [PMID: 14987448]

Perkinton, MS, Sihra, TS & Williams, RJ (1999) Ca(2+)-permeable AMPA receptors induce phosphorylation of cAMP response element-binding protein through a phosphatidylinositol 3-kinase-dependent stimulation of the mitogen-activated protein kinase signaling cascade in neurons. *J Neurosci,* 19, 5861-74.
[http://dx.doi.org/10.1523/JNEUROSCI.19-14-05861.1999] [PMID: 10407026]

Petr, GT, Sun, Y, Frederick, NM, Zhou, Y, Dhamne, SC, Hameed, MQ, Miranda, C, Bedoya, EA, Fischer, KD, Armsen, W, Wang, J, Danbolt, NC, Rotenberg, A, Aoki, CJ & Rosenberg, PA (2015) Conditional deletion of the glutamate transporter GLT-1 reveals that astrocytic GLT-1 protects against fatal epilepsy while neuronal GLT-1 contributes significantly to glutamate uptake into synaptosomes. *J Neurosci,* 35, 5187-201.
[http://dx.doi.org/10.1523/JNEUROSCI.4255-14.2015] [PMID: 25834045]

Petroff, OA (2002) GABA and glutamate in the human brain. *Neuroscientist,* 8, 562-73.
[http://dx.doi.org/10.1177/1073858402238515] [PMID: 12467378]

Plitman, E, Nakajima, S, de la Fuente-Sandoval, C, Gerretsen, P, Chakravarty, MM, Kobylianskii, J, Chung, JK, Caravaggio, F, Iwata, Y, Remington, G & Graff-Guerrero, A (2014) Glutamate-mediated excitotoxicity in schizophrenia: a review. *Eur Neuropsychopharmacol,* 24, 1591-605.
[http://dx.doi.org/10.1016/j.euroneuro.2014.07.015] [PMID: 25159198]

Poddar, R, Deb, I, Mukherjee, S & Paul, S (2010) NR2B-NMDA receptor mediated modulation of the tyrosine phosphatase STEP regulates glutamate induced neuronal cell death. *J Neurochem,* 115, 1350-62.
[http://dx.doi.org/10.1111/j.1471-4159.2010.07035.x] [PMID: 21029094]

Popoli, M, Yan, Z, McEwen, BS & Sanacora, G (2011) The stressed synapse: the impact of stress and glucocorticoids on glutamate transmission. *Nat Rev Neurosci,* 13, 22-37.
[http://dx.doi.org/10.1038/nrn3138] [PMID: 22127301]

Ramaswamy, P, Aditi Devi, N, Hurmath Fathima, K & Dalavaikodihalli Nanjaiah, N (2014) Activation of NMDA receptor of glutamate influences MMP-2 activity and proliferation of glioma cells. *Neurol Sci,* 35, 823-9.
[http://dx.doi.org/10.1007/s10072-013-1604-5] [PMID: 24374786]

Reiman, EM (2014) Alzheimer's disease and other dementias: advances in 2013. *Lancet Neurol,* 13, 3-5.
[http://dx.doi.org/10.1016/S1474-4422(13)70257-6] [PMID: 24331781]

Riaza Bermudo-Soriano, C, Perez-Rodriguez, MM, Vaquero-Lorenzo, C & Baca-Garcia, E (2012) New perspectives in glutamate and anxiety. *Pharmacol Biochem Behav,* 100, 752-74.
[http://dx.doi.org/10.1016/j.pbb.2011.04.010] [PMID: 21569789]

Riedel, G, Platt, B & Micheau, J (2003) Glutamate receptor function in learning and memory. *Behav Brain Res,* 140, 1-47.
[http://dx.doi.org/10.1016/S0166-4328(02)00272-3] [PMID: 12644276]

Robert, SM & Sontheimer, H (2014) Glutamate transporters in the biology of malignant gliomas. *Cell Mol Life Sci,* 71, 1839-54.
[http://dx.doi.org/10.1007/s00018-013-1521-z] [PMID: 24281762]

Ron, D (2002) Translational control in the endoplasmic reticulum stress response. *J Clin Invest,* 110, 1383-8.
[http://dx.doi.org/10.1172/JCI0216784] [PMID: 12438433]

Ross, CA & Tabrizi, SJ (2011) Huntington's disease: from molecular pathogenesis to clinical treatment. *Lancet Neurol,* 10, 83-98.
[http://dx.doi.org/10.1016/S1474-4422(10)70245-3] [PMID: 21163446]

Rossi, DJ, Oshima, T & Attwell, D (2000) Glutamate release in severe brain ischaemia is mainly by reversed uptake. *Nature,* 403, 316-21.
[http://dx.doi.org/10.1038/35002090] [PMID: 10659851]

Rothstein, JD, Martin, LJ & Kuncl, RW (1992) Decreased glutamate transport by the brain and spinal cord in amyotrophic lateral sclerosis. *N Engl J Med,* 326, 1464-8.

[http://dx.doi.org/10.1056/NEJM199205283262204] [PMID: 1349424]

Scarr, E, Pavey, G, Sundram, S, MacKinnon, A & Dean, B (2003) Decreased hippocampal NMDA, but not kainate or AMPA receptors in bipolar disorder. *Bipolar Disord,* 5, 257-64.
[http://dx.doi.org/10.1034/j.1399-5618.2003.00024.x] [PMID: 12895203]

Schölzke, MN, Potrovita, I, Subramaniam, S, Prinz, S & Schwaninger, M (2003) Glutamate activates NF-kappaB through calpain in neurons. *Eur J Neurosci,* 18, 3305-10.
[http://dx.doi.org/10.1111/j.1460-9568.2003.03079.x] [PMID: 14686903]

Sen, P, Mukherjee, S, Ray, D & Raha, S (2003) Involvement of the Akt/PKB signaling pathway with disease processes. *Mol Cell Biochem,* 253, 241-6.
[http://dx.doi.org/10.1023/A:1026020101379] [PMID: 14619975]

Seo, JY, Kim, BR, Oh, J & Kim, JS (2018) Soybean-Derived Phytoalexins Improve Cognitive Function through Activation of Nrf2/HO-1 Signaling Pathway. *Int J Mol Sci,* 19, 19.
[http://dx.doi.org/10.3390/ijms19010268] [PMID: 29337893]

Sepers, MD & Raymond, LA (2014) Mechanisms of synaptic dysfunction and excitotoxicity in Huntington's disease. *Drug Discov Today,* 19, 990-6.
[http://dx.doi.org/10.1016/j.drudis.2014.02.006] [PMID: 24603212]

Shah, SA, Amin, FU, Khan, M, Abid, MN, Rehman, SU, Kim, TH, Kim, MW & Kim, MO (2016) Anthocyanins abrogate glutamate-induced AMPK activation, oxidative stress, neuroinflammation, and neurodegeneration in postnatal rat brain. *J Neuroinflammation,* 13, 286.
[http://dx.doi.org/10.1186/s12974-016-0752-y] [PMID: 27821173]

Shah, SA, Lee, HY, Bressan, RA, Yun, DJ & Kim, MO (2014) Novel osmotin attenuates glutamate-induced synaptic dysfunction and neurodegeneration *via* the JNK/PI3K/Akt pathway in postnatal rat brain. *Cell Death Dis,* 5e1026
[http://dx.doi.org/10.1038/cddis.2013.538] [PMID: 24481440]

Shi, R, Weng, J, Zhao, L, Li, XM, Gao, TM & Kong, J (2012) Excessive autophagy contributes to neuron death in cerebral ischemia. *CNS Neurosci Ther,* 18, 250-60.
[http://dx.doi.org/10.1111/j.1755-5949.2012.00295.x] [PMID: 22449108]

Smith, KE, Gibson, ES & Dell'Acqua, ML (2006) cAMP-dependent protein kinase postsynaptic localization regulated by NMDA receptor activation through translocation of an A-kinase anchoring protein scaffold protein. *J Neurosci,* 26, 2391-402.
[http://dx.doi.org/10.1523/JNEUROSCI.3092-05.2006] [PMID: 16510716]

Snyder, EM, Nong, Y, Almeida, CG, Paul, S, Moran, T, Choi, EY, Nairn, AC, Salter, MW, Lombroso, PJ, Gouras, GK & Greengard, P (2005) Regulation of NMDA receptor trafficking by amyloid-beta. *Nat Neurosci,* 8, 1051-8.
[http://dx.doi.org/10.1038/nn1503] [PMID: 16025111]

Son, Y, Byun, SJ & Pae, HO (2013) Involvement of heme oxygenase-1 expression in neuroprotection by piceatannol, a natural analog and a metabolite of resveratrol, against glutamate-mediated oxidative injury in HT22 neuronal cells. *Amino Acids,* 45, 393-401.
[http://dx.doi.org/10.1007/s00726-013-1518-9] [PMID: 23712764]

Song, HP, Wu, SQ, Hao, H, Chen, J, Lu, J, Xu, X, Li, P & Yang, H (2016) A chemical family-based strategy for uncovering hidden bioactive molecules and multicomponent interactions in herbal medicines. *Sci Rep,* 6, 23840.
[http://dx.doi.org/10.1038/srep23840] [PMID: 27025397]

Song, JH, Kang, KS & Choi, YK (2017) Protective effect of casuarinin against glutamate-induced apoptosis in HT22 cells through inhibition of oxidative stress-mediated MAPK phosphorylation. *Bioorg Med Chem Lett,* 27, 5109-13.
[http://dx.doi.org/10.1016/j.bmcl.2017.10.075] [PMID: 29122481]

Song, JH, Kim, SY, Hwang, GS, Kim, YS, Kim, HY & Kang, KS (2019) Sanguiin H-11 from Sanguisorbae

radix protects HT22 murine hippocampal cells against glutamate-induced death. *Bioorg Med Chem Lett,* 29, 252-6. a
[http://dx.doi.org/10.1016/j.bmcl.2018.11.042] [PMID: 30497912]

Song, JH, Lee, HJ & Kang, KS (2019) Procyanidin C1 Activates the Nrf2/HO-1 Signaling Pathway to Prevent Glutamate-Induced Apoptotic HT22 Cell Death. *Int J Mol Sci,* 20, 20. b
[http://dx.doi.org/10.3390/ijms20010142] [PMID: 30609764]

Spencer, PS, Nunn, PB, Hugon, J, Ludolph, AC, Ross, SM, Roy, DN & Robertson, RC (1987) Guam amyotrophic lateral sclerosis-parkinsonism-dementia linked to a plant excitant neurotoxin. *Science,* 237, 517-22.
[http://dx.doi.org/10.1126/science.3603037] [PMID: 3603037]

Speyer, CL, Hachem, AH, Assi, AA, Johnson, JS, DeVries, JA & Gorski, DH (2014) Metabotropic glutamate receptor-1 as a novel target for the antiangiogenic treatment of breast cancer. *PLoS One,* 9e88830
[http://dx.doi.org/10.1371/journal.pone.0088830] [PMID: 24633367]

Spoont, M (2015) JAMA PATIENT PAGE. Posttraumatic Stress Disorder (PTSD). *JAMA,* 314, 532.
[http://dx.doi.org/10.1001/jama.2015.8109] [PMID: 26241611]

Stein-Behrens, BA, Lin, WJ & Sapolsky, RM (1994) Physiological elevations of glucocorticoids potentiate glutamate accumulation in the hippocampus. *J Neurochem,* 63, 596-602.
[http://dx.doi.org/10.1046/j.1471-4159.1994.63020596.x] [PMID: 7913489]

Südhof, TC & Rothman, JE (2009) Membrane fusion: grappling with SNARE and SM proteins. *Science,* 323, 474-7.
[http://dx.doi.org/10.1126/science.1161748] [PMID: 19164740]

Sukprasansap, M, Chanvorachote, P & Tencomnao, T (2017) Cleistocalyx nervosum var. paniala berry fruit protects neurotoxicity against endoplasmic reticulum stress-induced apoptosis. *Food Chem Toxicol,* 103, 279-88.
[http://dx.doi.org/10.1016/j.fct.2017.03.025] [PMID: 28315776]

Sukprasansap, M, Chanvorachote, P & Tencomnao, T (2020) Cyanidin-3-glucoside activates Nrf2-antioxidant response element and protects against glutamate-induced oxidative and endoplasmic reticulum stress in HT22 hippocampal neuronal cells. *BMC Complement Med Ther,* 20, 46.
[http://dx.doi.org/10.1186/s12906-020-2819-7] [PMID: 32046712]

Takamori, S (2006) VGLUTs: 'exciting' times for glutamatergic research? *Neurosci Res,* 55, 343-51.
[http://dx.doi.org/10.1016/j.neures.2006.04.016] [PMID: 16765470]

Tandon, R (2013) Schizophrenia and other psychotic disorders in DSM-5. *Clin Schizophr Relat Psychoses,* 7, 16-9.
[http://dx.doi.org/10.3371/CSRP.TA.032513] [PMID: 23538289]

Tang, GH, Chen, ZW, Lin, TT, Tan, M, Gao, XY, Bao, JM, Cheng, ZB, Sun, ZH, Huang, G & Yin, S (2015) Neolignans from Aristolochia fordiana Prevent Oxidative Stress-Induced Neuronal Death through Maintaining the Nrf2/HO-1 Pathway in HT22 Cells. *J Nat Prod,* 78, 1894-903.
[http://dx.doi.org/10.1021/acs.jnatprod.5b00220] [PMID: 26226070]

Tapiero, H, Mathé, G, Couvreur, P & Tew, KD (2002) II. Glutamine and glutamate. *Biomed Pharmacother,* 56, 446-57.
[http://dx.doi.org/10.1016/S0753-3322(02)00285-8] [PMID: 12481981]

Taube, JS & Schwartzkroin, PA (1988) Mechanisms of long-term potentiation: EPSP/spike dissociation, intradendritic recordings, and glutamate sensitivity. *J Neurosci,* 8, 1632-44.
[http://dx.doi.org/10.1523/JNEUROSCI.08-05-01632.1988] [PMID: 2896764]

Tebartz van Elst, L, Maier, S, Fangmeier, T, Endres, D, Mueller, GT, Nickel, K, Ebert, D, Lange, T, Hennig, J, Biscaldi, M, Riedel, A & Perlov, E (2014) Disturbed cingulate glutamate metabolism in adults with high-functioning autism spectrum disorder: evidence in support of the excitatory/inhibitory imbalance hypothesis. *Mol Psychiatry,* 19, 1314-25.

[http://dx.doi.org/10.1038/mp.2014.62] [PMID: 25048006]

Thapar, A & Cooper, M (2016) Attention deficit hyperactivity disorder. *Lancet,* 387, 1240-50.
[http://dx.doi.org/10.1016/S0140-6736(15)00238-X] [PMID: 26386541]

Tian, X, Sui, S, Huang, J, Bai, JP, Ren, TS & Zhao, QC (2014) Neuroprotective effects of Arctium lappa L. roots against glutamate-induced oxidative stress by inhibiting phosphorylation of p38, JNK and ERK 1/2 MAPKs in PC12 cells. *Environ Toxicol Pharmacol,* 38, 189-98.
[http://dx.doi.org/10.1016/j.etap.2014.05.017] [PMID: 24956398]

Torp, R, Lekieffre, D, Levy, LM, Haug, FM, Danbolt, NC, Meldrum, BS & Ottersen, OP (1995) Reduced postischemic expression of a glial glutamate transporter, GLT1, in the rat hippocampus. *Exp Brain Res,* 103, 51-8.
[http://dx.doi.org/10.1007/BF00241964] [PMID: 7615037]

Trotman, M, Vermehren, P, Gibson, CL & Fern, R (2015) The dichotomy of memantine treatment for ischemic stroke: dose-dependent protective and detrimental effects. *J Cereb Blood Flow Metab,* 35, 230-9.
[http://dx.doi.org/10.1038/jcbfm.2014.188] [PMID: 25407270]

Vallano, A, Fernandez-Duenas, V, Garcia-Negredo, G, Quijada, MA, Simon, CP, Cuffi, ML, Carbonell, L, Sanchez, S, Arnau, JM & Ciruela, F (2013) Targeting striatal metabotropic glutamate receptor type 5 in Parkinson's disease: bridging molecular studies and clinical trials. *CNS Neurol Disord Drug Targets,* 12, 1128-42.
[PMID: 24040811]

Van Damme, P, Dewil, M, Robberecht, W & Van Den Bosch, L (2005) Excitotoxicity and amyotrophic lateral sclerosis. *Neurodegener Dis,* 2, 147-59.
[http://dx.doi.org/10.1159/000089620] [PMID: 16909020]

van Os, J & Kapur, S (2009) Schizophrenia. *Lancet,* 374, 635-45.
[http://dx.doi.org/10.1016/S0140-6736(09)60995-8] [PMID: 19700006]

Verkhratsky, A (2005) Physiology and pathophysiology of the calcium store in the endoplasmic reticulum of neurons. *Physiol Rev,* 85, 201-79.
[http://dx.doi.org/10.1152/physrev.00004.2004] [PMID: 15618481]

Volbracht, C, Chua, BT, Ng, CP, Bahr, BA, Hong, W & Li, P (2005) The critical role of calpain *versus* caspase activation in excitotoxic injury induced by nitric oxide. *J Neurochem,* 93, 1280-92.
[http://dx.doi.org/10.1111/j.1471-4159.2005.03122.x] [PMID: 15934947]

Vucic, S, Rothstein, JD & Kiernan, MC (2014) Advances in treating amyotrophic lateral sclerosis: insights from pathophysiological studies. *Trends Neurosci,* 37, 433-42.
[http://dx.doi.org/10.1016/j.tins.2014.05.006] [PMID: 24927875]

Wada, K (1998) [Epilepsy and glutamate transporters: study of mice lacking a glutamate transporter and other recent advances]. *Tanpakushitsu Kakusan Koso,* 43, 244-50.
[PMID: 9528356]

Wada, S, Yone, K, Ishidou, Y, Nagamine, T, Nakahara, S, Niiyama, T & Sakou, T (1999) Apoptosis following spinal cord injury in rats and preventative effect of N-methyl-D-aspartate receptor antagonist. *J Neurosurg,* 91 (Suppl.), 98-104.
[PMID: 10419375]

Wang, D, Guo, TQ, Wang, ZY, Lu, JH, Liu, DP, Meng, QF, Xie, J, Zhang, XL, Liu, Y & Teng, LS (2014) ERKs and mitochondria-related pathways are essential for glycyrrhizic acid-mediated neuroprotection against glutamate-induced toxicity in differentiated PC12 cells. *Braz J Med Biol Res,* 47, 773-9.
[http://dx.doi.org/10.1590/1414-431X20143760] [PMID: 25075574]

Wang, JQ, Fibuch, EE & Mao, L (2007) Regulation of mitogen-activated protein kinases by glutamate receptors. *J Neurochem,* 100, 1-11.
[http://dx.doi.org/10.1111/j.1471-4159.2006.04208.x] [PMID: 17018022]

Wen, L, Shi, D, Zhou, T, Tu, J, He, M, Jiang, Y & Yang, B (2020) Identification of two novel prenylated

flavonoids in mulberry leaf and their bioactivities. *Food Chem,* 315126236
[http://dx.doi.org/10.1016/j.foodchem.2020.126236] [PMID: 32000079]

Willard, SS & Koochekpour, S (2013) Glutamate signaling in benign and malignant disorders: current status, future perspectives, and therapeutic implications. *Int J Biol Sci,* 9, 728-42. a
[http://dx.doi.org/10.7150/ijbs.6475] [PMID: 23983606]

Willard, SS & Koochekpour, S (2013) Glutamate, glutamate receptors, and downstream signaling pathways. *Int J Biol Sci,* 9, 948-59. b
[http://dx.doi.org/10.7150/ijbs.6426] [PMID: 24155668]

Xu, D, Chen, H, Mak, S, Hu, S, Tsim, KWK, Hu, Y, Sun, Y, Zhang, G, Wang, Y, Zhang, Z & Han, Y (2016) Neuroprotection against glutamate-induced excitotoxicity and induction of neurite outgrowth by T-006, a novel multifunctional derivative of tetramethylpyrazine in neuronal cell models. *Neurochem Int,* 99, 194-205.
[http://dx.doi.org/10.1016/j.neuint.2016.07.006] [PMID: 27445088]

Xu, J, Kurup, P, Zhang, Y, Goebel-Goody, SM, Wu, PH, Hawasli, AH, Baum, ML, Bibb, JA & Lombroso, PJ (2009) Extrasynaptic NMDA receptors couple preferentially to excitotoxicity *via* calpain-mediated cleavage of STEP. *J Neurosci,* 29, 9330-43.
[http://dx.doi.org/10.1523/JNEUROSCI.2212-09.2009] [PMID: 19625523]

Xu, MF, Xiong, YY, Liu, JK, Qian, JJ, Zhu, L & Gao, J (2012) Asiatic acid, a pentacyclic triterpene in Centella asiatica, attenuates glutamate-induced cognitive deficits in mice and apoptosis in SH-SY5Y cells. *Acta Pharmacol Sin,* 33, 578-87.
[http://dx.doi.org/10.1038/aps.2012.3] [PMID: 22447225]

Yang, EJ, Kim, M, Woo, JE, Lee, T, Jung, JW & Song, KS (2016) The comparison of neuroprotective effects of isoliquiritigenin and its Phase I metabolites against glutamate-induced HT22 cell death. *Bioorg Med Chem Lett,* 26, 5639-43.
[http://dx.doi.org/10.1016/j.bmcl.2016.10.072] [PMID: 27815122]

Yang, EJ, Lee, JY, Park, SH, Lee, T & Song, KS (2013) Neuroprotective effects of neolignans isolated from Magnoliae Cortex against glutamate-induced apoptotic stimuli in HT22 cells. *Food Chem Toxicol,* 56, 304-12. a
[http://dx.doi.org/10.1016/j.fct.2013.02.035] [PMID: 23454146]

Yang, EJ, Park, GH & Song, KS (2013) Neuroprotective effects of liquiritigenin isolated from licorice roots on glutamate-induced apoptosis in hippocampal neuronal cells. *Neurotoxicology,* 39, 114-23. b
[http://dx.doi.org/10.1016/j.neuro.2013.08.012] [PMID: 24012889]

Yang, M, Xu, DD, Zhang, Y, Liu, X, Hoeven, R & Cho, WC (2014) A systematic review on natural medicines for the prevention and treatment of Alzheimer's disease with meta-analyses of intervention effect of ginkgo. *Am J Chin Med,* 42, 505-21.
[http://dx.doi.org/10.1142/S0192415X14500335] [PMID: 24871648]

Yang, Z & Klionsky, DJ (2010) Mammalian autophagy: core molecular machinery and signaling regulation. *Curr Opin Cell Biol,* 22, 124-31.
[http://dx.doi.org/10.1016/j.ceb.2009.11.014] [PMID: 20034776]

Yin, W-Y, Ye, Q, Huang, H-J, Xia, N-G, Chen, Y-Y, Zhang, Y & Qu, Q-M (2016) Salidroside protects cortical neurons against glutamate-induced cytotoxicity by inhibiting autophagy. *Mol Cell Biochem,* 419, 53-64.
[http://dx.doi.org/10.1007/s11010-016-2749-3] [PMID: 27357827]

Yu, H, Yuan, B, Chu, Q, Wang, C & Bi, H (2019) Protective roles of isoastilbin against Alzheimer's disease *via* Nrf2-mediated antioxidation and anti-apoptosis. *Int J Mol Med,* 43, 1406-16.
[http://dx.doi.org/10.3892/ijmm.2019.4058] [PMID: 30664148]

Yudkoff, M, Daikhin, Y, Nissim, I & Nissim, I (2000) Acidosis and astrocyte amino acid metabolism. *Neurochem Int,* 36, 329-39.
[http://dx.doi.org/10.1016/S0197-0186(99)00141-2] [PMID: 10733000]

Yue, R, Li, X, Chen, B, Zhao, J, He, W, Yuan, H, Yuan, X, Gao, N, Wu, G, Jin, H, Shan, L & Zhang, W (2015) Astragaloside IV Attenuates Glutamate-Induced Neurotoxicity in PC12 Cells through Raf-MEK-ERK Pathway. *PLoS One,* 10e0126603
[http://dx.doi.org/10.1371/journal.pone.0126603] [PMID: 25961569]

Zetterberg, H & Blennow, K (2015) Fluid markers of traumatic brain injury. *Mol Cell Neurosci,* 66, 99-102.
[http://dx.doi.org/10.1016/j.mcn.2015.02.003] [PMID: 25659491]

Zhang, BB, Hu, XL, Wang, YY, Li, JY, Pham, TA & Wang, H (2019) Neuroprotective Effects of Dammarane-Type Saponins from Panax notoginseng on Glutamate-Induced Cell Damage in PC12 Cells. *Planta Med,* 85, 692-700.
[PMID: 30791058]

Zhang, X, Chen, Y, Ikonomovic, MD, Nathaniel, PD, Kochanek, PM, Marion, DW, DeKosky, ST, Jenkins, LW & Clark, RS (2006) Increased phosphorylation of protein kinase B and related substrates after traumatic brain injury in humans and rats. *J Cereb Blood Flow Metab,* 26, 915-26.
[http://dx.doi.org/10.1038/sj.jcbfm.9600238] [PMID: 16234845]

Zhang, Y, Tan, F, Xu, P & Qu, S (2016) Recent Advance in the Relationship between Excitatory Amino Acid Transporters and Parkinson's Disease. *Neural Plast,* 20168941327
[http://dx.doi.org/10.1155/2016/8941327] [PMID: 26981287]

Zhang, Y, Wang, W, Hao, C, Mao, X & Zhang, L (2015) Astaxanthin protects PC12 cells from glutamate-induced neurotoxicity through multiple signaling pathways. *J Funct Foods,* 16, 137-51.
[http://dx.doi.org/10.1016/j.jff.2015.04.008]

Zhang, Z, Cui, W, Li, G, Yuan, S, Xu, D, Hoi, MP, Lin, Z, Dou, J, Han, Y & Lee, SM (2012) Baicalein protects against 6-OHDA-induced neurotoxicity through activation of Keap1/Nrf2/HO-1 and involving PKCα and PI3K/AKT signaling pathways. *J Agric Food Chem,* 60, 8171-82.
[http://dx.doi.org/10.1021/jf301511m] [PMID: 22838648]

Zhao, H, Ji, ZH, Liu, C & Yu, XY (2015) Neuroprotective Mechanisms of 9-Hydroxy Epinootkatol Against Glutamate-Induced Neuronal Apoptosis in Primary Neuron Culture. *J Mol Neurosci,* 56, 808-14.
[http://dx.doi.org/10.1007/s12031-015-0511-z] [PMID: 25854778]

BenthamBriefs in Biomedicine and Pharmacotherapy, 2021, *Vol. 1*, 397-420

CHAPTER 15

Genistein – A Natural Antioxidant and its Use in Treatment of Various Diseases

Estera Rintz[1], Lidia Gaffke[1], Karolina Pierzynowska[1], Magdalena Podlacha[1], Jagoda Mantej[1], Marta Bednarek[1], Zuzanna Cyske[1], Magdalena Bałuch[1], Patrycja Bielanska[1], Agnieszka Bilak[1], Julian Guzowski[1] and **Grzegorz Wegrzyn[*, 1]**

[1] *Department of Molecular Biology, Faculty of Biology, University of Gdansk, Wita Stwosza 59, 80-308 Gdansk, Poland*

Abstract: Genistein (5,7-dihydroxy-3-(4-hydroxyphenyl)chromen-4-one or 4',5,7-trihydroxyisoflavone) can be found in various plants, though soy is especially rich in this compound. It has multiple biological activities, but one of its major features is its antioxidative function. Either genistein-rich extracts from plants or synthetic genistein have been used in studies on the potential treatment of various conditions and diseases. They are as different as neurodegenerative diseases (including Alzheimer's disease and various genetic diseases), cancer, cardiovascular disorders, liver dysfunctions, and many others. Although for the treatment of various diseases the major mechanisms of genistein action can be based on modulation of specific biochemical pathways, its antioxidative function may contribute significantly to its therapeutic potential. These aspects are discussed in the light of development of genistein-based therapies for a battery of different disorders.

Keywords: Antioxidant, Cancer, Cardiovascular diseases, Genistein, Neurodegenerative diseases.

INTRODUCTION

Naturally occurring compounds and/or their novel derivatives are among the most intensively tested molecules in biomedical and pharmaceutical studies. For instance, from around 1940s to 2014, 49% of approved molecules for cancer treatment were either natural products or derived directly from them (Newman and Cragg 2016). Flavonoids are a class of natural compounds, with anti-oxidative and other actions in various diseases. Therefore, they are used for

---

[*] **Corresponding author Grzegorz Wegrzyn:** Department of Molecular Biology, Faculty of Biology, University of Gdansk, Wita Stwosza 59, 80-308 Gdansk, Poland; E-mail: grzegorz.wegrzyn@biol.ug.edu.pl

Pardeep Kaur, Rajendra G. Mehta, Robin, Tarunpreet Singh Thind and Saroj Arora (Eds.)

nutraceutical, medical, pharmaceutical or cosmetic applications (Panche *et al.* 2016). These substances are widely distributed in vascular plants, particularly in fruits, vegetables, seeds, nuts, grains, and spices. They contribute to attractive colors of leaves, flowers, and fruits, and play crucial roles in UV protection by rummaging reactive oxygen species (ROS), created by the photosynthetic electron transport system (Pietta 2000). Flavonoids are divided into several subgroups, including flavones, flavonols and isoflavones (Fig. **1**). All the flavonoids have the same base structure of the flavan core, while differing from each other in substituents in the aromatic carbon ring. Among the numerous classes of flavonoids, those specifically noteworthy to this review are isoflavones, in particular one of them – genistein (Fig. **2**).

Isoflavones are bioactive compounds which can be found in the members of the bean family, legumes, including soybeans, fava beans, chickpeas, and peanuts (Setchell *et al.* 2001). They occur in the form of three different types, and each kind being available in four synthetic structures. Soybean contains most of the isoflavones in forms of aglycones (genistein, daidzein, glycitein), β-glucosides, malonyl-β-glucosides, and acetyl-β-glucosides (Wang and Murphy 1994). Aglycones are the most bioavailable isoflavone forms to humans, most likely because their structure does not contain any sugars or other derivatives (Rahman Mazumder and Hongsprabhas 2016). Structures and functions of isoflavones are similar to that of 17-estradiol, the strongest mammalian estrogen, thus, they are also called phytoestrogens, revealing high levels of estrogenic activity (Boué *et al.* 2003). One of the most recognizable aglycone is genistein, having diverse biological activities. This isoflavone interacts with the estrogen receptor, significantly influencing the regulation of expression of many genes. In addition, nonhormonal mechanisms of genistein action consist of antioxidation, anti-inflammatory, and antiproliferative properties (Sarkar and Li 2002).

When different isoflavones were compared according to the level of deoxidation reactions in cell cultures, genistein enhanced inhibition of O_2^- generation more effectively than other compounds, suggesting its high antioxidant potential (Wei *et al.* 1995). Oxidative stress occurs during the generation of ROS, including superoxide (O_2^-), peroxyl (ROO·), alkoxyl (RO·), hydroxyl (HO·) radicals, and nitric oxide (NO·). Due to their high reactivity, they cause damages in cells, such as destruction of the cell membrane, DNA lesions, and inactivation of proteins.

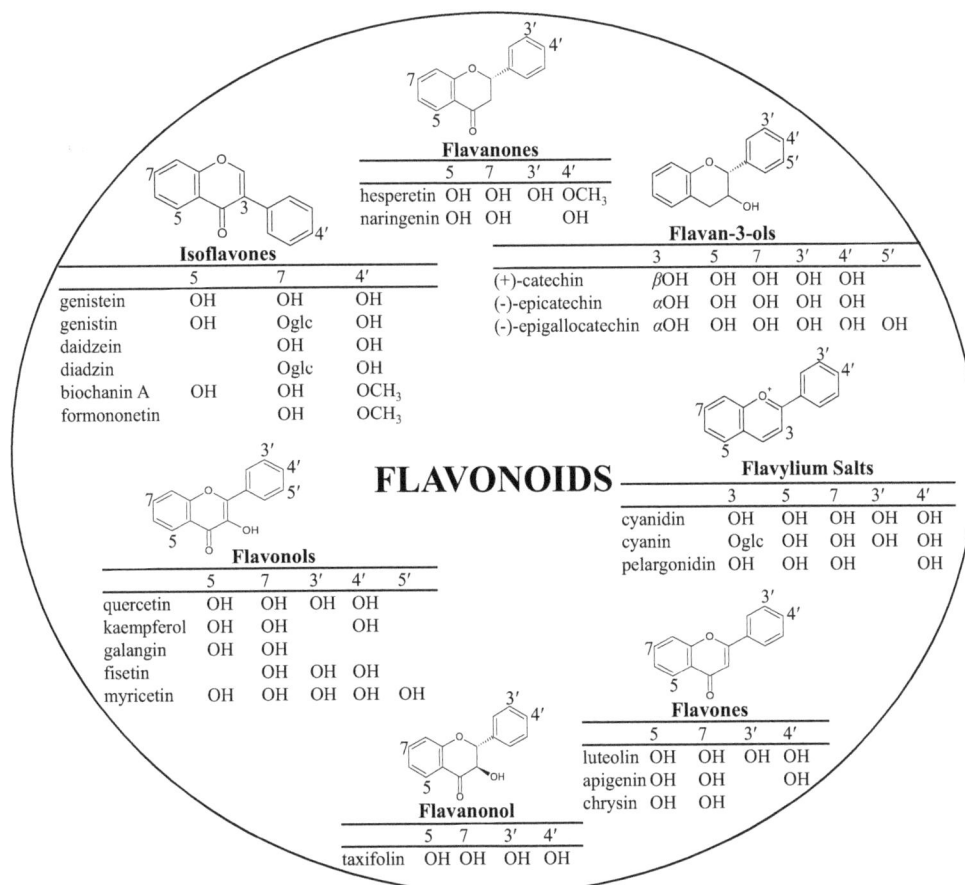

FLAVONOIDS

Flavanones

	5	7	3'	4'
hesperetin	OH	OH	OH	OCH₃
naringenin	OH	OH		OH

Flavan-3-ols

	3	5	7	3'	4'	5'
(+)-catechin	βOH	OH	OH	OH	OH	
(-)-epicatechin	αOH	OH	OH	OH	OH	
(-)-epigallocatechin	αOH	OH	OH	OH	OH	OH

Isoflavones

	5	7	4'
genistein	OH	OH	OH
genistin	OH	Oglc	OH
daidzein		OH	OH
diadzin		Oglc	OH
biochanin A	OH	OH	OCH₃
formononetin		OH	OCH₃

Flavonols

	5	7	3'	4'	5'
quercetin	OH	OH	OH	OH	
kaempferol	OH	OH		OH	
galangin	OH	OH			
fisetin		OH	OH	OH	
myricetin	OH	OH	OH	OH	OH

Flavylium Salts

	3	5	7	3'	4'
cyanidin	OH	OH	OH	OH	OH
cyanin	Oglc	OH	OH	OH	OH
pelargonidin	OH	OH	OH		OH

Flavones

	5	7	3'	4'
luteolin	OH	OH	OH	OH
apigenin	OH	OH		OH
chrysin	OH	OH		

Flavanonol

	5	7	3'	4'
taxifolin	OH	OH	OH	OH

Fig. (1). Structure of flavonoids [based on Pietta, 2000; modified].

Despite the existence of mechanisms controlling ROS, such as actions of antioxidants (tocopherols, ascorbic acid, and glutathione) or enzymes (superoxide dismutase - SOD, catalase or peroxidase), most of them are not sufficient to combat overwhelmed changes in several degenerative diseases caused by ROS (Pietta 2000, Gagné 2014). Genistein is an isoflavone with multiple antioxidant activities, and it is able to decrease levels of lipid peroxidation and ROS-mediated damages. Moreover, genistein is found to activate enzymes involved in deoxidation and to regulate the expression of antioxidation-related genes, like those coding for ERK1/2, and NF-κB (Gaur and Bhatia 2009). This review presents current knowledge on the properties of genistein, focusing on the use of this compound in the treatment of various diseases due to its antioxidative and anti-inflammatory activities.

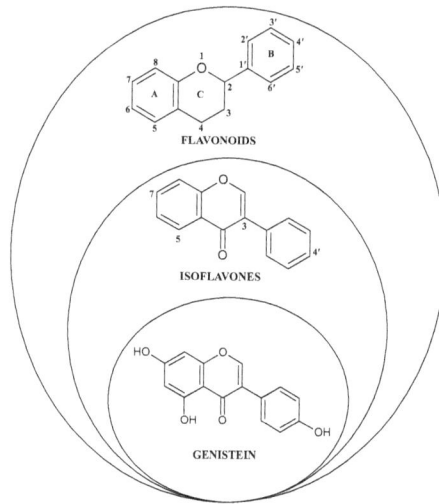

Fig. (2). Genistein classification.

USE OF GENISTEIN IN TREATMENT OF DISEASES

Neurodegenerative Diseases

There are thousands of neurodegenerative diseases for which no effective therapies are available. Among them, there are both rare genetic diseases or more commonly occurring disorders of the central nervous system (CNS).

According to data provided by the World Health Organization (WHO), nearly 44 million people currently suffer from Alzheimer's disease (AD) worldwide, with 7.7 million people annually. It is estimated that as many as 115 million people will suffer from AD in 2050. This disease is a neurodegenerative condition, which in the first stages manifests by short-term memory disorders and problems with orientation in new places. However, it is a progressive disorder, with time language deficits, aggression, lack of control over physiological functions appear, and the patient requires constant care (Devi *et al.* 2017). AD is the most common disorder related to dementia, it gradually leads to the exclusion of the patient from normal functioning in society, which is why it is so important to know as soon as possible all the factors leading to the formation of this disorder and to implement effective treatment already in the first stages of the disease.

Antioxidant properties of genistein (Jeon *et al.* 2014, Bingham *et al.* 1998) have been proposed to be useful in treatment of AD, and the first experiments were conducted using the mouse model (Ding *et al.* 2013). The results indicated that this isoflavone maintained the potential of the mitochondrial membrane, changed the glutathione/oxidized glutathione ratio and increased the level of glutathione peroxidase. In addition, increased production of manganese superoxide dismutase (mitochondria and brain) and downregulation of Nrf2 and HO-1 in the brain tissue were observed. In general, genistein can affect oxidative damage and can lead to preserving redox imbalance in the brain, and especially in mitochondria damaged by Aβ1-42. This may be due to the regulation of the Nrf2 / HO-1 pathway (Ding *et al.* 2013).

Low levels of acetylcholine and oxidative damage are one of the key players in pathogenesis of AD. Acetylcholine, a major neurotransmitter in the brain, is important for learning, memory, cognition and consciousness (Craig *et al.* 2011). Recently, one of the largely exploited therapeutic approaches in AD treatment involves the enhancement of the cholinergic neurotransmission by inhibiting cholinesterase (ChE) (Doody *et al.* 2001, Devi *et al.* 2017). It was demonstrated that genistein-O-alkylamine derivatives had significant acetylcholinesterase (AChE) inhibitory activity (Hong *et al.* 2019). After synthesis of a series of different compounds, antioxidant activity was determined by using the oxygen radical absorbance capacity-fluorescein assay, and multifunctional, nontoxic drug was suggested as a suitable candidate for the treatment of AD (Masliah *et al.* 1995).

Another important therapeutic target involved in cholesterol metabolism is apolipoprotein E (ApoE), the major apolipoprotein released by astrocytes and microglia. It participates in the transport of cholesterol between glial cells and neurons. Oxidative stress and the accompanying inflammation characteristic for ApoE$^{-/-}$ mice can promote the development of neurodegeneration. Despite the fact that ApoE$^{-/-}$ mice developed normally initially, in the fourth month of their life, dendritic changes appear (Park *et al.* 2016). The effect of neuroprotection in the cortex and hippocampus due to genistein supplementation in the diet (at a dose of 0.5 g/kg diet) of wild C57BL/6 (WT) and knockout ApoE (ApoE$^{-/-}$) mice which were fed high-fat diet for 24 weeks were investigated. As a result of supplementation, oxidative stress and neurological inflammation were suppressed in ApoE$^{-/-}$ mice (Park *et al.* 2016). Genistein influenced the formation of Aβ by reducing the production of APP processing enzymes (BACE1 and PS1) and by decreasing the level of hyperphosphorylated form of tau protein. This result from the inactivation of GSK-3β and JNK in the hippocampus and cortex (Park *et al.* 2016).

It is believed that oxidative stress, an imbalance between free radical generation and elimination, is involved in AD pathogenesis by disturbing mitochondrial functions, the pro-oxidant role of amyloid- (A) peptide, and redox active transition metals (Kairane *et al.* 2014). Several clinical studies indicate that estrogen therapy may have beneficial effects on the risk and symptoms of AD, and positive therapeutic effects result from reducing amyloid-mediated toxicity (Kim *et al.* 2001). Genistein increased Na,K-ATPase activity (otherwise impaired in AD) in the frontal cortex of the patients' brains, to the level almost for normal aging brain (Kairane *et al.* 2014). It was speculated that genistein, acting as an antioxidant, may change redox balance back towards the reduced state and help to up-regulate activity of Na,K-ATPase. This property would make it attractive substance to suppress the pathogenesis of AD (Kairane *et al.* 2014). Indirect evidence shows that estrogenic compounds (estradiol or phytoestrogens, such as genistein) may increase the expression of genes coding for antioxidant enzymes, leading to reduction of oxidative stress. This creates a possibility of using genistein to prevent the onset of AD (Viña *et al.* 2007). Recent studies have shown that an extremly high dose of genistein (150 mg/kg/day) can lead to the induction of the autophagy process in the rat model of sporadic streptozotocin-induced AD. Degradation of β-amyloid and hyperphosphorylated tau protein in the brain has been observed, while cell culture experiments have confirmed that it was indeed autophagy induction. What is more, the behavior of AD rats after genistein treatment was indistinguishable from healthy animals (Pierzynowska *et al.* 2019b). More detailed studies are required to determine whether this phytoestrogen fulfill also antioxidant-influence theory in this AD model.

Studies on the use of antioxidants as potential drugs for Huntington's disease (HD) have been reported. In experimental studies with animal models of HD, various compounds were tested, including co-enzyme Q10, l-carnitine, selenium, creatine, lipoic acid, pyruvate, vitamin E (Johri *et al.* 2012). However, genistein appeared to be particularly effective in the 3-nitropropionic acid (3-NPA)-induced HD rat model. Following 3-NPA injection into the brain, neurodegeneration occurs due to disturbed mitochondrial metabolism which result in reactive oxygen species release, disturbance of cellular energetics, and induction of apoptotic pathways. These disturbances cause symptoms that partially mimic those of the disease in humans. Genistein-treated rats with HD-like symptoms, induced with 3-NPA, had decreased levels of reactive oxygen species in the brain, expressed improved movement, and improved cognitive abilities (Menze *et al.* 2015, Menze *et al.* 2016). On the other hand, recent studies on the cellular models of HD, in which mutant huntingtin accumulated, indicated that genistein can effectively reduce level of such abnormal protein by stimulating the autophagy process (Pierzynowska *et al.* 2018, Pierzynowska *et al.* 2019a).

Parkinson's disease (PD) is another disease in which the antioxidant properties of genistein have been tested. PD is a neurodegenerative disorder that is characterised by progressive loss of neurons or their functions in the substantia nigra. Observed symptoms of this disease include resting tremor, distinctive posture, paralysis, reduced muscle strength, and their progression over time in characteristic for PD. Since genistein was found to scavenge oxygen-derived free radicals, this feature was linked with results showing that neurodegenetive disorders are accompanied with oxidative stress, and antioxidant effects of genistein on PD were studied using a fly model. It was found that genistein acted as an inhibitor of monoamine oxidase (MAO), reduced oxidative stress markers, increased dopamine content and increased the life span of PD flies. In addion, a delay in the loss of climbing ability in PD flies was evident (Siddique *et al.* 2018).

It was reported that genistein may inhibit microglial activation and consequently attenuate lipopolysaccharide-induced injury in dopaminergic neurons, limiting the production of nitric oxide and superoxide in cell cultures. Dose-dependent protection properties of genistein were observed, including abolition of LPS-induced neurotoxicity, microglial activation and proinflamatory factor release. Pretreatment of genistein (at 2.5 μM) significantly decreased production of nitricoxide (NO) and superoxide in LPS-treated cells. The obtained results indicated neuroprotective effect of genistein against oxidative insult on dopaminergic neurons, while no significant toxicity for primary cells have been shown (Wang *et al.* 2005).

An *in vitro* PD model study on rotenone-induced human cell death in SH-SY5Y cells overexpressing the mutated A53T α-synuclein were performed. Rotenone is a metabolite of dopamine, which produces peroxides and hydroxyl radicals that cause DNA oxidation and lipid peroxidation, leading to oxidative stress in mitochondria. In this model, genistein inhibited the death of cells by preventing the formation of oxidative stress in mitochondria. Incubation of genistein with rotenone for 24 h before treatment caused protection against apoptosis. Therefore, it was proposed that genistein is a promising drug for the treatment of PD against the anti-apoptotic effect caused by rotenone in the SH-SY5Y cell line (Wu *et al.* 2018).

Cancer

According to epidemiological evidence proved in many studies the consumption of soybeans in Asia is connected with lower risk of esophageal, breast and colorectal cancer (Recor *et al.* 1995, Morito *et al.* 2001). Genistein and other isoflavones are known as inhibitors of angiogenesis which can inhibit the unrestricted growth of cancer cells, most probably by restraining the activity of the substances which are responsible for cell survival (growth factors) and cell division. Numerous studies have revealed that genistein administration in moderate doses has an inhibitory effect on prostate cancer (Ye Won 2009), cervical cancer (Su-Hyeon 2009), brain cancer (Arabinda *et al.* 2009), breast cancer (Keiko *et al.* 2001, Takako *et al.* 2002, de Lemos 2001) and colon cancer.

Genistein has also been proven to sensitize some cells to radiation even though the timing of the use of phytoestrogen is also crucial (de Assis *et al.* 2006).

The major mechanism of action of the isoflavone genistein is inhibiton of tyrosine kinase. These kinases are less frequent than their Ser/Thr counterparts, but they take part in growth of almost all cells and in cascades of proliferation signals. Inhibition of DNA topoisomerase II is crucial in the cytotoxic activity of genistein too (Markovits *et al.* 1989, López-Lázaro *et al.* 2007). The study shows that the transition of normal lymphocytes from the resting (G0) phase to the G1 phase of the cell cycle is especially receptive to genistein. This fact prompted the scientists to consider isoflavone as a potentially immunosuppressive substance (Traganos 1992).

Studies on rodents have shown that genistein is effective in treating leukemia and it can be used in consolidation with some different anti-leukemic drugs to improve their effectiveness (Raynal *et al.* 2008). It is believed that soybeans are able to suppress mammary tumors in rodents (Barnes *et al.* 1990), and dietary meals based on toasted soybean could decrease activity of omithine decarboxylase and increase the activity of three substances: glutathione transferase, catalase, and protein kinase C. All the changes have positive effect regarding cancer chemo-prevention (Webb *et al.* 1992). Foti *et al.* (2005) made a comparison of protective effects of genistein and daidzein in a cell model (Jurkat T-cell and peripheral blood lymphocytes) administrated with hydrogen peroxide. In the two occurrences a decrease in malonaldehyde (MDA) production was noticed. These findings seem to assure that genistein is as efficient as daidzein in defending cells against oxidative damage, especially regarding the DNA structure. The experiment on mice suffering from L1210 leukemia have proved that genistein is effective in leukemia treatment and that it could be administered in consolidation with some other anti-leukemic medicines to increase their efficiency. These conclusions indicate that genistein may be potentially useful in increasing the clinical efficacy of 5-AZA-CdR during leukemia treatment (Raynal 2008).

Female Sprague-Dawley (SD) rats were given genistein s.c. or with the vehicle, dimethylsulfoxide (DMSO) postpartum. The animals which were administered genistein neonatally as compared to DMSO had reinforced latency and lowered the occurrence and multiplicity of DMBA-induced mammary adenocarcinomas (Coral *et al.* 1995). It is believed that genistein treatment neonatally expends its chemo-prevention action by acting straightly to reinforce maturation of terminal ductal structures and by modifying the endocrine system so that it lowers cell proliferation in the mammary gland (Coral *et al.* 1995). Different experiments proved that mammary tumors in rodents could be blocked by soybeans (Barnes *et al.* 1990).

Many studies assessed the results of genistein on the development of breast cancer (Constantinou *et al.* 1990, Barnes *et al.* 1990, Buckley *et al.* 1993). Reduction of cell proliferation and the reduction of the growth of a wide range of cultured cells such as leukemia, breast and prostate cancer, and lymphoma were presented. Genistein has also been proved to reduce the growth of MDA-MB-231 breast cancer cells and the inhibition has been dose- dependent.

Rao *et al.* (Rao 1997) presented the results of genistein on azoxymethane-induced (AOM) colon carcinogenesis and its modulatory effectiveness on levels of 8-isoprostane, cyclooxygenase (COX) and 15-hydroxyprostaglandin F2α dehydrogenase (15-PGDH) activity in colorectal mucosa and male colon F34 tumors. Genistein administration significantly increased non-invasive and total colon adenocarcinoma, but this did not affect the occurrence of colorectal adenocarcinoma or the incidence of invasive adenocarcinoma. In addition, genistein significantly inhibited activity of 15-PGDH and the levels of 8-is--prostane in the colon mucosa and tumors. On the contrary genistein had no valid effect on activity of synthetic COX as it was measured by the amount of prostaglandin and thromboxane B2 formed from arachidonic acid. These observations imply that biological effect of genistein may be organ specific, reducing the development of cancer in some organs, but showing no or even tumor enhancing effect in other places.

It was also demonstrated that the genistein-topotecan combination was potentially effective in LNCaP prostate cancer cells (Hormann *et al.* 2008). LNCaP cells were treated with changeable concentrations of genistein, topotecan and genistein-topotecan combination. Cellular death in LNCaP cells was noticed after using both genistein and topotecan, however genistein-topotecan combination was significantly more effective than either genistein or topotecan alone (Hormann *et al.* 2008).

Park *et al.* (2010) made an investigation on effectiveness of genistein soy isoflavone on antioxidant enzymes present in DU145 prostate cancer cells. Genistein essentially decreased the levels of reactive oxygen species and encouraged the expression of antioxidant enzymes such as manganese superoxide dismutase (MnSOD) and catalase, the enzymes which were connected with AMP activated protein kinase (AMPK) and phosphatase. Activated expression of catalase, MnSOD and PTEN was diminished by pretreatment with a pharmacological inhibitor of AMPK, showing that the effectiveness of genistein depends principally on AMPK. Additionally, PTEN was proven to be essential for genistein to function showing that this substance activates antioxidant enzymes through the activation of AMPK and raised expression of PTEN (Park *et al.* 2010).

Autoimmunological Diseases

The antioxidant properties of genistein have been confirmed in both *in vitro* and *in vivo* experiments, as well as in human studies, and suggest its potential use in autoimmunological diseases (Zhang *et al.* 2015). In fact, this phytoestrogen also limits the development of inflammation, which manifests in inhibiting the secretion of pro-inflammatory cytokines, as well as reactive forms of oxygen and nitrogen (Valsecchi *et al.* 2008).

Genistein has a significant number of effects on immune system cells. One of the described examples include intestinal epithelial cells, which are the first to contact with active isoflavone molecules. The malfunctions in the structure of tight-junctions which they are a part of, result in the development of inflammatory disorders, such as Crohn's disease and food allergies. Genistein has been shown to inhibit TNF-α – induced IL-8 production in this type of cell line. Another type of cells that express receptors for estrogens, are dendritic cells. Genistein can regulate their function and downregulate the expression of IL-6, which is dependent on TLR-signaling in autologous monocyte-derived dendritic cells. In addition, genistein inhibits MHC class II molecules activity, and affects p53 protein, which in turn suppress NF-κB gene expression. Many *in vitro* studies have confirmed that this isoflavone also limits the activity of macrophages by inhibiting the ROS and granular release. In turn, in activated mouse macrophages and human chondrocytes, its ability to inhibit cyclooxygenase COX-2 and thus block the release of prostaglandins, was observed. Other *in vitro* studies with J774 and RAW 264.7 macrophages, showed that genistein modulates the NF-κB–signaling pathway and as a result inhibited iNOS enzymatic activity (Masilamani *et al.* 2012). The mechanism by which genistein inhibits the aggregation of human platelets remains unclear. The most likely pathway seems to be the modification of phosphodiesterase activity. The anti-aggregatory effects of flavonoids may also be related to release of H_2O_2, which acts as a secondary messenger in platelets, while increasing the activity of phospholipase C and arachidonic acid. One of the factors taken into account as responsible for platelet aggregation and thrombosis, are production of free radicals, like NO. Genistein scavenges these free radicals. Therefore, the antioxidant properties of genistein are beyond doubt, and thus may be one of the mechanisms responsible for the broad spectrum of its impact on the immune system (Gottstein *et al.* 2003).

The interest of researchers in genistein as an exogenous estrogen is growing not only in the context of hormonal disorders, but also in inflammatory diseases. Ovariectomized mice are used to mimic a decline in estrogen levels in women. Estrogen deficiency leads to a number of changes in the immune system, such as CD28 or T cells deficits. The use of genistein in the ovariectomized mouse model resulted in suppression of humoral and cellular immunity, induction of thymic atrophy and decreation of thymocytes number. It was also demonstrated that genistein limited T cell proliferation and serum IgG1, but did not affect antigen presentation function of splenic CD11c+DCs (Masilamani *et al.* 2012).

Oxidative stress is one of the factors causing the deterioration of the patients affected with rheumatoid arthritis (RA). It is an autoimmune disease (MacGregor *et al.* 2000), with chronic inflammation leading to cartilage, bone and joint injuries, which ultimately makes it difficult or impossible to move (Shah *et al.* 2011). The current therapies are based on the search for high efficacy, less toxicity and antioxidant compounds (Cerhan *et al.* 2003). Genistein could be a new potential candidate for RA treatment. This isoflavone inhibited NF-κB activation and protected cells against ROS (Ruiz-Larrea *et al.* 1997). Small doses of genistein treatment could lead to activated proteins involved in antioxidative processes *in vitro*. In addition, this isoflavone increased expression of suppressor genes PTEN. This compound has also capability to activate several molecules involved in cell signaling, such as endothelial NO synthase (Park *et al.* 2010, Zhang *et al.* 2012). The use of a diet rich in genistein reduced the risk of collagen-induced arthritis and inhibited production of Th1 cytokines from splenocytes in Sprague-Dawley rats (MacGregor *et al.* 2000).

Another important property of genistein is the ability to modulate the activity of enzymes involved in glucose metabolism, which reduces the risk of type-1 insulin–dependent diabetes in mouse model. The main symptom of the diabetes mellitus is the chronic high glucose level (Wild *et al.* 2004). Disorders in body's sugar administration lead to many other diseases including retinopathy, nephropathy and neuropathy. Hyperglycemia is a state that involves a number of adverse changes in the organism, like the intensification of oxidative stress by NAD(P)H oxidase, the infiltration of macrophages and the release of ROS (Sasser *et al.* 2007). In addition, infiltration leads to over production of pro-inflammatory cytokines, such as TGF-β, TNF-α (Wada *et al.* 2000, Chow *et al.* 2004, Tesch 2010). Genistein has anti-inflammatory effects, which lead to reduced levels of MCP-1 excretion and ICAM-1 protein expression in diabetic mice. Significantly reduced level of TBARs (index of oxidative stress) and renal NAD(P)H oxidase subunit gp91phox expression were observed in genistein-treated diabetic mice. In the light of its anti-inflammatory and antioxidant properties, genistein is a reno-protective compound (Elmarakby *et al.* 2011). Genistein also alleviates peripheral neuropathy in a streptozotocin model of diabetic mice (Valsecchi *et al.* 2011). Administration of genistein led to reduced levels of pro-inflammatory cytokine and ROS over production. In addition, it restored the content of the nerve growth factor (NGF), glutathione (GSH) and the ratio of reduced to oxidized glutathione (GSH/GSSG). In the same model, the increased activity of antioxidant enzymes and decreased levels of ROS and lipoperoxide levels in brain and liver tissues, were noticed. Administration of genistein to mice resulted in restoration of iNOS and eNOS contents and SOD activity in the thoracic aorta (Valsecchi *et al.* 2011).

Genistein has promising therapeutic properties in experimental auto-immune encephalomyelitis (EAE) in a mouse model of multiple sclerosis (Masilamani *et al.* 2012). Subcutaneous injection of this isoflavone (200 mg/kg body weight) modulates activity of glycoprotein 35-55 peptide, which plays an important role in the progression of this disease. Beneficial properties of genistein are observed not only at molecular level, inhibiting the activity of enzymes utilizing ATP but also at the cellular level inducing apoptosis and inhibiting cell proliferation, suppressing osteoclast and lymphocyte properties. Genistein treatment significantly decreased the level of pro-inflammatory cytokines, such as IFN-γ and IL-12 in CNS. Moreover, the production of IFN-γ has been reduced in ConA-driven splenocytes. IFN-γ activates microglia to act as effector cells that damage CNS cells through phagocytosis and the release of cytotoxic factors including glutamate, NO, peroxide and pro-inflammatory cytokines (De Paula *et al.* 2008). In turn, Castro *et al.* (2012) observed the beneficial effects of the genistein analogue named 7-O-tetradecanoyl-genistein (TDG) in relieving symptoms of EAE. In TDG and genistein-treated groups, a decrease in the number of cells producing IL-17 has been observed. IL-17 acts through the formation of ROS, which inhibits the activity of tight junction proteins and activates endothelial contractile machinery. Animals treated with TDG showed a delayed onset of the disease, lowered maximum severity results, improved histological changes and early recovery.

Genistein could possess protective actions against other chronic autoimmune diseases besides those mentioned above. One of them is psoriasis, which is a chronic autoimmune skin disease. The characteristic symptoms such as erythematous plaques is caused by multifactorial diseases including extensive inflammation which leads to oxidative stress. Genistein reduced oxidative stress in *in vitro* model of psoriasis (Jurzak and Adamczyk 2013, Smolińska *et al.* 2018).

Another important example is Hashimoto thyroiditis (HT). Chronic lymphocytic thyroiditis or HT is an autoimmune disease, characterized by T and B cells infiltrating to the thyroid gland, and humoral immune response for TPO, Tg-antibody production. Growing evidence suggests that excessive iodine intake attenuates antioxidant reactions in experimental models. Several lines of evidence suggest that oxidative stress is significantly elevated in hypothyroid patients with positive antithyroperoxidase antibody (TPO-Ab) (Rostami *et al.* 2013). Zhang *et al.* (2015) demonstrated that genistein-treated patients had significantly increased

T4, FT4 levels, as well as reduction in serum TSH, TPO-Ab and TgAb levels. The genistein administration was not only effective, but also safe in HT patients. The most likely positive and well-tolerated effects of genistein observed in patients were mediated by regulating the function of Th1 cells.

Another important issue that cannot be overlooked is organ transplantation. The immunological suppression mediated by isoflavones has been found to be beneficial for organ transplant recipients as a high isoflavone diet or intravenous injection of genistein improves cardiac transplantation survival in Lewis rats (Masilamani *et al.* 2012). Similarly, intraperitoneal genistein injection reduced the number of activated macrophages infiltrating the transplanted aorta. Soy protein diets containing isoflavones improved endothelial function in renal transplant patients, whose deterioration is considered a cardiovascular risk factor connected with transplantation (Masilamani *et al.* 2012).

Cardiovascular Diseases

Potential therapeutic effects of genistein in cardiovascular diseases have been suggested relatively long ago (Park *et al.* 2005). It was speculated that genistein may cause a decrease in the cholesterol level with beneficial effects on blood circulation. Hypotheses that such activity of this isoflavone may arise from antioxidant properties, tyrosine kinase inhibition or improved vascular reactivity have been presented (Park *et al.* 2005). However, doubts about the efficacy of the use of isoflavones in treatment of cardiovascular diseases have been expressed at the beginning of 21st century (Park *et al.* 2005). These doubts were corroborated by studies on effect of genistein on the progression and composition of atherosclerotic lesions in the innominate arteries of *apoE$^{-/-}$* mice, as no significant differences in plasma cholesterol, body weight, and average lesion were observed in treated and untreated animals (Averill *et al.* 2009).

Despite the above mentioned doubts, early studies indicated that genistein may cause restoration of nitric oxide-mediated relaxation in chronically hypoxic rat pulmonary arteries (Karamsetty *et al.* 2001). Further studies confirmed beneficial effects of genistein in patients with coronary heart disease (Cruz *et al.* 2008). Moreover, subsequent experimental studies indicated that genistein caused salutary effects on isoproterenol-induced cardiac hypertrophy in rats. This isoflavone prevented increase in heart weight to body weight ratio, left ventricular mass, myocardial 1-OH proline, fibrosis, myocyte size and myocardial oxidative stress, apparently due to inhibition of activity of inducible nitric oxide synthase (Maulik *et al.* 2012). Furthermore, the use of genistein-rich diet in experiments with rats resulted in increased activities of antioxidant enzymes and nitrite/nitrate content, as well as mitigation of increased lipid peroxidation in animals subjected to myocardial infarction (Hagen *et al.* 2012). Therefore, isoflavone-mediated prevention of oxidative stress-related cardiovascular diseases could be suggested. Finally, recent studies indicated that genistein may ameliorate ischemic cardiomyopathy by improving antioxidant capacities through upregulation of Nrf2 activity (Li and Zhang 2017).

Liver Diseases

The antioxidant activity of genistein has also been tested in liver diseases. Studies performed in rats with liver fibrosis induced by carbon tetrachloride (CCl_4) indicated that genistein significantly reduced liver fibrosis and necrosis. In addition to the positive effect of genistein on the tissue's oxidative profile, a significant, negative effect on the level of inflammatory markers was also noted (Demiroren *et al.* 2014). This isoflavone was also tested against fatty liver disease for high fructose-fed rat (model of insulin resistance). It turned out that administration of genistein to rats prevented lipid accumulation as well as liver damage. It was observed that genistein (in addition to anti-inflammatory activity) prevented liver oxidative damage by activating the antioxidant profile, which leads to a significant decrease in fatty liver (Mohamed Salih *et al.* 2009).

Non-alcoholic fatty steatohepatitis (NASH) is another disease in which the antioxidant properties of this isoflavone have been tested. Studies on the rat model of this disease have shown that markers of oxidative stress (malondialdehyde) in liver were significantly reduced in the group of rats treated with genistein relative to control groups. Significantly lower steatosis, inflammatory cells and ballooning degeneration in liver were also reported as effects of genistein treatment (Yalniz *et al.* 2007).

Liver damage can also be caused by excessive alcohol consumption, which is now one of major global health problems. Studies on the use of genistein in alcoholic liver disease (ALD) on a mouse model have shown that genistein, compared to other flavonoids, was characterized by the greatest activity in alleviating liver fibrosis caused by alcohol. At the biochemical level, the authors pointed to the inhibition of lipid peroxidation, and thus the improvement of oxidative status in liver by genistein (Zhao *et al.* 2018). These phenomena (reduction of lipid peroxidation, activation of the antioxidant systems, reduction of liver fibrosis along with improvement of its function) were observed also in combination therapy of genistein with taurine and epigallocatechin gallate in rat liver fibrosis model induced by alcohol (Zhuo *et al.* 2012).

Other Diseases

Research on the use of genistein in assisting the treatment of the singlet oxygen-induced cerebral stroke is the first in a series of studies conducted on the use of this isoflavone in brain diseases. These studies indicated that cerebral stroke treatment of mice with genistein reduced cerebral lesion compared to control mice (Trieu *et al.* 1999). Sudden or progressive brain disease is another of a series of diseases for which the antioxidant properties of genistein have been tested. Studies conducted on scopolamine-induced amnesia in mice have shown that genistein significantly improved memory and that this phenomenon is based on both protection against the oxidative stress damage in the hippocampus and improvement of cholinergic neurotransmission (Lu *et al.* 2018). Oxidative stress is also considered one of the important aspects of cerebral ischemia. In a male rat model, with transient global cerebral ischemia induced *via* temporarily occluding four vessels, treatment of this isoflavone reduced the levels of reactive oxygen species and ischemia-induced apoptotic neuronal death within the hippocampus of rats (Liang *et al.* 2008). Similar studies were performed on the mouse model of cerebral ischemia induced by transient occlusion of the central cerebral artery. In these experiments, reduced levels of reactive oxygen species in the brains of mice were also observed, along with enhanced activity of antioxidant enzyme superoxide dismutase, and the reversal of mitochondrial dysfunction, which prevented cytochrome c from flowing out of mitochondria and prevented programmed nerve cell death (Qian *et al.* 2012).

Diabetes is another example of a disease in which genistein could potentially be helpful. Oxidative stress is one of the symptoms accompanying diabetes and hence the hypothesis regarding the beneficial effect of genistein in this disease was proposed. Studies conducted in diabetic mice indicated that genistein reduced the level of reactive oxygen species and lipo-peroxide and increased the activity of antioxidant enzymes in the brain and liver of mice in addition to alleviating diabetic peripheral painful neuropathy and inflammation (Valsecchi *et al.* 2011). This isoflavone was also tested in the diabetes associated cognitive decline (DACD) model. The DACD refers to patients with type 2 diabetes characterized by cognitive impairment. The symptoms observed in these patients, such as decline in cognitive function, weak episodic memory, cognitive inflexibility and poor psycho-motoric activity, make this disease to resemble Alzheimer's disease. Genistein studies were performed on a mouse model of this disease induced by streptozotocin. Decreased hyperglycemia and significant cognitive improvement, and at the molecular level reduced oxidative stress, inflammation and increased acetylcholinesterase activity were observed in genistein-treated mice (Rajput and Sarkar 2017).

Nephrotic syndrome is one of chronic diseases accompanied by severe oxidative stress. Studies on the influence of soy protein and genistein on the oxidative profile were conducted on the nephrotic rat model. Results indicated significantly increased total antioxidant capacity and catalase activity in the group of rats that were fed with genistein and soy protein. In addition, results of renal histology showed significant improvement in this group of animals (Javanbakht *et al.* 2014).

Interesting studies have been conducted on the antioxidant effects of genistein and another flavonoid, equol, on sperm DNA integrity. Oxidative damage in sperm was induced by hydrogen peroxide. The results indicated that genistein significantly protected sperm DNA from oxidative damage and it was the strongest antioxidant from the tested groups of compounds (equol, ascorbic acid, and alpha-tocopherol). In addition, given in combination with equol, genistein was more protective than when these two compounds were added separately (Sierens *et al.* 2002).

Genistein antioxidant activity was also tested in lipopolysaccharide-induced periodontitis (injected to the distal part of the gums) mice model. Such studies were also carried out *in vitro* on human gingival fibroblasts (hGFs) and RAW 264.7 macrophages models. The results of studies on cell cultures showed that stimulation of hGFs *via* lipopolysaccharide significantly reduced mitochondrial activity, whereas in the presence of genistein this activity was restored to a level similar to the control. In addition to the antioxidant property, this study also examined the anti-inflammatory properties, which were confirmed. A genistein-mediated periodontitis mouse-model study showed a marked improvement in the gums' condition, reduction of alveolar bone loss and periodontal tissue degradation along with inhibition of gingivitis (Bhattarai *et al.* 2017).

CONCLUDING REMARKS

Genistein has various biological activities, including antioxidative functions, which can be employed in development of therapies for many different diseases. These include neurodegenerative diseases, cancer, cardiovascular disorders, liver dysfunctions, and many others. Although for treatment of various diseases the major mechanisms of genistein action can be based on modulation of specific biochemical pathways, its antioxidative function may contribute significantly to its therapeutic potential.

CONFLICT OF INTEREST

The authors declare no conflict of interest.

ACKNOWLEDGEMENT

None Declared

CONSENT FOR PUBLICATION

None

REFERENCES

Averill, MM, Bennett, BJ, Rattazzi, M, Rodmyre, RM, Kirk, EA, Schwartz, SM & Rosenfeld, ME (2009) Neither antioxidants nor genistein inhibit the progression of established atherosclerotic lesions in older apoE deficient mice. *Atherosclerosis,* 203, 82-8.
[http://dx.doi.org/10.1016/j.atherosclerosis.2008.06.017] [PMID: 18667203]

Barnes, S, Grubbs, C, Setchell, KD & Carlson, J (1990) Soybeans inhibit mammary tumors in models of breast cancer. *Prog Clin Biol Res,* 347, 239-53.
[PMID: 2217394]

Bhattarai, G, Poudel, SB, Kook, SH & Lee, JC (2017) Anti-inflammatory, anti-osteoclastic, and antioxidant activities of genistein protect against alveolar bone loss and periodontal tissue degradation in a mouse model of periodontitis. *J Biomed Mater Res A,* 105, 2510-21.
[http://dx.doi.org/10.1002/jbm.a.36109] [PMID: 28509410]

Bingham, SA, Atkinson, C, Liggins, J, Bluck, L & Coward, A (1998) Phyto-oestrogens: where are we now?
Br J Nutr, 79, 393-406.
[http://dx.doi.org/10.1079/BJN19980068] [PMID: 9682657]

Boué, SM, Wiese, TE, Nehls, S, Burow, ME, Elliott, S, Carter-Wientjes, CH, Shih, BY, McLachlan, JA & Cleveland, TE (2003) Evaluation of the estrogenic effects of legume extracts containing phytoestrogens. *J Agric Food Chem,* 51, 2193-9.
[http://dx.doi.org/10.1021/jf021114s] [PMID: 12670155]

Castro, SB, Junior, CO, Alves, CC, Dias, AT, Alves, LL, Mazzoccoli, L, Mesquita, FP, Figueiredo, NS, Juliano, MA, Castañon, MC, Gameiro, J, Almeida, MV, Teixeira, HC & Ferreira, AP (2012) Immunomodulatory effects and improved prognosis of experimental autoimmune encephalomyelitis after O-tetradecanoyl-genistein treatment. *Int Immunopharmacol,* 12, 465-70.
[http://dx.doi.org/10.1016/j.intimp.2011.12.025] [PMID: 22245971]

Cerhan, JR, Saag, KG, Merlino, LA, Mikuls, TR & Criswell, LA (2003) Antioxidant micronutrients and risk of rheumatoid arthritis in a cohort of older women. *Am J Epidemiol,* 157, 345-54.
[http://dx.doi.org/10.1093/aje/kwf205] [PMID: 12578805]

Chow, F, Ozols, E, Nikolic-Paterson, DJ, Atkins, RC & Tesch, GH (2004) Macrophages in mouse type 2 diabetic nephropathy: correlation with diabetic state and progressive renal injury. *Kidney Int,* 65, 116-28.
[http://dx.doi.org/10.1111/j.1523-1755.2004.00367.x] [PMID: 14675042]

Constantinou, A, Kiguchi, K & Huberman, E (1990) Induction of differentiation and DNA strand breakage in human HL-60 and K-562 leukemia cells by genistein. *Cancer Res,* 50, 2618-24.
[PMID: 2158395]

Craig, LA, Hong, NS & McDonald, RJ (2011) Revisiting the cholinergic hypothesis in the development of Alzheimer's disease. *Neurosci Biobehav Rev,* 35, 1397-409.
[http://dx.doi.org/10.1016/j.neubiorev.2011.03.001] [PMID: 21392524]

Cruz, MN, Agewall, S, Schenck-Gustafsson, K & Kublickiene, K (2008) Acute dilatation to phytoestrogens and estrogen receptor subtypes expression in small arteries from women with coronary heart disease. *Atherosclerosis,* 196, 49-58.
[http://dx.doi.org/10.1016/j.atherosclerosis.2007.01.038] [PMID: 17367797]

Das, A, Banik, NL & Ray, SK (2010) Flavonoids activated caspases for apoptosis in human glioblastoma T98G and U87MG cells but not in human normal astrocytes. *Cancer,* 116, 164-76.
[PMID: 19894226]

De Assis, S & Hilakivi-Clarke, L (2006) Timing of dietary estrogenic exposures and breast cancer risk. *Ann N Y Acad Sci,* 1089, 14-35.
[http://dx.doi.org/10.1196/annals.1386.039] [PMID: 17261753]

de Lemos, ML (2001) Effects of soy phytoestrogens genistein and daidzein on breast cancer growth. *Ann Pharmacother,* 35, 1118-21.
[http://dx.doi.org/10.1345/aph.10257] [PMID: 11573864]

De Paula, ML, Rodrigues, DH, Teixeira, HC, Barsante, MM, Souza, MA & Ferreira, AP (2008) Genistein down-modulates pro-inflammatory cytokines and reverses clinical signs of experimental autoimmune encephalomyelitis. *Int Immunopharmacol,* 8, 1291-7.
[http://dx.doi.org/10.1016/j.intimp.2008.05.002] [PMID: 18602076]

Deardorff, WJ, Feen, E & Grossberg, GT (2015) The use of cholinesterase inhibitors across all stages of Alzheimer's disease. *Drugs Aging,* 32, 537-47.
[http://dx.doi.org/10.1007/s40266-015-0273-x] [PMID: 26033268]

Demiroren, K, Dogan, Y, Kocamaz, H, Ozercan, IH, Ilhan, S, Ustundag, B & Bahcecioglu, IH (2014) Protective effects of L-carnitine, N-acetylcysteine and genistein in an experimental model of liver fibrosis. *Clin Res Hepatol Gastroenterol,* 38, 63-72.
[http://dx.doi.org/10.1016/j.clinre.2013.08.014] [PMID: 24239319]

Devi, KP, Shanmuganathan, B, Manayi, A, Nabavi, SF & Nabavi, SM (2017) Molecular and therapeutic targets of genistein in Alzheimer's disease. *Mol Neurobiol,* 54, 7028-41.
[http://dx.doi.org/10.1007/s12035-016-0215-6] [PMID: 27796744]

Ding, J, Yu, HL, Ma, WW, Xi, YD, Zhao, X, Yuan, LH, Feng, JF & Xiao, R (2013) Soy isoflavone attenuates brain mitochondrial oxidative stress induced by β-amyloid peptides 1-42 injection in lateral cerebral ventricle. *J Neurosci Res,* 91, 562-7.
[http://dx.doi.org/10.1002/jnr.23163] [PMID: 23239252]

Doody, RS, Stevens, JC, Beck, C, Dubinsky, RM, Kaye, JA, Gwyther, L, Mohs, RC, Thal, LJ, Whitehouse, PJ, DeKosky, ST & Cummings, JL (2001) Practice parameter: management of dementia (an evidence-based review). Report of the Quality Standards Subcommittee of the American Academy of Neurology. *Neurology,* 56, 1154-66.
[http://dx.doi.org/10.1212/WNL.56.9.1154] [PMID: 11342679]

AA1, Elmarakby, AS, Ibrahim & J, Faulkner (2011) Tyrosine kinase inhibitor, genistein, reduces renal inflammation and injury in streptozotocin-induced diabetic mice. *Vascular Pharmacology,* 55, 149-56.

Foti, P, Erba, D, Riso, P, Spadafranca, A, Criscuoli, F & Testolin, G (2005) Comparison between daidzein and genistein antioxidant activity in primary and cancer lymphocytes. *Arch Biochem Biophys,* 433, 421-7.
[http://dx.doi.org/10.1016/j.abb.2004.10.008] [PMID: 15581598]

Gagné, F (2014) *Biochemical Ecotoxicology.*Academic Press, Cambridge, Massachusetts, USA.

Gaur, A & Bhatia, A (2009) Genistein: A multipurpose isoflavone. *International Journal of Green Pharmacy,* 3, 176.
[http://dx.doi.org/10.4103/0973-8258.56270]

Gottstein, N, Ewins, BA, Eccleston, C, Hubbard, GP, Kavanagh, IC, Minihane, AM, Weinberg, PD & Rimbach, G (2003) Effect of genistein and daidzein on platelet aggregation and monocyte and endothelial function. *Br J Nutr,* 89, 607-16.
[http://dx.doi.org/10.1079/BJN2003820] [PMID: 12720581]

Hagen, MK, Ludke, A, Araujo, AS, Mendes, RH, Fernandes, TG, Mandarino, JM, Llesuy, S, Vogt de Jong, E & Belló-Klein, A (2012) Antioxidant characterization of soy derived products *in vitro* and the effect of a soy diet on peripheral markers of oxidative stress in a heart disease model. *Can J Physiol Pharmacol,* 90, 1095-

103.
[http://dx.doi.org/10.1139/y2012-028] [PMID: 22808939]

Hong, C, Guo, HY, Chen, S, Lv, JW, Zhang, X, Yang, YC, Huang, K, Zhang, YJ, Tian, ZY, Luo, W & Chen, YP (2019) Synthesis and biological evaluation of genistein-O-alkylamine derivatives as potential multifunctional anti-Alzheimer agents. *Chem Biol Drug Des,* 93, 188-200.
[http://dx.doi.org/10.1111/cbdd.13414] [PMID: 30299583]

Hörmann, V, Kumi-Diaka, J, Durity, M & Rathinavelu, A (2012) Anticancer activities of genistein-topotecan combination in prostate cancer cells. *J Cell Mol Med,* 16, 2631-6.
[http://dx.doi.org/10.1111/j.1582-4934.2012.01576.x] [PMID: 22452992]

Hwang, YW, Kim, SY, Jee, SH, Kim, YN & Nam, CM (2009) Soy food consumption and risk of prostate cancer: a meta-analysis of observational studies. *Nutr Cancer,* 61, 598-606.
[http://dx.doi.org/10.1080/01635580902825639] [PMID: 19838933]

Javanbakht, MH, Sadria, R, Djalali, M, Derakhshanian, H, Hosseinzadeh, P, Zarei, M, Azizi, G, Sedaghat, R & Mirshafiey, A (2014) Soy protein and genistein improves renal antioxidant status in experimental nephrotic syndrome. *Nefrologia,* 34, 483-90.
[PMID: 25036062]

Jeon, S, Park, YJ & Kwon, YH (2014) Genistein alleviates the development of nonalcoholic steatohepatitis in ApoE(-/-) mice fed a high-fat diet. *Mol Nutr Food Res,* 58, 830-41.
[http://dx.doi.org/10.1002/mnfr.201300112] [PMID: 24214843]

Johri, A & Beal, MF (2012) Antioxidants in Huntington's disease. *Biochim Biophys Acta,* 1822, 664-74.
[http://dx.doi.org/10.1016/j.bbadis.2011.11.014] [PMID: 22138129]

Jurzak, M & Adamczyk, K (2013) Influence of genistein on c-Jun, c-Fos and Fos-B of AP-1 subunits expression in skin keratinocytes, fibroblasts and keloid fibroblasts cultured *in vitro. Acta Pol Pharm,* 70, 205-13.
[PMID: 23614275]

Kairane, C, Mahlapuu, R, Ehrlich, K, Zilmer, M & Soomets, U (2014) The effects of different antioxidants on the activity of cerebrocortical MnSOD and Na,K-ATPase from post mortem Alzheimer's disease and age-matched normal brains. *Curr Alzheimer Res,* 11, 79-85.
[http://dx.doi.org/10.2174/15672050113106660179] [PMID: 24156257]

Karamsetty, MR, Klinger, JR & Hill, NS (2001) Phytoestrogens restore nitric oxide-mediated relaxation in isolated pulmonary arteries from chronically hypoxic rats. *J Pharmacol Exp Ther,* 297, 968-74.
[PMID: 11356918]

Kim, H, Bang, OY, Jung, MW, Ha, SD, Hong, HS, Huh, K, Kim, SU & Mook-Jung, I (2001) Neuroprotective effects of estrogen against beta-amyloid toxicity are mediated by estrogen receptors in cultured neuronal cells. *Neurosci Lett,* 302, 58-62.
[http://dx.doi.org/10.1016/S0304-3940(01)01659-7] [PMID: 11278111]

Kim, SH, Kim, SH, Kim, YB, Jeon, YT, Lee, SCh & Song, YS (2009) Genistein inhibits cell growth by modulating various mitogen-activated protein kinases and AKT in cervical cancer cells. *Ann N Y Acad Sci,* 1171, 495-500.
[http://dx.doi.org/10.1111/j.1749-6632.2009.04899.x] [PMID: 19723095]

Lamartiniere, CA, Moore, JB, Brown, NM, Thompson, R, Hardin, MJ & Barnes, S (1995) Genistein suppresses mammary cancer in rats. *Carcinogenesis,* 16, 2833-40.
[http://dx.doi.org/10.1093/carcin/16.11.2833] [PMID: 7586206]

Leoni, V, Solomon, A & Kivipelto, M (2010) Links between ApoE, brain cholesterol metabolism, tau and amyloid beta-peptide in patients with cognitive impairment. *Biochem Soc Trans,* 38, 1021-5.
[http://dx.doi.org/10.1042/BST0381021] [PMID: 20658997]

Li, Y & Zhang, H (2017) Soybean isoflavones ameliorate ischemic cardiomyopathy by activating Nrf2-mediated antioxidant responses. *Food Funct,* 8, 2935-44.

[http://dx.doi.org/10.1039/C7FO00342K] [PMID: 28745354]

Liang, HW, Qiu, SF, Shen, J, Sun, LN, Wang, JY, Bruce, IC & Xia, Q (2008) Genistein attenuates oxidative stress and neuronal damage following transient global cerebral ischemia in rat hippocampus. *Neurosci Lett,* 438, 116-20.
[http://dx.doi.org/10.1016/j.neulet.2008.04.058] [PMID: 18467029]

López-Lazaro, M, Willmore, E & Austin, CA (2007) Cells lacking DNA topoisomerase II β are resistant to genistein. *J Nat Prod,* 70, 763-7.
[http://dx.doi.org/10.1021/np060609z] [PMID: 17411092]

Lu, C, Wang, Y, Xu, T, Li, Q, Wang, D, Zhang, L, Fan, B, Wang, F & Liu, X (2018) Genistein ameliorates scopolamine-induced amnesia in mice through the regulation of the cholinergic neurotransmission, antioxidant system and the ERK/CREB/BDNF signaling. *Front Pharmacol,* 9, 1153.
[http://dx.doi.org/10.3389/fphar.2018.01153] [PMID: 30369882]

MacGregor, AJ, Snieder, H, Rigby, AS, Koskenvuo, M, Kaprio, J, Aho, K & Silman, AJ (2000) Characterizing the quantitative genetic contribution to rheumatoid arthritis using data from twins. *Arthritis Rheum,* 43, 30-7.
[http://dx.doi.org/10.1002/1529-0131(200001)43:1<30::AID-ANR5>3.0.CO;2-B] [PMID: 10643697]

Markovits, J, Linassier, C, Fossé, P, Couprie, J, Pierre, J, Jacquemin-Sablon, A, Saucier, JM, Le Pecq, JB & Larsen, AK (1989) Inhibitory effects of the tyrosine kinase inhibitor genistein on mammalian DNA topoisomerase II. *Cancer Res,* 49, 5111-7.
[PMID: 2548712]

Martorell, M, Forman, K, Castro, N, Capó, X, Tejada, S & Sureda, A (2016) Potential therapeutic effects of oleuropein aglycone in Alzheimer's disease. *Curr Pharm Biotechnol,* 17, 994-1001.
[http://dx.doi.org/10.2174/1389201017666160725120656] [PMID: 27455905]

Masilamani, M, Wei, J & Sampson, HA (2012) Regulation of the immune response by soybean isoflavones. *Immunol Res,* 54, 95-110.
[http://dx.doi.org/10.1007/s12026-012-8331-5] [PMID: 22484990]

Masliah, E, Mallory, M, Ge, N, Alford, M, Veinbergs, I & Roses, AD (1995) Neurodegeneration in the central nervous system of apoE-deficient mice. *Exp Neurol,* 136, 107-22.
[http://dx.doi.org/10.1006/exnr.1995.1088] [PMID: 7498401]

Maulik, SK, Prabhakar, P, Dinda, AK & Seth, S (2012) Genistein prevents isoproterenol-induced cardiac hypertrophy in rats. *Can J Physiol Pharmacol,* 90, 1117-25.
[http://dx.doi.org/10.1139/y2012-068] [PMID: 22808991]

Mecocci, P, Bladström, A & Stender, K (2009) Effects of memantine on cognition in patients with moderate to severe Alzheimer's disease: post-hoc analyses of ADAS-cog and SIB total and single-item scores from six randomized, double-blind, placebo-controlled studies. *Int J Geriatr Psychiatry,* 24, 532-8.
[http://dx.doi.org/10.1002/gps.2226] [PMID: 19274640]

Menze, ET, Esmat, A, Tadros, MG, Abdel-Naim, AB & Khalifa, AE (2015) Genistein improves 3-NP--induced memory impairment in ovariectomized rats: impact of its antioxidant, anti-inflammatory and acetylcholinesterase modulatory properties. *PLoS One,* 10e0117223
[http://dx.doi.org/10.1371/journal.pone.0117223] [PMID: 25675218]

Menze, ET, Esmat, A, Tadros, MG, Khalifa, AE & Abdel-Naim, AB (2016) Genistein improves sensorimotor gating: Mechanisms related to its neuroprotective effects on the striatum. *Neuropharmacology,* 105, 35-46.
[http://dx.doi.org/10.1016/j.neuropharm.2016.01.007] [PMID: 26764242]

Morito, K, Hirose, T, Kinjo, J, Hirakawa, T, Okawa, M, Nohara, T, Ogawa, S, Inoue, S, Muramatsu, M & Masamune, Y (2001) Interaction of phytoestrogens with estrogen receptors α and β. *Biol Pharm Bull,* 24, 351-6.
[http://dx.doi.org/10.1248/bpb.24.351] [PMID: 11305594]

Newman, DJ & Cragg, GM (2016) Natural products as sources of new drugs from 1981 to 2014. *J Nat Prod,*

79, 629-61.
[http://dx.doi.org/10.1021/acs.jnatprod.5b01055] [PMID: 26852623]

Panche, AN, Diwan, AD & Chandra, SR (2016) Flavonoids: an overview. *J Nutr Sci,* 5e47
[http://dx.doi.org/10.1017/jns.2016.41] [PMID: 28620474]

Park, CE, Yun, H, Lee, EB, Min, BI, Bae, H, Choe, W, Kang, I, Kim, SS & Ha, J (2010) The antioxidant effects of genistein are associated with AMP-activated protein kinase activation and PTEN induction in prostate cancer cells. *J Med Food,* 13, 815-20.
[http://dx.doi.org/10.1089/jmf.2009.1359] [PMID: 20673057]

Park, D, Huang, T & Frishman, WH (2005) Phytoestrogens as cardioprotective agents. *Cardiol Rev,* 13, 13-7.
[http://dx.doi.org/10.1097/01.crd.0000126084.68791.32] [PMID: 15596022]

Park, SH, Kim, JH, Choi, KH, Jang, YJ, Bae, SS, Choi, BT & Shin, HK (2013) Hypercholesterolemia accelerates amyloid β-induced cognitive deficits. *Int J Mol Med,* 31, 577-82.
[http://dx.doi.org/10.3892/ijmm.2013.1233] [PMID: 23314909]

Park, YJ, Ko, JW, Jeon, S & Kwon, YH (2016) Protective effect of genistein against neuronal degeneration in ApoE$^{-/-}$ mice fed a high-fat diet. *Nutrients,* 8e692
[http://dx.doi.org/10.3390/nu8110692] [PMID: 27809235]

Pierzynowska, K, Gaffke, L, Hać, A, Mantej, J, Niedziałek, N, Brokowska, J & Węgrzyn, G (2018) Correction of Huntington's disease phenotype by genistein-induced autophagy in the cellular model. *Neuromolecular Med,* 20, 112-23.
[http://dx.doi.org/10.1007/s12017-018-8482-1] [PMID: 29435951]

Pierzynowska, K, Gaffke, L, Cyske, Z & Węgrzyn, G (2019) Genistein induces degradation of mutant huntingtin in fibroblasts from Huntington's disease patients. *Metab Brain Dis,* 34, 715-20. a
[http://dx.doi.org/10.1007/s11011-019-00405-4] [PMID: 30850940]

Pierzynowska, K, Podlacha, M, Gaffke, L, Majkutewicz, I, Mantej, J, Węgrzyn, A, Osiadły, M, Myślińska, D & Węgrzyn, G (2019) Autophagy-dependent mechanism of genistein-mediated elimination of behavioral and biochemical defects in the rat model of sporadic Alzheimer's disease. *Neuropharmacology,* 148, 332-46. b
[http://dx.doi.org/10.1016/j.neuropharm.2019.01.030] [PMID: 30710571]

Pietta, PG (2000) Flavonoids as antioxidants. *J Nat Prod,* 63, 1035-42.
[http://dx.doi.org/10.1021/np9904509] [PMID: 10924197]

Poirier, J (2000) Apolipoprotein E and Alzheimer's disease. A role in amyloid catabolism. *Ann N Y Acad Sci,* 924, 81-90.
[http://dx.doi.org/10.1111/j.1749-6632.2000.tb05564.x] [PMID: 11193807]

Profenno, LA, Porsteinsson, AP & Faraone, SV (2010) Meta-analysis of Alzheimer's disease risk with obesity, diabetes, and related disorders. *Biol Psychiatry,* 67, 505-12.
[http://dx.doi.org/10.1016/j.biopsych.2009.02.013] [PMID: 19358976]

Qian, Y, Guan, T, Huang, M, Cao, L, Li, Y, Cheng, H, Jin, H & Yu, D (2012) Neuroprotection by the soy isoflavone, genistein, *via* inhibition of mitochondria-dependent apoptosis pathways and reactive oxygen induced-NF-κB activation in a cerebral ischemia mouse model. *Neurochem Int,* 60, 759-67.
[http://dx.doi.org/10.1016/j.neuint.2012.03.011] [PMID: 22490611]

Rafii, MS & Aisen, PS (2009) Recent developments in Alzheimer's disease therapeutics. *BMC Med,* 7, 7.
[http://dx.doi.org/10.1186/1741-7015-7-7] [PMID: 19228370]

Rahman Mazumder, MA & Hongsprabhas, P (2016) Genistein as antioxidant and antibrowning agents in *in vivo* and *in vitro*: A review. *Biomed Pharmacother,* 82, 379-92.
[http://dx.doi.org/10.1016/j.biopha.2016.05.023] [PMID: 27470376]

Rajput, MS & Sarkar, PD (2017) Modulation of neuro-inflammatory condition, acetylcholinesterase and antioxidant levels by genistein attenuates diabetes associated cognitive decline in mice. *Chem Biol Interact,* 268, 93-102.

[http://dx.doi.org/10.1016/j.cbi.2017.02.021] [PMID: 28259689]

Rao, CV, Wang, CX, Simi, B, Lubet, R, Kelloff, G, Steele, V & Reddy, BS (1997) Enhancement of experimental colon cancer by genistein. *Cancer Res,* 57, 3717-22.
[PMID: 9288778]

Raynal, NJ, Charbonneau, M, Momparler, LF, Momparler, RL & Momparler, RL (2008) Synergistic effect of 5-Aza-2'-deoxycytidine and genistein in combination against leukemia. *Oncol Res,* 17, 223-30.
[http://dx.doi.org/10.3727/096504008786111356] [PMID: 18980019]

Recor, IR, Dreosti, IE & McInerey, JK (1995) The antioxidant activity of genistein *in vitro. Nutritional Biochemistry,* 6, 481-5.
[http://dx.doi.org/10.1016/0955-2863(95)00076-C]

Rostami, R, Aghasi, MR, Mohammadi, A & Nourooz-Zadeh, J (2013) Enhanced oxidative stress in Hashimoto's thyroiditis: inter-relationships to biomarkers of thyroid function. *Clin Biochem,* 46, 308-12.
[http://dx.doi.org/10.1016/j.clinbiochem.2012.11.021] [PMID: 23219737]

Ruiz-Larrea, MB, Mohan, AR, Paganga, G, Miller, NJ, Bolwell, GP & Rice-Evans, CA (1997) Antioxidant activity of phytoestrogenic isoflavones. *Free Radic Res,* 26, 63-70.
[http://dx.doi.org/10.3109/10715769709097785] [PMID: 9018473]

Sakamoto, T, Horiguchi, H, Oguma, E & Kayama, F (2010) Effects of diverse dietary phytoestrogens on cell growth, cell cycle and apoptosis in estrogen-receptor-positive breast cancer cells. *J Nutr Biochem,* 21, 856-64.
[http://dx.doi.org/10.1016/j.jnutbio.2009.06.010] [PMID: 19800779]

Mohamed Salih, S, Nallasamy, P, Muniyandi, P, Periyasami, V & Carani Venkatraman, A (2009) Genistein improves liver function and attenuates non-alcoholic fatty liver disease in a rat model of insulin resistance. *J Diabetes,* 1, 278-87.
[http://dx.doi.org/10.1111/j.1753-0407.2009.00045.x] [PMID: 20923528]

Sarkar, FH & Li, Y (2002) Mechanisms of cancer chemoprevention by soy isoflavone genistein. *Cancer Metastasis Rev,* 21, 265-80.
[http://dx.doi.org/10.1023/A:1021210910821] [PMID: 12549765]

Sasser, JM, Sullivan, JC, Hobbs, JL, Yamamoto, T, Pollock, DM, Carmines, PK & Pollock, JS (2007) Endothelin A receptor blockade reduces diabetic renal injury *via* an anti-inflammatory mechanism. *J Am Soc Nephrol,* 18, 143-54.
[http://dx.doi.org/10.1681/ASN.2006030208] [PMID: 17167119]

Setchell, KDR (2001) Soy isoflavones--benefits and risks from nature's selective estrogen receptor modulators (SERMs). *J Am Coll Nutr,* 20 (Suppl.), 354S-62S.
[http://dx.doi.org/10.1080/07315724.2001.10719168] [PMID: 11603644]

Shah, D, Wanchu, A & Bhatnagar, A (2011) Interaction between oxidative stress and chemokines: possible pathogenic role in systemic lupus erythematosus and rheumatoid arthritis. *Immunobiology,* 216, 1010-7.
[http://dx.doi.org/10.1016/j.imbio.2011.04.001] [PMID: 21601309]

Shepardson, NE, Shankar, GM & Selkoe, DJ (2011) Cholesterol level and statin use in Alzheimer disease: I. Review of epidemiological and preclinical studies. *Arch Neurol,* 68, 1239-44.
[http://dx.doi.org/10.1001/archneurol.2011.203] [PMID: 21987540]

Siddique, YH, Naz, F, Jyoti, S & Ali, F (2018) Effect of Genistein on the Transgenic Drosophila Model of Parkinson's Disease. *J Diet Suppl*
[http://dx.doi.org/10.1080/19390211.2018.1472706] [PMID: 29969325]

Sierens, J, Hartley, JA, Campbell, MJ, Leathem, AJ & Woodside, JV (2002) *in vitro* isoflavone supplementation reduces hydrogen peroxide-induced DNA damage in sperm. *Teratog Carcinog Mutagen,* 22, 227-34.
[http://dx.doi.org/10.1002/tcm.10015] [PMID: 11948633]

Smolińska, E, Moskot, M, Jakóbkiewicz-Banecka, J, Węgrzyn, G, Banecki, B, Szczerkowska-Dobosz, A,

Purzycka-Bohdan, D & Gabig-Cimińska, M (2018) Molecular action of isoflavone genistein in the human epithelial cell line HaCaT. *PLoS One,* 13e0192297
[http://dx.doi.org/10.1371/journal.pone.0192297] [PMID: 29444128]

Tesch, GH (2010) Macrophages and diabetic nephropathy. *Semin Nephrol,* 30, 290-301.
[http://dx.doi.org/10.1016/j.semnephrol.2010.03.007] [PMID: 20620673]

Traganos, F, Ardelt, B, Halko, N, Bruno, S & Darzynkiewicz, Z (1992) Effects of genistein on the growth and cell cycle progression of normal human lymphocytes and human leukemic MOLT-4 and HL-60 cells. *Cancer Res,* 52, 6200-8.
[PMID: 1330289]

Trieu, VN, Dong, Y, Zheng, Y & Uckun, FM (1999) *In vivo* antioxidant activity of genistein in a murine model of singlet oxygen-induced cerebral stroke. *Radiat Res,* 152, 508-16.
[http://dx.doi.org/10.2307/3580147] [PMID: 10523874]

Tsao, R (2010) Chemistry and biochemistry of dietary polyphenols. *Nutrients,* 2, 1231-46.
[http://dx.doi.org/10.3390/nu2121231] [PMID: 22254006]

Uranga, RM & Keller, JN (2010) Diet and age interactions with regards to cholesterol regulation and brain pathogenesis. *Curr Gerontol Geriatr Res,* 2010219683
[http://dx.doi.org/10.1155/2010/219683] [PMID: 20396385]

Valsecchi, AE, Franchi, S, Panerai, AE, Rossi, A, Sacerdote, P & Colleoni, M (2011) The soy isoflavone genistein reverses oxidative and inflammatory state, neuropathic pain, neurotrophic and vasculature deficits in diabetes mouse model. *Eur J Pharmacol,* 650, 694-702.
[http://dx.doi.org/10.1016/j.ejphar.2010.10.060] [PMID: 21050844]

Valsecchi, AE, Franchi, S, Panerai, AE, Sacerdote, P, Trovato, AE & Colleoni, M (2008) Genistein, a natural phytoestrogen from soy, relieves neuropathic pain following chronic constriction sciatic nerve injury in mice: anti-inflammatory and antioxidant activity. *J Neurochem,* 107, 230-40.
[http://dx.doi.org/10.1111/j.1471-4159.2008.05614.x] [PMID: 18691380]

Viña, J, Lloret, A, Vallés, SL, Borrás, C, Badía, MC, Pallardó, FV, Sastre, J & Alonso, MD (2007) Effect of gender on mitochondrial toxicity of Alzheimer's Abeta peptide. *Antioxid Redox Signal,* 9, 1677-90.
[http://dx.doi.org/10.1089/ars.2007.1773] [PMID: 17822363]

Wada, T, Furuichi, K, Sakai, N, Iwata, Y, Yoshimoto, K, Shimizu, M, Takeda, SI, Takasawa, K, Yoshimura, M, Kida, H, Kobayashi, KI, Mukaida, N, Naito, T, Matsushima, K & Yokoyama, H (2000) Up-regulation of monocyte chemoattractant protein-1 in tubulointerstitial lesions of human diabetic nephropathy. *Kidney Int,* 58, 1492-9.
[http://dx.doi.org/10.1046/j.1523-1755.2000.00311.x] [PMID: 11012884]

Wang, H & Murphy, PA (1994) Isoflavone content in commercial soybean foods. *J Agric Food Chem,* 42, 1666-73.
[http://dx.doi.org/10.1021/jf00044a016]

Wang, X, Chen, S, Ma, G, Ye, M & Lu, G (2005) Genistein protects dopaminergic neurons by inhibiting microglial activation. *Neuroreport,* 16, 267-70.
[http://dx.doi.org/10.1097/00001756-200502280-00013] [PMID: 15706233]

Webb, TE, Stromberg, PC, Abou-Issa, H, Curley, RW, Jr & Moeschberger, M (1992) Effect of dietary soybean and licorice on the male F344 rat: an integrated study of some parameters relevant to cancer chemoprevention. *Nutr Cancer,* 18, 215-30.
[http://dx.doi.org/10.1080/01635589209514222] [PMID: 1296195]

Wei, H, Bowen, R, Cai, Q, Barnes, S & Wang, Y (1995) Antioxidant and antipromotional effects of the soybean isoflavone genistein. *Proc Soc Exp Biol Med,* 208, 124-30.
[http://dx.doi.org/10.3181/00379727-208-43844] [PMID: 7892286]

Wild, S, Roglic, G, Green, A, Sicree, R & King, H (2004) Global prevalence of diabetes: estimates for the year 2000 and projections for 2030. *Diabetes Care,* 27, 1047-53.

[http://dx.doi.org/10.2337/diacare.27.5.1047] [PMID: 15111519]

Wu, HC, Hu, QL, Zhang, SJ, Wang, YM, Jin, ZK, Lv, LF, Zhang, S, Liu, ZL, Wu, HL & Cheng, OM (2018) Neuroprotective effects of genistein on SH-SY5Y cells overexpressing A53T mutant α-synuclein. *Neural Regen Res,* 13, 1375-83.
[http://dx.doi.org/10.4103/1673-5374.235250] [PMID: 30106049]

Yalniz, M, Bahcecioglu, IH, Kuzu, N, Poyrazoglu, OK, Bulmus, O, Celebi, S, Ustundag, B, Ozercan, IH & Sahin, K (2007) Preventive role of genistein in an experimental non-alcoholic steatohepatitis model. *J Gastroenterol Hepatol,* 22, 2009-14.
[http://dx.doi.org/10.1111/j.1440-1746.2006.04681.x] [PMID: 17914984]

Zhang, T, Wang, F, Xu, HX, Yi, L, Qin, Y & Chang, H (2012) Activation of nuclear factor erythroid 2-related factor 2 and PPARgamma plays a role in the genistein-mediated attenuation of oxidative stress-induced endothelial cell injury. *Br J Nutr,* 3, 1-13.
[PMID: 22716961]

Zhang, YJ, Gan, RY, Li, S, Zhou, Y, Li, AN, Xu, DP & Li, HB (2015) Antioxidant phytochemicals for the prevention and treatment of chronic diseases. *Molecules,* 20, 21138-56.
[http://dx.doi.org/10.3390/molecules201219753] [PMID: 26633317]

Zhao, L, Zhang, N, Yang, D, Yang, M, Guo, X, He, J, Wu, W, Ji, B, Cheng, Q & Zhou, F (2018) Protective effects of five structurally diverse flavonoid subgroups against chronic alcohol-induced hepatic damage in a mouse model. *Nutrients,* 10e1754
[http://dx.doi.org/10.3390/nu10111754] [PMID: 30441755]

Zhuo, L, Liao, M, Zheng, L, He, M, Huang, Q, Wei, L, Huang, R, Zhang, S & Lin, X (2012) Combination therapy with taurine, epigallocatechin gallate and genistein for protection against hepatic fibrosis induced by alcohol in rats. *Biol Pharm Bull,* 35, 1802-10.
[http://dx.doi.org/10.1248/bpb.b12-00548] [PMID: 23037169]

Industrial Prospects of Antioxidants

Diksha Sharma[1], Manju[2], Jyoti Lakhanpal[2], Amandeep Kaur[2], Suman Kumari[2] and Rohit Rai[2,*]

[1] *Department of Biotechnology, CT Institute of Pharmaceutical Sciences, CT Group of Institutions, Jalandhar, Punjab, India*

[2] *Faculty of Applied Medical Sciences, Lovely Professional University, Phagwara, Punjab, India*

Abstract: The highly reactive free radical species generated through abiotic stress lead to the degradation of essential biomolecules like proteins, carbohydrates, lipids and nucleic acids, thus deregulating a series of cellular functions. Several pathological conditions like wrinkling of skin, ageing, asthma, arthritis, carcinogenesis, cardiovascular diseases, cataract, AIDS, autoimmune disorders, Parkinson's dementia, Alzheimer's disease, *etc.*, are the manifestations of free radical toxicity. Apart from these clinical influences, free radicals are associated with spoilage of food resulting through oxidation of fats, oils and lipid content. Antioxidants have enormous potential to neutralize the effect of toxic moieties. Antioxidants can be natural or synthetic with the former taken directly from fruits, vegetables, herbs and spices. Synthetic antioxidants can also inhibit oxidation reactions but their use has been quoted as unsafe for humans. Therefore, expedition on innocuous antioxidants of natural origin has intensified in recent past. The scientific studies have demonstrated the potential of natural antioxidants as: (i) natural preservative for long term storage of ready to eat food products without compromising with their commercial and sensory values; (ii) an anti-ageing, anti-wrinkle agent in the cosmeceutical products; (iii) a medicinal ingredient preventing vesicular calcification and lipid peroxidation responsible for various diseases; (iv) a protective probe against several cardiovascular, neurodegenerative and autoimmune disorders. Owing to such a wide array of industrial applications, natural antioxidants are expected to capture the market in future generating high revenue of billions of dollars. Therefore, through this chapter we focus on bioprospecting diverse sources of natural antioxidant compounds and their industrial prospects.

Keywords: Alzheimer's disease, Anti-carcinogen, Antioxidants, Cardiovascular diseases, Cosmeceutical properties, Flavonoids, Health supplement, Medicinal value, Parkinson's dementia, Reactive oxygen species, Therapeutic aspects.

* **Corresponding author Rohit Rai:** Faculty of Applied Medical Sciences, Lovely Professional University, Phagwara, Punjab, India. E-mail: rohitraisharma44@gmail.com

INTRODUCTION

Antioxidants are the substances that delay oxidation of carbohydrates, lipids, proteins, and DNA due to oxidative stress at low concentrations (Niki 2004). The oxidative stress is a situation of disparity between reactive oxygen species (ROS) and the protective antioxidant barriers causing several pathological conditions like ageing, cataract, diabetes, asthma, carcinogenesis, arthritis, AIDS, autoimmune diseases, neurodegenerative diseases, Alzheimer's disease, Parkinson's disease and cardiovascular dysfunctions (Bakir *et al.* 2020, Gupta and Sharma 2006, Sindhi *et al.* 2013). ROS possess unpaired electrons in their valence shells and react swiftly with the cell membranes leading to their deterioration and death (Kajarabille and Latunde-Dada 2019). To counter the action of these free radicals, living systems produce antioxidants or these may be incorporated through diet. Broadly antioxidants can be grouped into: a) First line; b) Second line; c) Third line defense antioxidants (Sindhi *et al.* 2013). The first category of antioxidants comprise catalase, glutathione reductase, superoxide dismutase and minerals (Cu, Zn, Se, *etc.*) Second line defense antioxidants cover vitamin C and E, albumins, carotenoids, flavonoids, glutathione, *etc.* The third group of antioxidants include set of enzymes that mediate repair of impaired DNA and proteins, and oxidized lipids and peroxides (Ighodaro and Akinloye 2018, Irshad and Chaudhuri 2002, Sindhi *et al.* 2013). All the above mentioned classes operate either through enzymatic processes or non-enzymatic processes where the former group reduces the amount of antioxidants thus serving the protective function and latter group prevents lipid peroxidation and metal catalyzed radical reactions (Ighodaro and Akinloye 2018, Palozza and Krinsky 1992). Several scientific studies have indicated the significant industrial applications of this elite group of compounds, therefore, through this book chapter we present a cumulative survey of medicinal, pharmacological, therapeutic and food applications of the antioxidants.

SOURCES OF ANTIOXIDANTS

The compounds with antioxidant properties can be derived from natural products and in many cases, these compounds can be semi-synthetic or fully synthetic.

Natural Antioxidants

The natural antioxidants also known as primary antioxidants are present in both plants and animals with plants being the major sources of these compounds. On the other hand, only smaller amounts of these compounds are derived from animals thus making them an insignificant source of natural antioxidants. Vegetables, fruits, cereals, legumes, herbs, spices, tea, coffee, wine and beer are considered the richest sources of antioxidants. Various antioxidants and their sources have been summarized in Table **1**.

Table 1. Antioxidants from natural sources.

Source		Antioxidants
Fruits	Blackcurrant	Vitamin C, lutein, β carotene, anthocyanin, m-coumaric acid acid
	Grapes	Gallic acid, catechins, epicatechins, ellagic acid, myricetin, quercetin, kaempferol, anthocyanins, flavonols, trans-resveratrol
	Strawberry	Vitamin C, anthocyanin, ellagic acid, glycosides, ellagitannins
	Bilberry	Vitamin C, anthocyanins, carotenoids, derivatives of hydroxycinnamic acid
	Cranberry	Peonidin, cyanidin, flavanones, procyanidin, quercetin, myricetin, derivatives of hydroxycinnamic acid
	Blackberry	Anthocyanin, flavonols, ellagic acid, procyanidin, epicatechin
	Crowberry	Vitamin C, lutein, β carotene, flavanols, procyanidins, cinnamic acid, trans-resveratrol, p-coumaric acid
	Chokeberry	Anthocyanins, chlorogenic acid, neochlorogenic acid, epicatechins
	Cherry	Anthocyanins, hydroxycinnamic acid
	Plums	Catechins, hydroxycinnamic acid
	Pears	Catechins, hydroxycinnamic acid
	Kiwi	Catechins, hydroxycinnamic acid
	Apple	Epicatechin, procyanidin B2, chlorogenic acid, phlorizin, phloretin--xyloglucoside
	Lemons	Vitamin C, hesperetin, naringenin, eriodictyol
	Oranges	Vitamin C, hesperetin, naringenin, eriodictyol
	Grapefruits	Vitamin C, hesperetin, naringenin, eriodictyol, lycopene
	Papaya	β carotene, tocopherols, lycopene
	Guava	Lycopene, protocatechuic acid, quercetin, ferulic acid, ascorbic acid, gallic acid, caffeic acid

Source		Antioxidants
Vegetables	Tomatoes	Lycopene, quercetin, lutein, β carotene
	Onion	Flavonoids, phenolics
	Carrot	Vitamin C, β carotene
	Pumpkin	α carotene, β carotene, β cryptoxanthin
	Parsley	Flavones
	Cabbage	Choline, β carotene, lutein, zeaxanthin, kaempferol, quercetin, apigenin
	Kale	β carotene, vitamin C, flavonoids, polyphenols
	Broccoli	Glucobrassicin, zeaxanthin, β carotene, kaempferol
	Cauliflower	Choline, vitamin C, glutathione, chlorogenic acid, ferulic acid
	Spinach	Zeaxanthin and lutein
	Red paprika	β carotene, capsanthin, zeaxanthin and lutein
	Potato	Carotenoids, phenolics, flavonoids, vitamin C and E
	Lettuce	Phenolic acids, flavonoids, anthocyanins, vitamin A and C
Others	Cereal grains	Phenolic acids, flavonoids, stilbenes, coumarines and tannins
	Almonds	Vitamin E
	Hazelnuts	Vitamin E
	Apricots	β carotene, vitamin A, C and E, flavonoids
	Tea (mainly green)	Polyphenols, thearubigins, epicatechins, catechins
	Wheat bran	Phytic acids, polyphenols, vitamin A, C and E
	Fish	Catalase, glutathione, superoxide dismutase, tocopherols, ubiquinones
	Chicken liver	CoQ_{10} coenzyme
	Wine	Quercetin, isorhamnetin, kaempferol, myricetin, resveratrol
	Beer	Superoxide dismutase, catalase, and peroxidases

List compiled from (Anttonen and Karjalainen 2005, Augustyniak *et al.* 2010, Benvenuti *et al.* 2016, Benvenuti *et al.* 2004, Chaovanalikit and Wrolstad 2004, Gorinstein *et al.* 2001, Hägg 1996, Halliwell and Gutteridge 2007, Halvorsen *et al.* 2002, Kahkonen *et al.* 1999, Knoblich *et al.* 2005, Kopsell and Kopsell 2006, Kurilich and Juvik 1999, Lachman *et al.* 2003, Lu and Foo 2000, Manach *et al.* 2004, Olsson *et al.* 2004, Pastrana-Bonilla *et al.* 2003, Reyes Carmona *et al.* 2005, Sikora *et al.* 2008, Siriwoharn and Wrolstad 2004, Stewart *et al.* 2005, Taruscio *et al.* 2004, Vallejo *et al.* 2003, Wu *et al.* 2004, Yanishlieva-Maslarova and Heinonen 2001, Zadernowski *et al.* 1991).

Synthetic Antioxidants

Several experimental studies have suggested the potential of synthetic compounds also known as secondary antioxidants in therapies. Different groups of synthetic antioxidants contain nitroxides, spin traps, Mn-porphyrin superoxide dismutase mimics (like M40403 and M40419, AEOL-10113 and AEOL-10150), salens (*e.g.* EUK134), GPX mimetics (ebselen, BXT51072), coenzyme Q analogues (*e.g.* ibedenone) or aminosterols (lazaroids) (Chatterjee *et al.* 2004, Day 2008, Esposito and Cuzzocrea 2009, Kavanagh and Kam 2001, Pandolfo 2008). However, health risks associated with synthetic antioxidants limit their use for human applications (Table **2**).

Agro-industrial Residues as Source of Antioxidants

The agricultural and industrial sector produces bulk of residues every year leading to several ecological issues, however, these side streams can be utilized for extraction of biologically active compounds which can be used for numerous industrial applications like functional foods, cosmeceuticals, food additives, nutra-/pharmaceuticals, *etc* (Fierascu *et al.* 2019). The details of some agro-industrial residues and antioxidant compounds studded in them are compiled in Table **3**.

Table 2. General characteristics, applications and health concerns of synthetic antioxidants.

Synthetic Antioxidant	Properties	Applications	Health Effect	Reference
Butylated hydroxytoluene (BHT)	It is a phenolic antioxidant having low molecular weight 220.34 g/mol and chemical formula $C_{15}H_{24}O$. The lipid soluble antioxidant is produced from chemical reaction between *p*-cresol and isobutylene catalysed by sulphuric acid or hydroxymethylation or aminomethylation of 2,6-di-te-t-butylphenol followed by hydrogenolysis	It is used most commonly as a food additive to maintain freshness and prevent food spoilage. It is also used in turbine and gear oils, jet fuels, hydraulic fluids, transforming oils, pharmaceuticals, cosmetics, metalworking fluids, rubber and embalming fluids	When fed at high concentrations, it can act as tumour promoter	(Babich 1982, Burton and Ingold 1981, Fiege *et al.* 2000, Kaczmarski *et al.* 1999, Ramesh *et al.* Yehye *et al.* 2015, Shahidi, 2000)

Synthetic Antioxidant	Properties	Applications	Health Effect	Reference
Butylated hydroxyanisole (BHA)	It is a phenolic antioxidant having molecular weight 180.11 g/mol and chemical formula $C_{11}H_{16}O_2$. The lipid soluble antioxidant is a product of chemical reaction between 4-methoxyphenol and isobutylene	It is used to preserve edible fats and fat-containing food products by preventing the phenomenon of rancidification. Hence, it is used primarily as an antioxidant in food products, food packaging, cosmetics, animal feed, petroleum products and rubber	It has been prohibited in various areas owing to its carcinogenic properties	(Additives *et al.* 2018, Botterweck *et al.* 2000, Branen 1975, Burton and Ingold 1981, Ito *et al.* 1983, Lam *et al.* 1979, Verhagen *et al.* 1991)
Propyl gallates	It is an n-propyl ester soluble in ethyl ether, ethanol, oil, aqueous solution of PEG (polyethylene glycol), lard, ethers of acetyl alcohol and slightly soluble in water. Its molecular weight is 212.20 g/mol with chemical formula $C_{10}H_{12}O_5$. It is formed by the condensation reaction between gallic acid and propanol	It is used to prevent oxidation of oils and fat containing products like cosmetics, hair products, adhesives and lubricants	It acts as an antagonist of oestrogen with little or no carcinogenic effects	(Abdo *et al.* 1983, Amadasi *et al.* 2009, Eler *et al.* 2009, Georgieva *et al.* 2013, Hirose *et al.* 1993, Nakagawa *et al.* 1996)

(Table 2) cont.....

Synthetic Antioxidant	Properties	Applications	Health Effect	Reference
EDTA (Ethylene-diamin--tetraacetic acid)	It is an aminopoly-carboxylic acid having molecular weight 292.24 g/mol and chemical formula $[CH_2N(CH_2CO_2H)_2]_2$ It is prepared from sodium cyanide, formaldehyde and ethylenediamine.	EDTA along with vitamins and minerals possess antioxidant properties. It can be used for the treatment of diabetes and cardiovascular diseases. It can also be used to treat heavy metal toxicity. Calcium disodium EDTA can be used as antioxidant in vegetables, emulsified sauces, legumes and fish products	At high doses, EDTA can sequester essential metal ions and can inhibit their metabolic activity. It can also lead to health conditions like diarrhoea, vomiting and urinary disturbances	(González-Cuevas *et al.* 2011, Hart 2000, Lanigan and Yamarik 2002, Van De Sande *et al.* 2014)

Table 3. Antioxidant compounds derived from agro-industrial residues.

Residue	Antioxidant compounds	References
Apple seeds	Ellagic acid, ferulic acid, caffeic acid, gallic acid, phloridzin, protocatechuic acid	(Gunes *et al.* 2019)
Rapeseed cake	Sinapic acid, sinapine and canolol	(Zago *et al.* 2015)
Citrus peel	Phenolics, flavonoids, ascorbic acid, carotenoids	(Li *et al.* 2006)
Avocado seeds	Epicatechin, catechins, procyanidin B1 & B2, rans-5-O-caffeoyl-D-quinic acid	(Tremocoldi *et al.* 2018)
Tomato peel	Lycopene, rutin, naringenin, quercetin	(Choudhari and Ananthanarayan 2007)
Coconut shell	Phenolics	(Rodrigues *et al.* 2008)
Grape marc	Phenolics	(Castrica *et al.* 2019)
Grape skin	Epicatechin, caffeic acid, rutin, catechins, gallate, gallic acid, p-coumaric acid	(Liu *et al.* 2018)
Rice bran oil	Tocopherol	(Pestana-Bauer *et al.* 2012)
Pistachio hulls	Anacardic acid, gallic acid, penta-O-galloyl-β-D-glucose	(Ersan *et al.* 2018)
Mango peel	Carotene	(Sanchez 2009)
Banana peel	Caffeic acid	(Vu *et al.* 2018)

(Table 3) cont.....

Residue	Antioxidant compounds	References
Garlic waste	Ethanol extract	(Kallel and Ellouz Chaabouni 2017)
Onion waste	Phenolics	(Larrosa *et al.* 2002)
Meat industry waste	Gelatin and heparin	(Baiano 2014)
Squid waste	Astaxanthin	(Veeruraj *et al.* 2019)
Shrimp shells	Astaxanthin and carotenoprotein	(Xu *et al.* 2020)

INDUSTRIAL PROSPECTS OF ANTIOXIDANTS

Antioxidants and Food Industry

Public demand for healthy food is being fulfilled by adding unsaturated and polyunsaturated fats in the commercial food articles. The customer feedback for quality of food largely depends on its appearance, aroma and taste (Hashemi *et al.* 2020). Heat processing and long-term storage of food articles perish lipids, oils, and fats through oxidation reactions and breakdown of oxidation products which in turn leads to compromised nutritional and sensory quality of the food (Hofstrand 2008, Sindhi *et al.* 2013). The inhibition of oxidation processes is therefore necessary for food producers as well as consumers and can be attained in several ways like using lower temperatures, reduction in oxygen pressure, using suitable packaging material, preventing oxygen access and inactivating enzymes mediating oxidation reactions. An alternative method for shielding against oxidation is the addition of antioxidants in food items rich in unsaturated fatty acids that not only increases shelf life of food articles but also contains them from undergoing rancidity, therefore, acting as potential food preservatives (Sindhi *et al.* 2013). Several synthetic and natural compounds imparting antioxidant properties have been into practice and these may be categorized as following:

Free Radical Scavengers: These chain-breaking inhibitors function by reacting with free radicals *via* donating one electron to them. This inhibits the propagation step of lipid oxidation, generating antioxidant radicals of low reactivity which can't proceed further to react with lipids. The scavenging potential of such agents depends upon pH, bond dissociation energy between oxygen and a phenolic free radical, delocalization and reduction potential of the antioxidant radicals (Gordon 1990). Tocopherols, butylated hydroxytoluene, lignans, carotenoids, ascorbic acids, ubiquinone, butylated hydroxyanisole, propyl gallate, tertiary-butylhydroqunine, flavanoids and amino acids are some compounds that act as radical scavengers.

Singlet Oxygen Quenchers: This type of quenching can be either physical or chemical with the former involving deactivation of singlet oxygen through electron and/or charge transfer and latter involving oxidation of quencher thus producing oxidation products. Examples of this category include tocopherols, carotene, ascorbic acid, amino acids, peptides and phenolics (Becker *et al.* 2004).

Metal Chelators: Metal chelating agents can intensify oxidation stability by blocking pro-oxidant metal ions, therefore, restricting the generation of chain activators inhibiting the metal dependent hemolytic fission of hydroperoxides. Various chelating agents present in food include EDTA, citric acid, phosphoric acid, maillard reaction compounds, lignans, polyphenols, ascorbic acid and amino acids (Kähkönen *et al.* 1999, Kajimoto *et al.* 1997).

Inhibitors of Lipoxygenase: Lipoxygenases catalyze the oxidation of polyunsaturated fatty acids and lipids containing a 1,4-pentadiene structure producing lipid hydroperoxides. This forms secondary oxidation products which give off-flavors, thus leading to food deterioration. Flavonoids have been reported for their potential lipoxygenase inhibitory activity (Dohi *et al.* 1991, Lyckander and Malterud 1996, Richard Forget *et al.* 1995).

Photosensitizer Deactivation: Photoactivated sensitizer works by transferring electrons or energy to triplet oxygen, forming reactive oxygen species but transferring energy from the sensitizer to quencher results in energy dissipation. Example includes, carotenoids (Ghorbani *et al.* 2018, Jakus and Farkas 2005).

The natural sources such as herbs and spices (thyme, sage, pepper, oregano, clove, nutmeg, rosemary, cinnamon, *etc.*), and plant extracts (grapeseed and tea) contain ample amount of antioxidant compounds which operate through the above mentioned mechanisms.

Medicinal and Pharmacological Aspects of Antioxidants

The normal molecules in the body have paired electrons in their outer shell and the molecules with unpaired electrons in their outermost shell are known as free radicals. These molecules result from the combination of oxygen in the bloodstream with a diverse group of chemicals present in polluted air (Hamid *et al.* 2010). Deteriorating effects of these free radicals can however be controlled by supplementing antioxidants that act as potential medicinal and pharmacological agents.

The most significant vitamin in the human diet, Vitamin E represents two groups of closely related structures named tocopherols and tocotrienols. These compounds are found in a broad range of eatables and exhibit strong antioxidant properties. Though, vitamin E constitutes a large family of compounds, tocopherols consisting of 4 isomers namely alpha, beta, gamma and delta (α, β, γ and Δ, respectively) are the most dominant compounds (Dietrich *et al.* 2003). It occurs naturally in the form of phenolic benzopyrans, displaying antioxidants properties in vivo as well as in vitro. Alpha and delta tocopherols are considered to be the vital lipid-soluble antioxidants equipped with radical-scavenging properties in membranes and plasma, hence, protecting biological membranes from oxidative damage (lipid peroxidation) (Wei Yao *et al.* 2009). In a study, anti-inflammatory and anti-carcinogenic activities of different isoforms of tocopherols in the lungs and colon were demonstrated (Yang *et al.* 2010). As tocopherols are involved in trapping reactive nitrogen species, reducing oxidative damage, and inhibiting arachidonic metabolism, the compounds establish themselves as effective antioxidant and anti-inflammatory agents (Patel *et al.* 2007, Woodson *et al.* 1999). Along with this, in multiple studies, vitamin E is considered to have anti-vascular calcification properties by lowering lipid peroxidation, and improving coronary reserves by stimulating endothelial nitric oxide synthase activities (eNOS) (Chao *et al.* 2019, Peralta-Ramirez *et al.* 2014, Ülker *et al.* 2003). The α-tocopherol also plays an important role in protecting glutathione peroxidase (GPX4)-deficient cells from apoptosis and necrosis (Herrera and Barbas 2001). Higher level of serum tocopherols has also been found associated with reduced risks of type II diabetes (Reunanen *et al.* 1998). There are also reports for pro-oxidant role of α-tocopherols, however, exact mechanism behind this behavior is still unknown (Sies and Stahl 1995). As compared to other antioxidants, the anti-oxidant property of α- tocopherols is less but in combination with other natural antioxidants, its impact is increased. Hence, this antioxidant compound can be utilized for several pharmacological and clinical applications in combinations with other antioxidants.

Vitamin C also referred to as ascorbic acid is a water soluble ketolactone. It functions as an oxygen scavenger and protects biological system against lipid peroxidation by trapping peroxyl radicals in the aqueous phase. Both the names (vitamin C or ascorbic acid) denote to its antiscorbutic properties attributing to its role in collagen synthesis in the connective tissues. Ascorbic acid is considered to be an excellent antioxidant and reducing agent due to its ability to donate one or two electrons, hence, all of the biochemical and physiological functions are mainly due to its electron donor action (Du *et al.* 2012b). Ascorbate is mainly involved in enzymatic reactions catalyzed by Fe^{2+}-oxoglutarate dependent dioxygenases and mediate modification of hydroxylases in collagen metabolism (Arrigoni and De Tullio 2002, Du *et al.* 2012a). Further, it undergoes pH-dependent auto-oxidation which makes it an efficient radical scavenger of superoxide, hydroxyl & peroxyl radicals, and singlet oxygen. Several studies have suggested that high doses of ascorbic acid can limit the risk of numerous health conditions related to heart, ageing, neurons *etc*. In vitro studies have revealed that ascorbate scavenges free radicals thus preventing oxidation of LDL in cell system strongly (Carr *et al.* 2000). In the presence of redox active ions such as iron and copper, vitamin C behaves like a pro-oxidant that mediate synthesis of hydroxyl radicals leading to oxidation of lipids, proteins and DNA (Verma *et al.* 2007). In individuals suffering from hypovitaminosis C, considerate levels of cholesterol have been observed in liver and serum along with induced dyslipidemia and atherogenic changes (Chambial *et al.* 2013). Due it its radical trapping ability, vitamin C seems to be highly beneficial for either preventing or treating clinical conditions like diabetes, sepsis and hormone production (Wilson 2009).

Carotenoids, being ubiquitous in nature, mainly provide pigmentation to animals, plants and micro-organisms but crucially also serve as an antioxidant. These are lipophilic isoprenoids, naturally synthesized by many plants, bacteria, algae, and fungi. The polyene backbone of carotenoids consists of conjugated C=C bonds and attributes to their antioxidant effect. They mainly act as scavengers of reactive oxygen species (ROS), singlet molecular oxygen, and reactive nitrogen species (RNS) (Hernandez-Ortega *et al.* 2012). Various epidemiological studies have revealed that carotene-rich diet is directly correlated with diminished risk of various degenerative disorders, including cardiovascular diseases and different forms of cancer (Stahl and Sies 2003). Due to its unique structure, it performs reactions in protecting lipophilic network and scavenges reactive species generated through photo-oxidative processes. A study in past has shown how carotenoids extracted from pepper exhibit significant analgesic and anti-inflammatory effects (Hernández-Ortega *et al.* 2012). Few oxidative metabolites of carotenoids, such as zeaxanthin, lutein,and meso-zeaxanthin referred to as macular pigment (MP) serve in ocular protective role *via* defending the biological system against age-related macular degeneration (AMD) (Arunkumar *et al.* 2018).

Flavonoids, the most common and active chemical constituent occurring naturally in food comprise of significant antioxidant and chelating properties. The antioxidant ability of flavonoids resides mainly in their ability to donate hydrogen atoms. Since they possess activities of both hydrophilic and lipophilic systems, they scavenge free radicals generated through lipid peroxidation (Sharififar *et al.* 2009). A recent report has shown that flavonoids can increase the expression of glyoxalase-1 and glyoxalase-2 in the glyoxalase pathway, which in turn is beneficial for retaining cellular functions in cerebellar neurons (Frandsen and Narayanasamy 2017). In past, various mechanisms have been proposed to elucidate anti-inflammatory action of flavonoids comprising radical scavenging, regulation of cellular activities in inflamed cells, inhibition or induction of large number of mammalian enzyme systems, and modifications in the generation of pro-inflammatory components (García-Lafuente *et al.* 2009). Recent studies suggest that flavonoids attenuate the inflammatory response and are therefore considered efficient in modulating the expression of pro-inflammatory genes (García-Lafuente *et al.* 2009, Guardia *et al.* 2001). Being antioxidant in nature, several isoforms of flavonoids inhibit ROS production by modulating human neutrophils' oxidative burst which in turn minimizes hazardous effects of the uncontrolled inflammatory response (Freitas *et al.* 2014, Ribeiro *et al.* 2013). Besides anti-inflammatory properties, flavonoids have been researched for its potential in anticancer studies. Various forms of flavonoids, from the dietary sources, either individually or in combination reduce the risk of cancer or limit the cellular damage. Various combinations of flavonoids produce synergistic anticancer action as observed in the studies of human ovarian carcinoma cells and breast cancer cells (Lopez-Lazaro 2002, Ren *et al.* 2003). Due to structural alterations, different forms of flavonoids show different activities such as antifungal and antimicrobial activities (Cushnie and Lamb 2005, Orhan *et al.* 2010). Anthocyanin, a potential iron chelator acts as a cardioprotective agent and prevents cardiotoxicity caused *via* formation of oxygen free radicals by doxorubicin (van Acker *et al.* 1996). Conclusively, flavonoids can be employed as potential agents in functional foods and dietary supplements for treating many health conditions or lowering the risk of such conditions.

Lipoic acid (1, 2-dithiolane-3-pentanoic acid) is a therapeutic drug having antioxidant properties and act as cofactor in mitochondrial oxidative metabolism (Biewenga *et al.* 1997a). The reduced form of lipoic acid is known as dihydrolipoic acid (DHLA), which has better antioxidant properties than lipoic acid. Lipoic acid shows mainly four types of antioxidant activity *i.e.* chelation of iron, scavenging reactive oxygen species, repair of oxidative damaged biomolecules and regeneration of endogenous antioxidant like vitamin C and vitamin E (Biewenga *et al.* 1997b, Scott *et al.* 1994). Lipoic acid causes chelation of Fe^{2+} and Cu^{2+} while DHLA causes Cd^{2+} chelation. DHLA can also show antioxidant activity by reduction of Fe^{3+} to Fe^{2+} (Biewenga *et al.* 1997b). Thus they prevent the arrival or delay of pathologies and also participate in damage repair mechanism. In Germany lipoic acid has been approved for effective management of diabetes associated risks like neuropathy. Lipoic acid improves the blood circulation, glucose metabolism and conduction of nerve impulses (Smith *et al.* 2004).

Antioxidant Supplements and Human Health

The oxidative stress derestricts series of cellular functions leading to various pathological disorders such as atherosclerosis, arthritis, autoimmune diseases, cancer, cardiovascular diseases and diabetes. It also leads to numerous neurodegenerative disorders for example Alzheimer's disease (AD), Parkinson's dementia (PD) (Sindhi *et al.* 2013). As oxidative stress is an important part of several human diseases, use of antioxidants is intensely studied, predominantly for the treatment of stroke, atherosclerosis and neurodegenerative diseases. (Hamid *et al.* 2010). Antioxidants diminish damaging effects of free radicals on cells and are therefore being considered for treatment of several forms of brain injuries (Sindhi *et al.* 2013). These antioxidants are broadly used as a therapeutic agent in the cure of various health conditions.

Atherosclerosis, an artery associated disease, is caused because of oxidative modification of low-density lipoproteins (LDL) (Niki 2004, Steinberg *et al.* 1989). This implies that the antioxidants which are capable of inhibiting LDL oxidation could be effective in fighting with atherosclerosis. However, some animal based studies have also shown inconsistency of antioxidants in treating atherosclerosis and even in some studies, negative effects have also been observed (Noguchi and Niki 2000). Such results suggest that LDL oxidation being mediated by several processes may require antioxidants with different mechanisms to be effective. For instance, vitamin E is the major antioxidant active against LDL oxidation mediated by free radicals but it is quite possible that vitamin E can not suppress the non-radical mediated LDL oxidation for which, vitamin C supplementation is a most suitable therapy (Niki 2004). The anti-atherogenic effect has been well illustrated for α tocopherols which inhibit monocyte-endothelial adhesion, cytokine release, platelet adhesion and aggregation, and scavenger receptor expression (Keaney *et al.* 1999).

The patients undergoing conventional cancer treatment are often recommended with antioxidant supplements which are believed to boost up the benefits of treatment, reduce side effects and improve overall health, however, the substantial evidences for any of these aspects are largely indirect (Burstein *et al.* 1999, Kelly *et al.* 2000, VandeCreek *et al.* 1999). Several compounds having antioxidant properties such as lanthanide, selenium, flavonoids, lycopene and glutathione are also known for their potential to act as anticancer agents. Therapeutic radioisotopes of lanthanides are being used in radioimmuno and photodynamic therapies (Kostova 2005). Flavonoids, good scavengers of free radicals are considered to bear potential anticarcinogenic effects. Nearly 28 primary and secondary flavonoids have been reported with anti-leukemic properties (Jain *et al.* 1994, Sindhi *et al.* 2013). Lycopene, another class of antioxidants, is known to be helpful in preventing cancer of colon, rectum, cervical, pancreas, ovaries, esophagus, oral cavity and large bowel (Sharoni *et al.* 2000). The antioxidant compounds like vitamin C and E have been found effective in treating patients with hepatocellular carcinoma (Singal *et al.* 2011).

Red blood cells (RBCs) are involved primarily in the transport of oxygen and carbon dioxide and are therefore at high risk of oxidative injuries due to regular encounter with intracellular ROS. The naturally occurring enzymes like superoxide dismutase and catalase accumulate over the membrane of RBCs and provide defense against oxidative stress (Li 2009). Premature infants are generally at high risk of developing retinopathy of prematurity, necrotizing enterocolitis, periventricular leukomalacia, and bronchopulmonary dysplasia, which can be suppressed by supplementation of enzymatic and non-enzymatic antioxidants (Lee and Davis 2011).

Rheumatoid arthritis (RA), characterized by progressive, erosive and chronic polyarthritis, manifests into destroyed articular cartilage and bone. Some past studies have shown the involvement of ROS in RA, where enhanced oxidative stress has been found associated with the development of this disease (Karatas *et al.* 2003, Mahajan and Tandon 2004). The anti-inflammatory role of superoxide dismutase and vitamin E has been strongly proposed in therapeutic studies which demonstrate controlled symptoms of arthritis in first month and better control of disease by the end of second month (Beharka *et al.* 2002, Helmy *et al.* 2001, Salvemini *et al.* 2001).

Cardiovascular diseases (CVDs) and coronary heart diseases (CHDs) are highly associated with consumption of alcohol and tobacco, physical inactivity, and high fat diets are one of the leading causes of deaths worldwide (Nothlings *et al.* 2008, Wang *et al.* 2016). Intake of leguminous foods, which are rich sources of antioxidant compounds like phenolics, phenolic acids, flavonoids, coumarins, hydrolysable and condensed tannins, stilbenes and lignins, have a promising effect on the reduction of CVDs and CHDs (Dauchet *et al.* 2005, Naczk and Shahidi 2004). The cardioprotective effect of these antioxidants may be attributed to their ability of limiting the generation of secondary intracellular ROS following H_2O_2 exposure (Angeloni *et al.* 2007, Park *et al.* 2009). Further, studies have demonstrated that pretreatment of cardiomyocytes with dietary antioxidants induces the expression of catalase, superoxide dismutase, and glutathione peroxidase which in turn prevent cardiomyocytes from undergoing oxidative stress induced programmed cell death (PCD) (Li and Förstermann 2009).

The brain is highly susceptible to oxidative injuries because it has high metabolic rate and increased concentration of polyunsaturated lipids which can undergo peroxidation. The neurodegenerative diseases such as Parkinson's disease (PD) and Alzheimer's disease (AD) are primarily the resultant of oxidative stress induced neuronal apoptosis and it is a well-known fact that these diseases can not be cured, therefore, there is need to design therapies to prevent them (Zhao 2009). In this direction, the use of antioxidants would be an appropriate step owing to their innate tendency to subdue oxidative stress. Flavonoids, polyphenols and nicotine are some of the natural antioxidants that can have a protecting role against AD and PD. Ginkgo biloba extract (EGb) being a rich source of flavonoids, ginkgolides and biolobalids may be useful in protecting brain against hypoxic damage and interrupting synthesis of ROS in cerebellar neurons (Ishige *et al.* 2001, Ni *et al.* 1996). The synergistic effect of flavonoid and terpenes to protect cerebellar granule cells from oxidative damage and apoptosis induced by hydroxyl radicals has been reported (Chen *et al.* 1999, Xin *et al.* 2000). Green tea polyphenols and catechins are also known to play a protective role in neurodegenerative disorders (Nanjo *et al.* 1996, Nie *et al.* 2001). The clinical trials with vitamin E and combinations of vitamin E, C and ubiquinone have shown great benefits for treating AD. Several other naturally occurring antioxidants like lipoic acid, β-carotene, creatine, melatonin and curcumin are also known for their potential to suppress AD (Grundman *et al.* 2002).

Cosmeceutical Aspects of Antioxidants

It is well illustrated that oxidation reactions produce free radicals that trigger chain reactions and damage skin cells resulting in wrinkling, elastosis, pigmentation, drying and photoaging of the skin. Therefore, the trend of incorporating antioxidants in cosmetics is increasing because these antioxidants can terminate chain reactions producing free radicals. Many plants produce natural antioxidant products which are highly capable of controlling oxidative stress mediated by sunlight and oxygen. An apt example of which can be turmeric that is in use since ancient times. The extracts from plants such as rosemary, green tea, basil grape, grape seed, tomato, blueberry, milk thistle, pine bark and acerola seed are used either single or in combinations in many cosmetic formulations (Kusumawati and Indrayanto 2013). These plant extracts are rich in natural antioxidant compounds like polyphenols, stibens, flavonols, flavonoids, carotenoids, essential oils, *etc.* (Andreassi *et al.* 2004, Baliga and Katiyar 2006). The natural and pure compounds like kojic acid, resveratrol and quercetin have been used in the formulations of various commercial products (Gediya *et al.* 2011, Kusumawati and Indrayanto 2013, Pouillot *et al.* 2011).

CONCLUSION AND FUTURE PERSPECTIVES

The reactions of ROS with food constituents generate several unwanted volatile compounds and carcinogens. These unwanted compounds combined with oxidative stress promotes tissue injuries and diseases in humans. Recent studies have revealed that occurrence of such diseases can be restricted by supplementing antioxidants in diet which interact with and stabilize ROS thus neutralizing their toxicity. Further, various aspects of antioxidants such as their medicinal uses, pharmacological upshots, therapeutic attributes and potential to act as food preservatives make them an important industrial candidate that could generate billions of dollars as a revenue. The unpredictable changes in the synthetic antioxidants during processing and storage restrict their use and may be detrimental to the consumer health. Since, modern consumer demands natural products without synthetic additives, therefore, antioxidants of natural origin will be in high demand in future. However, it is necessary to study changes and interactions of natural antioxidant compounds to validate their potentials and establish them as a suitable industrial candidate.

CONFLICT OF INTEREST

Authors declare no conflict of interest.

ACKNOWLEDGEMENT

No funding has been received from any agency for this work. However, we acknowledge the contribution of all the authors.

CONSENT FOR PUBLICATION

None

REFERENCES

Andreassi, M, Stanghellini, E, Ettorre, A, Di Stefano, A & Andreassi, L (2004) Antioxidant activity of topically applied lycopene. *J Eur Acad Dermatol Venereol,* 18, 52-5.
[http://dx.doi.org/10.1111/j.1468-3083.2004.00850.x] [PMID: 14678532]

Angeloni, C, Spencer, JP, Leoncini, E, Biagi, PL & Hrelia, S (2007) Role of quercetin and its in vivo metabolites in protecting H9c2 cells against oxidative stress. *Biochimie,* 89, 73-82.
[http://dx.doi.org/10.1016/j.biochi.2006.09.006] [PMID: 17045724]

Anttonen, MJ & Karjalainen, RO (2005) Environmental and genetic variation of phenolic compounds in red raspberry. *J Food Compos Anal,* 18, 759-69.
[http://dx.doi.org/10.1016/j.jfca.2004.11.003]

Arrigoni, O & De Tullio, MC (2002) Ascorbic acid: much more than just an antioxidant. *Biochimica et Biophysica Acta (BBA)-. General Subjects,* 1569, 1-9.
[http://dx.doi.org/10.1016/S0304-4165(01)00235-5]

Arunkumar, R, Calvo, CM, Conrady, CD & Bernstein, PS (2018) What do we know about the macular pigment in AMD: the past, the present, and the future. *Eye (Lond),* 32, 992-1004.
[http://dx.doi.org/10.1038/s41433-018-0044-0] [PMID: 29576617]

Augustyniak, A, Bartosz, G, Cipak, A, Duburs, G, Horáková, L, Luczaj, W, Majekova, M, Odysseos, AD, Rackova, L, Skrzydlewska, E, Stefek, M, Strosová, M, Tirzitis, G, Venskutonis, PR, Viskupicova, J, Vraka, PS & Zarković, N (2010) Natural and synthetic antioxidants: an updated overview. *Free Radic Res,* 44, 1216-62.
[http://dx.doi.org/10.3109/10715762.2010.508495] [PMID: 20836663]

Baiano, A (2014) Recovery of biomolecules from food wastes--a review. *Molecules,* 19, 14821-42.
[http://dx.doi.org/10.3390/molecules190914821] [PMID: 25232705]

Bakir, S, Catalkaya, G, Ceylan, FD, Khan, H, Guldiken, B, Capanoglu, E & Kamal, MA (2020) Role of dietary antioxidants in neurodegenerative diseases: Where are we standing? *Curr Pharm Des,* 26, 714-29.
[http://dx.doi.org/10.2174/1381612826666200107143619] [PMID: 31914905]

Baliga, MS & Katiyar, SK (2006) Chemoprevention of photocarcinogenesis by selected dietary botanicals. *Photochem Photobiol Sci,* 5, 243-53.
[http://dx.doi.org/10.1039/B505311K] [PMID: 16465310]

Becker, EM, Nissen, LR & Skibsted, LH (2004) Antioxidant evaluation protocols: Food quality or health effects. *Eur Food Res Technol,* 219, 561-71.
[http://dx.doi.org/10.1007/s00217-004-1012-4]

Beharka, AA, Wu, D, Serafini, M & Meydani, SN (2002) Mechanism of vitamin E inhibition of cyclooxygenase activity in macrophages from old mice: role of peroxynitrite. *Free Radic Biol Med,* 32, 503-11.
[http://dx.doi.org/10.1016/S0891-5849(01)00817-6] [PMID: 11958951]

Benvenuti, S, Bortolotti, E & Maggini, R (2016) Antioxidant power, anthocyanin content and organoleptic performance of edible flowers. *Sci Hortic (Amsterdam),* 199, 170-7.
[http://dx.doi.org/10.1016/j.scienta.2015.12.052]

Benvenuti, S & Pellati, F (2004) Polyphenols, anthocyanins, ascorbic acid, and radical scavenging activity of Rubus, Ribes, and Aronia. *J Food Sci,* 69, FCT164-9.
[http://dx.doi.org/10.1111/j.1365-2621.2004.tb13352.x]

Biewenga, GP, Haenen, GR & Bast, A (1997) The pharmacology of the antioxidant lipoic acid. *Gen Pharmacol,* 29, 315-31. a
[http://dx.doi.org/10.1016/S0306-3623(96)00474-0] [PMID: 9378235]

Biewenga, GP, Haenen, GR & Bast, A (1997) The pharmacology of the antioxidant lipoic acid. *Gen Pharmacol,* 29, 315-31. b
[http://dx.doi.org/10.1016/S0306-3623(96)00474-0] [PMID: 9378235]

Burstein, HJ, Gelber, S, Guadagnoli, E & Weeks, JC (1999) Use of alternative medicine by women with early-stage breast cancer. *N Engl J Med,* 340, 1733-9.
[http://dx.doi.org/10.1056/NEJM199906033402206] [PMID: 10352166]

Carr, AC, Zhu, BZ & Frei, B (2000) Potential antiatherogenic mechanisms of ascorbate (vitamin C) and alpha-tocopherol (vitamin E). *Circ Res,* 87, 349-54.
[http://dx.doi.org/10.1161/01.RES.87.5.349] [PMID: 10969031]

Castrica, M, Rebucci, R, Giromini, C, Tretola, M, Cattaneo, D & Baldi, A (2019) Total phenolic content and antioxidant capacity of agri-food waste and by-products. *Ital J Anim Sci,* 18, 336-41.
[http://dx.doi.org/10.1080/1828051X.2018.1529544]

Chambial, S, Dwivedi, S, Shukla, KK, John, PJ & Sharma, P (2013) Vitamin C in disease prevention and cure: an overview. *Indian J Clin Biochem,* 28, 314-28.
[http://dx.doi.org/10.1007/s12291-013-0375-3] [PMID: 24426232]

Chao, CT, Yeh, HY, Tsai, YT, Chuang, PH, Yuan, TH, Huang, JW & Chen, HW (2019) Natural and non-natural antioxidative compounds: potential candidates for treatment of vascular calcification. *Cell Death Discov,* 5, 145.
[http://dx.doi.org/10.1038/s41420-019-0225-z] [PMID: 31754473]

Chaovanalikit, A & Wrolstad, R (2004) Total anthocyanins and total phenolics of fresh and processed cherries and their antioxidant properties. *J Food Sci,* 69, FCT67-72.
[http://dx.doi.org/10.1111/j.1365-2621.2004.tb17858.x]

Chatterjee, PK, Patel, NS, Kvale, EO, Brown, PA, Stewart, KN, Mota-Filipe, H, Sharpe, MA, Di Paola, R, Cuzzocrea, S & Thiemermann, C (2004) EUK-134 reduces renal dysfunction and injury caused by oxidative and nitrosative stress of the kidney. *Am J Nephrol,* 24, 165-77.

[http://dx.doi.org/10.1159/000076547] [PMID: 14752229]

Chen, C, Wei, T, Gao, Z, Zhao, B, Hou, J, Xu, H, Xin, W & Packer, L (1999) Different effects of the constituents of EGb761 on apoptosis in rat cerebellar granule cells induced by hydroxyl radicals. *Biochem Mol Biol Int,* 47, 397-405.
[http://dx.doi.org/10.1080/15216549900201423] [PMID: 10204076]

Choudhari, SM & Ananthanarayan, L (2007) Enzyme aided extraction of lycopene from tomato tissues. *Food Chem,* 102, 77-81.
[http://dx.doi.org/10.1016/j.foodchem.2006.04.031]

Cushnie, TP & Lamb, AJ (2005) Antimicrobial activity of flavonoids. *Int J Antimicrob Agents,* 26, 343-56.
[http://dx.doi.org/10.1016/j.ijantimicag.2005.09.002] [PMID: 16323269]

Dauchet, L, Amouyel, P & Dallongeville, J (2005) Fruit and vegetable consumption and risk of stroke: a meta-analysis of cohort studies. *Neurology,* 65, 1193-7.
[http://dx.doi.org/10.1212/01.wnl.0000180600.09719.53] [PMID: 16247045]

Day, BJ (2008) Antioxidants as potential therapeutics for lung fibrosis. *Antioxid Redox Signal,* 10, 355-70.
[http://dx.doi.org/10.1089/ars.2007.1916] [PMID: 17999627]

Dietrich, M, Block, G, Norkus, EP, Hudes, M, Traber, MG, Cross, CE & Packer, L (2003) Smoking and exposure to environmental tobacco smoke decrease some plasma antioxidants and increase γ-tocopherol in vivo after adjustment for dietary antioxidant intakes. *Am J Clin Nutr,* 77, 160-6.
[http://dx.doi.org/10.1093/ajcn/77.1.160] [PMID: 12499336]

Dohi, T, Anamura, S, Shirakawa, M, Okamoto, H & Tsujimoto, A (1991) Inhibition of lipoxygenase by phenolic compounds. *Jpn J Pharmacol,* 55, 547-50.
[http://dx.doi.org/10.1016/S0021-5198(19)39925-1] [PMID: 1909391]

Du, J, Cullen, JJ & Buettner, GR (2012) Ascorbic acid: chemistry, biology and the treatment of cancer. *Biochimica et Biophysica Acta (BBA)-. Rev Can,* 1826, 443-57. a

Du, J, Cullen, JJ & Buettner, GR (2012) Ascorbic acid: chemistry, biology and the treatment of cancer. *Biochim Biophys Acta,* 1826, 443-57. b
[PMID: 22728050]

Erşan, S, Güçlü Üstündağ, Ö, Carle, R & Schweiggert, RM (2018) Subcritical water extraction of phenolic and antioxidant constituents from pistachio (Pistacia vera L.) hulls. *Food Chem,* 253, 46-54.
[http://dx.doi.org/10.1016/j.foodchem.2018.01.116] [PMID: 29502842]

Esposito, E & Cuzzocrea, S (2009) Superoxide, NO, peroxynitrite and PARP in circulatory shock and inflammation. *Front Biosci,* 14, 263-96.
[http://dx.doi.org/10.2741/3244] [PMID: 19273067]

Fierascu, RC, Fierascu, I, Avramescu, SM & Sieniawska, E (2019) Recovery of Natural Antioxidants from Agro-Industrial Side Streams through Advanced Extraction Techniques. *Molecules,* 24, 4212.
[http://dx.doi.org/10.3390/molecules24234212] [PMID: 31757027]

Frandsen, J & Narayanasamy, P (2017) Flavonoid Enhances the Glyoxalase Pathway in Cerebellar Neurons to Retain Cellular Functions. *Sci Rep,* 7, 5126.
[http://dx.doi.org/10.1038/s41598-017-05287-z] [PMID: 28698611]

Freitas, M, Ribeiro, D, Tomé, SM, Silva, AM & Fernandes, E (2014) Synthesis of chlorinated flavonoids with anti-inflammatory and pro-apoptotic activities in human neutrophils. *Eur J Med Chem,* 86, 153-64.
[http://dx.doi.org/10.1016/j.ejmech.2014.08.035] [PMID: 25151578]

García-Lafuente, A, Guillamón, E, Villares, A, Rostagno, MA & Martínez, JA (2009) Flavonoids as anti-inflammatory agents: implications in cancer and cardiovascular disease. *Inflamm Res,* 58, 537-52.
[http://dx.doi.org/10.1007/s00011-009-0037-3] [PMID: 19381780]

Gediya, SK, Mistry, RB, Patel, UK, Blessy, M & Jain, HN (2011) Herbal plants: used as a cosmetics. *J Nat Prod Plant Resour,* 1, 24-32.

Ghorbani, B, Pakkish, Z & Khezri, M (2018) Nitric oxide increases antioxidant enzyme activity and reduces chilling injury in orange fruit during storage. *N Z J Crop Hortic Sci,* 46, 101-16.
[http://dx.doi.org/10.1080/01140671.2017.1345764]

Gordon, M (1990) *The mechanism of antioxidant action in vitro Food antioxidants.*Springer.

Gorinstein, S, Martín-Belloso, O, Park, Y-S, Haruenkit, R, Lojek, A, Číž, M, Caspi, A, Libman, I & Trakhtenberg, S (2001) Comparison of some biochemical characteristics of different citrus fruits. *Food Chem,* 74, 309-15.
[http://dx.doi.org/10.1016/S0308-8146(01)00157-1]

Grundman, M, Grundman, M & Delaney, P (2002) Antioxidant strategies for Alzheimer's disease. *Proc Nutr Soc,* 61, 191-202.
[http://dx.doi.org/10.1079/PNS2002146] [PMID: 12133201]

Guardia, T, Rotelli, AE, Juarez, AO & Pelzer, LE (2001) Anti-inflammatory properties of plant flavonoids. Effects of rutin, quercetin and hesperidin on adjuvant arthritis in rat. *Farmaco,* 56, 683-7.
[http://dx.doi.org/10.1016/S0014-827X(01)01111-9] [PMID: 11680812]

Gunes, R, Palabiyik, I, Toker, OS, Konar, N & Kurultay, S (2019) Incorporation of defatted apple seeds in chewing gum system and phloridzin dissolution kinetics. *J Food Eng,* 255, 9-14.
[http://dx.doi.org/10.1016/j.jfoodeng.2019.03.010]

Gupta, VK & Sharma, SK (2006) *Plants as natural antioxidants*

Hägg, M (1996) Year) Published. Vitamins E, C, thiamine, riboflavin, α-and β-carotene in finnish and imported foods. *Proceedings of the technical workshop on trace elements, natural antioxidants and contaminants,* Helsinki-EspooAugust 25-26, 1995187-203.

Halliwell, B & Gutteridge, J (2007) Antioxidant defences: endogenous and diet derived. *Free Radic Biol Med,* 4, 79-186.

Halvorsen, BL, Holte, K, Myhrstad, MC, Barikmo, I, Hvattum, E, Remberg, SF, Wold, AB, Haffner, K, Baugerød, H, Andersen, LF, Moskaug, Ø, Jacobs, DR, Jr & Blomhoff, R (2002) A systematic screening of total antioxidants in dietary plants. *J Nutr,* 132, 461-71.
[http://dx.doi.org/10.1093/jn/132.3.461] [PMID: 11880572]

Hamid, A, Aiyelaagbe, O, Usman, L, Ameen, O & Lawal, A (2010) Antioxidants: Its medicinal and pharmacological applications. *African Journal of pure and applied chemistry,* 4, 142-51.

Hashemi, M, Hashemi, M, Daneshamooz, S, Raeisi, M, Jannat, B, Taheri, S & Noori, S (2020) An overview on antioxidants activity of polysaccharide edible films and coatings contains essential oils and herb extracts in meat and meat products. *Adv Anim Vet Sci,* 8, 198-207.
[http://dx.doi.org/10.17582/journal.aavs/2020/8.2.198.207]

Helmy, M, Shohayeb, M, Helmy, MH & el-Bassiouni, EA (2001) Antioxidants as adjuvant therapy in rheumatoid disease. A preliminary study. *Arzneimittelforschung,* 51, 293-8.
[PMID: 11367869]

Hernández-Ortega, M, Ortiz-Moreno, A, Hernández-Navarro, MD, Chamorro-Cevallos, G, Dorantes-Alvarez, L & Necoechea-Mondragón, H (2012) Antioxidant, antinociceptive, and anti-inflammatory effects of carotenoids extracted from dried pepper (Capsicum annuum L.). *J Biomed Biotechnol,* 2012524019
[http://dx.doi.org/10.1155/2012/524019] [PMID: 23091348]

Hernández-Ortega, M, Ortiz-Moreno, A, Hernández-Navarro, MD, Chamorro-Cevallos, G, Dorantes-Alvarez, L & Necoechea-Mondragón, H (2012) Antioxidant, antinociceptive, and anti-inflammatory effects of carotenoids extracted from dried pepper (Capsicum annuum L.). *J Biomed Biotechnol,* 2012524019
[http://dx.doi.org/10.1155/2012/524019] [PMID: 23091348]

Herrera, E & Barbas, C (2001) Vitamin E: action, metabolism and perspectives. *J Physiol Biochem,* 57, 43-56.
[http://dx.doi.org/10.1007/BF03179812]

Hofstrand, D (2008) Domestic perspectives on food *versus* fuel. *AgMRC Renew Energy News Lett,* 7, 1e6.

Ighodaro, O & Akinloye, O (2018) First line defence antioxidants-superoxide dismutase (SOD), catalase (CAT) and glutathione peroxidase (GPX): Their fundamental role in the entire antioxidant defence grid. *Alex J Med,* 54, 287-93.
[http://dx.doi.org/10.1016/j.ajme.2017.09.001]

Irshad, M & Chaudhuri, PS (2002) Oxidant-antioxidant system: role and significance in human body. *Indian J Exp Biol,* 40, 1233-9.
[PMID: 13677624]

Ishige, K, Schubert, D & Sagara, Y (2001) Flavonoids protect neuronal cells from oxidative stress by three distinct mechanisms. *Free Radic Biol Med,* 30, 433-46.
[http://dx.doi.org/10.1016/S0891-5849(00)00498-6] [PMID: 11182299]

Jain, M, Miller, AB & To, T (1994) Premorbid diet and the prognosis of women with breast cancer. *J Natl Cancer Inst,* 86, 1390-7.
[http://dx.doi.org/10.1093/jnci/86.18.1390] [PMID: 8072032]

Jakus, J & Farkas, O (2005) Photosensitizers and antioxidants: a way to new drugs? *Photochem Photobiol Sci,* 4, 694-8.
[http://dx.doi.org/10.1039/b417254j] [PMID: 16121279]

Kähkönen, MP, Hopia, AI, Vuorela, HJ, Rauha, J-P, Pihlaja, K, Kujala, TS & Heinonen, M (1999) Antioxidant activity of plant extracts containing phenolic compounds. *J Agric Food Chem,* 47, 3954-62.
[http://dx.doi.org/10.1021/jf990146l] [PMID: 10552749]

Kajarabille, N & Latunde-Dada, GO (2019) Programmed Cell-Death by Ferroptosis: Antioxidants as Mitigators. *Int J Mol Sci,* 20, 4968.
[http://dx.doi.org/10.3390/ijms20194968] [PMID: 31597407]

Kajimoto, G, Yamaguchi, M, Kusano, T, Goda, K & Yamamoto, J (1997) Antioxidant effects of barley aqueous extract on the oxidative deterioration of oil. *Nippon Shokuhin Kogyo Gakkaishi,* 44, 788-94.
[http://dx.doi.org/10.3136/nskkk.44.788]

Kallel, F & Ellouz Chaabouni, S (2017) Perspective of garlic processing wastes as low cost substrates for production of high added value products: A review. *Environ Prog Sustain Energy,* 36, 1765-77.
[http://dx.doi.org/10.1002/ep.12649]

Karatas, F, Ozates, I, Canatan, H, Halifeoglu, I, Karatepe, M & Colakt, R (2003) Antioxidant status & lipid peroxidation in patients with rheumatoid arthritis. *Indian J Med Res,* 118, 178-81.
[PMID: 14700353]

Kavanagh, RJ & Kam, PC (2001) Lazaroids: efficacy and mechanism of action of the 21-aminosteroids in neuroprotection. *Br J Anaesth,* 86, 110-9.
[http://dx.doi.org/10.1093/bja/86.1.110] [PMID: 11575384]

Keaney, JF, Jr, Simon, DI & Freedman, JE (1999) Vitamin E and vascular homeostasis: implications for atherosclerosis. *FASEB J,* 13, 965-75.
[http://dx.doi.org/10.1096/fasebj.13.9.965] [PMID: 10336880]

Kelly, KM, Jacobson, JS, Kennedy, DD, Braudt, SM, Mallick, M & Weiner, MA (2000) Use of unconventional therapies by children with cancer at an urban medical center. *J Pediatr Hematol Oncol,* 22, 412-6.
[http://dx.doi.org/10.1097/00043426-200009000-00005] [PMID: 11037851]

Knoblich, M, Anderson, B & Latshaw, D (2005) Analyses of tomato peel and seed byproducts and their use as a source of carotenoids. *J Sci Food Agric,* 85, 1166-70.
[http://dx.doi.org/10.1002/jsfa.2091]

Kopsell, DA & Kopsell, DE (2006) Accumulation and bioavailability of dietary carotenoids in vegetable crops. *Trends Plant Sci,* 11, 499-507.

[http://dx.doi.org/10.1016/j.tplants.2006.08.006] [PMID: 16949856]

Kostova, I (2005) Synthetic and natural coumarins as cytotoxic agents. *Curr Med Chem Anticancer Agents,* 5, 29-46.
[http://dx.doi.org/10.2174/1568011053352550] [PMID: 15720259]

Kurilich, AC & Juvik, JA (1999) Quantification of carotenoid and tocopherol antioxidants in Zea mays. *J Agric Food Chem,* 47, 1948-55.
[http://dx.doi.org/10.1021/jf981029d] [PMID: 10552476]

Kusumawati, I & Indrayanto, G (2013) *Natural antioxidants in cosmetics Studies in natural products chemistry.*Elsevier.

Lachman, J, Pronek, D, Hejtmánková, A, Dudjak, J, Pivec, V & Faitová, K (2003) Total polyphenol and main flavonoid antioxidants in different onion (Allium cepa L.) varieties. *Hortic Sci,* 30, 142-7.
[http://dx.doi.org/10.17221/3876-HORTSCI]

Larrosa, M, Llorach, R, Espín, JC & Tomás-Barberán, FA (2002) Increase of antioxidant activity of tomato juice upon functionalisation with vegetable byproduct extracts. *Lebensm Wiss Technol,* 35, 532-42.
[http://dx.doi.org/10.1006/fstl.2002.0907]

Lee, JW & Davis, JM (2011) Future applications of antioxidants in premature infants. *Curr Opin Pediatr,* 23, 161-6.
[http://dx.doi.org/10.1097/MOP.0b013e3283423e51] [PMID: 21150443]

Li, B (2009) *An antioxidant metabolon at the red blood cell membrane.*Concordia University.

Li, B, Smith, B & Hossain, MM (2006) Extraction of phenolics from citrus peels: II. Enzyme-assisted extraction method. *Separ Purif Tech,* 48, 189-96.
[http://dx.doi.org/10.1016/j.seppur.2005.07.019]

Li, H & Förstermann, U (2009) *Resveratrol: a multifunctional compound improving endothelial function.*Springer.

Liu, Q, Tang, GY, Zhao, CN, Feng, XL, Xu, XY, Cao, SY, Meng, X, Li, S, Gan, RY & Li, HB (2018) Comparison of Antioxidant Activities of Different Grape Varieties. *Molecules,* 23, 2432.
[http://dx.doi.org/10.3390/molecules23102432] [PMID: 30249027]

López-Lázaro, M (2002) Flavonoids as anticancer agents: structure-activity relationship study. *Curr Med Chem Anticancer Agents,* 2, 691-714.
[http://dx.doi.org/10.2174/1568011023353714] [PMID: 12678721]

Lu, Y & Foo, LY (2000) Antioxidant and radical scavenging activities of polyphenols from apple pomace. *Food Chem,* 68, 81-5.
[http://dx.doi.org/10.1016/S0308-8146(99)00167-3]

Lyckander, IM & Malterud, KE (1996) Lipophilic flavonoids from Orthosiphon spicatus prevent oxidative inactivation of 15-lipoxygenase. *Prostaglandins Leukot Essent Fatty Acids,* 54, 239-46.
[http://dx.doi.org/10.1016/S0952-3278(96)90054-X] [PMID: 8804120]

Mahajan, A & Tandon, VR (2004) Antioxidants and rheumatoid arthritis. *J Indian Rheumatol Assoc,* 12, 139-42.

Manach, C, Scalbert, A, Morand, C, Rémésy, C & Jiménez, L (2004) Polyphenols: food sources and bioavailability. *Am J Clin Nutr,* 79, 727-47.
[http://dx.doi.org/10.1093/ajcn/79.5.727] [PMID: 15113710]

Naczk, M & Shahidi, F (2004) Extraction and analysis of phenolics in food. *J Chromatogr A,* 1054, 95-111.
[http://dx.doi.org/10.1016/S0021-9673(04)01409-8] [PMID: 15553136]

Nanjo, F, Goto, K, Seto, R, Suzuki, M, Sakai, M & Hara, Y (1996) Scavenging effects of tea catechins and their derivatives on 1,1-diphenyl-2-picrylhydrazyl radical. *Free Radic Biol Med,* 21, 895-902.
[http://dx.doi.org/10.1016/0891-5849(96)00237-7] [PMID: 8902534]

Ni, Y, Zhao, B, Hou, J & Xin, W (1996) Protection of cerebellar neuron by Ginkgo-biloba extract against apoptosis induced by hydroxyl radicals. *Neuron Sci Letter,* 214, 115-8.
[http://dx.doi.org/10.1016/0304-3940(96)12897-4]

Nie, G, Wei, T, Shen, S & Zhao, B (2001) *Polyphenol protection of DNA against damage Methods in enzymology.*Elsevier.

Niki, E (2004) Antioxidants and atherosclerosis. *Biochem Soc Trans,* 32, 156-9.
[http://dx.doi.org/10.1042/bst0320156] [PMID: 14748738]

Noguchi, N & Niki, E (2000) Phenolic antioxidants: a rationale for design and evaluation of novel antioxidant drug for atherosclerosis. *Free Radic Biol Med,* 28, 1538-46.
[http://dx.doi.org/10.1016/S0891-5849(00)00256-2] [PMID: 10927179]

Nöthlings, U, Schulze, MB, Weikert, C, Boeing, H, van der Schouw, YT, Bamia, C, Benetou, V, Lagiou, P, Krogh, V, Beulens, JW, Peeters, PH, Halkjaer, J, Tjønneland, A, Tumino, R, Panico, S, Masala, G, Clavel-Chapelon, F, de Lauzon, B, Boutron-Ruault, MC, Vercambre, MN, Kaaks, R, Linseisen, J, Overvad, K, Arriola, L, Ardanaz, E, Gonzalez, CA, Tormo, MJ, Bingham, S, Khaw, KT, Key, TJ, Vineis, P, Riboli, E, Ferrari, P, Boffetta, P, Bueno-de-Mesquita, HB, van der A, DL, Berglund, G, Wirfält, E, Hallmans, G, Johansson, I, Lund, E & Trichopoulo, A (2008) Intake of vegetables, legumes, and fruit, and risk for all-cause, cardiovascular, and cancer mortality in a European diabetic population. *J Nutr,* 138, 775-81.
[http://dx.doi.org/10.1093/jn/138.4.775] [PMID: 18356334]

Olsson, ME, Gustavsson, KE, Andersson, S, Nilsson, A & Duan, RD (2004) Inhibition of cancer cell proliferation in vitro by fruit and berry extracts and correlations with antioxidant levels. *J Agric Food Chem,* 52, 7264-71.
[http://dx.doi.org/10.1021/jf030479p] [PMID: 15563205]

Orhan, DD, Ozçelik, B, Özgen, S & Ergun, F (2010) Antibacterial, antifungal, and antiviral activities of some flavonoids. *Microbiol Res,* 165, 496-504.
[http://dx.doi.org/10.1016/j.micres.2009.09.002] [PMID: 19840899]

Palozza, P & Krinsky, NI (1992) *Antioxidant effects of carotenoids in Vivo and in Vitro: An overview Methods in enzymology.*Elsevier. [38]

Pandolfo, M (2008) Drug Insight: antioxidant therapy in inherited ataxias. *Nat Clin Pract Neurol,* 4, 86-96.
[http://dx.doi.org/10.1038/ncpneuro0704] [PMID: 18256680]

Park, S, Kim, MY, Lee, DH, Lee, SH, Baik, EJ, Moon, CH, Park, SW, Ko, EY, Oh, SR & Jung, YS (2009) Methanolic extract of onion (Allium cepa) attenuates ischemia/hypoxia-induced apoptosis in cardiomyocytes *via* antioxidant effect. *Eur J Nutr,* 48, 235-42.
[http://dx.doi.org/10.1007/s00394-009-0007-0] [PMID: 19234663]

Pastrana-Bonilla, E, Akoh, CC, Sellappan, S & Krewer, G (2003) Phenolic content and antioxidant capacity of muscadine grapes. *J Agric Food Chem,* 51, 5497-503.
[http://dx.doi.org/10.1021/jf030113c] [PMID: 12926904]

Patel, A, Liebner, F, Netscher, T, Mereiter, K & Rosenau, T (2007) Vitamin E chemistry. Nitration of non-alpha-tocopherols: products and mechanistic considerations. *J Org Chem,* 72, 6504-12.
[http://dx.doi.org/10.1021/jo0706832] [PMID: 17636958]

Peralta-Ramírez, A, Montes de Oca, A, Raya, AI, Pineda, C, López, I, Guerrero, F, Diez, E, Muñoz-Castañeda, JR, Martinez, J, Almaden, Y, Rodríguez, M & Aguilera-Tejero, E (2014) Vitamin E protection of obesity-enhanced vascular calcification in uremic rats. *Am J Physiol Renal Physiol,* 306, F422-9.
[http://dx.doi.org/10.1152/ajprenal.00355.2013] [PMID: 24370590]

Pestana-Bauer, VR, Zambiazi, RC, Mendonça, CR, Beneito-Cambra, M & Ramis-Ramos, G (2012) γ-Oryzanol and tocopherol contents in residues of rice bran oil refining. *Food Chem,* 134, 1479-83.
[http://dx.doi.org/10.1016/j.foodchem.2012.03.059] [PMID: 25005970]

Pouillot, A, Polla, LL, Tacchini, P, Neequaye, A, Polla, A & Polla, B (2011) Natural antioxidants and their effects on the skin. *Formulating, packaging, and marketing of natural cosmetic products,* 239-57.

Ren, W, Qiao, Z, Wang, H, Zhu, L & Zhang, L (2003) Flavonoids: promising anticancer agents. *Med Res Rev,* 23, 519-34.
[http://dx.doi.org/10.1002/med.10033] [PMID: 12710022]

Reunanen, A, Knekt, P, Aaran, RK & Aromaa, A (1998) Serum antioxidants and risk of non-insulin dependent diabetes mellitus. *Eur J Clin Nutr,* 52, 89-93.
[http://dx.doi.org/10.1038/sj.ejcn.1600519] [PMID: 9505151]

Reyes Carmona, J, Yousef, GG, Martínez Peniche, RA & Lila, MA (2005) Antioxidant capacity of fruit extracts of blackberry (Rubus sp.) produced in different climatic regions. *J Food Sci,* 70, s497-503.
[http://dx.doi.org/10.1111/j.1365-2621.2005.tb11498.x]

Ribeiro, D, Freitas, M, Tomé, SM, Silva, AM, Porto, G & Fernandes, E (2013) Modulation of human neutrophils' oxidative burst by flavonoids. *Eur J Med Chem,* 67, 280-92.
[http://dx.doi.org/10.1016/j.ejmech.2013.06.019] [PMID: 23871908]

Richard Forget, F, Gauillard, F, Hugues, M, Jean Marc, T, Boivin, P & Nicolas, J (1995) Inhibition of horse bean and germinated barley lipoxygenases by some phenolic compounds. *J Food Sci,* 60, 1325-9.
[http://dx.doi.org/10.1111/j.1365-2621.1995.tb04583.x]

Rodrigues, S, Pinto, GA & Fernandes, FA (2008) Optimization of ultrasound extraction of phenolic compounds from coconut (Cocos nucifera) shell powder by response surface methodology. *Ultrason Sonochem,* 15, 95-100.
[http://dx.doi.org/10.1016/j.ultsonch.2007.01.006] [PMID: 17400017]

Salvemini, D, Mazzon, E, Dugo, L, Serraino, I, De Sarro, A, Caputi, AP & Cuzzocrea, S (2001) Amelioration of joint disease in a rat model of collagen-induced arthritis by M40403, a superoxide dismutase mimetic. *Arthritis Rheum,* 44, 2909-21.
[http://dx.doi.org/10.1002/1529-0131(200112)44:12<2909::AID-ART479>3.0.CO;2-#] [PMID: 11762952]

Sánchez, C (2009) Lignocellulosic residues: biodegradation and bioconversion by fungi. *Biotechnol Adv,* 27, 185-94.
[http://dx.doi.org/10.1016/j.biotechadv.2008.11.001] [PMID: 19100826]

Scott, BC, Aruoma, OI, Evans, PJ, O'Neill, C, Van der Vliet, A, Cross, CE, Tritschler, H & Halliwell, B (1994) Lipoic and dihydrolipoic acids as antioxidants. A critical evaluation. *Free Radic Res,* 20, 119-33.
[http://dx.doi.org/10.3109/10715769409147509] [PMID: 7516789]

Sharififar, F, Dehghn-Nudeh, G & Mirtajaldini, M (2009) Major flavonoids with antioxidant activity from Teucrium polium L. *Food Chem,* 112, 885-8.
[http://dx.doi.org/10.1016/j.foodchem.2008.06.064]

Sharoni, Y, Danilenko, M & Levy, J (2000) Molecular mechanisms for the anticancer activity of the carotenoid lycopene. *Drug Dev Res,* 50, 448-56.
[http://dx.doi.org/10.1002/1098-2299(200007/08)50:3/4<448::AID-DDR28>3.0.CO;2-U]

Sies, H & Stahl, W (1995) Vitamins E and C, beta-carotene, and other carotenoids as antioxidants. *Am J Clin Nutr,* 62 (Suppl.), 1315S-21S.
[http://dx.doi.org/10.1093/ajcn/62.6.1315S] [PMID: 7495226]

Sikora, E, Cieślik, E, Leszczyńska, T, Filipiak-Florkiewicz, A & Pisulewski, PM (2008) The antioxidant activity of selected cruciferous vegetables subjected to aquathermal processing. *Food Chem,* 107, 55-9.
[http://dx.doi.org/10.1016/j.foodchem.2007.07.023]

Sindhi, V, Gupta, V, Sharma, K, Bhatnagar, S, Kumari, R & Dhaka, N (2013) Potential applications of antioxidants–A review. *J Pharm Res,* 7, 828-35.
[http://dx.doi.org/10.1016/j.jopr.2013.10.001]

Singal, AK, Jampana, SC & Weinman, SA (2011) Antioxidants as therapeutic agents for liver disease. *Liver Int,* 31, 1432-48.
[http://dx.doi.org/10.1111/j.1478-3231.2011.02604.x] [PMID: 22093324]

Siriwoharn, T & Wrolstad, R (2004) Polyphenolic composition of Marion and Evergreen blackberries. *J Food Sci,* 69, FCT233-40.
[http://dx.doi.org/10.1111/j.1365-2621.2004.tb06322.x]

Smith, AR, Shenvi, SV, Widlansky, M, Suh, JH & Hagen, TM (2004) Lipoic acid as a potential therapy for chronic diseases associated with oxidative stress. *Curr Med Chem,* 11, 1135-46.
[http://dx.doi.org/10.2174/0929867043365387] [PMID: 15134511]

Stahl, W & Sies, H (2003) Antioxidant activity of carotenoids. *Mol Aspects Med,* 24, 345-51.
[http://dx.doi.org/10.1016/S0098-2997(03)00030-X] [PMID: 14585305]

Steinberg, D, Carew, TE, Fielding, C, Fogelman, AM, Mahley, RW, Sniderman, AD & Zilversmit, DB (1989) Lipoproteins and the pathogenesis of atherosclerosis. *Circulation,* 80, 719-23.
[http://dx.doi.org/10.1161/01.CIR.80.3.719] [PMID: 2670321]

Stewart, AJ, Mullen, W & Crozier, A (2005) On-line high-performance liquid chromatography analysis of the antioxidant activity of phenolic compounds in green and black tea. *Mol Nutr Food Res,* 49, 52-60.
[http://dx.doi.org/10.1002/mnfr.200400064] [PMID: 15602765]

Taruscio, TG, Barney, DL & Exon, J (2004) Content and profile of flavanoid and phenolic acid compounds in conjunction with the antioxidant capacity for a variety of northwest Vaccinium berries. *J Agric Food Chem,* 52, 3169-76.
[http://dx.doi.org/10.1021/jf0307595] [PMID: 15137871]

Tremocoldi, MA, Rosalen, PL, Franchin, M, Massarioli, AP, Denny, C, Daiuto, ER, Paschoal, JAR, Melo, PS & Alencar, SM (2018) Exploration of avocado by-products as natural sources of bioactive compounds. *PLoS One,* 13e0192577
[http://dx.doi.org/10.1371/journal.pone.0192577] [PMID: 29444125]

Ülker, S, McKeown, PP & Bayraktutan, U (2003) Vitamins reverse endothelial dysfunction through regulation of eNOS and NAD(P)H oxidase activities. *Hypertension,* 41, 534-9.
[http://dx.doi.org/10.1161/01.HYP.0000057421.28533.37] [PMID: 12623955]

Vallejo, F, Tomás Barberán, F & García Viguera, C (2003) Phenolic compound contents in edible parts of broccoli inflorescences after domestic cooking. *J Sci Food Agric,* 83, 1511-6.
[http://dx.doi.org/10.1002/jsfa.1585]

van Acker, SA, van den Berg, DJ, Tromp, MN, Griffioen, DH, van Bennekom, WP, van der Vijgh, WJ & Bast, A (1996) Structural aspects of antioxidant activity of flavonoids. *Free Radic Biol Med,* 20, 331-42.
[http://dx.doi.org/10.1016/0891-5849(95)02047-0] [PMID: 8720903]

VandeCreek, L, Rogers, E & Lester, J (1999) Use of alternative therapies among breast cancer outpatients compared with the general population. *Altern Ther Health Med,* 5, 71-6.
[PMID: 9893318]

Veeruraj, A, Liu, L, Zheng, J, Wu, J & Arumugam, M (2019) Evaluation of astaxanthin incorporated collagen film developed from the outer skin waste of squid Doryteuthis singhalensis for wound healing and tissue regenerative applications. *Mater Sci Eng C,* 95, 29-42.
[http://dx.doi.org/10.1016/j.msec.2018.10.055] [PMID: 30573252]

Verma, RS, Mehta, A & Srivastava, N (2007) In vivo chlorpyrifos induced oxidative stress: attenuation by antioxidant vitamins. *Pestic Biochem Physiol,* 88, 191-6.
[http://dx.doi.org/10.1016/j.pestbp.2006.11.002]

Vu, HT, Scarlett, CJ & Vuong, QV (2018) Phenolic compounds within banana peel and their potential uses: A review. *J Funct Foods,* 40, 238-48.
[http://dx.doi.org/10.1016/j.jff.2017.11.006]

Wang, B, Yan, Y, Tian, Y, Zhao, W, Li, Z, Gao, J, Peng, R & Yao, Q (2016) Heterologous expression and characterisation of a laccase from Colletotrichum lagenarium and decolourisation of different synthetic dyes. *World J Microbiol Biotechnol,* 32, 40.

[http://dx.doi.org/10.1007/s11274-015-1999-7] [PMID: 26867601]

Wei Yao, W, Mei Peng, H & Webster, RD (2009) Electrochemistry of α-tocopherol (vitamin E) and α-tocopherol quinone films deposited on electrode surfaces in the presence and absence of lipid multilayers. *J Phys Chem C,* 113, 21805-14.
[http://dx.doi.org/10.1021/jp9079124]

Wilson, JX (2009) Mechanism of action of vitamin C in sepsis: ascorbate modulates redox signaling in endothelium. *Biofactors,* 35, 5-13.
[http://dx.doi.org/10.1002/biof.7] [PMID: 19319840]

Woodson, K, Albanes, D, Tangrea, JA, Rautalahti, M, Virtamo, J & Taylor, PR (1999) Association between alcohol and lung cancer in the alpha-tocopherol, beta-carotene cancer prevention study in Finland. *Cancer Causes Control,* 10, 219-26.
[http://dx.doi.org/10.1023/A:1008911624785] [PMID: 10454067]

Wu, X, Beecher, GR, Holden, JM, Haytowitz, DB, Gebhardt, SE & Prior, RL (2004) Lipophilic and hydrophilic antioxidant capacities of common foods in the United States. *J Agric Food Chem,* 52, 4026-37.
[http://dx.doi.org/10.1021/jf049696w] [PMID: 15186133]

Xin, W, Wei, T, Chen, C, Ni, Y, Zhao, B & Hou, J (2000) Mechanisms of apoptosis in rat cerebellar granule cells induced by hydroxyl radicals and the effects of EGb761 and its constituents. *Toxicology,* 148, 103-10.
[http://dx.doi.org/10.1016/S0300-483X(00)00200-6] [PMID: 10962128]

Xu, J, Wei, R, Jia, Z & Song, R (2020) Characteristics and bioactive functions of chitosan/gelatin-based film incorporated with ε-polylysine and astaxanthin extracts derived from by-products of shrimp (Litopenaeus vannamei). *Food Hydrocoll,* 100105436
[http://dx.doi.org/10.1016/j.foodhyd.2019.105436]

Yang, CS, Lu, G, Ju, J & Li, GX (2010) Inhibition of inflammation and carcinogenesis in the lung and colon by tocopherols. *Ann N Y Acad Sci,* 1203, 29-34.
[http://dx.doi.org/10.1111/j.1749-6632.2010.05561.x] [PMID: 20716280]

Yanishlieva-Maslarova, N & Heinonen, I (2001) Sources of natural antioxidants: vegetables, fruits, herbs, spices and teas. Antioxidants in food *practical applications,* 66-210.

Zadernowski, R, Nowak, H & Kozlowska, H (1991) Year) Published. Natural antioxidants from rapeseed. Rapeseed in a Changing World *8th International Rapeseed Congress,* July 9–11Saskatoon883-7.

Zago, E, Lecomte, J, Barouh, N, Aouf, C, Carré, P, Fine, F & Villeneuve, P (2015) Influence of rapeseed meal treatments on its total phenolic content and composition in sinapine, sinapic acid and canolol. *Ind Crops Prod,* 76, 1061-70.
[http://dx.doi.org/10.1016/j.indcrop.2015.08.022]

Zhao, B (2009) Natural antioxidants protect neurons in Alzheimer's disease and Parkinson's disease. *Neurochem Res,* 34, 630-8.
[http://dx.doi.org/10.1007/s11064-008-9900-9] [PMID: 19125328]

CHAPTER 17

Antioxidants in Cancer Prevention and Combination Therapy

Safura Nisar[1,#], **Basharat Ahmad Bhat**[1,#], **Umar Mehraj**[1], **Hina Qayoom**[1], **Wajahat Rashid Mir**[1] and **Manzoor Ahmad Mir**[1,*]

[1] *Department of Bioresources, School of Biological Sciences, University of Kashmir, Srinagar-190006, J&K, India*

Abstract: Combination therapy, also known as polytherapy, is a form of treatment that involves the use of several drugs. In fact, the term applies to the use of various treatments to cure a particular illness, with pharmaceutical therapies being the most common. Non-medical treatment, such as the use of a mixture of medications and psychotherapy to relieve depression, may also be used. Polypharmacy, which applies to the usage of multiple medications, is also a related term. When referring to prescription combination treatment, the term polymedicine is also used. The antioxidant protection mechanism, which is responsible for reducing a wide variety of oxidants like reactive oxygen species (ROS), lipid peroxides, and metals, *etc.,* maintains redox homeostasis. Antioxidants are used to guard against the harmful consequences of oxidation and as nutritional additives to counteract the negative effects of stress. Antioxidants are compounds that may prevent or delay cell damage induced by free radicals, which are reactive molecules produced by the body in response to external environmental and other stress. Free-radical scavengers is a term used to describe them. Antioxidants may come from either natural or synthetic sources. Many plant-based foods are thought to have high levels of antioxidants. Plant-based antioxidants are phytonutrients that contribute to disease prevention. These phytonutrients as single entity or in combination have demonstrated beneficial effects in several models and might protect against cancer.

Keywords: Antioxidants, Cancer, Carotenoids, Chemotherapy, Combinational therapy, Free-radicals, Homeostasis, Immunity, Oxidative stress, Reactive oxygen species, Scavengers, Therapeutics, Tumor, Zeaxanthin.

INTRODUCTION

Antioxidants are the constituents that are present abundantly in foods. At small

* **Corresponding author Manzoor Ahmad Mir:** Department of Bioresources, School of Biological Sciences, University of Kashmir, Srinagar-190006, J&K, India;
E-mails: mirmanzoor110@gmail.com and drmanzoor@kashmiruniversity.ac.in
Equal First Author Contribution

Pardeep Kaur, Rajendra G. Mehta, Robin, Tarunpreet Singh Thind and Saroj Arora (Eds.)

concentrations as compared to that of an oxidizable substrate, these compounds substantially delays or averts the oxidation of that substrate. Food manufacturers often use food-grade antioxidants to maintain products' nutritious value while preventing deterioration of their quality. (Senanayake *et al.* 2005, Guo 2013). Biochemists and health practitioners also have an interest in antioxidants because these can help the body defend itself from harm caused by the reactive oxygen (ROS), nitrogen (RNS), and chlorine (RCS) species (Pisoschi and Pop 2015, Winterbourn *et al.* 2016). A number of reactive species including, oxygen radicals, are generated continuously under certain physiological conditions, resulting in severe oxidative damage (Sgherri *et al.* 2018). This free radical generation leads to the development of an efficient defense system in all biological organisms. Therefore, it is assumed that with the evolution of aerobic organisms, there is a development of defense systems with varied functions of antioxidants (Di Meo and Venditti 2020).

Butylated hydroxyanisole (BHA), propyl gallate (PG), butylated hydroxytoluene (BHT), and tert-butyl hydroquinone (TBHQ) are some of the most commonly found antioxidants in foods (Fig. **1 A-D**).

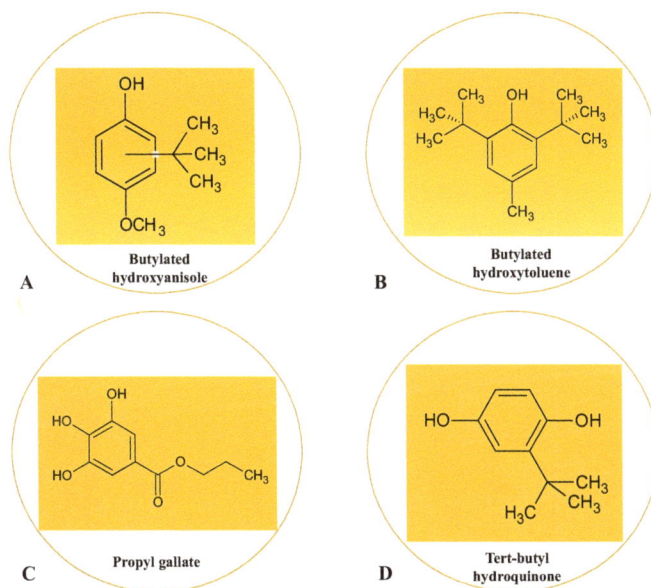

Fig. (1). (A-D) This figure represents the commonly used antioxidants in food like **(A)** Butylated hydroxyanisole (BHA), **(B)** Butylated hydroxytoluene (BHT), **(C)** Propyl gallate (PG) and **(D)** Tert-butylhydroquinone (TBHQ).

The class of phenolic or polyphenolic compounds contains the most potent dietary antioxidants. Phenolic compounds occurring in foods belong to the phenylpropanoids (C6-C3) family and are derivative forms of cinnamic acid. These compounds are formed from the phenylalanine, and to a lesser degree, from tyrosine in certain plants, by way of phenylalanine ammonia lyase's (PAL) mechanism of action, or its corresponding tyrosine lyase (Peter 2012, Cooper and Nicola 2014, Cseke *et al.* 2016) as depicted in the Fig. (**2**).

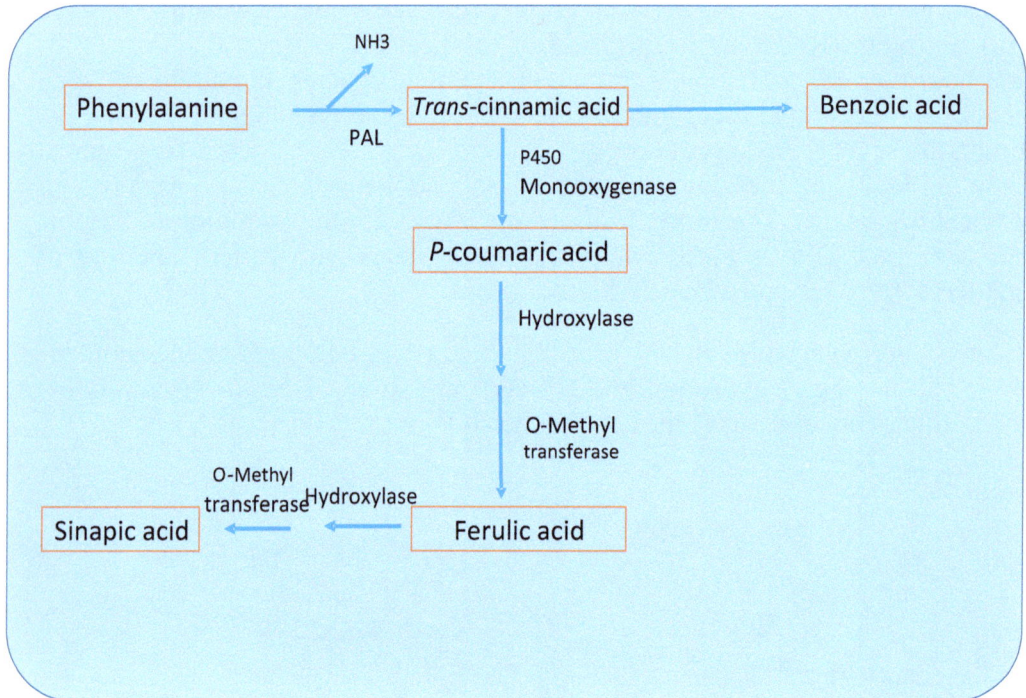

Fig. (2). Biosynthesis of phenylpropanoids and phenolic acids.

Following the loss of a two-carbon moiety, benzoic acid derivatives can be produced from C6–C3 compounds. The participation of malonyl coenzyme A in the condensation of C6–C3 compounds results in the production of chalcones, which can then cyclize under acidic conditions to create flavonoids and isoflavonoids (Fig. **3**) (Vermerris and Nicholson 2007, Hoda *et al.* 2019).

Oxidants and Antioxidants: Basic Concepts

The production and action of ROS acting as oxidants (molecules that have a propensity to donate the oxygen to the other molecules) are accountable for much of oxygen's potentially deleterious outcomes. (Husain *et al.* 2012, Sies and Jones 2020, Saed-Moucheshi *et al.* 2014). ROS are formed in the human body on a continuous basis as a result of natural physiological processes. Free radicals formed as a result of different reactions (Husain *et al.* 2012, Sies and Jones 2020) are shown in Fig. (**4**).

Continued activation of free radicals damages cellular biomolecules containing proteins, carbohydrates, lipids and nucleic acids. Reactions involved in free radical attack on lipids and the types of damage resulted from such actions (Lobo *et al.* 2010, Phaniendra *et al.* 2015) are illustrated in the Fig. (**5**).

Many of such effects have drawn in a number of degenerative diseases; for example, cataracts due to the effects on protein, cancer due to the effects on DNA, atherosclerosis due to the effects on lipids (Phaniendra *et al.* 2015, Sivanandham 2011). It should be known that free radicals are not always harmful. They also provide useful purpose in humans; for instance, free radicals play a key part in destructing microbes that are disease causing *via* phagocytosis by specialized blood cells (Lobo *et al.* 2010, Halliwell and Gutteridge 2015).

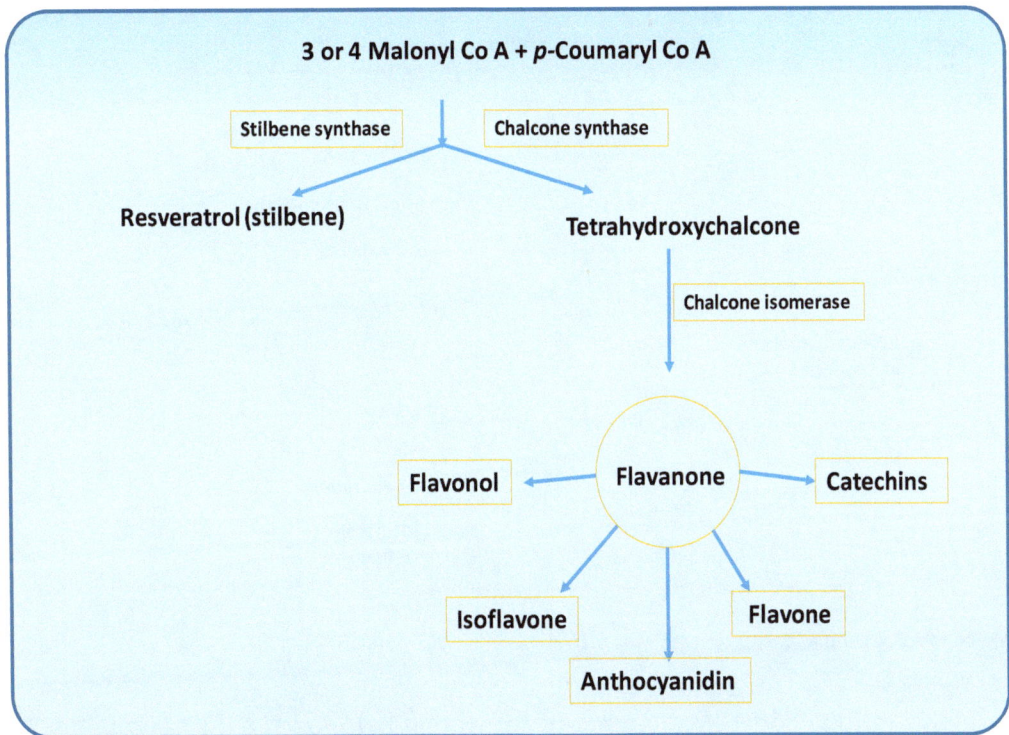

Fig. (3). Biosynthesis of flavonoids.

Enzymatic free radical formation

$$\text{Xanthine} + O_2 + H_2O \xrightarrow{\text{Xanthine oxidase}} \text{Urate} + O_2^{-\bullet} + 2H^+$$

$$\text{NADPH} + 2O_2 \xrightarrow{\text{NADPH oxidase}} \text{NADP}^+ + 2O_2^{-\bullet} + H^+$$

$$\text{NADPH} + 2 \text{ Quinone} \xrightarrow{\text{Cytochrome P450 reductase}} \text{NADP}^+ + 2 \text{ semiquinone} + H^+$$

Non-enzymatic free radical formation

$$Fe^{2+} + H_2O_2 \longrightarrow Fe^{3+} + {}^{\bullet}OH + OH^-$$

$$Fe^{3+} + O_2^{\bullet} \longrightarrow Fe^{2+} + O_2$$

Lipid oxidation by radical attack

$$LH + {}^{\bullet}OH \longrightarrow L^{\bullet} + H_2O$$

$$L^{\bullet} + O_2 \longrightarrow LOO^{\bullet}$$

$$LOO^{\bullet} + LH \longrightarrow LOOH + L^{\bullet} \longrightarrow \text{chain reaction}$$

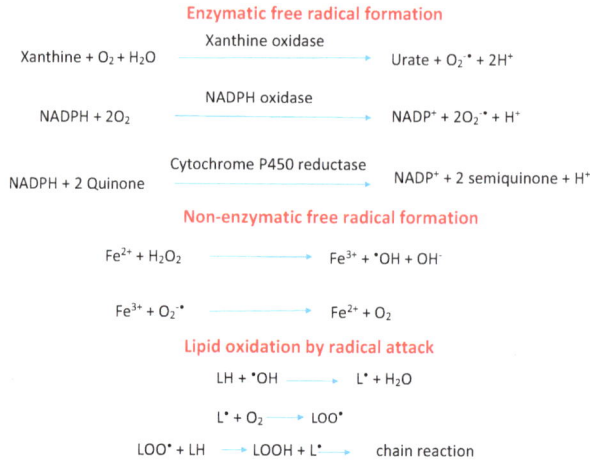

Fig. (4). Reactions that trigger the formation of free radicals.

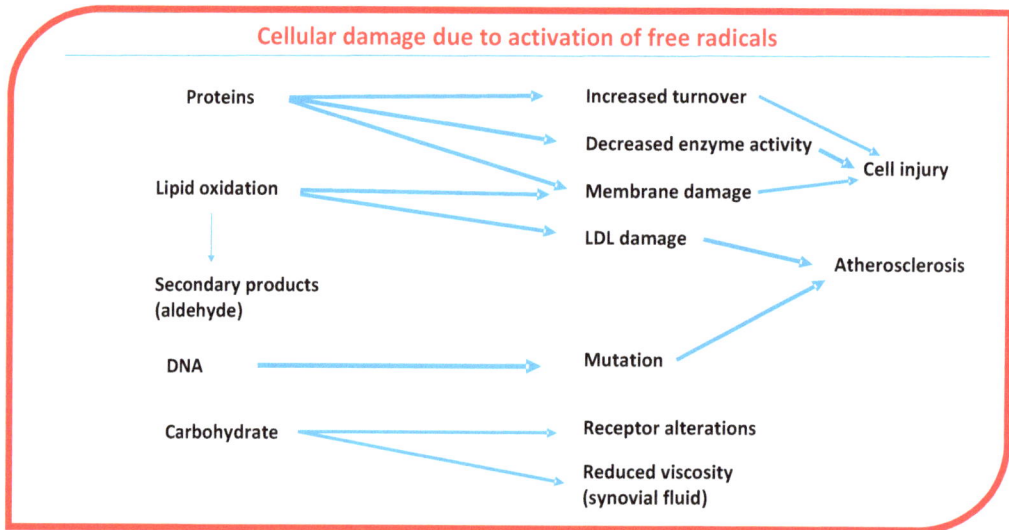

Fig. (5). Number of cellular damages due to the activation of the free radicals.

Antioxidants in food come in a number of forms that help to keep diseases at bay. All of these are essential nutrients in significant amounts needed by our body (Langseth 1995, Suleman *et al.* 2019). The epidemiological as well as clinical studies have provided evidence that antioxidants occur in cereals, fruits and vegetables (Kaur and Kapoor 2001, Miller *et al.* 2000). All of these are chief contributing factors in reducing the incidence of both chronic as well as degenerative diseases, especially among the people whose diet is rich in specific foods containing natural antioxidants (Willcox *et al.* 2004, Liu *et al.* 2018,

Landete 2013). Natural antioxidants in plants can be extracted and added as a component into food formulation either to enhance the stability or to increase the antioxidant activity (Pokorný *et al.* 2001, da Silva *et al.* 2016).

Tocopherols: Edible oils and oilseeds, a rich source of unsaponifiable matter contain a variety of active ingredients that are used to prevent or control many deteriorative processes (O'brien 2008, Nagaraj 2009). Tocopherols and tocotrienols, collectively referred to as tocols, are non-triacylglycerol components in oils and oilseeds. Oils and oilseeds contain phenolics and flavonoids, sterols, phospholipids, carotenoids, and triterpene alcohols as well as the phytic acid family of compounds. Tocopherols are widely present in plant species, and are monophenolic and lipophilic compounds as shown in Fig. (**6**).

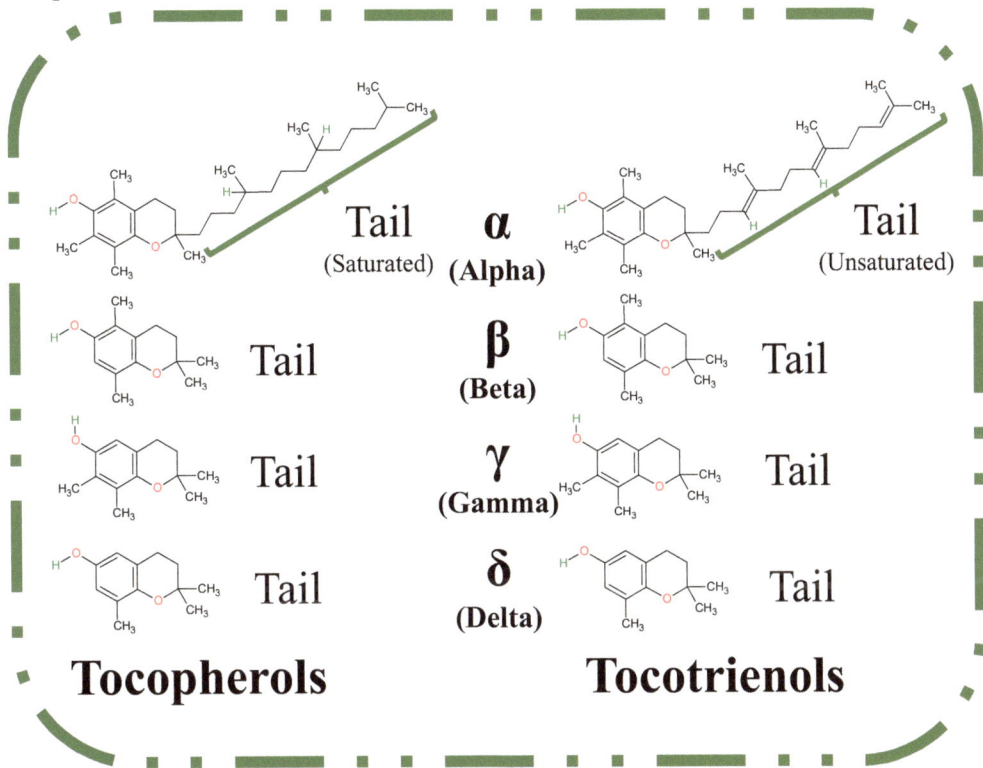

Fig. (6). Tocopherols as monophenolic and lipophilic compounds.

There are almost eight different tocopherols possessing the vitamin E activity of which all or some are present in various edible oil sources. The tocopherols and tocotrienols are classified into different groups depending upon the quantity and location of methyl groups on the chromane ring; as: alpha, beta, gamma and delta (Shahidi 2000, Sen *et al.* 2007, Singh *et al.* 2013). The alpha-tocopherol with respect to vitamin E activity is the most powerful compound present.

Spices and herbs: The spices and herbs are used in diets since times immemorial to enhance their taste and aroma. Some studies show that sage, mace and black pepper inhibited oxidation of frozen meat (Bilderback 2007, Staub 2008). Even extracts of rosemary, sage and thyme retarted oxidation. Among the herbs and spices rosemary and sage extracts are most important plants with their increased application in food formulations (Berdahl and McKeague 2015, Shahidi 2000, Bubonja-Sonje *et al.* 2011).

Teas and tea extracts: Teas of various types, such as non-fermented (green), semi-fermented (oolong), and fermented (black), are consumed all over the world. The extracts from such teas are now commercially accessible as the antioxidants to prevent degradation of food lipids (Pasrija and Anandharamakrishnan 2015, Luximon-Ramma *et al.* 2005, Rahman 2016). Tea is one such material that contains very high content of polyphenolics. The antioxidant action of green tea often exceeds that of black tea and its extracts. Green tea extracts may even exert a pro-oxidant activity under photo-oxidative conditions, due to the presence of chlorophyll that acts as a photosensitizer (Wang *et al.* 2003, Rahman 2016).

Interactions between Different Antioxidants

Antioxidants, along with their individual effects, can interact with other as well in synergistic ways showing pronounced effects. Antioxidants have sparing effect as well where one antioxidant protects another against any oxidative stress (Langseth 1995, Simioni *et al.* 2018). For example, after interacting with a free radical, vitamin C enhances the antioxidant activity of vitamin E through rejuvenating the active form of the vitamin. There are a number of beneficial interactions being demonstrated in all biological systems. One more evidence is ubiquinol, a fat-soluble antioxidant created in the human body, might also generate vitamin E (Burton 1994). Vitamin E will also shield the beta-carotene molecule from degradation, reducing the amount of this antioxidant in the body. Selenium and vitamin E have a synergistic impact (Burton 1994). Any one of these nutrients, when supplemented, may help to alleviate symptoms induced by a deficiency of other. Though anyone of them cannot replace each other fully. Consequently, the interaction of all such combinations of different antioxidants might have more effect than using a single antioxidant in larger quantities (Rock *et al.* 1996). The synergistic action of vitamin E and C has been depicted in the Fig. (**7**).

Antioxidants and the Prevention of Cancer

Cancer is the culmination of a multistep phase that takes years, if not decades, to develop. The Fig. (**8**) summarises a modern theoretical approach to the mechanism through which regular cells may transformed into cancerous cells.

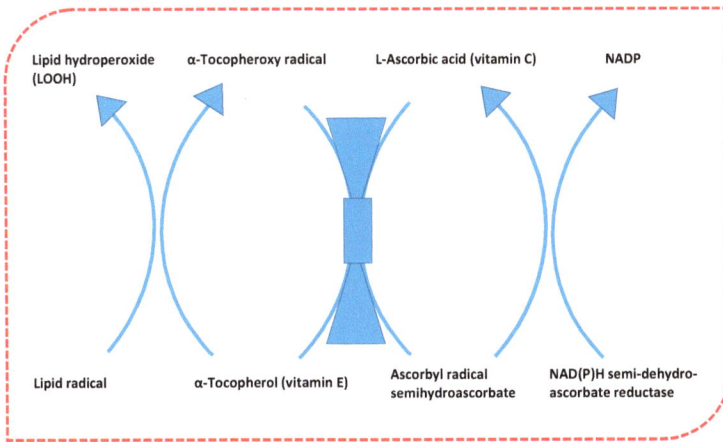

Fig. (7). The synergistic action of vitamin E and C.

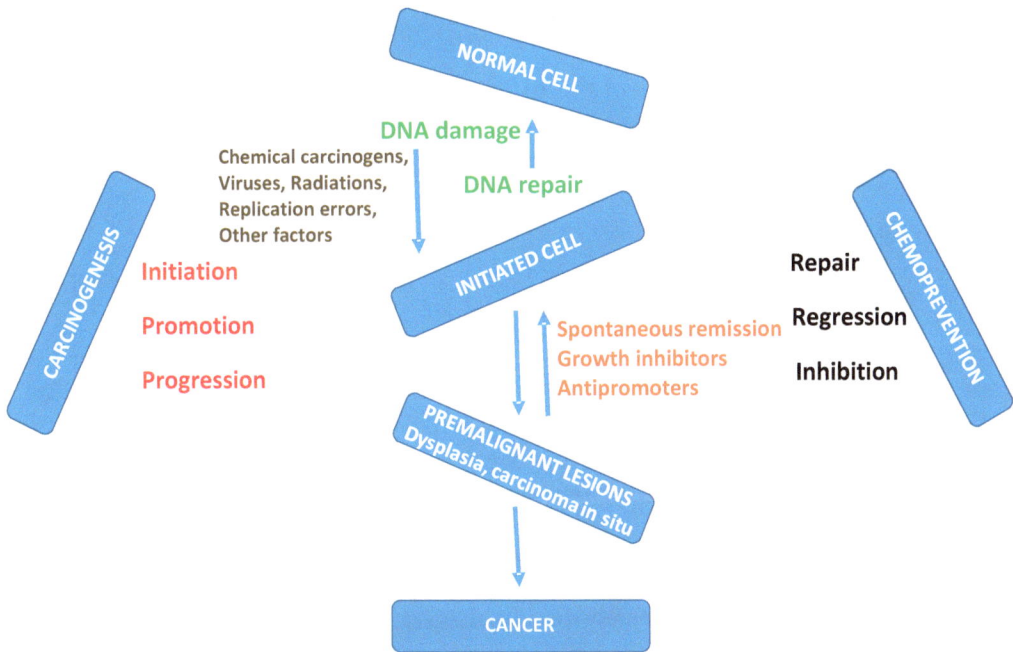

Fig. (8). The process by which normal cells are transformed into the cancerous cells.

DNA damage is thought to be one of the most important aspects in the growth of cancer. Oxidative stress is responsible for a significant portion of this injury. A predictor of mutagenic damage to DNA would be very useful in estimating the incidence of cancer in communities, as well as in tracking the results of chemoprevention. The majority of the damage is caused by oxidation. The likelihood of cancer increases when oxidative lesions grow with age. The DNA repair enzymes clear up the majority of this destruction. One of the first steps in carcinogenesis is the permanent genetic alteration as a result of DNA damage when a cell divides even before its DNA is repaired. Rapidly dividing cells are more susceptible to carcinogenesis than cells that divide slowly because there is less opportunity for DNA repair prior to cell division. Free radicals play a very crucial part in the growth of many cancers (Valko *et al.* 2006, Willcox *et al.* 2004, Black *et al.* 2020).

To conclude it is evident that cancer is less prone to occur in individuals who consume a lot of fruits and vegetables. Since vitamin C and carotenoids are mostly found in fruits and vegetables and are believed to contribute in the cancer-protection (Gaziano *et al.* 2009). Vitamin E can be found in fruits and vegetables as well as the other nutrients such as folate, which is a vitamin B complex. Also the fiber may protect against cancer to a large extent (Donaldson 2004, Key *et al.* 2004).

There is an increasing accord that antioxidant combinations can be more effective rather than single entities over an extended period. The antioxidants might be of high importance in boosting the quality of life *via* inhibiting the commencement of degenerative ailments (Key *et al.* 2004). Still much of the research and scientific understanding is needed to know the beneficial health properties of the antioxidants and for potential cost in health care delivery.

CONCEPT OF COMBINATIONAL THERAPY

The use of two or more treatments, including medications, to manage a disorder or illness is referred to as combinational therapy. It is also called as multimodality therapy. In recent years, there has been a greater emphasis on antioxidants as possible therapies in restoring the normal physiology of cells.

Antioxidant Combination Therapy

There are number of diseases whose pathophysiology is associated to the oxidative stress, for example; cancer, chronic obstructive pulmonary disease (COPD), Duchenne muscular dystrophy, neurodegenerative disorders such as Alzheimer's disease, hypertension, stroke, diabetes, metabolic syndrome *etc.* Several *in vitro* and *in vivo* studies have been performed using a wide variety of antioxidants (Rovira-Llopis *et al.* 2014). Although a number of experiments have been carried out in order to assess the efficiency of clinical trials but with unsatisfactory results. For example, it has been reported that hemodialysis patient's treatment with vitamin E showed no reduction in the oxidative stress induced protein modification and lipid peroxidation but observed a reduction in oxidative stress with improved endothelial functions (Wray *et al.* 2012). Papparella *et al.* (2007) showed that vitamin C prevent the zidovudine-induced cardiovascular disease (CVD) in rats and demonstrated beneficial antioxidant therapy by vitamin C *via* inhibition of NADPH oxidase activity. However, Sesso *et al.* (2008) found that vitamin C and E therapies have no protective effects in several clinical trials on cardiovascular patients. One more antioxidant therapy with vitamin E in Alzheimer's patients showed no improvement in cognitive defects while such therapy showed a reduction in lipid peroxidation and β-amyloid depositions in mice models (Sung *et al.* 2004).

The global burden of cancer is increasing drastically. The main reasons for this cancer burden are life-style and dietary factors that results in carcinogenesis *via* oxidative stress and ultimately produce mutagenic DNA damage as a result of the ROS and nitrogen reactive species leading to aberrant cell signaling pathways as well as the loss of redox control (Jones *et al.* 2006). Despite the utilization of antioxidant remedies in treating several diseases including cancer, a number of clinical trials have been performed and are yet ongoing in order to evade this dreadful disease. Some of these cancer prevention clinical trials using antioxidants as single entity or in combination have been summarized briefly in Table **1** below. Apart from this there are several completed or ongoing clinical trials for analysing the efficiency of antioxidants in treating cancer (Jones *et al.* 2008). Some completed and ongoing antioxidants clinical trials in cancer treatment are presented in Table **2**. Numerous natural antioxidants have been discovered to be effective at replenishing antioxidant levels in the body, which are often reduced during chemotherapy, resulting in less adverse outcomes and longer survival period in patients. As a result, targeted phytonutrient therapies utilising antioxidants or their precursors could be effective in mitigating drug toxicity and thereby enhancing therapeutic effectiveness (Singh *et al.* 2018).

Table 1. Clinical trials of antioxidants in the cancer treatment.

S. No.	Antioxidant Therapy	Type of Cancer	Primary Outcome	Clinical Trial	Reference
1.	Aspirin and β-carotene or in the combination	Prostate, Colon, Rectum, Lung, Lymphoma, Leukemia, Bladder, Brain, Melanoma, Stomach	Reduced total cancer incidence and cardiovascular diseases (CVD)	Physician Health Study (PHS), USA	Cook *et al.* (2000)
2.	β-carotene and retinol in the combination	Lung cancer	Reduced lung cancer incidence	Beta-Carotene and Retinol Efficacy Trial (CARET), USA	Omenn *et al.* (1996)

(Table 1) cont.....

S. No.	Antioxidant Therapy	Type of Cancer	Primary Outcome	Clinical Trial	Reference
3.	α-tocopherol and β-carotene or in the combination	Lung, Esophagus, Stomach, Pancreas	Reduced lung cancer incidence	Alpha-tocopherol and beta-carotene (ATBC) study, Finland	The Alpha-Tocopherol Beta Carotene Cancer Prevention Study Group (1994), Rautalahti *et al.* (1999), Wright *et al.* (2007), Malila *et al.* (2002)
4.	Retinol, zinc, molybdenum, selenium, α-tocopherol, β-carotene	Esophagus, Stomach	Reduced gastric and esophageal cancer mortality	Linxian Study, China	Blot *et al.* (1993), Qiao *et al.* (2009)
5.	Vitamin A, β-carotene, aspirin either alone or in the combination	Breast, Lung, Colon *etc.*	Reduced cancer incidence and cardiovascular disease	Women's Health Study (WHS), USA	Li *et al.* (1989), Lee *et al.* (2005)
6.	Vitamin E	Prostate, Lung, Oral/Pharynx, Colon/rectum, Breast, Melanoma	Reduced cancer incidence and cardiovascular disease	Health Outcomes Prevention Evaluation (HOPE) and HOPE the Ongoing Outcomes (HOPE-TOO) studies, International	Lonn *et al.* (2005)
7.	Vitamin E and β-carotene	All types of cancer, Lung, Stomach *etc.*	Reduced cardiovascular incidence	Heart Protection Study (HPS), United Kingdom	Heart Protection Study Collaborative Group (2002)
8.	α-tocopherol, β-carotene, selenium, zinc	All cancer types including prostate	Reduced cancer incidence and cardiovascular disease	Supplementation en Vitamines et Minéraux Antioxydants (SU.VI.MAX) study, France	Hercberg *et al.* 2004 Meyer *et al.* (2005)
9.	Vitamin C, vitamin E, β-carotene either alone or in the combination	All cancer types	Reduced cardiovascular incidence	Women's Antioxidant Cardiovascular Study (WASC), USA	Lin *et al.* (2009)
10.	Multivitamin and β-carotene	All cancer types including prostate, colon/rectum, lung *etc.*,	Reduced cancer incidence and cardiovascular disease	Physician Health Study II (PHS II), USA	Gaziano *et al.* (2009)

(Table 1) cont.....

S. No.	Antioxidant Therapy	Type of Cancer	Primary Outcome	Clinical Trial	Reference
11.	Selenium and vitamin E either alone or in the combination	Prostate, Lung, Colon/rectum	Reduced prostate cancer	Selenium and Vitamin E Cancer Prevention Trial (SELECT), USA	Lippman *et al.* 2009

Table 2. Completed and ongoing clinical trials of antioxidant in cancer treatment (Goodman *et al.* 2011).

S. No.	Antioxidant Therapy	Clinical trial	Primary Outcome	Status of The Clinical Trial
1.	Selenium	selenium for avoiding cancer in patients with prostate neoplasia, USA	Reduced prostate cancer	Study completed
2.	Selenium in low, medium and high dose	Selenium for the inhibition of cancer, United Kingdom	Reduced total cancer incidence	Study completed
3.	Vitamin E, selenium as well as soy protein	Vitamin E, selenium, as well as soy proteins in combating cancer in high-grade prostatic intraepithelial patients neoplasia, Canada	Reduced prostate cancer incidence	Study completed
4.	Apigenin in combination with the epigallocatechin	Bioflavonoid supplementation in the diet to avoid neoplasia recurrence, Germany	Recurrence rate of colorectal neoplasia	Ongoing
5.	Selenium	Selenium in combating prostate cancer, USA	Reduced prostate cancer	Ongoing
6.	Selenium and vitamin E separately and in the combination	Bangladesh Vitamin E and Selenium Trial (BEST), Bangladesh	Reduced skin cancer	Study completed

Cancer cells are believed to be killed by chemotherapy medications that induce a high degree of oxidative stress. However, oxidative stress can minimise chemotherapy's overall effectiveness (Chio and Tuveson 2017). Since oxidative stress delays the mechanism of cell replication, which is why chemotherapy destroys cancer cells, thus slower cell replication may indicate poorer chemotherapy efficacy (Conklin 2000, Halliwell 2007). One approach to this problem is to add specific antioxidants at sufficient doses to mitigate oxidative stress and thus make chemotherapy care more effective. Chemotherapy and antioxidants have a more complicated relationship than just fostering and preventing oxidative stress. Chemotherapy, on the other hand, works by a variety of pathways, and antioxidants have a variety of impacts on the body. In chemotherapy, evey antioxidant has a unique interaction, and this influence will also vary depending on the dose (O'Connor 2015). Antioxidants can have some advantage when used in conjunction with some forms of chemotherapy, according to current evidence. The randomised clinical study testing the safety and effectiveness of supplying antioxidants to chemotherapy has indeed been used because of the possibility for favourable outcomes (Drisko *et al.* 2003, Firuzi *et al.* 2011).

CONCLUSION

Antioxidants are a class of chemical compounds that biochemists and health practitioners are interested in since they enable the body defend itself against harm caused by reactive oxygen, nitrogen, and chlorine species. A wide-ranging variety of antioxidants found in foods contribute to the disease control and prevention. These antioxidants are also required as essential nutrients for our body. Plants contain several antioxidants with varied actions and have been extensively studied in recent years. Antioxidants are one of the most important components that play a critical role in maintaining the functions and integrity of the cell. They play a very vital role in disease prevention especially cancer and can degenerate premalignant lesions or inhibit the development of cancer. There have been a great deal of clinical studies carried out and still the process is ongoing. Many of these antioxidant compounds as single entity or in combination have demonstrated beneficial effects in several models which could protect against the cancers *via* mechanisms other than their properties. Although there is a growing accord that combination therapy of antioxidants is more effective as shown in certain clinical trials using several antioxidants either singly or in combination for long-term effects. Antioxidants can play a critical role in enhancing quality of life by mitigating degenerative diseases and according to many pieces of evidence, antioxidants provide several benefits when combined with certain types of chemotherapeutics.

CONSENT FOR PUBLICATION

Not acceptable.

CONFLICT OF INTEREST

The authors have no conflicts of interest to declare.

ACKNOWLEDGEMENT

This chapter was framed and initiated by Manzoor A Mir. It has been written by Safura Nisar, Basharat Ahmad Bhat and edited and compiled by Dr. Manzoor A Mir. The authors are very thankful to Dr. Manzoor A Mir for his assistance in the preparation of this manuscript.

REFERENCES

Berdahl, DR & McKeague, J (2015) *Rosemary and sage extracts as antioxidants for food preservation Handbook of antioxidants for food preservation.*Elsevier.

Bilderback, L (2007) *The complete idiot's guide to spices and herbs.*Penguin.

Black, HS, Boehm, F, Edge, R & Truscott, TG (2020) The Benefits and Risks of Certain Dietary Carotenoids that Exhibit both Anti- and Pro-Oxidative Mechanisms-A Comprehensive Review. *Antioxidants, 9*, 264.
[http://dx.doi.org/10.3390/antiox9030264] [PMID: 32210038]

Blot, WJ, Li, JY, Taylor, PR, Guo, W, Dawsey, S, Wang, GQ, Yang, CS, Zheng, SF, Gail, M & Li, GY (1993) Nutrition intervention trials in Linxian, China: supplementation with specific vitamin/mineral combinations, cancer incidence, and disease-specific mortality in the general population. *J Natl Cancer Inst, 85*, 1483-92.
[http://dx.doi.org/10.1093/jnci/85.18.1483] [PMID: 8360931]

Bubonja-Sonje, M, Giacometti, J & Abram, M (2011) Antioxidant and antilisterial activity of olive oil, cocoa and rosemary extract polyphenols. *Food Chem, 127*, 1821-7.
[http://dx.doi.org/10.1016/j.foodchem.2011.02.071]

Burton, GW (1994) Vitamin E: molecular and biological function. *Proc Nutr Soc, 53*, 251-62.
[http://dx.doi.org/10.1079/PNS19940030] [PMID: 7972139]

Chio, IIC & Tuveson, DA (2017) ROS in cancer: the burning question. *Trends Mol Med, 23*, 411-29.
[http://dx.doi.org/10.1016/j.molmed.2017.03.004] [PMID: 28427863]

Conklin, KA (2000) Dietary antioxidants during cancer chemotherapy: impact on chemotherapeutic effectiveness and development of side effects. *Nutr Cancer, 37*, 1-18.
[http://dx.doi.org/10.1207/S15327914NC3701_1] [PMID: 10965514]

Cook, NR, Le, IM, Manson, JE, Buring, JE & Hennekens, CH (2000) Effects of beta-carotene supplementation on cancer incidence by baseline characteristics in the Physicians' Health Study (United States). *Cancer Causes Control, 11*, 617-26.
[http://dx.doi.org/10.1023/A:1008995430664] [PMID: 10977106]

Cooper, R & Nicola, G (2014) *Natural Products Chemistry: Sources, Separations and Structures.*CRC Press.
[http://dx.doi.org/10.1201/b17244]

Cseke, LJ, Kirakosyan, A, Kaufman, PB, Warber, S, Duke, JA & Brielmann, HL (2016) *Natural products from plants.*CRC press.
[http://dx.doi.org/10.1201/9781420004472]

da Silva, BV, Barreira, JC & Oliveira, MBP (2016) Natural phytochemicals and probiotics as bioactive ingredients for functional foods: Extraction, biochemistry and protected-delivery technologies. *Trends Food Sci Technol, 50*, 144-58.
[http://dx.doi.org/10.1016/j.tifs.2015.12.007]

Di Meo, S & Venditti, P (2020) Evolution of the Knowledge of Free Radicals and Other Oxidants. *Oxid Med Cell Longev*, 20209829176
[http://dx.doi.org/10.1155/2020/9829176] [PMID: 32411336]

Donaldson, MS (2004) Nutrition and cancer: a review of the evidence for an anti-cancer diet. *Nutr J, 3*, 19.
[http://dx.doi.org/10.1186/1475-2891-3-19] [PMID: 15496224]

Drisko, JA, Chapman, J & Hunter, VJ (2003) The use of antioxidant therapies during chemotherapy. *Gynecol Oncol, 88*, 434-9.
[http://dx.doi.org/10.1016/S0090-8258(02)00067-7] [PMID: 12648599]

Firuzi, O, Miri, R, Tavakkoli, M & Saso, L (2011) Antioxidant therapy: current status and future prospects. *Curr Med Chem, 18*, 3871-88.
[http://dx.doi.org/10.2174/092986711803414368] [PMID: 21824100]

Gaziano, JM, Glynn, RJ, Christen, WG, Kurth, T, Belanger, C, MacFadyen, J, Bubes, V, Manson, JE, Sesso,

HD & Buring, JE (2009) Vitamins E and C in the prevention of prostate and total cancer in men: the Physicians' Health Study II randomized controlled trial. *JAMA,* 301, 52-62.
[http://dx.doi.org/10.1001/jama.2008.862] [PMID: 19066368]

Goodman, M, Bostick, RM, Kucuk, O & Jones, DP (2011) Clinical trials of antioxidants as cancer prevention agents: past, present, and future. *Free Radic Biol Med,* 51, 1068-84.
[http://dx.doi.org/10.1016/j.freeradbiomed.2011.05.018] [PMID: 21683786]

Guo, M (2013) *Functional foods: principles and technology.*Elsevier.

Halliwell, B (2007) Oxidative stress and cancer: have we moved forward? *Biochem J,* 401, 1-11.
[http://dx.doi.org/10.1042/BJ20061131] [PMID: 17150040]

Halliwell, B & Gutteridge, JM (2015) *Free radicals in biology and medicine.*Oxford University Press, USA.
[http://dx.doi.org/10.1093/acprof:oso/9780198717478.001.0001]

(2002) MRC/BHF Heart Protection Study of antioxidant vitamin supplementation in 20,536 high-risk individuals: a randomised placebo-controlled trial. *Lancet,* 360, 23-33.
[http://dx.doi.org/10.1016/S0140-6736(02)09328-5] [PMID: 12114037]

Hercberg, S, Galan, P, Preziosi, P, Bertrais, S, Mennen, L, Malvy, D, Roussel, AM, Favier, A & Briançon, S (2004) The SU.VI.MAX Study: a randomized, placebo-controlled trial of the health effects of antioxidant vitamins and minerals. *Arch Intern Med,* 164, 2335-42.
[http://dx.doi.org/10.1001/archinte.164.21.2335] [PMID: 15557412]

Hoda, M, Hemaiswarya, S & Doble, M (2019) *Phenolic Phytochemicals: Sources, Biosynthesis, Extraction, and Their Isolation Role of Phenolic Phytochemicals in Diabetes Management.*Springer.
[http://dx.doi.org/10.1007/978-981-13-8997-9]

Husain, N, Kumar, A & Radicals, F (2012) Reactive oxygen species and natural antioxidants: a review. *Adv Biores,* 3, 164-75.

Jones, DP (2006) Redefining oxidative stress. *Antioxid Redox Signal,* 8, 1865-79.
[http://dx.doi.org/10.1089/ars.2006.8.1865] [PMID: 16987039]

Jones, DP (2008) Radical-free biology of oxidative stress. *Am J Physiol Cell Physiol,* 295, C849-68.
[http://dx.doi.org/10.1152/ajpcell.00283.2008] [PMID: 18684987]

Kaur, C & Kapoor, HC (2001) Antioxidants in fruits and vegetables–the millennium's health. *Int J Food Sci Technol,* 36, 703-25.
[http://dx.doi.org/10.1046/j.1365-2621.2001.00513.x]

Key, TJ, Schatzkin, A, Willett, WC, Allen, NE, Spencer, EA & Travis, RC (2004) Diet, nutrition and the prevention of cancer. *Public Health Nutr,* 7, 187-200.
[http://dx.doi.org/10.1079/PHN2003588] [PMID: 14972060]

Landete, JM (2013) Dietary intake of natural antioxidants: vitamins and polyphenols. *Crit Rev Food Sci Nutr,* 53, 706-21.
[http://dx.doi.org/10.1080/10408398.2011.555018] [PMID: 23638931]

Langseth, L (1995) *Oxidants, antioxidants, and disease prevention.*ILSI Europe.

Lee, IM, Cook, NR, Gaziano, JM, Gordon, D, Ridker, PM, Manson, JE, Hennekens, CH & Buring, JE (2005) Vitamin E in the primary prevention of cardiovascular disease and cancer: the Women's Health Study: a randomized controlled trial. *JAMA,* 294, 56-65.
[http://dx.doi.org/10.1001/jama.294.1.56] [PMID: 15998891]

Lin, J, Cook, NR, Albert, C, Zaharris, E, Gaziano, JM, Van Denburgh, M, Buring, JE & Manson, JE (2009) Vitamins C and E and beta carotene supplementation and cancer risk: a randomized controlled trial. *J Natl Cancer Inst,* 101, 14-23.
[http://dx.doi.org/10.1093/jnci/djn438] [PMID: 19116389]

Lippman, SM, Klein, EA, Goodman, PJ, Lucia, MS, Thompson, IM, Ford, LG, Parnes, HL, Minasian, LM, Gaziano, JM, Hartline, JA, Parsons, JK, Bearden, JD, III, Crawford, ED, Goodman, GE, Claudio, J,

Winquist, E, Cook, ED, Karp, DD, Walther, P, Lieber, MM, Kristal, AR, Darke, AK, Arnold, KB, Ganz, PA, Santella, RM, Albanes, D, Taylor, PR, Probstfield, JL, Jagpal, TJ, Crowley, JJ, Meyskens, FL, Jr, Baker, LH & Coltman, CAJ, Jr (2009) Effect of selenium and vitamin E on risk of prostate cancer and other cancers: the Selenium and Vitamin E Cancer Prevention Trial (SELECT). *JAMA,* 301, 39-51.
[http://dx.doi.org/10.1001/jama.2008.864] [PMID: 19066370]

Liu, Z, Ren, Z, Zhang, J, Chuang, C-C, Kandaswamy, E, Zhou, T & Zuo, L (2018) Role of ROS and nutritional antioxidants in human diseases. *Front Physiol,* 9, 477.
[http://dx.doi.org/10.3389/fphys.2018.00477] [PMID: 29867535]

Li, JY, Ershow, AG, Chen, ZJ, Wacholder, S, Li, GY, Guo, W, Li, B & Blot, WJ (1989) A case-control study of cancer of the esophagus and gastric cardia in Linxian. *Int J Cancer,* 43, 755-61.
[http://dx.doi.org/10.1002/ijc.2910430502] [PMID: 2714880]

Lobo, V, Patil, A, Phatak, A & Chandra, N (2010) Free radicals, antioxidants and functional foods: Impact on human health. *Pharmacogn Rev,* 4, 118-26.
[http://dx.doi.org/10.4103/0973-7847.70902] [PMID: 22228951]

Lonn, E, Bosch, J, Yusuf, S, Sheridan, P, Pogue, J, Arnold, JM, Ross, C, Arnold, A, Sleight, P, Probstfield, J & Dagenais, GR (2005) Effects of long-term vitamin E supplementation on cardiovascular events and cancer: a randomized controlled trial. *JAMA,* 293, 1338-47.
[http://dx.doi.org/10.1001/jama.293.11.1338] [PMID: 15769967]

Luximon-Ramma, A, Bahorun, T, Crozier, A, Zbarsky, V, Datla, KP, Dexter, DT & Aruoma, OI (2005) Characterization of the antioxidant functions of flavonoids and proanthocyanidins in Mauritian black teas. *Food Res Int,* 38, 357-67.
[http://dx.doi.org/10.1016/j.foodres.2004.10.005]

Malila, N, Taylor, PR, Virtanen, MJ, Korhonen, P, Huttunen, JK, Albanes, D & Virtamo, J (2002) Effects of alpha-tocopherol and beta-carotene supplementation on gastric cancer incidence in male smokers (ATBC Study, Finland). *Cancer Causes Control,* 13, 617-23.
[http://dx.doi.org/10.1023/A:1019556227014] [PMID: 12296509]

Meyer, F, Galan, P, Douville, P, Bairati, I, Kegle, P, Bertrais, S, Estaquio, C & Hercberg, S (2005) Antioxidant vitamin and mineral supplementation and prostate cancer prevention in the SU.VI.MAX trial. *Int J Cancer,* 116, 182-6.
[http://dx.doi.org/10.1002/ijc.21058] [PMID: 15800922]

Miller, HE, Rigelhof, F, Marquart, L, Prakash, A & Kanter, M (2000) Antioxidant content of whole grain breakfast cereals, fruits and vegetables. *J Am Coll Nutr,* 19 (Suppl.), 312S-9S.
[http://dx.doi.org/10.1080/07315724.2000.10718966] [PMID: 10875603]

Nagaraj, G (2009) *Oilseeds: properties, processing, products and procedures.*New India Publishing.

O'brien, RD (2008) *Fats and oils: formulating and processing for applications.*CRC press.
[http://dx.doi.org/10.1201/9781420061673]

O'Connor, MJ (2015) Targeting the DNA damage response in cancer. *Mol Cell,* 60, 547-60.
[http://dx.doi.org/10.1016/j.molcel.2015.10.040] [PMID: 26590714]

Omenn, GS, Goodman, GE, Thornquist, MD, Balmes, J, Cullen, MR, Glass, A, Keogh, JP, Meyskens, FL, Jr, Valanis, B, Williams, JH, Jr, Barnhart, S, Cherniack, MG, Brodkin, CA & Hammar, S (1996) Risk factors for lung cancer and for intervention effects in CARET, the Beta-Carotene and Retinol Efficacy Trial. *J Natl Cancer Inst,* 88, 1550-9.
[http://dx.doi.org/10.1093/jnci/88.21.1550] [PMID: 8901853]

Papparella, I, Ceolotto, G, Berto, L, Cavalli, M, Bova, S, Cargnelli, G, Ruga, E, Milanesi, O, Franco, L, Mazzoni, M, Petrelli, L, Nussdorfer, GG & Semplicini, A (2007) Vitamin C prevents zidovudine-induced NAD(P)H oxidase activation and hypertension in the rat. *Cardiovasc Res,* 73, 432-8.
[http://dx.doi.org/10.1016/j.cardiores.2006.10.010] [PMID: 17123493]

Pasrija, D & Anandharamakrishnan, C (2015) Techniques for extraction of green tea polyphenols: a review.

Food Bioprocess Technol, 8, 935-50.
[http://dx.doi.org/10.1007/s11947-015-1479-y]

Peter, KV (2012) *Handbook of herbs and spices.*Elsevier.

Phaniendra, A, Jestadi, DB & Periyasamy, L (2015) Free radicals: properties, sources, targets, and their implication in various diseases. *Indian J Clin Biochem,* 30, 11-26.
[http://dx.doi.org/10.1007/s12291-014-0446-0] [PMID: 25646037]

Pisoschi, AM & Pop, A (2015) The role of antioxidants in the chemistry of oxidative stress: A review. *Eur J Med Chem,* 97, 55-74.
[http://dx.doi.org/10.1016/j.ejmech.2015.04.040] [PMID: 25942353]

Pokorný, J, Yanishlieva, N & Gordon, M (2001) *Antioxidants in food: practical applications.*Elsevier.

Qiao, YL, Dawsey, SM, Kamangar, F, Fan, JH, Abnet, CC, Sun, XD, Johnson, LL, Gail, MH, Dong, ZW, Yu, B, Mark, SD & Taylor, PR (2009) Total and cancer mortality after supplementation with vitamins and minerals: follow-up of the Linxian General Population Nutrition Intervention Trial. *J Natl Cancer Inst,* 101, 507-18.
[http://dx.doi.org/10.1093/jnci/djp037] [PMID: 19318634]

Rahman, I (2016) *Comparative analysis of phytochemical constituents, antibacterial and antioxidant activity of green tea: camellia sinensis.*Brac University.

Rautalahti, MT, Virtamo, JR, Taylor, PR, Heinonen, OP, Albanes, D, Haukka, JK, Edwards, BK, Kärkkäinen, PA, Stolzenberg-Solomon, RZ & Huttunen, J (1999) The effects of supplementation with alpha-tocopherol and beta-carotene on the incidence and mortality of carcinoma of the pancreas in a randomized, controlled trial. *Cancer,* 86, 37-42.
[http://dx.doi.org/10.1002/(SICI)1097-0142(19990701)86:1<37::AID-CNCR7>3.0.CO;2-F]   [PMID: 10391561]

Rock, CL, Jacob, RA & Bowen, PE (1996) Update on the biological characteristics of the antioxidant micronutrients: vitamin C, vitamin E, and the carotenoids. *J Am Diet Assoc,* 96, 693-702.
[http://dx.doi.org/10.1016/S0002-8223(96)00190-3] [PMID: 8675913]

Rovira-Llopis, S, Bañuls, C, Apostolova, N, Morillas, C, Hernandez-Mijares, A, Rocha, M & Victor, VM (2014) Is glycemic control modulating endoplasmic reticulum stress in leukocytes of type 2 diabetic patients? *Antioxid Redox Signal,* 21, 1759-65.
[http://dx.doi.org/10.1089/ars.2014.6030] [PMID: 25000244]

Saed-Moucheshi, A, Shekoofa, A & Pessarakli, M (2014) Reactive oxygen species (ROS) generation and detoxifying in plants. *J Plant Nutr,* 37, 1573-85.
[http://dx.doi.org/10.1080/01904167.2013.868483]

Sen, CK, Khanna, S & Roy, S (2007) Tocotrienols in health and disease: the other half of the natural vitamin E family. *Mol Aspects Med,* 28, 692-728.
[http://dx.doi.org/10.1016/j.mam.2007.03.001] [PMID: 17507086]

Senanayake, SN, Wanasundara, PJP & Shahidi, F (2005) Antioxidants: Science, Technology, and Applications. *Bailey's Industrial Oil and Fat Products,* 1-61.

Sesso, HD, Buring, JE, Christen, WG, Kurth, T, Belanger, C, MacFadyen, J, Bubes, V, Manson, JE, Glynn, RJ & Gaziano, JM (2008) Vitamins E and C in the prevention of cardiovascular disease in men: the Physicians' Health Study II randomized controlled trial. *JAMA,* 300, 2123-33.
[http://dx.doi.org/10.1001/jama.2008.600] [PMID: 18997197]

Sgherri, C, Pinzino, C & Quartacci, MF (2018) Reactive oxygen species and photosynthetic functioning: Past and present. *Reactive Oxygen Species in Plants: Boon or Bane–Revisiting the Role of ROS,* 137-55.

Shahidi, F (2000) Antioxidants in food and food antioxidants. *Food/nahrung,* 44, 158-63.

Sies, H & Jones, DP (2020) Reactive oxygen species (ROS) as pleiotropic physiological signalling agents. *Nat Rev Mol Cell Biol,* 21, 363-83.

[http://dx.doi.org/10.1038/s41580-020-0230-3] [PMID: 32231263]

Simioni, C, Zauli, G, Martelli, AM, Vitale, M, Sacchetti, G, Gonelli, A & Neri, LM (2018) Oxidative stress: role of physical exercise and antioxidant nutraceuticals in adulthood and aging. *Oncotarget, 9,* 17181-98.
[http://dx.doi.org/10.18632/oncotarget.24729] [PMID: 29682215]

Singh, K, Bhori, M, Kasu, YA, Bhat, G & Marar, T (2018) Antioxidants as precision weapons in war against cancer chemotherapy induced toxicity - Exploring the armoury of obscurity. *Saudi Pharm J, 26,* 177-90.
[http://dx.doi.org/10.1016/j.jsps.2017.12.013] [PMID: 30166914]

Singh, VK, Beattie, LA & Seed, TM (2013) Vitamin E: tocopherols and tocotrienols as potential radiation countermeasures. *J Radiat Res (Tokyo), 54,* 973-88.
[http://dx.doi.org/10.1093/jrr/rrt048] [PMID: 23658414]

Sivanandham, V (2011) Free radicals in health and diseases-a mini review. *Pharmacologyonline, 1,* 1062-77.

Staub, J (2008) *75 Exceptional Herbs.*Gibbs Smith.

Suleman, M, Khan, A, Baqi, A, Kakar, MS & Ayub, M (2019) 2. Antioxidants, its role in preventing free radicals and infectious diseases in human body. *Pure Appl Biol, 8,* 380-8. [PAB].

Sung, S, Yao, Y, Uryu, K, Yang, H, Lee, VM, Trojanowski, JQ & Praticò, D (2004) Early vitamin E supplementation in young but not aged mice reduces Abeta levels and amyloid deposition in a transgenic model of Alzheimer's disease. *FASEB J, 18,* 323-5.
[http://dx.doi.org/10.1096/fj.03-0961fje] [PMID: 14656990]

(1994) The effect of vitamin E and beta carotene on the incidence of lung cancer and other cancers in male smokers. *N Engl J Med, 330,* 1029-35.
[http://dx.doi.org/10.1056/NEJM199404143301501] [PMID: 8127329]

Valko, M, Rhodes, CJ, Moncol, J, Izakovic, M & Mazur, M (2006) Free radicals, metals and antioxidants in oxidative stress-induced cancer. *Chem Biol Interact, 160,* 1-40.
[http://dx.doi.org/10.1016/j.cbi.2005.12.009] [PMID: 16430879]

Vermerris, W & Nicholson, R (2007) *Phenolic compound biochemistry.*Springer Science & Business Media.

Wang, H, Provan, G, Helliwell, K & Ransom, W (2003) The functional benefits of flavonoids: The case of tea.*Phytochemical Functional Foods* CRC Press and Woodhead Publishing Limited 128-59.
[http://dx.doi.org/10.1533/9781855736986.1.128]

Willcox, JK, Ash, SL & Catignani, GL (2004) Antioxidants and prevention of chronic disease. *Crit Rev Food Sci Nutr, 44,* 275-95.
[http://dx.doi.org/10.1080/10408690490468489] [PMID: 15462130]

Winterbourn, CC, Kettle, AJ & Hampton, MB (2016) Reactive oxygen species and neutrophil function. *Annu Rev Biochem, 85,* 765-92.
[http://dx.doi.org/10.1146/annurev-biochem-060815-014442] [PMID: 27050287]

Wray, DW, Nishiyama, SK, Harris, RA, Zhao, J, McDaniel, J, Fjeldstad, AS, Witman, MA, Ives, SJ, Barrett-O'Keefe, Z & Richardson, RS (2012) Acute reversal of endothelial dysfunction in the elderly after antioxidant consumption. *Hypertension, 59,* 818-24.
[http://dx.doi.org/10.1161/HYPERTENSIONAHA.111.189456] [PMID: 22353612]

Wright, ME, Virtamo, J, Hartman, AM, Pietinen, P, Edwards, BK, Taylor, PR, Huttunen, JK & Albanes, D (2007) Effects of alpha-tocopherol and beta-carotene supplementation on upper aerodigestive tract cancers in a large, randomized controlled trial. *Cancer, 109,* 891-8.
[http://dx.doi.org/10.1002/cncr.22482] [PMID: 17265529]

SUBJECT INDEX

Xenobiotic Metabolism 1

Z